www.bma.org.uk/library

D1345540

BRITISH MEDICAL ASSOCIATION

0921774

Oxford Textbook of
Women and Mental Health

Oxford Textbooks in Psychiatry

Oxford Textbook of
Women and Mental Health

Edited by

Dora Kohen

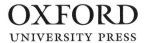

OXFORD

UNIVERSITY PRESS

OXFORD
UNIVERSITY PRESS

Great Clarendon Street, Oxford OX2 6DP

Oxford University Press is a department of the University of Oxford.
It furthers the University's objective of excellence in research, scholarship,
and education by publishing worldwide in

Oxford New York

Auckland Cape Town Dar es Salaam Hong Kong Karachi
Kuala Lumpur Madrid Melbourne Mexico City Nairobi
New Delhi Shanghai Taipei Toronto

With offices in

Argentina Austria Brazil Chile Czech Republic France Greece
Guatemala Hungary Italy Japan Poland Portugal Singapore
South Korea Switzerland Thailand Turkey Ukraine Vietnam

Oxford is a registered trade mark of Oxford University Press
in the UK and in certain other countries

Published in the United States
by Oxford University Press Inc., New York

© Oxford University Press, 2010

The moral rights of the authors have been asserted

Database right Oxford University Press (maker)

First published 2010

All rights reserved. No part of this publication may be reproduced,
stored in a retrieval system, or transmitted, in any form or by any means,
without the prior permission in writing of Oxford University Press,
or as expressly permitted by law, or under terms agreed with the appropriate
reprographics rights organization. Enquiries concerning reproduction
outside the scope of the above should be sent to the Rights Department,
Oxford University Press, at the address above

You must not circulate this book in any other binding or cover
and you must impose this same condition on any acquirer

British Library Cataloguing in Publication Data is available

Library of Congress Cataloging-in-Publication Data

Oxford textbook of women and mental health / edited by Dora Kohen.
      p. ; cm.
   Includes bibliographical references.
      ISBN 978–0–19–921436–5 (hardback : alk. paper)
1. Women—Mental health—Textbooks.   I. Kohen, Dora, 1946– II. Title:
Textbook of women and mental health.
   [DNLM: 1. Mental Disorders.   2. Women's Health.   3. Mental Health.
WM 140 O985 2010]
      RC451.4.W6O94 2010
      616.890082—dc22   2009053042

Typeset in Minion
by Glyph International, Bangalore, India
Printed by CPI Antony Rowe, UK
ISBN 978–0–19–921436–5

10 9 8 7 6 5 4 3 2 1

Oxford University Press makes no representation, express or implied, that the drug
dosages in this book are correct. Readers must therefore always check the product
information and clinical procedures with the most up-to-date published product
information and data sheets provided by the manufacturers and the most recent codes of
conduct and safety regulations. The authors and the publishers do not accept responsibility
or legal liability for any errors in the text or for the misuse or misapplication of material in
this work. Except where otherwise stated, drug dosages and recommendations are for the
non-pregnant adult who is not breast-feeding

Foreword

Questions—and some answers

This important book goes to the heart of much post-modern psychiatry, and the scholarly chapters expose the ambiguities of terms used by policy makers to characterize women's mental health services. What *is* mental health *promotion*, and how is it distinguished from *mental disorder prevention*? They each have overlapping properties but are derived from 'different conceptual principles and frame works of understanding', as the WHO (2005) has aptly summarized. What 'mainstreaming' means—and how such attempts to integrate and routinize such services cope with rapid changes in culture and gender roles in a multi-faith world? Are women-only services delivered by women-only health workers basic needs, or are they wants, preferences, and desires? We pay lip service to 'personalized' health care, but is 'individualized' care the same thing? Not according to the relationship-based Medicine of the Person concept developed by Paul Tournier.

How can revised classifications of mental disorder, whether in DSM-5 or ICD-11, capture these gender-specific relationship-based facets? The Royal College of Psychiatrists' Perinatal Specialist Section has recommended that the familiar diagnostic terms 'puerperal psychosis' and 'post-natal depression' should no longer be separately delineated, and that a mandatory pre- and post-partum onset specifier be introduced for all mental disorders. Such nosological scientific mainstreaming paradoxically could disadvantage women and the development of the women-only services currently advocated by policy makers if the established link of mood disorder to childbirth, symbolized by the 'puerperal' or 'post-natal' nosological specifier, is lost.

The reader will be stimulated to reflect on the answers to these questions within a local National Health Service (NHS) context. Thus a culturally sensitive psychiatry and a women's mental health service does 'begin at home'; and most chapters reflect the structures of the NHS in the UK, with its systems of commissioning and competition for resources.

Society is indeed changing in its core structures, with more serial marriages, lone parenting, same-sex relationships, and the way in which transmission of knowledge occurs between generations. Britain has one of the highest divorce rates in Europe. The roles of women and men, and the circumstances for the development of children are changing—and changing fast. Some women regard childbearing and optimal parenthood as a threat to autonomy, economic viability, and to individualized choice. Yet Layard and Dunn (2007) have concluded, as does this author, that parenthood is an awesome responsibility and that parents should therefore plan for 'long-term commitment' to each other as well as to the welfare of their child. Yet the proposal that 'relationship disorders' should be coded in hospital statistics rarely gains popular credence, despite the evidence that bonding problems adversely effect child development and that relationship difficulties can be ameliorated with psychological assistance.

Training issues

The insight of continental philosophers (Buber, Levinas, Merleau-Ponty, and Kirkegaard) to the understanding that personhood is achieved in relationship to others has been neglected; British medicine has also been impoverished by the lack of a developmental dynamic and humanistic perspective which is more prominent on the continent. Thus mental health and psychiatry training in reproductive health and in women's health programmes is surprisingly weak. Obstetricians and gynaecologists may for example have had no postgraduate training in these subjects and yet failure to provide accessible *specialist* perinatal liaison mental health services can have tragic consequences.

This book shows clearly that mental disorder in women, including perinatal disorder is still, alas, judged harshly by society; women are expected to remain strong and to multi-task with impunity. Furthermore in-depth discussion about the health promoting benefits of consensual sexual activity, strategies to maintain a creative and loving relationship, and the relevance of religious and spiritual beliefs are overlooked.

An understanding of women's mental health requires therefore a conceptual framework that exceeds the conventions of a narrow bio-medical scientific approach (the medical model), is sensitive to the dynamics of relationship-driven mental disorders, and recognizes that most women most of the time are in relationships with men, and many with their own or others' children. To encompass this broad public and personal health agenda requires a breadth of training and personal maturity in the health professional; or a team that, in its entirety, is able to understand the bio-social and psycho-spiritual facets of the woman's disorder.

There are two current theoretical approaches, which assist this multi-professional process, and which provide the theoretical framework, without which the consideration of women's mental health becomes a personal lottery of loosely formed ideas and prejudices. The first is derived from philosophical ideas of linguistic analysis which recognized that the understanding of diverse values (such as gender and sex roles, or autonomy, and patriarchy) as well as the contribution of scientific facts are both vital for any comprehensive care programme that is shared with the service user.

The second is the integrative diagnostic assessment developed by the World Psychiatric Association which combines the descriptive with the ideographic approach and emphasizes the need to contextualize the individual's symptoms and to engage the user in the management process. This socio-cultural envelope draws less on the intricacies of philosophy than on the track record of sociology (of gender, sex roles, and feminism) and the socio-anthropological studies of women's health, which were pioneered by Margaret Mead, Scheper Hughes, and Carol MacCormack.

Professional assumptions

Professor Kohen has commendably succeeded in encouraging her authors to highlight how a consideration of women's mental health may challenge the personal assumptions of professionals, whose hidden prejudices and values become exposed. Readers will be urged to reflect on the endemic nature of domestic violence; the cultural confusion of changing gender roles; the lower status and threat to autonomy of motherhood in high income countries; the doubling of rates of depression and anxiety in divorced women compared with those who are married; and the adverse effect of all these factors on child development. In low and middle income countries, the link between adverse mental health in women, poverty and low school attainment, and a 1 in 16 life time risk of maternal mortality in parts of Africa should override any reluctance to consider reproductive health as a specific priority in a postmodern feminist society.

Of the eight UN Millennium Development Goals, three are specifically related to women's mental health: gender equality, reduction of child mortality by two-thirds by 2015, and reduction of maternal mortality by three-quarters. At the conclusion of the International Consensus Statement of Women's Mental Health, the 139 WPA member societies were each urged to implement its recommendations and to distribute them to their members. The WPA now needs to determine the impact of this consensus statement, and the extent to which psychiatrists, and their professional organizations, are effectively advocating the scaling up of maternal, newborn, and child health (MNCH) services and greater gender equality—and, when necessary, challenging religious assumptions that may disadvantage women.

The Royal College of Psychiatrists has recently mainstreamed its international outreach and should work with the College of Obstetricians and Gynaecologists to encourage NHS collaborative links with maternity services in low and middle income countries and so support an infrastructure at community level. Silo thinking in world organizations, including WHO and WPA and national colleges, has increased the likelihood that the well-being of the newborn and gender-specific women's mental health can be overlooked.

The triple jeopardy of old age, femininity, and dementia can similarly be overlooked; at least a third of women suffer from mental disorder in their old age and may not have children or other family members to care for them.

Pastoral work, lunch clubs, drop-in centres, practice choirs, and charitable agencies, such as Methodist Homes for the Aged (MHA), Help the Aged, and Age Concern, will relieve, not just the burden of mental disorder on the elderly person, but also reduce the frequency of depression in carers (mostly women) and younger family members.

Societal responses

In the UK greater thought should now be given to sustaining marriage (through, for example, tax incentives) and supporting parenthood—but not at all costs. The churches and other voluntary organizations should consider modernizing and secularizing their naming ceremonies (baptism) and provide greater support to families and children at risk.

I have spent over 30 years conducting studies on post-natal and antenatal mental disorder, and have been a strong advocate for improved services for women, but these activities were driven by the clinical priorities that confronted me first in Uganda, and then subsequently in Scotland and Stoke-on-Trent. I have never regarded these studies, or their conceptual framework, as confined to women's health to the exclusion of men and their families. The renowned Charles Street Day Hospital, 'opposite the bus station in Hanley', was deliberately named a 'parent and baby' and not a 'mother and baby' unit. Likewise the Edinburgh Postnatal Depression Scale (EPDS), now translated into over 25 languages, has not only withstood the test of time but is used to highlight the impact of mental disorder on the father and the impact of depression on the development of the infant. The most complex clinical managements, in my experience, were when both parents had mental disorder; when the grandparents, though healthy, were unhelpful, and if absent or themselves unwell, were unsupportive.

Women and men

Women's and men's health are partially interlocked; what is required of clinicians is a relationship-based personalized biosocial/psychospiritual assessment, which considers 'meaning and purpose' (spiritual/existential needs) and, when relevant, the world-views and beliefs of the family.

Greater attention to women's mental health is thus a political, economic, humanitarian, and human rights priority. It is scandalous that we accept a 1 in 16 lifetime risk of dying in childbirth in sub-Saharan Africa; that governments do not speak out against all forms of domestic violence; and that the availability of cost-effective treatments for common mental disorders (which disrupt family life and threaten the well-being of the children) are so often lost between competing priorities.

Globalization, and the influx of migrants with different world-views and religious beliefs, make it essential that those advocating improved mental health for women demonstrate not only that there is 'no health without mental health', but that there is also 'no reproductive health without mental health.'

Taking these slogans seriously will raise profound questions about the future directions for psychiatry. Psychiatry is at a crossroad; the issues raised by the contributors to this scholarly volume will ensure that this debate continues, and any new routes are more clearly sign-posted. Psychiatry, psychiatrists, and other mental health workers are bio-psycho-social scientists, who accept the limitations for research of a 'patchy reductionism', and yet also make available skills as healers of the body, mind, and spirit. Such a complex vocation requires thorough training, a personal sense of meaning and purpose as well as an inherent curiosity about women as well as men—and especially about those factors that make for harmonious relationships.

This excellent book about women and mental health provides pointers to the direction ahead, and to the need to make yet more explicit the evidence base and the diverse values, which will underpin these public health priorities.

John Cox
Secretary General
World Psychiatric Association (2002–2008)
Cheltenham, January 2010

This book is dedicated to the memory of Dora Kohen who died in 2009 and had worked so tirelessly to improve the well-being of families throughout the world.

Contents

List of contributors

Dr Adil Akram
Academic Clinical Fellow in Psychiatry,
St George's, University of London,
South West London & St George's Mental Health
NHS Trust
London, UK

Dr Kristian Aleman
Clinical Psychologist, Psychodynamic Psychotherapist,
Psychoanalyst and Doctor of Psychology;
Member of the International Psychoanalytical
Association,
Stockholm, Sweden

Dr. Alaa Al-Sheikh
Locum Consultant Psychiatrist in Learning Disability,
Middlesex, UK

Dr Giles Berrisford
Consultant Perinatal Psychiatrist,
Birmingham and Solihull Mental Health
Foundation Trust,
Birmingham, UK

Professor Antonia Bifulco
Professor in Health and Social Care,
Lifespan Research Group,
Department of Health and Social Care,
Royal Holloway, University of London,
London, UK

Dr Stefan Borgwardt
Psychiatric Outpatient Department,
University Hospital Basel,
Switzerland

Dr Rebecca Cashmore
Leicester Eating Disorder Service,
Leicester Partnership Trust,
Brandon Mental Health Unit,
Leicester, UK

Dr Neerja Chowdhary
Psychiatrist, Sangath,
Goa, India

Dr Heather A. Church
Registrar in Psychiatry,
St Patrick's University Hospital,
Dublin, Ireland

Dr Irene Cormac
Consultant Forensic Psychiatrist,
Nottinghamshire Healthcare NHS Trust,
Nottingham, UK

Professor John Cox
Professor Emeritus,
Keele University, UK

Dr Ed Day
Senior Lecturer in Addiction Psychiatry,
University of Birmingham,
Department of Psychiatry,
Birmingham, UK

Professor Timothy G. Dinan
Chair of Psychiatry,
Department of Psychiatry,
University College Cork,
Ireland

Dr Ronald Doctor
Consultant Psychiatrist in Psychotherapy,
West London Mental Health NHS Trust,
West Middlesex Hospital,
Isleworth,
Middlesex, UK

Dr Peter Fitzgerald
Lecturer, Department of Psychiatry,
University College Cork,
Ireland

Dr Trevor Friedman
Consultant Liaison Psychiatrist, Brandon Unit,
Leicester General Hospital,
Leicester, UK

Dr Eilish Gilvarry
Drug and Alcohol Service, Newcastle upon Tyne;
Consultant Psychiatrist in Addiction,
Northumberland, Tyne and Wear NHS Trust,
Newcastle upon Tyne, UK

Professor Vivette Glover
Professor of Perinatal Psychobiology,
Imperial College London,
London, UK

Dr Michael Göpfert
Consultant Child and Adolescent Psychiatrist,
Alderhey Children's NHS Foundation Trust,
Liverpool;
Honorary Clinical Lecturer,
University of Liverpool,
Liverpool, UK

Dr Jessica Heron
Perinatal Research Programme Lead,
Birmingham & Solihull Mental Health NHS
Foundation Trust,
Honorary Research Fellow in Perinatal
Psychiatry,
Department of Psychiatry,
University of Birmingham,
Birmingham, UK

Judith Horrocks
Research Officer,
Leeds Institute of Health Sciences,
University of Leeds,
Leeds, UK

Professor Allan House
Professor of Liaison Psychiatry,
Leeds Institute of Health Sciences,
University of Leeds,
Leeds, UK

Dr Ian Jones
Senior Lecturer in Perinatal Psychiatry,
Department of Psychological Medicine,
Cardiff University,
Cardiff, UK

Dr Andrew Kent
Reader in Psychiatry,
St George's, University of London
London, UK

Professor Levent Küey
Associate Professor of Psychiatry,
Secretary General of World Psychiatric Association,
Istanbul Bilgi University, Department of Psychology,
Istanbul, Turkey

Geetha Kumeravelu
Consultant Psychiatrist,
Northgate Hospital,
Morpeth, UK

Dr Jona Lewin
Consultant Psychiatrist and Honorary Senior Lecturer,
Imperial College London;
Coombe Wood Perinatal Service,
Park Royal Centre for Mental Health,
London, UK

Professor James V. Lucey
Clinical Professor of Psychiatry,
Trinity College, Dublin University;
Medical Director, St Patrick's University Hospital,
Dublin, Ireland

Professor Anthony Maden
Professor of Forensic Psychiatry,
Imperial College London, UK

Dr Sarah Majid
Specialist Registrar in Psychotherapy,
Halliwick Unit, St Ann's Hospital,
London, UK

Dr Jane McCarthy
Consultant Psychiatrist in Learning Disabilities,
Estia Centre, Institute of Psychiatry,
King's College London,
London, UK

Nora McClelland
Department of Sociological Studies,
University of Sheffield,
Sheffield, UK

Dr Daniel McQueen
Specialist Registrar in Psychotherapy,
Cassel Hospital, Richmond, Surrey, and
Psychotherapy Service,
Lakeside Mental Health Unit,
West Middlesex University Hospital,
Isleworth, UK

Dr Patricia Moran
Chartered Psychologist,
Research Co-ordinator and Tutor,
Metanoia Institute,
London, UK

Dr Mervat Nasser
Consultant Psychiatrist and Senior Research Fellow
Health Service and Population Research Department
Institute of Psychiatry, King's College,
London, UK

Professor Karen Newbigging
Principal Lecturer and Senior Researcher,
International School of Communities,
Rights and Inclusion, University of Central Lancashire,
Preston, UK

Professor Gregory O'Brien
Professor in Developmental Psychiatry,
Northumbria University;
Associate Medical Director,
Northumberland Tyne and Wear NHS Trust;
Consultant Psychiatrist,
Northgate Hospital,
Morpeth, UK

Dr T.G. O'Connor
Department of Psychiatry,
University of Rochester Medical Center,
Rochester,
New York, USA

Kieran O'Donnell
Institute of Reproductive and Developmental Biology,
Imperial College London,
London, UK

Professor Bob Palmer
Consultant Psychiatrist,
Leicester Adult Eating Disorders Service,
Leicestershire and Rutland Partnership NHS Trust;
Honorary Professor of Psychiatry,
Department of Health Sciences,
University of Leicester,
Leicester, UK

Dr Dimitrios Paschos
Consultant Psychiatrist in Learning Disabilities,
Estia Centre, Institute of Psychiatry,
King's College London,
London, UK

Professor Vikram Patel
Professor of International Mental Health &
Wellcome Trust
Senior Clinical Research Fellow in Tropical
Medicine,
Centre for Global Mental Health,
London School of Hygiene & Tropical
Medicine,
London, UK

Professor Jenifer Paul
Former National Lead for Gender Equality and
Women's Mental Health,
Care Services Improvement Partnership (now National
Mental Health Development Unit),
UK

Dr Marlon Pflüger
Psychiatric Outpatient Department,
University Hospital Basel,
Switzerland

Professor David Pilgrim
Professor of Mental Health Policy,
Department of Social Work,
Faculty of Health,
University of Central Lancashire,
Preston, UK

Professor Anita Riecher-Rössler
Psychiatric Outpatient Department,
University Hospital Basel,
Switzerland

Dr Emma Robertson Blackmore
University of Rochester Medical Center,
Rochester,
New York, USA

Dr John Roche
Honorary Clinical Lecturer in Psychiatry,
University of Birmingham,
Department of Psychiatry,
Birmingham, UK

Professor Vedat Şar
Department of Psychiatry,
Istanbul Faculty of Medicine,
University of Istanbul;
Director, Clinical Psychotherapy Unit and
Dissociative Disorders Program,
Istanbul Medical Faculty Hospital,
Istanbul, Turkey

Professor Mary V. Seeman
Graduate Coordinator,
Institute of Medical Science;
Professor Emerita, Department of Psychiatry,
University of Toronto,
Canada

Dr Joanne Stubley
Tavistock Trauma Service,
Adult Department,
Tavistock Clinic,
London, UK

Dr Nora Turjanski
Consultant Liaison Psychiatrist and
Perinatal Psychiatrist
Royal Free Hospital,
London, UK

Dr Erin Turner
Consultant Psychiatrist,
Early Intervention Service Birmingham and
Solihull Mental Health Foundation Trust,
Birmingham, UK

Dr Gillian Wainscott
Consultant Perinatal Psychiatrist,
Birmingham and Solihull Mental Health NHS
Foundation Trust,
Birmingham, UK

Dr James Wilson
Lecturer in Philosophy and Health,
University College London,
London, UK

Dr Lisa Wootton
Consultant Forensic Psychiatrist,
South London and Maudsley NHS Foundation Trust;
Visiting Research Associate,
Institute of Psychiatry,
King's College London,
London, UK

CHAPTER 1

Stigma, women, and mental health

Levent Küey

Introduction

People with mental disorders have been discriminated against and stigmatized worldwide throughout history. Since the pioneering studies carried out in the 1950s, the stigma attached to 'mental illness' has been widely researched and documented. In early studies, stigma was found to be very general and shared by all social subgroups (Rabkin 1974). Furthermore, research had revealed that patients with mental health problems were regarded with fear, distrust, and dislike more than virtually any other disabled group. Scientific efforts to help understand and tackle these phenomena enhanced the development of anti-stigma programmes that exist in many countries. Yet fewer attempts have been made to understand stigma-related problems in the context of women's mental health, and this would have to be considered a relatively new field of research and conceptualization in psychiatry. It is a field where we have more hypotheses and questions than evidence and answers. Since other sections in this book will cover various aspects of women's mental health, this chapter will mainly focus on stigmatization and discrimination issues relating to women's mental health. This is a subject that deserves volumes of writing, but here, some basic perspectives and reflections are highlighted.

Stigma

Humans are social beings. Human existence and survival relies on a net of interactions with their fellow beings. This reality presents an inevitable basis for social groupings and, in turn, generates the categorization of ingroups and outgroups in the minds of people; at least, so far in human history.

The categorization of 'ingroup' versus 'outgroup' or 'us' versus 'them' or 'me' versus 'the other' has also been

the source of discrimination and stigmatization throughout history. Race, ethnicity, and religion-based prejudice and discrimination have caused vast human suffering in almost all societies across the world; as has gender-based discrimination. Indeed, many acts of mass violence have been executed in the name of such group differences. Besides its multiple socioeconomic, cultural, and political dimensions, the process of discrimination covers various dimensions of sociopsychological dynamics. In almost all societies, these multiple sources of stigmatization and discrimination lead to each society creating its own 'scapegoats'. Paradoxically, the same psychosocial phenomena creating discrimination also set the ground for 'subidentities' or 'group identities' for their members. Since human beings seek higher levels of social integration to survive, they need social identities to complement their personal identities. These personally incorporated social identities, which can be constructed based on differences in sex, gender, age, ethnicity, belief systems, etc., are also sources of perceived and/or personal stigma.

In fact, some of these variables have been perceived as justifications for stigmatization, irrespective of mental problems or disorders. History is full of depressing accounts of the devastating consequences of discrimination based on the marginalization of groups—due to any of the aforementioned variables. However, such discrimination is not only part of history—such discrimination still exists and gender role-based discrimination is a prominent form of discrimination which results in the underprivileged status of women across the world.

It is a broadly accepted idea that 'social power relations' determine the stratification of 'us' and 'them' groupings. In other words, whether a group is to be designated as the 'other' and labelled with prejudice and discrimination will heavily depend on the *zeitgeist* of the current 'social power'. Gender roles and mental health-related stigma could be considered in this context.

From a perspective of a person, what happens when a human meets a fellow human designated to be 'the other' in that society? How does stereotype-based ignorance lead to stigma and discrimination? Could meeting 'the other' alternatively lead to enrichment motivated by a hospitality-based acknowledgement? How could hospitality, found in the writings of Levinas and Derrida, as openness to the other, irrespective of social labels imposed on her/him (George 2009), lead to enrichment? The hypothetical vicious circles presented in Figs. 1.1 and 1.2 are assumed to be the two options here.

Stigmatization and mental health

Stigmatization in the field of mental health could be conceptualized within a multi-perspective approach. Its

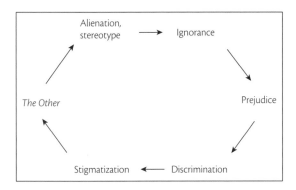

Fig. 1.1 Meeting 'the other': routes to stigmatization.

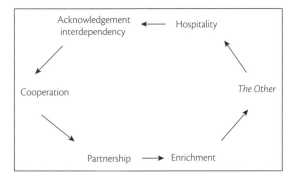

Fig. 1.2 Meeting 'the other': routes to enrichment.

relationship with adjacent concepts, such as stereotype, ignorance, prejudice, discrimination, devaluation, and disgrace, should be taken into consideration. One approach considers stigma as an amalgam of ignorance (lack of knowledge), prejudice (negative attitudes), and discrimination (excluding and avoiding behaviours) (Rose *et al.* 2007). As a further effort to differentiate these concepts, the following formulation (Hinshaw 2007) is clarifying: *stereotypes* are considered to reflect the cognitive aspect of social categorization of members of ingroups and outgroups. The emotional aspect of differentiation is reflected in *prejudices* toward the outgroups, and *discrimination* refers to the behavioural patterns directed to the well-being of outgroups, and consequently, giving harm to them.

In an elaborative stepwise explanation of the process of stigmatization related to mental disorders (Link and Phelan 2001; Link *et al.* 2004), the labelling of individuals with mental disorders is considered to be the first phase. Later, stereotyping attitudes connected to this specific label will be triggered. As a result of this stereotyping, the next phase will entail the construction of the categories of 'us' versus 'them'. Together with this categorization, as well as the emotional reactions of the perceivers, such as fear, anxiety, anger, and pity, and complementary emotional responses, such as shame, alienation, and embarrassment, discrimination against 'them' is induced.

A similar conceptual model that was used in a programme against stigmatization of schizophrenia in nearly 20 countries, over the past 10 years, defines stigma in general as a vicious circle (Sartorius 2006). The starting point of this vicious circle is marking an individual with the label of a mental disorder. This yields a negative content loading associated with the present psychopathology of the person. These attributions and loadings, along with the already lowered quality of life of the person, can become an additional source of stigmatization. The stigmatization and discrimination causing disadvantage will follow. These, in turn, set the basis for low self-esteem, disability, and less biological and psychological resistance to be internalized by the individual and this process will result in a heavy reinforcement of the initial marking.

Whenever there is stigmatization, it targets the person as a whole, covering all of his/her various demographic (e.g. age, sex, socioeconomic status) and psychosocial variables (e.g. gender role, race, ethnicity, religion), and physical health features (e.g. height, weight). It seems that the psychological and sociocultural processes producing discrimination and stigmatization are more 'holistic' than our prevailing psychiatric understanding and clinical practice (Küey 2008). Besides, stigmatization disregards the heterogeneity of the intergroup characteristics within the discriminated group. This causes transference of stigma from one focus to another. It seems that whenever a person is stigmatized because of one of his/her characteristics, this discrimination is almost spontaneously generalized to that person's being as a whole, disregarding any variations in the individual's features. Hence, the stigma attached to mental disorders in general forms the basis of the stigma towards women with mental health problems. Moreover, stigmatizers, recipients of stigma, and destigmatizers all interact in the process of stigmatization.

In the field of mental health, the process of stigmatization is based on the categorical differentiation of 'normality' versus 'abnormality'. In general, whatever is considered to be 'abnormal' in that particular society or community has a higher possibility of being stigmatized.

Stigmatization and women with mental ill health

The kind of stigma witnessed against those with mental disorders in general forms the basis for the stigma towards women with mental ill health, with the stigma related to gender differences then intensifying this discriminatory process. In other words, any stigma conceptualized in the context of understanding, explaining, or the management and treatment of patients with mental illness can only be understood in the context of both the stigma against mental disorders in general and the discrimination against women in general. Being a woman with mental ill health puts the person under a double burden of discrimination. Stigma towards women with mental disorders thus works in two ways, reinforcing each other.

Case study: depression and women

A brief discussion of a case sample could help to demonstrate the double burden of discrimination that women with mental ill health face.

> My husband had been used to my submissive behaviour for more than 20 years. That is what he had expected and what he got. Now, since I had started to look after my own interests and express my negative feelings or ideas more freely than before, and my hostile feelings against his mother, he is surprised by this transformation in my attitude and behaviour. He says, 'you had been an angel for so many years, and now you are becoming a witch'. Well, I say, I was not an angel but a dummy not to defend

my own rights, and of course, I do not wish to be taken as a witch!

A lady of 42 years, who had married at 18, and had two sons of 22 and 18, was diagnosed as having dsythymia, chronic depression, recurrent episodes of major depression, and suicidal risk in many psychiatric consultations for nearly 10 years. She had been having antidepressive treatment and psychodynamically-oriented psychotherapy for the last two years and for the last four months had not had any symptoms of depression. She began to express her aggressivity towards others, and although a novice to start with, she improved her own safe coping styles of expressing aggression; she now feels happier and no longer has suicidal ideas. She plans to go to university, an ambition she had dreamt of for many years and had postponed until her son went to university. She wants to study catering and become a pastry cook; 'It is the first time in my life that I am considering my own goals, in spite of my usual worries about my husband and sons' well-being'.

The phase of the treatment where she began to gain resourcefulness and overcome her long-lasting learned helplessness is also the period at which she was stigmatized and labelled as 'becoming a witch'. It is noteworthy that the suffering she experienced during her enduring depressive states was not stigmatized but was 'normalized' by her husband. In her depressive states, characterized with intrinsic submissiveness, she was regarded as 'being an angel', whereas once she began being aggressive towards the external world she was labelled as 'evil'. Stigmatization of women in mental ill health and women in psychiatric treatment is not free from the socially accepted norms of being 'a normal woman'.

The attitudes and behaviour of many women are stigmatized with reference to the 'accepted and expected norms of normal woman', in especially non-Western societies. These norms are characterized by submissiveness, non-assertiveness, altruism, introjections of guilt, being a good wife, mother, and housekeeper. Thus, in mild to moderate depressive states where women can still undertake the responsibilities of their gender roles, they are considered to be within the limits of the norms, i.e. 'normal'. As a consequence, if the treatment is efficient and the woman has no depressive symptomology then paradoxically, the stigmatization process starts against her: 'you're becoming evil'. No wonder why, in many instances, a successful treatment of depression in married women is frequently followed by marital conflicts and clinicians may face the complaints of the husband. For prevention, a family/systematic approach is usually necessary, starting from the very first days of the therapeutic interventions.

Conclusions

Stigmatization is the expression of discrimination and puts the stigmatized person in a position of 'the other'. Thus, it is strongly related to the values and social criteria of 'normality' of gender roles and identities. The cultural and social norms and perceptions of 'normality' and 'abnormality' in the context of mental health, profoundly determine the process, the level, and the target person of stigmatization.

In women with mental ill health, stigmatization is not only limited to the psychopathological state in question; since stigmatization disregards heterogeneity of inner group differences, even the normal emotional or behavioural responses of the 'labelled' could be stigmatized. The narratives of many female mental health service users have revealed the heavy burden of this experience. Furthermore, stigma surrounding these women has played a discouraging role in their recovery processes.

From a clinical perspective, another important component when we consider problems related to stigma is the clinician's diagnostic and treatment practices of women. The overdiagnosing of depressive disorders and overmedication during natural life cycles in women are just two examples of more recently addressed issues which seem to be related to stigma. Another widely seen stigmatizing practice is the fact that most research, especially in the field of drug trials, does not take gender differences into account.

On the other hand, it was argued in a recent study that men could have characteristics such as stoicism and personal stigma associated with mental health problems that mitigate against self-recognition and acceptance of emotional problems and thus pose barriers to help-seeking for such problems. These factors are thought to be more potent in cultural groups where gender inequality is marked (Jude *et al.* 2008).

Much remains to be understood about how the characteristics of stigma towards mental disorders are differentiated by the biological sex of the stigmatizer and the stigmatized. In fact, it is the gender roles that determine these attitudes and behaviour not the biological sex. It has been determined that strict gender-role adherence, rather than biological sex, accounts for the variance in the attitudes of the community towards mental illness (Hinkelman and Granello 2003). Additionally, as stated in a recent study, factors associated with stigma appear to vary by gender and therefore gender differences need to be considered in initiatives aiming at stigma reduction (Wang *et al.* 2007).

There are more hypotheses and questions than evidence and answers in this field. How is and how much of the stigma towards people with mental illness is determined by gender? What are the cross-gender differences in the processes of stigmatizing and being stigmatized? What could be the specific areas in mental health and illnesses where gender, as a variable, determines the degree and the nature of the stigma towards people with mental illness? Questions such as these indicate just some of the aspects of this subject that require further research and discussion.

References

George SK (2009). Hospitality as openness to the other – Levinas, Derrida and the Indian hospitality ethos. *Journal of Human Values*, **15**, 29–47.

Hinkelman L and Granello DH (2003). Biological sex, adherence to traditional gender roles, and attitudes toward persons with mental illness: an exploratory investigation. *Journal of Mental Health Counseling*, **25**, 259–70.

Hinshaw SP (2007). *The Mark of Shame: Stigma of Mental Illness and an Agenda for Change*, pp. 140–56. Oxford University Press, Oxford.

Judd F *et al.* (2008). How does being female assist help-seeking for mental health problems? *Australian and New Zealand Journal of Psychiatry*, **42**, 24–9.

Küey L (2008). The impact of stigma on somatic treatment and care for people with comorbid mental and somatic disorders. *Current Opinion in Psychiatry*, **21**, 403–11.

Link BG and Phelan JC (2001). Conceptualizing stigma. *Annual Review of Sociology*, **27**, 363–85.

Link BG *et al.* (2004). Measuring mental illness stigma. *Schizophrenia Bulletin*, **30**, 511–41.

Rabkin J (1974). Public attitudes toward mental illness: a review of the literature. *Schizophrenia Bulletin*, **10**, 9–33.

Rose D *et al.* (2007). 250 labels used to stigmatise people with mental illness. *BMC Health Services Research*, **7**, 97.

Sartorius N (2006). Lessons from a 10-year global programme against stigma and discrimination because of an illness. *Psychology, Health and Medicine*, **11**, 383–8.

Wang J *et al.* (2007). Gender specific correlates of stigma toward depression in a Canadian general population sample. *Journal of Affective Disorders*, **103**, 91–7.

CHAPTER 2

Gender-based violence and mental health

Neerja Chowdhary and Vikram Patel

Introduction

Violence against women is a subject that has generated considerable global attention from health professionals and policy makers, underlining its importance in the lives of women, their families, and society at large. There are various forms that violence against women can take and different terms that are used to describe the experience. We begin this chapter by describing key definitions of gender-based violence. According to Article 1 of the United Nations Declaration on Violence Against Women (1993), violence against women can be understood as:

> Any act of gender-based violence that results in, or is likely to result in, physical, sexual or psychological harm or suffering to women, including threats of such acts, coercion or arbitrary deprivations of liberty, whether occurring in public or private life.

A definition that may prove to be more useful in the development of programmes to reduce violence by focusing on the social determinants, particularly the structural determinant of gender disadvantage of women is:

> Gender-based violence is violence involving men and women, in which the female is usually the victim; and which is derived from unequal power relationships between men and women. Violence is directed specifically against a woman because she is a woman, or affects women disproportionately. It includes, but is not limited to, physical, sexual and psychological harm (including intimidation, suffering, coercion, and/or deprivation of liberty within the family, or within the general community). It includes that violence which is perpetrated or condoned by the state.
>
> UNPFA (2005)

Violence against women within the family is often described under the broad term of domestic violence.

This encompasses various forms of violence and includes spousal abuse, bride burning or dowry-related violence, marital rape, forced prostitution, and denial of contraceptive use. Intimate partner violence (IPV) is a term used to describe violence that women experience in the context of an intimate relationship; IPV has unique significance in the lives of women due to its occurrence within what should have been a trusting adult relationship, and the shroud of secrecy and social isolation that are often an intrinsic part of this experience.

The important role that violence against women plays in the progress and development of countries throughout the world is reflected in its integration in two global policy instruments: the Millennium Development Goals (MDGs) and the Human Development Index (HDI). The MDGs are the priority goals agreed by the international community and reflect the areas that are crucial for national and global development. Violence against women is identified as a potential major obstacle in achieving these goals, in particular the goals on maternal and child health, gender equality, and combating HIV. A recent World Health Organization (WHO 2005a). report concluded that:

> Unless prevention and awareness of violence against women is integrated into all MDGs, sustainable development will continue to suffer – and the ambitious Goals agreed to by the international community will remain unattainable.

The Human Development Report measures social and economic development in countries around the world on the basis of three broad indicators: life expectancy, educational attainment, and income. The gender-related development index (GDI) is a related composite measure which specifically takes note of inequality of achievement between men and women. Hence the greater the gender disparity in a number of opportunities and achievements, the lower a country's GDI compared with its HDI. The 2007/2008 GDI ranks for 157 countries and areas reveals that low- and middle-income countries (LAMIC) tend to have lower GDI than high-income countries (HIC) (UNDP 2007). Thus it can be seen that gender disadvantage and gender-based violence, although universal phenomena, exact a higher toll in terms of development and economic burden in the poorer regions of the world. These are also regions where health services, including mental health services, are scarce and distributed in an inefficient and inequitable manner.

In this chapter, we will present an overview of the relationship between gender-based violence and mental health, particularly in the context of IPV. Thus, we will not discuss issues around child sexual abuse or violence against women by persons not intimately related to the woman, issues which are covered elsewhere in this book (see Chapter 31). We will describe the public health importance of IPV, the mental health problems that predispose to the perpetration of violence, the association of violence with mental illness in women, and the specific mental health outcomes in women exposed to violence. Finally, we consider implications of these findings for reducing the burden of mental illness in women through interventions that have been found to have an impact in reducing violence and its adverse mental health consequences.

The public health importance of intimate partner violence

The universality of the phenomenon of intimate partner violence has been firmly established through a large number of surveys in several countries. One notable, and recent, example was the WHO Multi-Country Study on Women's Health and Domestic Violence against Women (WHO 2005b). This study collected data through standardized population-based household surveys from over 24 000 women from 15 sites in ten countries around the world. The main findings were that between 15–71% of ever-partnered women reported physical or sexual violence, or both, by an intimate partner at some point in their lives. The prevalence rate in most sites varied between 30–50%. Figure 2.1 illustrates the wide variation in prevalence between study sites. The difference in the prevalence of violence reported across studies and sites may reflect true regional variations, but may also be partly attributable to various factors such as differences in the definitions of violence used in the study, the study design, and sampling differences. In addition, in many cultures the experience of violence is under-reported by women due to shame, guilt, and fear of retribution.

The experience of violence has myriad effects on a woman's health—physical, sexual, and, very importantly, psychological (Campbell 2002). We discuss specific mental health consequences in more detail later in

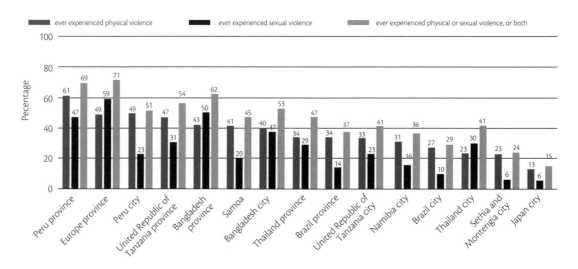

Fig. 2.1 Prevalence of lifetime physical and sexual violence by an intimate partner, by site. Reproduced with permission (WHO 2005b).

this chapter. The increased risk of premature mortality in women exposed to IPV is attributable to the direct effects of an assault and resulting injuries—due to other health consequences of IPV—and suicide. Apart from being a cause of acute trauma and injury, violence also leads to effects on a woman's health long after the violence has ceased. Chronic pain syndromes, gastrointestinal problems, hypertension, and chest pain have all been linked to IPV.

Sexual violence, in addition, is associated with a range of gynaecological problems such as pain during intercourse, sexually transmitted infections, pelvic pain, and urinary tract infections (Chowdhary and Patel 2008). Transmission of HIV infection is associated with IPV through various pathways such as trauma to the genital tract, difficulty in negotiating use of condoms in violent relationships, and the greater likelihood of violent men having multiple sexual partners and therefore being at a greater risk of acquiring and transmitting HIV. Also, women in violent relationships are more likely to engage in transactional sex and other sexual risk-taking behaviour (WHO 2004). Violence during pregnancy can have adverse effects on reproductive health of the woman as well as adverse perinatal outcomes such as increased maternal and infant mortality, increased risk of low birthweight babies, and preterm labour.

IPV has considerable economic implications. In the USA, for example, it has been estimated that IPV costs the economy $5.8–12.6 billion on an annual basis, i.e. up to 0.125% of the gross domestic product (Waters 2004). This estimate includes direct costs, for example for legal and medical services, as well as indirect costs, such as lost productivity. As a percentage of the gross domestic product, estimates of the costs of IPV are considerably higher in LAMIC. The costs of domestic violence against women in Chile and Nicaragua, based only on the lost productivity of affected women, is around $1.73 billion in Chile, i.e. 1.6% of the gross domestic product, and $32.7 million in Nicaragua, i.e. 2.0% of the gross domestic product.

The use of disability adjusted life years (DALYs) as a metric to assess the burden of disease allows for the estimation of the impact of health problems in a population, taking into account chronicity of illness, associated disability, and the risk of premature death. It provides a standard measure that can be used to compare health impact of various diseases and assist in setting priorities. IPV is a major risk factor for burden of disease in women. A study conducted in Victoria, Australia, for example, measured the burden of disease in women and then estimated the contribution of IPV as a risk factor for various health problems. The study revealed that IPV accounted for a larger proportion of the total burden of disease in women under the age of 45 years than any other risk factor and was responsible for an estimated 9% of the total disease burden. The greatest proportion of the disease burden was associated with mental health problems, of which depression and anxiety accounted for 60% of the burden, suicide 13%, tobacco use 10%, alcohol use 6%, and illicit drug use 6% (VicHealth 2004).

Mental health risk factors for intimate partner violence

Several factors have been consistently found to increase the risk of IPV, not least among which is the structural inequalities in power between men and women. These inequalities may manifest differently in different cultural settings, and may be reflected through indicators such as the levels of involvement of both sexes in economic and political spheres, in commerce, in the formation of public policy, and in access to appropriate healthcare. In some cultures, particularly in Asia, the preference for a male child is attributed to the value that sons carry forward the family name and contribute to the well-being of the family in greater measure than girls. These attitudes then play out in marital relationships where men use violence in order to maintain their position of power in the relationship, and families expect mothers to bear boy-children. The falling sex ratio in some Asian countries bears testimony to the impact of this form of gender inequality on the poorer prospects for a live-birth for a female baby compared to a male baby.

Social determinants of IPV include low family income, lower education levels of women and their partners, and spousal unemployment. In addition, mental health-related determinants are also potential risk factors for IPV, notably alcohol and drug misuse and mental illness in the woman or her partner. The association between mental illness in women and IPV is discussed in the next section. Men who witness domestic violence or are exposed to childhood sexual abuse are more likely to abuse their partners than those who have not had such experiences (Jewkes 2002). The WorldSAFE Study, a survey carried out in four developing countries, i.e. Chile, Egypt, Philippines, and India, found significant associations between regular alcohol consumption of the husband/partner, past witnessing of father beating mother, the woman's poor mental health, and poor family work status with any lifetime

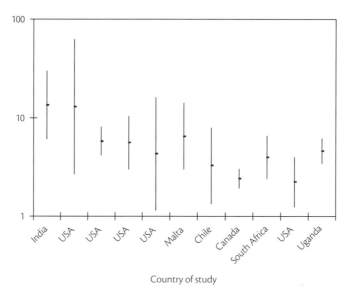

Country of study

Fig. 2.2 Odds ratio and 95% confidence intervals in studies describing the association between alcohol consumption and intimate partner violence. Adapted with permission (Gil-Gonzalez *et al.* 2006).

physical IPV (Jeyaseelan *et al.* 2004). A systematic review and meta-analysis was performed by Gil-Gonzalez and colleagues (2006) to assess the magnitude of the association between male alcohol consumption and IPV. Despite the heterogeneity in the 11 studies selected for the meta-analysis and the dearth of cohort studies, alcohol was associated with statistically significant risk excess for IPV in all the studies (Figure 2.2).

The precise mechanism by which spousal alcohol consumption increases the risk of IPV is not clear; it is likely that physiological, psychological, and environmental factors may all play a critical role. Alcohol intoxication increases the likelihood of violence by causing impaired judgement, perceptions, and impulse control. Even in the absence of intoxication, disinhibition and autonomic arousal may facilitate aggressive behaviour. Pathological intoxication, when aggression occurs within minutes of consuming moderate amounts of alcohol, has been implicated as a cause of alcohol-related violence. However, this diagnosis is of uncertain validity and behavioural disturbances are usually attributable to additional factors such as hypoglycaemia and head injury. Alcohol withdrawal, too, is associated with irritability and violence. Furthermore, the coexistence of substance abuse with mental disorder significantly increases the risk of violent behaviour. Pathological jealousy is frequently associated with chronic alcohol use and can lead to violence and even homicide directed

against the allegedly unfaithful spouse, the so-called 'crimes of passion'.

Mental health of women who are exposed to intimate partner violence

The relationship between violence and mental illness is multi-directional and complex. For most women, history of violence precedes mental illness and substance abuse; depression results from the experience of violence while substance abuse may be the consequence of unhealthy coping styles for symptoms of depression and anxiety. However, in some instances, mental illness in the woman may also be associated with the risk of IPV. It is well established, for example, that women with schizophrenia, especially in the presence of paranoid symptoms and at times of acute exacerbations, are at greater risk to suffer IPV. Depressive illnesses, when associated with irritability, delusions, morbid preoccupations, and hopelessness, can predispose to violence, though this is not as common as with schizophrenia. There is modest evidence to suggest that women with mental illness are more likely to be involved in unsafe and abusive relationships, thus increasing their risk of being exposed to gender-based violence.

A meta-analysis of studies on the prevalence of mental health problems in women exposed to IPV reported a prevalence of 47.6% depression, 17.9%

suicidality, 63.8% post-traumatic stress disorder (PTSD), 18.5% alcohol abuse, and 8.9% drug abuse (Golding 1999). When these associations were examined further, a dose–response relationship was found between the severity of IPV and the risk for depression and PTSD, suggesting a causal association between IPV and mental illness in women. Thus, the well-recognized increased risk of depression and PTSD in women in the general population may, at least in part, be attributed to the greater risk of exposure to IPV.

Though the diagnostic construct of PTSD across cultural settings is controversial, some authors have considered it useful to describe the intrusive memories and hyperarousal that women who are exposed to IPV experience. PTSD is associated with greater severity of violence especially when there is threat to life, sexual violence, use of a weapon, and multiple experiences of violence through adulthood and childhood including childhood sexual abuse. Women exposed to IPV may develop depression and PTSD as co-morbid mental health conditions. Apart from depression and PTSD, other psychiatric disorders described in women exposed to IPV include anxiety disorders, obsessive–compulsive disorder, and eating disorders. Alcohol and substance abuse have been found to occur more frequently in these women. The pathway for this association may be the use of alcohol and other substances to cope with the symptoms of depression/PTSD or as a means to cope with the reality of the violence in their lives.

Apart from clear-cut psychiatric disorders, women exposed to IPV experience long-term psychological sequelae such as low self-esteem, deliberate self-harm, a chronic sense of unhappiness, and somatic complaints such as insomnia, headache, and abdominal pains. The low self-esteem, social isolation, and limited choices that accompany IPV may contribute to the development of depression. IPV is an independent risk factor for suicidal behaviour in women (Chowdhary and Patel 2008), with or without the presence of a depressive illness; this increased risk is probably mediated by factors such as low self-esteem, helplessness, and hopelessness (Gielen *et al.* 2005). For example, in a study from Goa, India (Pereira *et al.* 2007), one woman describes:

> I had thoughts of committing suicide. I had even gone to jump in the well. This was last year. And then my husband came and pulled me. He used to always abuse and lift his hands (to slap) and kick me. If I said anything he used to beat me. I don't know what happened to me that day. I would have jumped in the well that day.

Given the complex nature of the association between violence and mental health and the interplay of diverse factors such as socioeconomic status, levels of gender disadvantage, and women's disempowerment which differ across countries, it is inappropriate to generalize findings across countries, especially if one wants to plan culturally-specific preventive and intervention strategies. For example, the view held by many women in India that 'wife-beating' is a husband's right and justified in a variety of circumstances, such as the neglect of household chores and failure to obey the husband, may mitigate the adverse effects of violence on a woman's mental health (Jejeebhoy 1998). Thus, it is relevant to ask whether there are associations between IPV and mental illness in women in LAMIC. We reviewed studies from LAMIC which described the prevalence of mental health problems in women exposed to IPV. Among the 11 studies which met our inclusion criteria, the prevalence of IPV ranged from 9.4–77%. All the studies reported a significant association between IPV and the risk of mental disorder (depression, unhappiness, mental distress) with odds ratios ranging from 1.67–10.30. Hence, the evidence from literature in the LAMIC does not differ greatly from that in HIC with comparable rates of mental disorders in women exposed to IPV across settings; however, the implications of this association may differ across settings.

It is important to understand the culture-specific contexts of abuse, as the meaning that the woman attributes to the violence can determine both the psychological consequences as well as help-seeking behaviour. Women cope with the experience in various ways including the use of denial, minimizing the abuse, and even placating the abuser. Where violence is identified as being linked to alcohol, women overlook the violence and blame alcohol use for their husbands' behaviour. Women who suffer violence from a spouse who is suspicious, sometimes eroticize the experience and explain it as an index of his love. Many women cite biological determinism as the reason for the violence they suffer. They see themselves as being emotionally and physically weak, needing to be protected by men, and hence belonging to men who look after them who thus have a right to beat them. They do not question this state of affairs and accept it as their 'fate' which has to be borne. Some authors have argued that this also reflects the internalization of the structural inequalities between men and women. In addition, for many women living in dire poverty, the violence they suffer parallels their daily struggle to make ends meet (Geetha 1998). Whether these perceptions act as protective mechanisms against the development of mental health problems is questionable, but they do pose a barrier in terms of health seeking and may make accessing and accepting healthcare interventions difficult.

Prevention and intervention programmes for intimate partner violence

Given the public health implications of IPV for women's health, and the well-being of their families and society, interventions need to operate at many diverse levels. We consider, briefly, interventions both for the prevention of IPV as well as addressing the specific mental health needs of women exposed to IPV. There are three levels at which intervention programmes can be targeted: the individual, the healthcare system, and the community (Ramsey *et al.* 2005).

Individual level interventions

Psychological interventions have been found to be effective in reducing the risk of IPV and the risk of depression in women exposed to IPV. These can be provided in individual or group setting and employ different approaches such as psychoeducational programmes, cognitive behaviour therapy, feminist-oriented counselling, and grief resolution-oriented counselling. While these interventions are typically recommended to treat depression and low self-esteem in women who have left abusive relationships, they could also play a useful role in addressing the mental health needs of women attempting to cope with life with a violent partner. In one randomized controlled trial in Colombia, abused women were given cognitive behaviour therapy along with lectures and structured exercises, involving for example, role play. The control group attended unstructured support group meetings. While the frequency and intensity of abuse decreased markedly in both groups, women who received the intervention showed significant improvement in measures of communication skills, handling of aggression and assertiveness, and their feelings towards their partners as compared to women in the control group (Ramsey *et al.* 2005).

It is important to understand protective factors as well in planning prevention and intervention programmes. One such factor is social support; strengthening social support can improve self-esteem and make a woman feel valued apart from providing practical assistance to deal with the violence, such as a safe temporary refuge to escape from heightened violence.

Hence, encouraging a woman who is isolated and alone to rebuild her social network and re-establish contact with, for example, a favourite relative, friend, or neighbour, is an important step in helping women cope with violence. In addition, it is useful to provide women with advice regarding safety behaviours such as: hiding money, clothes, and keys for use when needed; making an exit plan in the event of feeling threatened; informing neighbours to call the police in case there is a call for help or a disturbance; and establishing a danger code with others.

Group interventions, which focus on educating participants about issues around violence, build self-esteem, and assist in development of concrete plans in coping with their situation, have been found to be effective in reducing IPV and have a beneficial impact on perceived supports and locus of control. An example of a community level intervention which empowers women is described later (see Box 2.3). Individual level advocacy for women who seek help from professional services or who are in a shelter has been shown to be beneficial in reducing subsequent IPV, increasing social support, and improving quality of life. The main aim of advocacy interventions are to respond to the individual woman's needs and coordinate support services so that the woman can remain independent and safe. There are few studies which examine the impact of interventions to empower women who are exposed to IPV on their mental health. One such study in Hong Kong evaluated the effects of empowerment training for pregnant women who were exposed to IPV. The intervention comprised of advice in the areas of safety, choice making and problem solving, and empathic understanding. Women who received the intervention reported significantly less psychological abuse, less minor physical violence, and improved mental health status as compared to those who received standard care (Tiwari *et al.* 2005).

Health system interventions
Primary care

In countries where the public health system is reasonably well developed, primary healthcare provides an easily accessible and stigma-free setting where women with IPV can seek help. However, the vast majority of women do not seek help for the IPV, but for the health complaints resulting from IPV. The primary care physician may follow two steps for the effective detection and management of IPV in women. The first step is routine screening of married or cohabiting women who attend the clinic followed by provision of simple advice

Box 2.1   Integrating mental healthcare in IPV services: the Dilaasa model

A public hospital-based crisis centre for women exposed to IPV was established in Bombay, India in 2001. The centre, called Dilaasa (meaning reassurance in Hindi) provides social and psychological support to women who face violence in a setting that is easily accessible to a large number of women. Training of hospital staff in the detection and sensitive handling of women exposed to IPV, and collaboration with medical personnel, legal experts, and other non-governmental organizations (NGOs) are part of the centre's activities. The interventions provided consist of individual counselling, assistance with registration of complaints, legal assistance, overnight shelter, and medical and psychiatric care. In a one-year period from April 2006 to March 2007, 197 women sought counselling at the centre and 105 women were referred to the centre from other hospital departments. It is notable that almost all these 105 women were admitted either with history of self-harm (in the form of poisoning or burns) or medically unexplained symptoms, indicative of the mental health issues which were relevant in these admissions. While Dilaasa is an NGO initiative, staff from within the hospital, for example, nurses, are recruited and trained to provide the counselling services with the aim of better integration of the intervention into the public hospital system (Deosthali *et al.* 2005).

on reducing risk for IPV. Routine assessment of mental health is strongly recommended for all women who are exposed to IPV. A systematic review of interventions for IPV at the level of primary healthcare, while concluding that information on evidence-based approaches for prevention of IPV in the primary care setting is seriously lacking, provides evidence in support of the efficacy of advocacy counselling, staying in a shelter, personal and vocational counselling, and prenatal counselling to reduce further violence (Wathen and MacMillan 2003). Thus, well-established referral pathways between primary care and such intervention programmes outside the formal health sector are strongly recommended.

Reproductive healthcare

Integration of violence prevention and screening into reproductive health programmes has been advocated as a means of reaching out to the large number of women

who access such services. A UNFPA (United Nations Population Fund) pilot programme tested a guide for integration of services for the prevention and assessment of gender-based violence into reproductive health services in ten countries in five regions (UNFPA and AIDOS 2003). These programmes involved displaying information material in the clinic, asking women directly about IPV, and provision of referral to on-site or off-site intervention programmes. Evaluation of the programme in four of the pilot countries (Lebanon, Mozambique, Nepal, and Romania) revealed beneficial effects in terms of greater capacity among health facility staff to service the needs of clients who have experienced IPV; an increase in the number of health facilities providing screening and on-site treatment; and the establishment of referral services, though their effectiveness was uneven. Links were also established among medical and non-medical services and an increase in the number of abused women who chose to speak about their experiences was reported.

Mental healthcare

It is essential to integrate interventions to improve the detection and management of mental disorders in women accessing IPV shelters or services, and interventions to detect and provide advice on reducing exposure to IPV in women attending mental health services. Despite the strong inter-relationship between mental illness and IPV, only a minority of women reporting IPV obtain mental healthcare. The utilization of mental health services by these women is subject to various barriers including the controlling behaviour of partners and the double stigma of IPV and mental illness which preclude seeking mental healthcare, failure of healthcare staff to recognize mental health problems in women with history of violence, failure of mental health professionals to screen for presence of IPV among their patients, and lack of coordinated services among the various healthcare providers. Apart from regular screening and intervention services directed at helping women at the individual level, mental health professionals need to respond to the issue of domestic violence by providing training to other healthcare workers in identifying and responding to women, development of partnerships with women's organizations in the government and non-government sector that work with women in abusive relationships, and promoting public education campaigns that address societal attitudes and cultural norms. Box 2.1 describes a programme that integrates mental health care in an IPV service. There is also a need to address interventions for men who are violent

Box 2.2   Guidelines for mental health professionals in the management of IPV

- Routinely ask all women attending the clinic for their experience of IPV. This can be very effective when done in the context of a trusting therapeutic relationship, assurance of confidentiality, and in a respectful and non-judgemental fashion

- Acknowledge and validate disclosure. Disclosure of IPV is a difficult step and it is important to acknowledge this, at the same time accepting non-disclosure

- Offer education and support. Inform the woman of the effects of violence on herself and the family and discuss various options that she may have

- Empower women to make their own decision about their plans about the future of the relationship and avoid imposing value judgements related to the woman's decision

- Provide treatment for mental health problems arising as a consequence of violence

- Discuss safety measures that the woman can institute to protect herself and her children

- Offer referral to shelter, legal services, and women's organizations

- Assess level of social support and encourage help seeking

- Documentation in a clear and precise fashion is mandatory

- Offer help to the woman for the abusive partner, especially for treatment of alcohol/substance abuse.

and in advocating for reforms in the legal and law enforcement sectors. Legally mandated batterer intervention programmes use educational classes or treatment groups which consist of psychoeducational, cognitive behavioural, and self-help models. These programmes have been found to produce small but significant benefits, particularly when employed as part of an overall violence prevention strategy. A full list of recommendations on the role of mental health professionals in the management of IPV is presented in Box 2.2.

The Women, Co-occurring Disorders, and Violence Study (WCDVS), sponsored by the Substance Abuse and Mental Health Service Administration (SAMHSA), is a multi-site cooperative study to evaluate new service models for women with co-occurring mental health and substance use disorders and a history of physical and/or sexual abuse (McHugo *et al.* 2005). The WCDVS is based on the premise of the co-occurrence of mental illness and substance abuse problems in the life of women who are exposed to IPV. The nine sites selected for the study used diverse trauma-focused intervention models which emphasized skill building techniques, psychoeducation, and cognitive behavioural models. These were integrated with mental health and substance abuse services. Six-month project outcomes revealed that despite wide variability in study sites, women showed improvement from the baseline in all outcomes of mental ill-health, alcohol use, drug use, and post-traumatic symptoms. In sites where the intervention was most integrated (i.e. addressed mental health, substance abuse, and trauma issues together within individual and group counselling for IPV), the results were more favourable. The key messages learnt from this study, and other efforts towards integration in mental health services, are that it is feasible to assist women who have these complicated co-occurring problems by using integrated models, that such integrated models in a trauma-informed context are more effective than treatment as usual, and that the full involvement of women with the lived experiences of IPV in all aspects of policy, planning, implementation, and evaluation improve the quality of these interventions.

Community level and policy interventions

The link between IPV and parameters of gender disadvantage such as poverty and lack of education has been firmly established. It is reasonable to expect, therefore, that interventions that focus on increasing educational levels and reducing poverty will empower women and hence be effective in reducing violence. Education improves social networks, enhances self-confidence, increases capacity to use resources and information available, and can improve economic status. For adult women, literacy programmes and non-formal educational programmes, and microfinance interventions may serve such an empowerment function that in turn can reduce IPV exposure (Box 2.3).

The recognition of IPV as a global issue with widespread public health implications makes it important for countries and political leaders to address it as a priority in planning public policy and healthcare initiatives. Each country, through its mechanisms of legislature and judiciary, is responsible for combating gender discrimination. International policy instruments such as the Convention on the Elimination of All Forms of

---

Box 2.3   Empowering women through micro-credit: the IMAGE trial

The Intervention with Microfinance for AIDS and Gender Equity (IMAGE) study conducted in South Africa evaluated an intervention that combined microfinance with a gender-focused participatory learning programme. The microfinance component of the intervention consisted of the provision of loans to poor women for the development of income-generating activities using the group lending model where businesses were run by individual women but groups of five women guaranteed each other's loans. A participatory learning and action curriculum called Sisters For Life was integrated into fortnightly loan meetings. This consisted of training on topics such as gender roles, cultural beliefs, relationships, IPV, HIV, along with wider community mobilization of youths and men in the intervention. Eight villages were pair-matched and randomly allocated to receive the intervention at study onset or three years later. The intervention was found to lead to significant improvements in economic well-being, social capital, and empowerment; furthermore, the risk for IPV was reduced to almost half (Pronyk *et al.* 2006).

Box 2.4   A pubic advocacy campaign to combat IPV

The White Ribbon Campaign (http://www.whiteribbon.ca/) which was initiated in Canada in 1991 is the largest effort of its kind in the world and is based on the idea that all men and boys must take responsibility for ending violence against women. Campaigns are led by both men and women in over 55 countries and wearing a white ribbon is a personal pledge never to commit, condone, or remain silent about violence against women. The objectives of the campaign are accomplished by:

- Educating young people, especially young men and boys, on the issue
- Encouraging people to speak out and challenging their beliefs and actions
- Raising public awareness
- Working in partnership with women's organizations, the corporate sector, the media, and other partners.

Discrimination against Women (CEDAW), adopted in 1979 by the United Nations General Assembly assists this process by setting up an agenda for national action to end discrimination against women. Accessibility of legal assistance to women who are exposed to IPV should be ensured. The role of legal advocates for women, use of civil protection orders, arrest of the abuser, and legally mandated batterer intervention programmes have all been found to have some usefulness at preventing further abuse. The role of men in advocacy is best exemplified in the White Ribbon Campaign (Box 2.4).

Conclusion

The far-reaching effects of IPV on women and society have gained recognition by international organizations and policy makers. IPV is a major cause of disease burden affecting economic growth and development of countries. While mental health problems such as alcohol dependence in the perpetrator and mental illness in women increase the risk of IPV, IPV in itself leads to mental illness. Depression, anxiety disorders, substance abuse, and increased suicide risk are not infrequently associated with IPV. Hence, it is mandatory for mental

health professionals to recognize this association and routinely question all women for the experience of IPV and offer interventions to reduce IPV and its consequences. Interventions to reduce violence can be in the form of individual counselling but these do not address the societal attitudes and gender disadvantage that exist to a greater or lesser degree in almost all cultural settings. Thus, educating women, empowering them financially, and involving men in violence prevention efforts are important strategies to reduce violence. Integrating these and other violence prevention programmes into already established healthcare systems, especially mental health systems, is perhaps the most effective method of ensuring accessibility of these services to women who might otherwise find it difficult to seek help. In addition, it is essential to integrate mental healthcare into programmes that provide assistance to women affected by IPV.

References

Campbell JC (2002). Health consequences of intimate partner violence. *Lancet*, **359**, 1331–6.

Chowdhary N and Patel V (2008). The effect of spousal violence on women's health: Findings from the Stree Arogya Shodh in Goa, India. *Journal of Postgraduate Medicine*, Oct–Dec; **54**(4), 306–12.

Deosthali P *et al.* (2005). *Establishing Dilaasa: Documenting the challenges.* Centre for Enquiry into Health and Allied Themes (CEHAT), Mumbai.

Geetha V (1998). On bodily love and hurt. In: M John and J Nair (eds) A *Question of Silence? The Sexual Economics of Modern India*. Kali for Women, New Delhi.

Gielen AC *et al*. (2005). Suicide risk and mental health indicators: Do they differ by abuse and HIV status? *Women's Health Issues*, **15**, 89–95.

Gil-Gonzalez D *et al*. (2006). Alcohol and intimate partner violence: do we have enough information to act? *European Journal of Public Health*, **16**, 279–85.

Golding JM (1999). Intimate partner violence as a risk factor for mental disorders: A meta-analysis. *Journal of Family Violence*, **14**, 99–132.

Jejeebhoy S (1998). Wife-beating in rural India: A Husband's Right? Evidence from survey data. *Economic and Political Weekly*, **33**, 855–62.

Jewkes R (2002). Intimate partner violence: causes and prevention. *Lancet*, **359**, 1423–9.

Jeyaseelan L *et al*. (2004). World studies of abuse in the family environment–risk factors for physical intimate partner violence. *International Journal of Injury Control and Safety Promotion*, **11**, 117–24.

McHugo GJ *et al*. (2005). Women, Co-occurring Disorders, and Violence Study: evaluation design and study population. *Journal of Substance Abuse Treatment*, **28**, 91–107.

Pereira B *et al*. (2007). The explanatory models of depression in low income countries: listening to women in India. *Journal of Affective Disorders*, **102**, 209–18.

Pronyk PM *et al*. (2006). Effect of a structural intervention for the prevention of intimate-partner violence and HIV in rural South Africa: a cluster randomised trial. *Lancet*, **368**, 1973–83.

Ramsey J *et al*. (2005). *Interventions to reduce violence and promote the physical and psychological well-being of women who experience partner violence: a systematic review of controlled evaluations*. Barts and The London, Queen Mary's School of Medicine and Dentistry, London.

Tiwari A *et al*. (2005). A randomised controlled trial of empowerment training for Chinese abused pregnant women in Hong Kong. *BJOG: An International Journal of Obstetrics & Gynaecology*, **112**, 1249–56.

UN Declaration on the Elimination of Violence Against Women (1993). General Assembly Resolution 48/104 of 20 December 1993. http://www.un.org/documents/ga/res/48/a48r104.htm

UNDP (2007). *Fighting Climate Change. Human Solidarity in a Divided World*. UNDP, New York.

UNFPA (2005). *State of the World Population 2005: The Promise of Equality: Gender Equity. Reproductive Health and the Millennium Development Goals*. UNFPA, New York.

UNFPA and AIDOS (2003). *Addressing Violence against Women: Piloting and Programming. Rome, Italy, 15–19 September 2003*. UNFPA, New York.

VicHealth (2004). *The Health Costs of Violence: Measuring the Burden of Disease caused by Intimate Partner Violence. A summary of findings*. Victorian Health Promotion Foundation, Carlton.

Waters H *et al*. (2004). *The Economic Dimensions of Interpersonal Violence*. World Health Organization, Department of Injuries and Violence Prevention, Geneva.

Wathen CN and MacMillan HL (2003). Interventions for violence against women: scientific review. *Journal of the American Medical Association*, **289**, 589–600.

WHO (2004). *Violence against Women and HIV/AIDS: Critical Intersections. Intimate Partner Violence and HIV/AIDS*. Information Bulletin Series Number 1. WHO, Geneva.

WHO (2005a). *Addressing violence against women and achieving the Millennium Development Goals*. WHO, Geneva.

WHO (2005b). *WHO multi-country study of women's health and domestic violence against women: summary report of initial results on prevalence, health outcomes and women's responses*. WHO, Geneva.

CHAPTER 3

Mind the gender gap: mental health in a post-feminist context

David Pilgrim

Introduction

Differences in mental health status (if any) between men and women remain an important matter of debate for two main reasons. First, methodological questions abound about measuring mental health and which inclusion criteria to utilize in empirical studies. Second, the gendered picture has been shaped, in part, by pre-empirical or non-empirical forces, which reflect interest work in the academy (first in relation to masculine assumptions in psychiatry and second in relation to the response of feminist scholars). Thus an exploration of the gender gap is a window into both the general challenges of doing mental health research and in understanding our current post-feminist discourse. This chapter will address both of these areas of understanding.

A couple more points can be made by way of introduction. The first is that the ambiguity of gender as a social variable, in predicting mental health status, is also shared by others (such as age and race) (Rogers and Pilgrim 2005). The least ambiguous predictor is social class—generally the poorer the person, the poorer their mental health, as with physical health. Basically, the poor are sicker in all respects and they die younger than richer citizens. They are consequently over-represented in psychiatric populations. But even in the case of class as a predictor of mental health status, a clear gradient in diagnosis does not apply to a few categories (such as bipolar disorder and obsessive–compulsive personality disorder).

A second contextualizing point is that the analysis of mental health in terms of single social variables is an academic convenience, in a highly complex world in flux. But, in the latter, people with or without mental health problems are not just old or young, black or white, men or women, etc. Social variables coexist in the open systems of real populations. This makes definitive deductions about single variable influences inherently open to challenge in relation to cohorts and when seeking to definitively formulate the genesis of a mental health problem or its maintenance in a particular patient. For example, women have lower incomes on average than men and are often employed more precariously. This being the case, if a gender gap is recorded in mental health status, it could be explained by the stressors associated with these labour market features or socioeconomic status (combined with domestic responsibilities, itself a form of division of labour).

Thus disaggregating the specific causal impact of single social variables (of in this case gender) is a risky task. A safer model is to posit multi-factorial formulations and talk in terms of risk and probability rather than in terms of certain causation. A fuller discussion of the mental health inequalities literature in relation to gender and other social variables can be found in Rogers and Pilgrim (2003, 2005). With these general points in mind, I now turn to the first main part of the chapter.

The gendered state of mental health

Mental health is undoubtedly gendered but in a complicated way. The following list illustrates this general point.

◆ Some diagnoses do not seem to be related to gender. For example, the major psychotic illnesses of schizophrenia and bipolar disorder are diagnosed in equal numbers in men and women

♦ Some diagnoses can only *logically* be diagnosed in women because they are gynaecological in nature (postnatal depression and postpartum psychosis). This statement is not contentious. However, what remains contentious is the ontological status of the emotional concomitants of pregnancy, menstruation, and the menopause (and the contested diagnoses in their wake). Should they be framed as ordinary variations in female experience or as psychopathology?

♦ Some diagnoses are not limited to women but male patients with the same labels are significantly *less common*. For example, 90% of those with a diagnosis of eating disorders are female. In accounting for these differences in incidence does it reveal biological or social differences between females and males? If eating disorders are sex-linked genetically, what is the mechanism involved? If they are socially determined, which societal forces encourage abnormal eating patterns in girls more than boys?

♦ Some diagnoses are *overwhelmingly male*, such as antisocial personality disorder (under DSM-IV or 'dissocial personality disorder' under ICD-10). Many sex offenders (the bulk of who are male) fulfil these criteria. Whether psychiatrized in prison or formally detained in secure psychiatric facilities, this subgroup of patients is overwhelmingly male. The diagnosis of personality disorder is generally contentious (independent of the question of gender) and the practical application of the label is gendered. If men are deemed more often to be antisocial, women receive the label of 'borderline personality disorder' and 'histrionic personality disorder' more often than men. Again what does this mean? Are men by objective criteria more 'psychopathic' than women and the latter more hysterically organized and emotionally labile? If so, are these patriarchal attributions from diagnosticians or do they reflect real behavioural tendencies in men and women? And if the answer to this is in the affirmative what does this say about the socialization of boys and girls and the way that the sexes have differential access to repertoires of action as adults?

♦ Some diagnoses have a slight preponderance in men (e.g. substance misuse). However, patterns in this are changing in relation to both legal and illegal drug use. In the case of tobacco use and of binge drinking in young Northern European women, the long-term consequences for physical morbidity (liver, lung, and cardiovascular disease) will be gendered in a different way in the future than in the past. This provides a clear example of how gendered behavioural norms mediate physical health outcomes. Where these rates of substance misuse are now converging between the sexes, questions are begged about why this is the case. At the turn of the 21st century, does it reflect a post-feminist context of greater social permissiveness for women than in the past, where sexual liberation is being expressed as personal indulgence? Does it reflect a (pathological) alternative to the demands from patriarchy of female passivity and restraint? For a discussion of the impact of changing norms about acceptable female behaviour, see deSwaan (1990) in relation to agoraphobia at the turn of the 20th century

♦ Some diagnoses are more likely in women, such as anxiety states, depression, and post-traumatic stress disorder. Most of these cases are not recorded in specialist mental health services but in primary care or in community surveys

♦ In old age the prevalence (but not the incidence) of both dementia and depression is higher in women. They live longer than men, creating that gap between incidence and prevalence. There are some sex differences in the incidence of some types of dementia

♦ There are sex differences in suicidal action. Men complete suicide more often than women and are prone to use more violent means.

If we scan these points, it soon becomes obvious why the overall statement about women suffering poorer mental health might be true. At the same time, this general picture can be problematized in a variety of ways. First, there are cross-national differences in diagnosis. Take eating disorders. These vary in prevalence internationally, being much higher in countries where food is supplied excessively rather than it being in short supply. In China, depression is diagnosed less often in women but more women are given a diagnosis of schizophrenia. This might itself reflect the disvaluing of females in Chinese culture and the greater tendency to coercively control female deviance (Pearson 1995).

Second, this question of control is implicated in inclusion criteria. If psychiatry is used inter alia for purposes of social control, then some aspects of antisocial deviance are medicalized. The best example here is of the diagnosis of antisocial personality disorder, with men not women being over-represented in secure facilities. Thus if the psychiatric system is reframed as part of the apparatus of State social control (rather than as part of the healthcare system) then that aspect will be male not female dominated, reflecting the penal population.

Third, the difference in lifetime prevalence can be accounted for by women living longer than men. This point is obvious in relation to dementia and old age depression but was a point of controversy in retrospective analyses by feminist scholars about asylum psychiatry in the Victorian period. I return to this point later when discussing differences in feminist scholarship about women and madness.

Explanations for sex differences in incidence

The earlier list indicates that the gendered nature of mental health reflects a complex pattern related to the differential incidence of types of diagnosed mental disorder. Here I set out some explanations for this pattern—some of these compete but some are not mutually exclusive.

Direct biological causation

One possibility is that there are measurable biological differences between males and females, which make the latter particularly susceptible to psychological abnormality, especially the manifestation of distress (fear and sadness). This biodeterminist position itself could reflect both genetic and biodevelopmental possibilities (females are genetically vulnerable and/or environmental impacts in utero or in early life differentially shape biological vulnerability). From its inception, psychiatry has presumed a gynaecological basis for mental instability: see the discussion of Rush and Maudsley by Russell (1995) and Prior (1999).

The crude biodeterminism of Kraepelinian psychiatry and its enmeshment with eugenics has indeed left us with a socially conservative body of knowledge (Pilgrim 2008). However, logically, genetic or biodevelopmental differences between the sexes could explain differences in health and psychological functioning, especially when the endocrine system is posited as a mediating variable. For example, the role of oestrogen as a protective factor against cardiovascular disease premenopause can be added to radical feminist explanations about the mediating role of testosterone in male aggression. In this regard, radical feminist and conservative biological psychiatrists find common cause in a form of bioreductionism.

Another example of gender essentialism can be found in Kleinian psychoanalysis and even in the environmentalist reaction of her colleagues such as Winnicott and Bowlby, who focused on the primary caregiving role of mothers and celebrated it as a source of mental health for offspring. Nurturance, unlike violence, is a laudable human tendency and so it could imply the inherent moral superiority of women—an ironic reversal of Freud's assumption that women have inferior superego development.

These biological explanations might suggest that women experience and express sympathetic nervous system arousal as distress, whereas the correlate in men is aggression, with this difference being mediated by hormonal sex differences. Another possibility is that there are (yet to be identified) sex differences in genetic susceptibility. For example, the very large discrepancy in the diagnosis of eating disorders could be accounted for in this way (though I am not aware of this evidence to date). This speculation, as opposed to solid proof, about biodeterminism has not prevented it being a powerful driving force in psychiatric knowledge.

Direct social causation

Intuitively for social determinists this is probably the most obvious explanation for sex differences; an excess in female mental health problems is because women are differentially affected by social stress (Dohrenwend, and Dohrenwend 1977; Gove 1984; Nazroo *et al.* 1998). This hypothesis is in line with evidence we have on two fronts. First, social stress is gendered because women are poorer on average than men and there remains in most societies a gendered division of domestic labour. These social features about income and the division of labour place extra stress on women, which increases the probability of distress.

An important note here is how sex partially determines socioeconomic status. Given that the latter is a good predictor of mental health status then it is because women are on average poorer than men that social stress leads to real differences in rates of distress. If this mediator of socioeconomic status is true then at the individual level it is this class position, not gender, which eventually explains symptom production (Rogers and Pilgrim 2003). In other words, poverty not sex could determine individual distress in a particular woman.

The second front to consider relates to differential rates of abuse in childhood and adulthood. Whilst both boys and girls are abused, the latter suffer more intrafamilial sexual victimization. The relevance of this is that girls are more likely than boys to experience personal betrayal (an important conceptual distinction from and additional to traumatization). At the same time boys are more likely than girls to be physically abused in families. This could account in part for learned aggression—brutalized children are at greater risk of relating to others aggressively (cf. the essentialist radical feminist argument about testosterone).

Arguments about rates of adult abuse remain heated. The standard feminist position is that intimate violence is a function of patriarchal power (enacted using physical force). Indeed it is not unusual for this conventional wisdom now to lead to domestic violence being conflated completely with male violence against women (e.g. Itzin 2006). However, the empirical picture is less clear cut than this. Men, as well as women, are victims in heterosexual relationships and intimate violence in gay and lesbian couples is as common as in heterosexual couples (Rogers and Pilgrim 2003). However, if domestic violence is only conflated with heterosexual female victimhood then it can then be invoked as an explanation for raised levels of psychiatric diagnosis and treatment in women (Mazza and Dennerstein 1996).

Methodological factors and help-seeking

These need to be considered in the context of the next section about the feminist discourse on patriarchy. If gender has been mainly conflated with women in social scientific investigations of mental health then we will tend to know much more about women than men. An example here is that female depression is now highly researched. The extensive body of work by Brown and his colleagues on this began in the 1970s as a study of *class* and depression (Brown and Harris 1978). However, because women were at home more and the researchers found female respondents easier to talk to, the study became one of gender (i.e. women) not class. Thereafter the peculiar biographical features of depressed *women* were elaborated, leaving us in the dark about depressed men (Bifulco *et al.* 1992; Bifulco and Moran 1998).

This tendency to focus on women itself is a function of feminist scholarship, leading to the paradox that the latter's objection to medical knowledge framing ordinary female experience as pathological may have become part of the problem rather than solution. If the research community differentially focuses on female service contact then it may contribute to the construction of women as particularly weak and vulnerable to mental abnormality (Broverman *et al.* 1970; Brodsky and Holdroyd 1975; Bury and Gabe 1990).

However, this is not only a discursive matter. There are real and measurable differences in help-seeking behaviour (Rickwood and Braithwaite 1994; Rogers *et al.* 1999). Women attend more primary care consultations than men. Consequently they present themselves more than men for assessment and diagnosis. Indeed, given that the reported incidence of 'common mental health problems' is significantly higher in women than men and this is a product of attendance for medical consultations, then this process could be the most persuasive explanation for gender differences in lifetime prevalence.

It could, of course, be that women are more distressed than men and so diagnosis is a simple direct read out of community incidence and it is not an artefact of attendance. However, this is not likely given what we know about the 'clinical iceberg' (the point prevalence of symptoms in community samples recurrently outstrips clinically recorded incidence). Gendered differences in help-seeking mean that the tip of the iceberg is female dominated.

Another methodological factor relates to what we *call* mental disorder. Should it be limited to madness, as was the case in relation to the Victorian focus on lunacy (in which case sex differences would be absent)? Should it focus on 'common mental problems' of anxiety and depression, as is the case with modern primary care-driven services (in which case women clearly predominate)? Should it focus on psychiatric inpatients (in which case men now predominate)? Should it include fecklessness, recurrent intoxication, and aspects of criminality where personal, especially sexual, gratification rather than acquisitive motives are evident? These psychosocial problems increasingly became medicalized in the 20th century and generally implicated men more than women. Thus, the shifting ambit of psychiatric nosology has meant that we find what we seek in different ways over time, depending what is and is not considered to be 'mental disorder'.

Patriarchal psychiatry

Many feminist writers have emphasized the way in which psychiatric knowledge is oppressively patriarchal (e.g. Chesler 1972; English and Ehrenreich 1976; Barrett and Roberts, 1978; Davis *et al.* 1985; Sheppard 1991; Barnes and Maple 1992; Ussher 1994; Russell 1995; Prior 1999). There is a minority discourse which draws attention to the resultant silencing of male patienthood. Also some feminist scholars have been alert to the dangers of ideology racing ahead of evidence. For example, the assumption about patriarchy in Victorian psychiatry led Showalter (1980) to argue that women were differentially oppressed by male doctors and detained at higher levels than men in the asylum system. However, Busfield (1994) in her analysis of asylum records demonstrated that the sex difference in asylum figures could be accounted for by higher female prevalence because of greater longevity.

Busfield (1996) went on to provide a critique of patriarchy in arguments about mental health on a few fronts.

First, it is not empirically self-evident that patriarchy is universal (it varies in presence and intensity over time and place).

Second, patriarchal relationships have provided a particular function in advanced industrial societies. As a result, capitalist relations are built inter alia upon a sexual division of labour. Consequently the personalistic arguments invoked to blame men for female oppression in intimate relationships can obscure the structural point that *both* men and women are victims of systemic features of their shared economic context.

Third (a point I emphasized in the introduction to this chapter), any social analysis, which relies analytically on only one form of intergroup oppression, in this case of sexism, will fail to account for differences *within* social groups. The patriarchal emphasis creates a singular focus on the difference between men and women. It diverts us from the evidence of large variations in psychological functioning *between men and between women and the overlap in the range of functioning across the gender divide*. These variations are a product of other interacting social factors (especially class, race, and age). A consequence of this picture is that binary oppositions (of the 'all women/all men' type) are logically and empirically untenable. What we find are tendencies in social groups, with large within-group differences and a large overlap of features between groups.

A final point to note about institutional psychiatry and gender is that contra Showalter's unfounded empirical claims about women in the asylum system, in more recent times it is clear now that there is indeed a gendered gradient in relation to coercion. Men now outnumber women in acute psychiatric units and it is men, not women, who are overwhelmingly detained in conditions of security. Indeed active steps have been taken in the United Kingdom context to close maximum secure psychiatric facilities such as Ashworth Hospital (Pilgrim 2007). Thus the *context* of psychiatric contact is important to consider, not just diagnostic differences between the sexes. The more coercive the context, the more that psychiatry is part of the coercive wing of the State apparatus. Men not women are over-represented in that wing.

Psychosocial explanations of within-group differences

An account has already been given of the multi-factorial determination of mental health problems and the dangers of single factor reductionism (whether this is biological or social). In the midst of this complexity there are also fine grain biographical differences in the life experience of people. Thus it is possible for a girl born into a very poor ethnic minority family to develop into adulthood showing no symptoms of mental distress. How is this possible? One explanation is that psychological resilience is wholly genetically determined. This is possible but unlikely given the evidence we have about interacting factors. The most obvious explanation resides in the quality of past and current relationships. A fuller account of this explanation for within-group differences is provided by Pilgrim *et al.* (2009) but here the main features of this explanation can be outlined:

◆ We all vary in our genetic, congenital, and environmental experience as we develop from conception

◆ Social group membership (race, gender, class, and age) raises or lowers our chances of remaining mentally healthy but cannot completely explain outcomes in individual cases

◆ These background biological and social factors affecting mental health status interact with *particular* biographical features in individuals

◆ The quality of our care in early life is vital in predicting individual mental health

◆ The quality of our intimate and social relationships in adulthood then interacts with the legacy of early life experience to maintain or jeopardize our mental health.

This model to explain within-group differences draws upon two types of evidence. The first is within the tradition of attachment theory (Bowlby 1951; Winnicott 1958), which spawned a large body of knowledge about childhood adversity and its short-term and long-term impact on mental health. The second refers to evidence from current interpersonal contexts. The work alluded to earlier of Brown and colleagues, despite its limited female focus, provides a good model to be tested empirically about how the legacy of childhood adversity interacts with current interpersonal factors, which may buffer a vulnerable person from symptom presentation or trigger that outcome.

Conclusion

This chapter has summarized the evidence and debates related to gender and mental health. By contrasting overall claims about sex differences in lifetime prevalence with the highly variegated picture about incidence, it was possible to put forward both unanswered questions and a range of explanations for that variability. The main conclusion is that single factor reductionism about gender and mental health should be avoided.

Instead we need to explore the many ambiguities about biopsychosocial interactionism. We have some answers already in this regard but there are still many begged questions. Given that feminist scholarship now may have become part of the problem rather than the solution in mental health research, we now are involved in a post-feminist discourse about mental health (and other psychosocial phenomena). This chapter reflects that new context.

References

Barnes M and Maple N (1992). *Women and Mental Health: Challenging the Stereotypes*. Venture Press, Birmingham.

Barrett M and Roberts H (1978). Doctors and their patients. In: H Smart and B Smart (eds) *Women, Sexuality and Social Control*. Routledge and Kegan Paul, London.

Bifulco A and Moran A (1998). *Wednesday's Child: Research into Women's Experience of Neglect and Abuse in Childhood and Adult Depression*. Tavistock, London.

Bifulco A *et al.* (1992). Mourning or inadequate care? Re-examining the relationship of maternal loss in childhood with adult depression and anxiety. *Development and Psychopathology*, **4**, 119–28.

Bowlby J (1951). *Maternal Care and Mental Health*. World Health Organization, Geneva.

Brodsky A and Holdroyd J (1975). Report of the task force on sex bias and sex role stereotyping in psychotherapeutic practice. *American Psychologist*, **30**, 1169–75.

Broverman D *et al.* (1970). Sex role stereotypes and clinical judgements of mental health. *Journal of Consulting and Clinical Psychology*, **34**, 1–7.

Brown GW and Harris TO (1978). *Social Origins of Depression*. Tavistock, London.

Brown GW *et al.* (1995). Loss, humiliation and entrapment among women developing depression: a patient and non-patient comparison. *Psychological Medicine*, **25**, 7–21.

Bury M and Gabe J (1990). Hooked? Media responses to tranquillizer dependency. In: P Abbott and G Payne (eds) *New Directions in the Sociology of Health*. Flamer Press, London.

Busfield J (1994). Is mental illness a female malady? Men, women and madness in nineteenth century England. *Sociology* **28**, 259–77.

Busfield J (1996). *Men, Women and Madness*, Macmillan, Basingstoke.

Cameron E and Bernardes J (1998). Gender and disadvantage in health: men's health for a change. *Sociology of Health and Illness*, **20**(5), 673–93.

Chesler P (1972). *Women and Madness*. Doubleday, New York.

Davis A *et al.* (1985). Women and mental health: a guide for the approved social worker. In: E Brook and A Davis (eds) *Women, the Family and Social Work*. Tavistock, London.

DeSwaan A (1990). *The Management of Normality*. Routledge, London.

Dohrenwend B and Dohrenwend BS (1977). Sex differences in mental illness: a reply to Gove and Tudor. *American Journal of Sociology*, **82**, 1336–41.

English B and Ehrenreich D (1976). *Complaints and Disorders: The Sexual Politics of Sickness*. Writers and Readers Publishing Cooperative, London.

Gove W (1984). Gender differences in mental and physical illness: the effects of fixed roles and nurturant roles. *Social Science and Medicine*, **19**(2), 77–91.

Itzin C (2006). *Tackling the health and mental health effects of domestic sexual violence and abuse*. Department of Health/Home Office, London.

Mazza D and Dennerstein L (1996). Psychotropic drug use by women: could violence account for the gender difference? *Journal of Psychosomatic Obstetrics and Gynaecology*, **17**(4), 229–34.

Nazroo JY *et al.* (1998). Gender differences in the prevalence of depression: artefact, alternative disorders, biology or roles? *Sociology of Health and Illness*, **20**(3), 3112–330.

Pearson V (1995). Goods on which one loses: women and mental health in China. *Social Science and Medicine*, **41**(8), 1159–73.

Pilgrim D (ed) (2007). *Inside Ashworth: Professional Accounts of Institutional Life*. Radcliffe Press, Oxford.

Pilgrim D (2008). The eugenic legacy in psychiatry and psychology. *International Journal of Social Psychiatry*, **54**(3), 272–84.

Pilgrim D *et al.* (2009). The centrality of personal relationships in the creation and amelioration of mental health problems. *Health*, **13**(2), 235–54.

Prior PM (1999). *Gender and Mental Health*. Macmillan, Basingstoke.

Rickwood DJ and Braithwaite VA (1994). Social psychological factors affecting help seeking for emotional problems. *Social Science and Medicine*, **39**(4), 563–72.

Rogers A and Pilgrim D (2003). *Mental Health and Inequality*. Palgrave, Basingstoke.

Rogers A and Pilgrim D (2005). *A Sociology of Mental Health and Illness*. Open University Press, Maidenhead.

Rogers A *et al.*(1999). *Demanding Patients?* Open University Press, Buckingham.

Russell D (1995). *Women, Madness and Medicine*. Polity, Cambridge.

Sheppard M (1991). General practice, social work and mental health sections: the social control of women. *British Journal of Social Work*, **21**, 663–83.

Showalter E (1980). Victorian women and insanity. In: A Scull (ed) *Madhouses. Mad-Doctors and Madmen*, pp. 313–38. Athlone Press, London.

Ussher J (1994). Women and madness – a voice in the dark of women's despair. *Feminism and Psychology*, **4**(2), 288–92.

Winnicott DW (1958). *Collected Works*. Hogarth Press, London.

CHAPTER 4

Women, ethnicity, and mental health

Mervat Nasser

Culture and psychopathology

Culture has been described as one of the most elusive terms in the history of modern thought. The term commonly refers to social heritage and encompasses ideas, beliefs, aesthetic perceptions, and values. The interaction between culture and variables such as gender, race, ethnicity, nationality, social class, literacy, or religion is, however, far from clear.

The interest in the impact of 'culture' on the 'human mind' began in the 18th century with the development of social theories of psychopathology that led to the study of the vulnerability of certain cultural groups to particular forms of mental illness and the general role played by cultural conditions in causing or shaping human distress.

In the early stages of transcultural psychiatric research, the main interest was with the notion of *cultural causality*, namely whether culture has a direct causative role in forming or generating psychopathology. These culture-specific conditions are often referred to as *culture-bound syndromes*, and were initially considered to be exotic forms of mental illness exclusive to certain geographical areas in the world, often remote from Western modernizing forces (Bhugra and Jacob 1977).

Central to the argument of the cultural specificity of psychopathology is the relativity of cultural normality and abnormality, which according to Kleinman (1977) can only be understood within the social and cultural context. This approach clearly emphasizes differences within societies, particularly those variable ways of perceiving and conceptualizing the world. This approach examines the mind through shared cultural categories and focuses on the relationship between public and private symbolism and how the individual makes sense of his/her own personal situation (Littlewood 1984). Under these conditions the different patterns of psychopathology are considered specific cultural preoccupations and impart culturally relevant meanings. The approach is an 'interpretative' one that searches for explanatory models for the disorders in question within cultures and clearly implies that cultures are *pathogenic*. The notion of cultural causality/specificity means that the disorder cannot be understood apart from its specific cultural or subcultural context and its aetiology symbolizes core meanings and behaviours that are considered norms of that culture (Cassidy 1982; Ritenbough 1982) However, this notion is problematic given the subjectivity of any cultural value system and its susceptibility to vary with time and changing social conditions (Nasser 1997).

On the other hand, culture may only contribute to the shaping of the symptom pattern and the final presentation of the psychopathology (Hare 1981). In this context, culture exercises a 'modelling' or 'plastering' effect on psychopathology i.e. *pathoplastic*.

In recent years the term 'ethnicity' has increasingly been in use, in an attempt to overcome some of the vagueness and difficulties that surround the definition of culture. Ethnicity, which is often confused with race or nationality, refers to a socially constructed phenomenon that implies shared and distinctive traditions that are maintained between generations and lead to a sense of a group identity.

Devereux introduced the term *ethnic disorder* in 1955 (Devereux 1955). The ethnic syndrome represents core contradictions and anxieties in any particular society, and its symptoms are considered exaggerations of normal attitudes and behaviours that are prevalent in the culture, again implying the causal nature of cultural conditions. The difference, however, between the traditional construct of culture-bound and ethnic disorder, is the fact that the latter could better embrace a broad array of cultural forces that are shared by a large number of societies, rather than a particular geographic locale. The notion of ethnic syndrome was advanced by Gordon (1990, 2001) in relation to the issue of the specificity of eating disorders to the Western culture and their emergence in other non-Western societies following changes in sociocultural conditions and identification with Western values. This means that the contribution of culture to psychopathology can not be considered meaningful in isolation of the changing nature of cultural conditions, and their impact on the individual. In view of this, the focus of this chapter will be on the interface between cultural change, gender, and individual identity and the impact of these variables on psychopathology.

Cultural change and cultural identity

Triandis (1989) made a distinction between the private self (the assessment of the self by the self) and the collective self (the assessment of the self by a referential group), and suggested that such distinction is essential for the measurement of the 'acculturation process' and the definition of 'cultural identity'. Acculturation commonly refers to the identification of a small (non-dominant) group with the values of larger (dominant) group. The process entails both cultural and psychological change in groups, families, and individuals following intercultural contact. The issue of one's cultural identity comes to the fore during this process where individuals attempt to sort out who they are in relation to these two ways of living.

The process of acculturation is normally considered when such culture-contact occurs during colonization and migration, and continues among ethnocultural communities in culturally plural societies (Berry 2003). The term 'Westernization' has often been used interchangeably with acculturation to refer specifically to identification with Western cultural norms for currently being the prevailing dominant culture. However, the process of identification with these values is now taking place through the integration of the whole world into a 'global superculture', facilitated by the adoption of many societies of market economy and the wide spread of deregulated media and information technologies.

And yet, the emphasis on 'value identification' in either terminology reduces the individual to a passive template open to mimicry and manipulation, and fails to take into account the true forces of change that impact on the individual and consequently shape cultural identity and psychopathology. These forces may include urbanization, social mobility, social isolation, the threat to national identity, as well as the disappearance of traditional structures of support and the familiar cultural idioms for articulating distress (Nasser and Katzman 1999). This is clearly illustrated in relation to certain disorders such as eating psychopathology where evidence of their increase was noted following urbanization, migration to the cities, and the nuclearization of the family structure (Selvini-Palazzoli 1985; Hoek *et al.* 1995; Nasser 1997).

The transition from state-controlled economies to markets brought with it a surge in consumerism. One of the main features of market economy is the selling via the media of the possibility of recreating the 'self' through refiguring of the body or 'body re-production' (Rathner 2001). It is clear now that the 'body' in our changing world has become a platform for expressing the individual's stress of cultural ambiguities and paradoxes. Forms of body reconstruction range from the adaptive to the pathological and are normally geared towards creating a new self/identity, one that is more suited to negotiate the new demands of sociocultural instability. In other words, it creates a new 'cultural identity' that has more congruency or 'consonance' with the new social setting and its new conditions (Skarderud and Nasser 2007).

Culture change and gender ambivalence

'Gender ambivalence' is a term coined by Silvertein and Perlick (1995) to describe the ambiguities in the female role during periods of historical and cultural transition. The economic transformation following the decline of communism and the adoption of market philosophy was found to affect women's perception of themselves and their social roles. The undermining of socialist collectivist structures in former communist Europe, the Kibbutz, China, and other countries that have experimented with socialist regimes, has been responsible for the change in the value system that took place in these societies. Under socialist policies women were, by and large, directed and protected in their education, health, employment, and child care. Women's sense of value appeared to derive from taking part in an overall social philosophy and their expectation of themselves seemed to be more reconciled with those of their society. In a profit-motivated economy some of these social provisions had to go. This created greater ambivalence about women's positions in the workplace and a subsequent increase in the rate of unemployment among highly qualified women in post-socialist countries (Nasser 1997; Catina and Joja 2001).

Another dimension to this is the rise in fundamentalist religion in a great number of societies. This was seen as an attempt fill the vacuum created by the death of communism, but in some instances has also been instrumental in supporting the new economic structures that promote home as the right place for women. This societal ambivalence about women's roles is likely to cause greater ambivalence among women themselves (Nasser 1997; Nasser and DiNicola 2001). This gender ambivalence is symptomatic of women's sense of devalued identity and low self-worth.

In the case of women belonging to different races or ethnic groups, this ambivalence becomes more magnified. This 'gender intensification' engenders emotional dilemmas centred on one's identity which often finds expression in a combination of psychological and somatic symptoms. This behaviour/symptomatology could in turn help women—paradoxically—to find a new identity/definition within the fluidity of societies caught in the grips of change (Nasser 2000; Nasser and DiNicola 2001).

Gender, culture, and psychopathology

In the statistics on mental health and illness, gender differences have long been apparent with more women than men being diagnosed with and treated for 'mental illness' (Ehrenreich and English 1974; Showalter 1985). Historically, some diagnoses such as hysteria, chlorosis, and neurasthenia were almost exclusively considered woman's illnesses (Brumberg 1982; Showalter 1985). Recent epidemiological data demonstrate a continuation of this preponderance of women both for overall diagnoses of mental health problems (Ussher 1991, 2000) and for particular diagnostic categories. Depression, for instance, appears to be twice as common in women as men whilst girls and women represent 95% of those diagnosed with eating disorders.

This clearly implies that 'being a woman' constitutes in itself a certain vulnerability to mental illness. However, this gender risk is commonly deduced from epidemiological data obtained through quantitative research methodologies, based on quantified variables to assess incidence and prevalence rate regardless of any cultural interpretation. Quantitative research also depends on the reliability and validity of instruments used as well as the nature of diagnostic manuals (ICD-10 and DSM-IV) through which caseness decisions are made, with the probability of error, misrepresentation, and cultural bias. Further, incidence and prevalence data, being derived either from community data or hospital rates of admissions and referrals, are inevitably influenced by the ways in which both users and providers of mental health care services interpret service users' experiences. For example, women have been found to seek help more often than men from primary care services when experiencing distress, a gender difference which may be due to differences in help-seeking and expressing emotional dis/content as much as to gender differences in levels of distress. However, the tendency towards presentation to medical services by women is not uniform as women from some minority racial/cultural groups were found to have little faith in conventional medical services and therefore tended to be underrepresented in statistical data (Cochrane and Sashidharan 1996; Nasser 1997; Malson and Nasser 2007).

There is a need therefore to look for different approaches to researching women's mental health that take into account gender differences between men and women in sociocultural context including differences in pay, social status, political power, burdens of domestic care and mothering, relationship inequalities and rates of domestic violence (Ussher 1991) as well as gender differences in social pressures and expectations (Malson 1998; Nasser 2000).

Brown and Harris's (1978, 1989) social theory of depression, for example, explains women's depression in terms of their experiences of adversity. Similarly, eating disorders are seen to be resulting from the societal pressures that are now placed on women in our modern times and convey conflicting cultural messages. However, these sociocultural explanations were often restricted to one culture, namely the Western culture. The living laboratory of other cultures remained untapped with little or no cross-fertilization between the feminist and the transcultural school of thought (Katzman and Lee 1997). Despite the fact that the issue of gender risk encountered in white/Western communities may even be intensified in certain situations in other cultures and minority groups, *other* women were for long considered largely immune from the turmoil facing their counterparts in the West. This presumed protection was attributed to rigidly enforced traditional familial expectations and clear-cut gender roles.

However, in order to illustrate the commonality of gender risk across different cultures and ethnicities, recent research of the following mental health problems will briefly be discussed: eating disorders, deliberate self-harm, and postnatal depression.

Eating disorders

Disordered eating behaviours were thought for a long time to be a phenomenon unique to Western culture (Prince 1983). The culture-boundedness/specificity of eating pathology was based on the perceived differences in aesthetic values and gender roles between West and non-West, and was supported by the apparent rarity of these disorders in other cultures.

However, recent epidemiological data show that eating psychopathology is now emerging in many of the societies that were initially thought to be free of such problems. In the 1990s, a surge of publications from different countries across the world suggested that eating disorders are increasingly becoming a global phenomenon. Recent research from the Middle East, the Far East, South America, and Africa, all indicate that eating disorders do exist in these societies with similar or even higher rates to those reported in the West (Nasser 1997; Gordon 2001).

However, the true observer could easily notice that disordered eating patterns were appearing against a background of 'cultural transition', marked by rapid market economies and their associated influence on the status of women. The impact of a global consumer culture, with its powerful mandates for cultivation of a certain type of body ideal, appears to play a significant role. Equally important, however, are the contradictory pressures that emerge when women begin to have access on a mass level to education and a role in public life, and struggles about sexual equality come to the foreground (Gordon 2001). This suggests that eating disorders—regardless of culture type—are symptomatic of gender ambivalence characteristic of any culture in the process of change (Nasser 2000; Nasser and DiNicola 2001; for further discussion, refer to Chapter 24 on the sociocultural dimension of eating disorders in this volume).

Deliberate self-harm

In psychiatric terminology, the act of deliberate self-harm (DSH) invites a multitude of clinical expressions including deliberate self-injury, self-inflicted violence, self-attack, deliberate non-fatal act, symbolic wounding, and parasuicide. Examples of these self-damaging behaviours include self-cutting, overdosing, or substance misuse.

The act of fasting or self-starvation in eating disorders is a form of body deprivation that in due course may lead to physical harm or even death, and the clinical literature is full of cases of eating disorders associated with a variety of self-harming behaviours.

Hospital-based analyses of admissions data, as well as surveys carried out in school settings, suggest that young Asian women born in the United Kingdom are at a higher risk for attempted suicide and self-harm behaviour as compared with white Caucasian and African-Caribbean young women (Merrill and Owens 1986, 1988; Mumford and Whitehouse 1988). As it is the case with eating disorders, the results of these studies have been considered a by-product of acculturation into Western cultures (Burke 1976; Merrill and Owens 1988; Hodes 1990). 'Culture clash' explanations have also been applied, referring to cultural and religious customs that place high demands on young Asian women living in the United Kingdom (Soni-Raleigh and Balarajan 1992). The high rates of deliberate self-harm among Asian women in Britain is also seen as an expression of disconnection and reaction to the sense of cultural alienation felt by this particular group (Bhugra 2002).

Hunter and Harvey (2002) compared rates of self-harm behaviour among indigenous populations in Australia, New Zealand, Canada, and the United Sates. They concluded that the vulnerability of the young populations to self-harm behaviour was attributed to the impact of cultural breakdown, demonstrating how young people are influenced by the cultural changes and the circumstances that surround them. In line with these findings, American Indian youths in Alaska were shown to have a higher vulnerability to life-threatening behaviours than their white counterparts (Frank and Lester 2002).

All of these studies show that the greatest incidence of self-harm was also found to be among women who were expected to conform to conflicting cultural expectations of gender role, drawing attention once again to the issue of 'gender ambivalence' and the combined risk of gender and culture change in both eating disorders and self-harm phenomena. The act of self-harm functions here as a medium for communicating the distress caused by the loss of the relationship between one's outer self and inner self, as well as the loss of the self in relation to others. It is a reaction to a sense of cultural confusion, disorganization, and disconnection (Nasser 2004).

Postpartum depression

Postpartum depression (PPD) is another psychiatric diagnosis that is commonly thought of as unique to Western culture. Reports of its prevalence in non-Western cultures and ethnicities appear to be highly variable, ranging from almost 0% to almost 60%. This variability might reflect a number of issues including cross-cultural variables, reporting style, differences in perception of mental health and its stigma, or differences in socioeconomic standards, including poverty and levels of social support.

Few cases of PPD were reported in countries like Singapore, Malta, Malaysia, Austria, and Denmark whereas in other countries such as Brazil, Guyana, Costa Rica, Italy, Chile, South Africa, Taiwan, and Korea, postpartum depressive symptoms were found to be very prevalent (Halbreich and Karkun 2006).

In another review, PPD was found to be a universal experience describing women throughout the world as experiencing degrees of sadness postnatally, which persist up to one year. The risk factors for PPD also share similar themes cross-culturally, with one notable exception—the impact that the sex of the infant had on PPD—for a higher value for male children over female offspring was reported in literature from China, Turkey, and India (Goldbort 2006).

Poor levels of social support/networks were found to have high correlations with rates of postpartum depression regardless of ethnicity (Surkan *et al.* 2006). Other risk factors were all studied in a sample of Arab women from the United Arab Emirates (UAE), using the Edinburgh Postnatal Depression Scale (EPDS). Higher depression scores were associated with not breastfeeding, giving birth to the first child, poor self-body image, and concern about weight, poor relationship with mother-in-law, and an older age at marriage (Green *et al.* 2006).

In a study carried out in Québec, Canada, the immigration variable was explored. The prevalence of depressive symptoms in mothers five months after giving birth was studied according to immigration status. Immigrant mothers were classified according to their ethnocultural (majority or minority) group and compared with Canadian-born mothers. The prevalence of high depressive symptoms was higher among immigrants from minority groups than among immigrants from majority groups and Canadian-born mothers. The study concluded a high correlation between minority status and depressive symptoms which clearly warrants further research (Mechakra-Tahiri *et al.* 2007). However, no relationship between 'acculturation' and perinatal health outcomes was found when PPD was studied in Hispanic women in the United States. Postpartum depressive symptoms were nonetheless found to correlate significantly with being a single mother (Beck 2006).

The results of these studies clearly suggest that 'social adversity' is by far the major risk for PPD, regardless of culture/ethnicity. This social adversity, as is the case in Western societies, includes social/economic disadvantage, poor social support, and single motherhood.

Conclusion

This chapter attempts to explore the complex relationship between gender, culture, and individual psychopathology. Women are generally considered to be more at risk of developing certain disorders such as depression, eating disorders, and deliberate self-harm. These psychopathologies appear to be connected to women's sense of identity and the perception of their gender roles, and therefore are likely to occur during times of change when gender roles are questioned and socially revised. The conflict over identity or self-definition produces 'gender ambivalence' and explains why women of all colours, cultures, and ethnicities seem to be under the same pressures and have similar predispositions to such disorders at times of social change and cultural transition, and may even be seen as means of negotiating the complex nature of the modernizing global environment.

References

American Psychiatric Association (1993). *Diagnostic and Statistical Manual of Mental Disorders, fourth edition.* American Psychiatric Association, Washington, DC.

Beck CT (2006). Acculturation: implications for prenatal research. *MCN: The American Journal of Maternal Child Nursing*, **31**, 114–20.

Berry JW (2003). Conceptual approaches to acculturation. In: K Chun, P Balls Organista, and G Marin (eds) *Acculturation*, pp. 17–37. American Psychological Association Press, Washington, DC.

Bhugra D (2002). Suicidal behaviour in South Asians in the UK. *Crisis*, **23**, 108–13.

Bhugra D and Jacob KS (1977). Culture-bound syndromes in troublesome disguises. In: D Bhughra and A Munro (eds) *Undiagnosed Psychiatric Syndromes*, pp. 296–334. Blackwell Science, Oxford.

Brown GW and Harris TO (1978). *Social Origins of Depression: A Study of Psychiatric Disorder in Women.* Tavistock Publications, London; Free Press, New York.

Brown GW and Harris TO (1989). Depression. In: GW Brown and TO Harris (eds) *Life Events and Illness*, pp. 49–93. Unwin Hyman, London.

Brumberg J (1982). Chlorotic girls, 1870-1920: a historical perspective on female adolescence. *Child Development*, **53**, 1468–77.

Burke AW (1976). Attempted suicide among Asian immigrants in Birmingham. *British Journal of Psychiatry*, **128**, 528–33.

Cassidy C (1982). Protein-energy malnutrition as a culture bound syndrome. *Culture, Medicine and Psychiatry*, **6**, 325–45.

Catina A and Joja O (2001). Emerging markets: submerging women. In: M Nasser *et al.* (eds) *Eating Disorders and Cultures in Transition*, pp. 111–27. Bruner–Routledge, East Sussex.

Cochrane R and Sashidharan SP (1996). Mental Health and ethnic minorities: a review of the literature and service implications. In: *Ethnicity and Health: reviews of literature and guidance for purchasers in the areas of cardiovascular disease, mental health and haemoglobinopathies. CRD Reports.* NHS Centre for reviews and dissemination social policy research unit, University of York.

Devereux G (1955). *Basic Problems of Ethnopsychiatry.* University of Chicago Press, Chicago, IL.

Dohn FA *et al.* (2002). Self-harm and substance use in a community sample of Black and White women with binge eating disorder or bulimia nervosa. *International Journal of Eating Disorders*, **32**, 389–400.

Ehrenreich B and English D (1974). Complaints and disorders: the sexual politics of sickness. In: *Glass Mountain Pamphlet No. 2.* Compendium, London.

Frank ML and Lester D (2002). Self-destructive behaviours in American Indian and Alaska Native high school youth. *American Indian & Alaskan Native Mental Health Research*, **10**, 24–32.

Goldbort J (2006). Transcultural analysis of postpartum depression. *MCN: The American Journal of Maternal Child Nursing*, **31**(2), 121–6.

Gordon R (1990). *Anorexia and Bulimia: Anatomy of A Social Epidemic.* Blackwell, Cambridge, MA.

Gordon R (2001). Eating disorders East and West: a culture-bound syndrome unbound. In: M Nasser *et al.* (eds) *Eating Disorders and Cultures in Transition*, pp. 1–24. Bruner–Routledge, East Sussex.

Green K *et al.* (2006). Postnatal depression among mothers in the United Arab Emirates: sociocultural and physical factors. *Psychology Health and Medicine*, **11**(4), 425–31.

Halbreich U and Karkun S (2006). Cross-cultural and social diversity of prevalence of postpartum depression and depressive symptoms. *Journal of Affective Disorders*, **91**(2–3), 97–111.

Hare E (1981). The two manias: a study of the modern concept of mania. *British Journal of Psychiatry*, **138**, 89–99.

Hodes M (1990). Overdosing as communication; A cultural perspective. *British Journal of Medical Psychology*, **63**, 319–33.

Hoek H *et al.* (1995). Impact of urbanisation on detection rates of eating disorders. *American Journal of Psychiatry*, **152**(9), 1272–85.

Hunter E and Harvey D (2002). Indigenous suicide in Australia, New Zealand, Canada, and the United States. *Emergency Medicine*, **14**, 14–23.

Katzman MA and Lee S (1997). Beyond body image: the integration of feminist and trans-cultural theories in understanding of self-starvation. *International Journal of Eating Disorders*, **22**, 385–94.

Kleinman A (1977). Depression, somatization and the "new cross-cultural psychiatry". *Social Science and Medicine*, **11**, 3–10.

Littlewood R (1984). The individual articulation of shared symbols. *Journal of Operational Psychiatry*, **15**, 17–24.

Malson H (1998). *The Thin Woman: Feminism, Post-structuralism and the Social Psychology of Anorexia Nervosa.* Routledge, London.

Malson H and Nasser M (2007). At risk by reason of gender. In: M Nasser *et al.* (eds) *The Female Body in Mind: The Interface Between the Female Body and Mental Health*, pp. 3–17. Routledge, East Sussex.

Marshall H and Yazdani A (2000). Young Asian women and self harm. In: J Ussher (ed) *Women's Health. Contemporary International Perspectives*, pp. 59–69. British Psychological Society, London.

Mechakra-Tahiri S *et al.* (2007). Self-rated health and postnatal depressive symptoms among immigrant mothers in Québec. *Women & Health*, **45**(4), 1–17.

Merrill J and Owens J (1986). Ethnic differences in self-poisoning: A comparison of Asian and white groups. *British Journal of Psychiatry*, **148**, 708–12.

Merrill J and Owens J (1988). Self-poisoning among four immigrant groups. *Acta Psychiatrica Scandinavica*, **77**, 77–80.

Mumford DB and Whitehouse AM (1988). Increased prevalence of bulimia nervosa among Asian schoolgirls. *British Medical Journal*, **297**, 718.

Nasser M (1997). *Culture and Weight Consciousness.* Brunner & Routledge, London.

Nasser M (2000). Gender, culture and eating disorders. In: JM Ussher (ed) *Women's Health: Contemporary International Perspectives*, pp. 379–87. British Psychological Society, London.

Nasser M (2004). Dying to live: eating disorders and self harm behaviour in the cultural context. In: J Levitt *et al.* (eds) *Self-harm Behaviour and Eating Disorders: Dynamics, Assessment and Treatment*, pp. 15–31. Brunner–Routledge, New York and Hove.

Nasser M and Katzman M (1999). Eating disorders: transcultural perspectives inform prevention. In: N Piran *et al.* (eds) *Preventing Eating Disorders. A Handbook of Interventions and Special Challenges*, pp. 26–44. Brunner/Mazel. Philadelphia, PA.

Nasser M *et al.* (2001). Changing bodies, changing cultures: an intercultural dialogue on the body as the final frontier. In: M Nasser *et al.* (eds) *Eating Disorders and Cultures in Transition*, pp. 171–94. Brunner & Routledge, London.

Prince R (1983). Is anorexia nervosa a culture-bound syndrome? *Transcultural Psychiatry Research and Review,* **20**, 299–300.

Rathner G (2001). Post-communism and the marketing of the thin ideal. In: M Nasser *et al.* (eds) *Eating Disorders and Cultures in Transition,* pp. 93–111. Bruner–Routledge, East Sussex.

Ritenbaugh C (1982). Obesity as a culture bound syndrome. *Culture, Medicine and Psychiatry,* **6**, 347–61.

Selvini-Palazzoli MS (1985). Anorexia nervosa, a syndrome of the affluent society. *Transcultural Psychiatry Research Review,* **22**(3), 199–205.

Skarderud F and Nasser M (2007). Re figuring identities; my body is what I am. In: M Nasser *et al.* (eds) *The Female Body in Mind: The Interface Between the Female Body and Mental Health,* pp. 17–29. Taylor & Francis Group, East Sussex.

Silverstein B and Perlick D (1995). *The Cost of Competence: Why Inequality Causes Depression, Eating Disorders and Illness in Women.* Oxford University Press, New York.

Soni-Raleigh V and Balarajan R (1992). Suicide and self-burning among Indians and West Indians in England and Wales. *British Journal of Psychiatry,* **161**, 365–68.

Showalter E (1985). The Female Malady: Women, Madness and English Culture, 1830–1980. Virago, London.

Surkan PJ *et al.* (2006). The role of social networks and support in postpartum women's depression: a multiethnic urban sample. *Maternal Child Health Journal,* **110**(4), 375–83.

Triandis HC (1989). The self and social behaviour in differing cultural context. *Psychological Review,* **96**, 506–20.

Ussher J (1991). *Women's Madness: Misogyny or Mental Illness.* Harvester Wheatsheaf, London.

Ussher JM (2000). Women's health contemporary concerns. In: JM Ussher (ed) *Women's Health: Contemporary International Perspectives,* pp. 1–26. British Psychological Society, London.

CHAPTER 5

Biological sex differences relevant to mental health

Peter Fitzgerald and Timothy G. Dinan

Introduction

Scientific interest in the effects of the female sex steroids on modulating mood and behaviour stems largely in the modern era from the well-recognized sex differences found in certain psychiatric disorders.

The finding across many cultures and ethnic backgrounds from large epidemiological studies that women have twice the prevalence rate for depression as men, that this only becomes apparent after the onset of puberty, and that after the menopause rates return to near parity between the sexes, is a strong finding implicating a role for female gonadal hormones in playing an active part in such discrepancy. Further epidemiological evidence for sex steroids' capability to impact on mood and behaviour comes from the high rate of mood disturbance and psychosis seen in the postpartum period, a time of dramatic and rapid change in gonadal steroid secretion, in addition to the occurrence of a discrete menstrual cycle-related mood disorder (the premenstrual or late luteal phase dysphoric disorder), for which removal of the ovaries has been noted to be curative. Some conditions which may not be associated with a sex difference in lifetime prevalence rates are nevertheless associated with marked differences in course or outcome between the sexes, such as the later age of onset of schizophrenia in females, who generally manifest a less severe disorder which is more responsive to treatment, and who display a second peak onset around the time of the menopause, all suggestive of a somewhat protective role for gonadal steroids in this disorder.

How do gonadal steroids have such widespread effects on the brain so as to explain these sex differences? While current knowledge is far from complete on this issue, this chapter will outline some key structural and functional differences between a female and male brain which arise due to the differential actions of the gonadal steroids. In particular, those central structures and systems which are believed to play an integral role in the psychiatric disorders for which a marked sex difference exists will be focused upon, including the limbic system, the various neurotransmitter systems such as serotonin, noradrenaline, and dopamine, and finally the neuroendocrine system involved in the stress response, the hypothalamic–pituitary–adrenal axis.

Brain morphology

Organizational/activational hypothesis of gonadal steroids

Phoenix was the first to propose an 'organizational' effect of prenatal steroids on structure and subsequent function of the brain, when he demonstrated that prenatal androgen exposure in female guinea pigs led to defeminization of reproductive behaviour in adulthood (Pheonix *et al.* 1959). He proposed that at specific 'developmental windows' (the timing of which differs across species) exposure of the developing brain to a differing hormonal milieu, dependent on underlying sex, resulted in permanently altered brain structure and this, in turn, led to altered function and behaviour later in life.

The notion that there were no significant structural or functional differences between male and female brains, however, was widely accepted in the scientific community up until the late 1960s and early 1970s when a series of classic studies pioneered by Pfaff and Raisman demonstrated that rat brain morphology was sexually dimorphic (i.e. the brain differed structurally and functionally as a product of sex) (Pfaff 1966;

Raisman and Field 1971). Further studies in birds high-lighted the importance of sexually dimorphic brain structures in orchestrating the later development of sex-specific behaviours in adulthood, such as the find-ing that administration of testosterone perinatally to the female zebra finch resulted in the later development of adult song behaviour (which normally only develops in males) (Schlinger and Arnold 1991), and this led to a renewed and sustained interest in the 'organizational role' of pre- and perinatal gonadal steroids on structure and subsequent function of the developing brain.

The capacity of steroids to act early in development to alter brain morphology in a sexually dimorphic manner, which consequently dictates components of adult behaviour, is now one of the most well-accepted tenets in behavioural neuroendocrinology (Rubinow *et al.* 2002). Organizational effects represent permanent changes in structure or function which, once set in motion, no longer require the presence of the steroid. This should be contrasted to the 'activational' proper-ties of gonadal steroids on the central nervous system (CNS) in adulthood (discussed further later), which are dependent on the continuing presence of the steroid but which may differ between the sexes due, in part, to discrete prior organizational effects on the underlying brain structure being 'activated'.

The 'organizing/activating' model of sex steroid modulation of the CNS is thus thought to underscore all of the differential effects which sex steroids have on the male and female brain.

Sexual differentiation

Sex is the classification of living things according to their reproductive organs. A developing fetus possesses a bipotential gonadal system until the sixth week of ges-tation, during which, if the fetus is to be male, testes develop and begin to produce androgens. Whether or not an indifferent gonadal system develops testes or not is determined by the presence or absence of the Y chro-mosome, and in particular, activation of a gene called SRY (sex-determining region of the Y chromosome) (Koopman *et al.* 1991). Activation of SRY induces a cascade of events that results in the development of the male gonadal system. In the absence of this gene, the bipotential gonad will go on to develop into an ovary.

Like the gonadal system, the developing brain is also bipotential. Its sexual differentiation is dependent upon the steroid hormone milieu determined by the differen-tiated gonads, and the period of time of maximum sensitivity of the CNS to the organizational effects of the sex steroids in humans is thought to lie between gestational weeks 14 and 16 (Finegan *et al.* 1988), and again in the perinatal period between the 34th to 41st weeks of gestation (Swaab and Hofman 1995). The majority of sex differences in the brain are therefore permanently established during these restricted devel-opmental windows (with the exception of those that occur after the onset of puberty: see later) and are driven by higher testosterone levels in males during these periods.

It is, however, not testosterone itself but, paradoxi-cally, oestrogen which masculinizes brain structure and this occurs in accordance with the aromatization hypothesis first proposed by Naftolin in 1975 (Naftolin *et al.* 1975). The brain is a major producer of oestradiol synthase (also known as P450 aromatase) which con-verts testosterone into oestradiol. Once converted, the oestrogen can bind to intracellular neuronal oestrogen receptors which then translocate to the nucleus. Here, they act as transcription factors for a multitude of genes which ultimately result in altered structure and func-tion of the neuron. The majority of neurons containing such steroid receptors are found in the hypothalamus and limbic system (Simerly *et al.* 1990), and the aro-matase enzyme is expressed at its highest levels in these areas during the 'developmental window' periods. Therefore, these are the structures which display the most evident sexual dimorphism, and, interestingly, they are also those areas of the brain which are believed to play an integral role in many of the psychiatric disor-ders for which a marked sex difference, in either course or prevalence, exists.

Neuroanatomical sex differences

The hypothalamus is located within the ventromedial portion of the diencephalon, and is a critical area for the maintenance of homeostasis in many bodily func-tions, including the stress response system, reproduc-tive capability, autonomic function, and circadian rhythms. It consists of a number of discrete nuclei, the main ones being the preoptic area (POA), suprachias-matic nucleus (SCN), paraventricular nucleus (PVN), ventromedial nucleus (VMN), and arcuate nucleus (ARC), each of which is involved in specialized func-tions. The limbic system is a functional neural system which includes the hippocampus and amygdala, and which plays a prominent role in learning, memory, and affective regulation. Both areas are intimately connected and each is capable of influencing activity in the other through several direct and indirect pathways.

Volumetric sex differences have been consistently found in many of these nuclei in preclinical animal studies, especially those located in the rostral area of the hypothalamus. Indeed in rodents, the POA is known as the sexually dimorphic nucleus (SDN-POA) as it is five to seven times larger in males than females (Gorski *et al.* 1978). Other nuclei which demonstrate volumetric sex differences include the anteroventral periventricular nucleus (AVPn), which is larger in females, and the bed nucleus of the stria terminalis (BNST), which displays opposing morphological heterogeneity dependent on whether the anterior portion (larger in females) or posteromedial segment (larger in males) is considered (Swaab and Hofman 1995). In the limbic system, the medial amygdaloid nucleus is larger in males, and neuronal somatic volume has been shown to vary across the oestrous cycle in females in response to an altered sex steroid milieu (Mizukami *et al.* 1983; Hines *et al.* 1992; Hermel *et al.* 2006).

In addition to modulating the number or size of neurons in a particular brain region, oestradiol has also been shown to regulate the patterns of connectivity between them (synaptic patterning). Its effect on the formation of dendritic spines is a good example of the organizational/activational role of oestrogen on CNS activity. In the neonatal period, oestradiol administration results in a dramatic increase in the dendritic spines of hypothalamic neurons, an effect which persists into adulthood. However, while in the adult hippocampus and hypothalamus the effect of oestradiol on dendritic spine formation remains stimulatory, its actions are transient and less pronounced, inducing up to a 30% increase in the density of dendritic spines at times during the oestrous cycle when its secretion is at peak levels, after which synaptic density returns to baseline numbers (Woolley and McEwen 1992; Calizo and Flanagan-Cato 2000). Sex differences in neuronal 'wiring' are widespread in the hypothalamic nuclei, most notably perhaps in the ARC, and are also significant in the limbic structures of the hippocampus and amygdala. In the ARC, females have twice as many dendritic spine synapses (which tend to be glutamatergic in nature) but much fewer somatic synapses (the majority of which are GABAergic) than males, thus functionally impacting on the degree of excitability as well as the nature of afferent input to the ARC between the sexes (McCarthy 2008).

With regard to human studies, postmortem and structural neuroimaging investigations have demonstrated sex differences supportive of those found in preclinical animal research. The ratio of grey to white matter thickness has been shown to be greater in females, who also have a larger hippocampus, caudate,

thalamus, dorsolateral, and orbitofrontal cortices (Filipek *et al.* 1994; Harasty *et al.* 1997; Goldstein *et al.* 2001; Allen *et al.* 2003; Haier et al. 2005). Men, on the other hand, have been shown to have larger volumes in the amygdala, the hypothalamus, and the medial prefrontal cortex (Allen *et al.* 1989; Zhou *et al.* 1995; Goldstein *et al.* 2001). Intriguingly, after puberty amygdala volume increases significantly more in adolescent boys than girls, whereas the opposite is found in relation to hippocampal growth (Giedd *et al.* 1997). This is consistent with a final organizational action of gonadal steroids on these structures, given previous non-human primate studies which demonstrated a preponderance of androgen receptors in the amygdala and of oestrogen receptors in the hippocampus (Clark *et al.* 1988; Sholl and Kim 1989) and as discussed further later, these areas are exquisitely sensitive to stress and modulation by stress hormones (Sapolsky 2003).

Furthermore, functional neuroimaging techniques have demonstrated both increased cerebral blood flow and cerebral glucose metabolism in females, and this has been shown to vary significantly with menstrual cycle phase indicating acute sex steroid effects (Baxter *et al.* 1987; Reiman *et al.* 1996).

Functional significance of sexually dimorphic brain morphology

The differences noted earlier between the male and female brain in terms of neural development, structure, and plasticity likely contribute to sex differences observed in certain psychiatric disorders.

For example, it is well recognized that sex differences exist in relation to emotional memory, in that women experience the remembering of emotional events in more detail and with greater intensity than men (Seidlitz and Diener 1998). Such differences have been theorized to contribute to the higher prevalence of depression (via a predisposition to ruminative thinking) and posttraumatic stress disorder noted in women (Davidson *et al.* 2002; Hamann 2005), and functional neuroimaging studies have consistently related enhanced emotional memory in females to differential activity and response in the amygdala between the sexes (Canli *et al.* 1999; Cahill *et al.* 2001, 2004).

The loss (or possible reversal) of sexual dimorphism in certain cerebral structures (e.g. anterior cingulate gyrus and the amygdala) involved in the processing of emotions has been demonstrated in schizophrenic patients (Goldstein *et al.* 2002; Gur *et al.* 2004). Functional studies have found that amygdala activation following an emotional stimulus is greater in male schizophrenic patients than female (Mendrek *et al.* 2005) who have also been shown to display much more widespread cerebral activation than females in response to aversive stimuli (Mendrek *et al.* 2007)—both findings the direct opposite to the sex differences observed in health. These findings, coupled with evidence for an abnormality in prenatal sex steroid levels in those with schizophrenia (Arato *et al.* 2004; Procopio *et al.* 2006) have led Mendrek (2007) to propose that aberrant organizational effects of gonadal steroids *in utero* may contribute to a predisposition to the disease, which may then further be acted upon by activational oestrogenic effects after reproductive maturity (see discussion later on oestrogen's impact on dopamine transmission) (Mendrek 2007).

It is well recognized that males and females differ in performance of certain cognitive functions, such as women excelling on tests of verbal fluency and verbal and working memory, while men perform better on spatial tasks. Oestrogen's effect on hippocampal synaptic patterning is thought to be integral to the sex differences noted in learning strategies, given this structure's central role in episodic, declarative, contextual and spatial learning and memory. As described earlier, oestrogen increases dendritic spine density on pyramidal neurons, thus increasing hippocampal neurons' sensitivity to excitation (Woolley *et al.* 1997). This leads to greater long-term potentiation (LTP), a hippocampal neuronal process involved in learning and memory, which has been shown to be at its peak when oestrogen is highest during the oestrous cycle (Warren *et al.* 1995), and which likely contributes to females' better performance in certain cognitive tasks.

Finally, the increase in cerebral blood flow in women compared to men may lead to better distribution of psychotropic medications in the brain at lower doses, and be a factor in why certain medications are more effective for treating psychiatric disorders in women versus men.

Sex differences in neurotransmission

In general, it has been found that female gonadal hormones can alter neural transmission by a number of mechanisms which involve (1) the synthesis, (2) the release, and (3) the action of neurotransmitters. We will describe briefly these effects for the neurotransmitter systems of serotonin, noradrenaline, and dopamine which have been implicated in the pathophysiology of affective or psychotic disorders for which sex differences exist.

The serotonin system

The serotonergic neural system projects from the dorsal raphe nuclei to nearly every area of the forebrain, with substantial input to the areas and brain structures involved in memory, mood, and cognition such as the hypothalamus, hippocampus, amygdala, and the prefrontal cortex.

The degree of serotonergic neural transmission involves the sum of many processes which include serotonin synthesis, neuronal firing, and subsequent receptor activation, in addition to the reuptake and degradation of the neurotransmitter. Serotonin (5-HT) synthesis is governed by tryptophan hydroxylase (TPH), the rate-limiting enzyme in the conversion of tryptophan to 5-hydroxytryptophan. Serotonin neural activity is largely determined by the inhibitory actions of the presynaptic 5-HT1A autoreceptor, which detects serotonin in the extracellular space and acts to rapidly decrease neuronal discharge. Serotonin reuptake or elimination from the synaptic cleft is accomplished by the presynaptic serotonin reuptake transporter (SERT), and finally, degradation of the neurotransmitter is accomplished by monoamine oxidases (MAOs), which can be found in both serotonin neurons and their target neurons.

The ovarian sex hormones have been found to regulate serotonergic tone via influencing each of the components discussed earlier and thus their modulation is quite complex in nature. Generally, however, they have an enhancing effect on serotonin neurotransmission.

Animal studies have demonstrated that oestrogen is capable of increasing tryptophan hydroxylase gene expression. In ovariectomized female macaque monkeys, the administration of oestrogen and/or progesterone resulted in a marked elevation of TPH mRNA in the dorsal raphe (Pecins-Thompson *et al.* 1996), while the same group demonstrated increased TPH protein levels in a similar study (Bethea *et al.* 2000). The ability of oestrogens to increase expression and activity of TPH, thus increasing 5-HT availability, has been consistently reported in the literature (Bethea *et al.* 2002; Smith *et al.* 2004).

Oestrogens have also been shown to affect the distribution and state of 5-HT receptors. Presynaptic 5-HT1A autoreceptors play an important inhibitory role on serotonin neurotransmission. Desensitization of these receptors is considered to be a pivotal part of the mechanism of action of agents which work via 5-HT reuptake inhibition. Oestrogen has been shown to desensitize 5-HT1A receptors in several animal studies. Le Saux and Di Paolo (2005) found that binding of a 5-HT1A agonist increased by 36% in the dorsal raphe of female rats which had undergone ovariectomy, and that this was reversed by the administration of oestrogen. In primates, oestrogen administration has been noted to decrease 5-HT1A mRNA (Lu and Beathea 2002).

Another serotonin receptor which has been shown to be oestrogen-regulated is the postsynaptic 5-HT2A receptor. Oestrogen has a stimulatory action on this receptor's density in the anterior frontal and cingulated cortex, as well as in the nucleus accumbens in rats (Fink et al. 1996). Positron emission tomography (PET) studies in humans have been consistent with this finding, showing increased 5-HT2A receptor binding following hormone therapy in postmenopausal healthy females (Kugaya et al. 2003; Moses-Kolko et al. 2003).

Though oestrogen has been found to decrease expression of the SERT gene, as demonstrated by the reduced SERT mRNA levels found in oestrogen treated ovariectomized primates (Pecins-Thompson et al. 1998), the hormone actually increases SERT protein density in brain-specific regions (Bethea et al. 2002). This apparent contradictory finding results from a reduction in SERT degradation due to the stabilizing effect which 5-HT binding has on the transporter, coupled with the greater 5-HT synthesis which oestrogen promotes.

Finally, further enhancement of 5-HT neurotransmission is inferred by the capability of oestrogen to decrease expression of the monoamine oxidase A (MAO-A) gene, which is the main enzyme responsible for degradation of the neurotransmitter (Gundlah et al. 2002).

It is of note that the 5-HT1A, SERT, and MAO-A genes all lack an oestrogen response element in them, therefore the signal pathway which results in oestrogen reducing their mRNA expression must be via an intermediate factor, with recent evidence suggesting this to be nuclear factor kappa B (NFκB) (Bethea et al. 2006).

The catecholamines: noradrenaline and dopamine systems

Noradrenergic neurons, which project predominantly from the locus ceruleus in the midpons to many of the brain areas involved in the regulation of emotional stability, have been found to contain an abundance of oestrogen receptors, stimulation of which promotes increased noradrenaline neurotransmission.

Similar to oestrogen's action on promoting 5-HT synthesis, the ovarian hormone also increases induction of tyrosine hydroxylase, the rate-limiting enzyme in the synthetic pathway of catecholamines (Pau et al. 2000). This action, coupled with the inhibitory effect of the

steroid on the expression of MAOs, results in the enhanced noradrenergic neurotransmission. Oestrogen has also been shown to alter the expression of many adrenergic receptors in animal models (Wilkinson et al. 1983; Karkanias et al. 1997; Etgen et al. 2001).A further layer of complexity in relation to the influence of ovarian steroids on neurotransmission is provided by the bidirectional communication between the noradrenergic and serotonergic neural systems, with activation of serotonergic neurons having an overall inhibitory effect on norepinephrine (NE) transmission, while activation of NE neurons have a stimulatory effect on serotonin transmission (Blier 2001). Thus the overall effect of an increased oestrogenic milieu on noradrenergic neurons is complex and multilayered.

Females also display enhanced dopamine (DA) neurotransmission compared to men, largely again due to the modulatory effects of gonadal steroids (Cyr et al. 2002). The density of the DA transporter (DAT), which functions to regulate synaptic DA availability, is higher in women compared with men (Mozley et al. 2001) and furthermore, young females have been shown to have higher striatal DA synthesis (Laakso et al. 2002). In animal studies, oestrogen has been shown to modulate DA receptors in the striatum and nucleus accumbens: ovariectomy of female rats was shown to result in a decrease in D2 receptor density (and also DAT density) within two weeks of the procedure while oestradiol treatment resulted in increased D2 receptor density (Le Saux et al. 2006; Le Saux and Paolo 2006). In humans, PET studies of sex differences in D2 receptors have been inconsistent, one demonstrating lower striatal receptor affinity in females (Pohjalainen et al. 1998) but another finding higher receptor-binding in the female cortex (Kaasinen et al. 2001). However, both studies were small and neither controlled for menstrual cycle status, which is of relevance given previous research that suggested D2 receptor availability varies across the menstrual cycle (Wong et al. 1988).

Functional significance of sexually dimorphic neurotransmitter systems

Abnormal serotonin neurotransmission is implicated in the pathology of mood and anxiety disorders, eating disorders, and schizophrenia, all of which have significant sex differences in either prevalence or course. Elucidating the cause and nature of sex differences in 5-HT function may thus serve to illuminate pathophysiological processes involved in these disorders and may impact on pharmacological therapies that target 5-HT neurotransmission. The modulation by sex hormones of these neurotransmission systems in a continuously fluctuating manner from the time of menarche to menopause may confer a greater risk for aberrant functioning of these systems with subsequent development of affective disorders, when compared to the relatively stable hormonal milieu of the male. Furthermore, as a result of oestrogenic enhancement of serotonergic tone in females, it has been suggested that young women with depression may be more responsive to selective serotonin reuptake inhibitor medication than tricyclic antidepressants compared to older women and men (Kornstein *et al.* 2000).

With regards to schizophrenia, oestrogen may be neuroprotective in its interaction with the DA system, principally via enhancing presynaptic dopaminergic tone in females of a reproductive age. This is thought to confer greater protection against developing the disorder, thus providing a biological rationale for the later age of onset seen in females and for the second peak in incidence seen around the time of the menopause when such protective factors are removed. In addition, the better response of females to antidopaminergic drug treatment may be due to the enhanced DA transmission in women (Seeman 1995).

Sex differences in the stress response system

Basic outline of the hypothalamic–pituitary–adrenal axis

The hypothalamic–pituitary–adrenal (HPA) axis forms the principal effector arm of the body's stress response system. It is activated in response to environmental stressors which threaten homeostasis, and it functions to mobilize adaptive behaviours and peripheral functions while inhibiting biologically costly behaviours (e.g. feeding, reproduction, growth) thus priming the body to adapt successfully to the environmental perturbation.

The principal molecular regulators of the HPA axis are corticotropin-releasing hormone (CRH) and arginine vasopressin (AVP), both of which are synthesized and secreted by neurons found in the hypothalamic paraventricular nucleus (PVN). Once secreted, these hormones travel to the anterior pituitary gland where they synergistically stimulate the synthesis and release of adrenocorticotropic hormone (ACTH). Circulating ACTH subsequently stimulates release of glucocorticoids from the adrenal cortex, which go on to have widespread actions on multiple systems throughout the body,

effected through binding to specific intracellular receptors known as the mineralcorticoid (or Type I) and glucocorticoid (or Type II) receptor. Glucocorticoids are also involved in regulating their own secretion by providing negative feedback control on the HPA axis at multiple levels, including the hippocampus, hypothalamus, and pituitary.

The finding of abnormalities in the regulation of the HPA axis in patients with mood and anxiety disorders, coupled with the fact that these disorders are clearly precipitated and perpetuated by stress, has led to extensive research in both animal and human models to attempt to identify differences in stress responsivity between the sexes which may convey a greater risk for females to develop affective disorders.

Animal studies

Sex differences in the response of the HPA axis to a variety of stressors have been consistently demonstrated in the animal study literature, with females displaying a more robust response characterized by a faster onset of glucocorticoid secretion when under stress, a faster rate of rise of adrenal steroids during stress, and a slower rate of recovery to baseline levels once the stress has terminated(Jones *et al.* 1972; Kant *et al.* 1983; Burgess and Handa 1992; Yoshimura *et al.* 2003)

Gonadal steroids have been shown to explain this sexually dimorphic response of the HPA axis to stress. Studies evaluating stress-responsiveness across the oestrous cycle of rodents have demonstrated that at times during the cycle when oestrogen is at its highest, the response of the HPA axis is at its greatest. (Raps *et al.* 1971; Viau and Meaney 1991) Though oestrogen administration has been consistently shown to increase baseline and stress-induced glucocorticoid secretion in rodent studies, the mechanism of action for this is still to be fully elucidated. Many studies have noted a stimulatory effect of oestrogen on ACTH levels (Viau and Meaney 1991; Burgess and Handa 1992; Young 1996) which is felt to probably reflect a greater central CRH response to stress, as supported by the discovery of an oestrogen response element on the human CRH gene (Vamvakopoulos and Chrousos 1993). However, recent research has suggested that gonadal steroids' enhancement of the stress response may, at least in part, be mediated through potentiation of peripheral adrenocortical responses also (Figueiredo *et al.* 2007).

Progesterone administration has also been shown to elicit greater stress responsiveness, primarily through antiglucocorticoid effects of the hormone which diminishes feedback control of the axis (Svec 1988).

Furthermore, androgens may contribute to the discussed sex differences in stress responsiveness by dampening the degree of HPA activation in males, as indicated by Bingaman and colleagues (1994) who observed increased hypothalamic CRH levels following castration of male rodents which could subsequently be reversed following administration of the non-aromatizable androgen, dihydrotestosterone.

The organizational role of gonadal steroids on the developing CNS should also be borne in mind, given that many of the areas which exhibit the most sexually dimorphic structure are also those areas involved in the central regulation of the HPA axis. For example, Choi and colleagues (2007) have recently shown that HPA axis responsivity to stress is modulated by afferent input from the BNST. This brain structure can function as a relay station between the limbic system and the PVN of the hypothalamus, and lesions induced in the anterior portion of it have been shown to result in attenuation of glucocorticoid response to stress in rats, while posterior BNST nuclei lesions result in elevated plasma ACTH and corticosterone response to acute restraint stress, increased stress-induced PVN c-fos mRNA, and elevated CRH and AVP mRNA expression in the hypothalamus (Choi *et al.* 2007). These data suggest that posterior BNST nuclei are involved in inhibition of the HPA axis, whereas the anteroventral BNST nuclei are involved in HPA axis excitation, and as outlined earlier, the anterior portion is much larger in females while males have a larger posterior BNST (Swaab and Hofman 1995). Similarly, stimulation of medial and central amygdaloid nuclei (which are larger in males) elicits corticosterone secretion, and ablation of these areas can block the HPA axis response to certain stimuli (e.g. restraint stress and fear conditioning) (Van de Kar *et al.* 1991).

Surprising data on relative resistance of the female hippocampus to the deleterious effects of long-term stress has been demonstrated in rodent and primate studies. The apical dendrites of male hippocampal neurons have consistently been observed to undergo reversible atrophy following chronic stress, a finding not demonstrated in females (Uno *et al.* 1989; Mizoguchi *et al.* 1992; Galea *et al.* 1997). The hippocampus plays an important role in modulating HPA axis responsivity by providing an additional target for feedback control by glucocorticoids due to its tonic inhibition of hypothalamic CRH and AVP secretion. According to the glucocorticoid cascade hypothesis (Sapolsky *et al.* 2000), chronic stress results in prolonged glucocorticoid stimulation of hippocampal neurons which, in turn, results in downregulation of their steroid receptors.

Such downregulation leads to a reduction in the hippocampal inhibition of the PVN neurons and renders the HPA axis less sensitive to glucocorticoid feedback. Thus prolonged hypercortisolism ensues which is deleterious to hippocampal neurons, and eventually results in their atrophy with further loss of feedback control. Female hippocampal resistance to such atrophy, together with the findings of greater impairment of spatial memory, escape learning, and enhancement of fear behaviours in males following acute or chronic stress, suggest that females display a relative resistance to the stress-induced neurobiological effects that are evident in males (Steenbergen *et al.* 1990; Heinsbroek *et al.* 1991; Luine 2002; Conrad *et al.* 2004; Altemus 2006).

Human data on sex differences in stress response

Consistent with preclinical animal research, the effect of oestrogen on human HPA axis reactivity has been shown to be stimulatory. Women receiving high-dose oestrogen therapy and pregnant women have demonstrated elevated levels of free cortisol, while oestrogen administration to men has also been observed to result in HPA axis hyper-responsiveness (Lindholm and Schultz-Moller 1973; Kirschbaum *et al.* 1996)

Despite these effects, however, the overall picture painted from human research thus far suggests that adult males respond to psychological stress with greater increases in cortisol compared to women, whereas females tend to display an enhanced stress response system to pharmacological challenge tests (Kudielka and Kirschbaum 2005). This discrepancy may lie in the fact that psychological stressors are central stimuli of the HPA axis which require processing at higher brain centres (such as the prefrontal cortex, hippocampus, and amygdala) prior to stimulating the PVN of the hypothalamus. Such neurocircuits display marked sexual dimorphism as outlined earlier, which functionally likely modulates their processing of stress and their impact on the HPA axis stress response. Pharmacological tests, however, bypass this higher-order cognitive processing and have a more direct route to various levels of the HPA axis dependent on the specific agent employed. It is of interest that when the effects of circulating sex steroids are removed (as when individuals are induced into a state of hypogonadism), then males display enhanced stress response to both pharmacological challenge tests and to psychological stressors (Putnam *et al.* 2005; Roca *et al.* 2005).

The Trier Social Stress Test (TSST) (Kirschbaum *et al.* 1993) is widely accepted as being the best psychological stressor for evaluating HPA axis responses (Dickerson and Kemeny 2004). It is a standardized laboratory stress test which consists of a three-minute preparation period followed by five minutes of public speaking and mental arithmetic tasks, and is thus characterized by elements of uncontrollability and social-evaluative threat. The TSST has been shown to elicit greater ACTH and free cortisol responses in men compared to women (Kirschbaum et al. 1999; Kudielka et al. 2004; Uhart et al. 2006). ACTH responses in males have been shown to be higher no matter what phase of the menstrual cycle the females are in, although free cortisol response levels are higher only when compared to women in the follicular phase (Rohleder et al. 2001; Wolf et al. 2001). This suggests that the luteal phase of the cycle may be associated with enhanced adrenal sensitivity to ACTH, a hypothesis in accordance with an earlier small study which observed a higher cortisol to ACTH ratio in the female participants (Roelfsema et al. 1993).

There is some suggestion that different types of psychological stress may result in a differential sex-specific HPA axis response also. Stroud and colleagues (2002) observed in their study that men had significantly higher free cortisol response to psychological stressors involving achievement challenges in comparison to females, who demonstrated significantly higher cortisol response to social rejection challenges, a finding of potential importance for depression in women yet which requires further study and replication.

Pharmacological challenges, as mentioned, have generally been shown to elicit greater response in the female HPA axis. Uhart and colleagues (2006) demonstrated greater ACTH and free cortisol responses to naloxone challenge in females compared to males (while also confirming in the same study that males had a greater response to a psychological stressor, the TSST). The administration of CRH, either alone or in combination with dexamethasone, has been found to elicit greater stress responses in females (Galluci et al. 1993; Heuser et al. 1994). A recent study by Putnam and colleagues (2005) controlled for the activational effects of gonadal steroids on the HPA axis responsivity to pharmacological challenge by inducing a state of hypogonadism in study participants (via several consecutive monthly gonadotropin-releasing hormone agonist [leuprolide] injections) and then subsequently administered a CRH challenge. Under such circumstances, male participants exhibited significantly greater ACTH and free cortisol responses than females, thus suggesting that sex differences in stress response are not entirely determined by the acute (or 'activational') effects of sex steroids.

As mentioned previously, it is well established that many of the sexual dimorphisms in brain structure and function are initiated by early, usually fetal, exposures to sex steroids which convey an organizational role on subsequent CNS development. The impact of such organization on stress responsiveness has been described in animal studies which have demonstrated neonatal oestrogenization of female rats is able to cause persistent and profound alterations in neurocircuitry involved in HPA axis regulation (elevated CRH and AVP mRNA in the PVN, reduced glucocorticoid receptor mRNA in the hippocampus) (Patchev et al. 1995; McCormick et al. 2002). Presumably, the higher stress responses to pharmacological challenge unmasked in the male participants of Uhart's study reflects such organizational activities of gonadal hormones during CNS development, an effect which is reversed when the activational properties of such hormones (which had been negated in the study by inducing hypogonadism) are taken into consideration.

Functional significance of sex differences in stress response

The literature discussed earlier suggests that a female's HPA axis, when viewed in isolation, is primed to respond to stress in a greater fashion than that of a male, and that this is mediated primarily through the acute effects of gonadal steroids on promoting a greater CRH drive while also reducing the feedback control of glucocorticoids on the stress axis.

The consistent finding of a greater response of the axis to psychological stress in males, together with the relative resistance to neurobiological effects of stress demonstrated by females, is therefore surprising given the higher female prevalence of stress-related disorders and the stimulating effect of female gonadal steroids on the HPA axis. It has recently been speculated that a possible way of reconciling these apparent contradictory findings is to consider the stress-induced neurobiological changes in males as adaptive in nature (Altemus 2006). Differential stress-induced activation of higher cognitive centres in a sexually dimorphic manner may allow males to mount a strong stress response when challenged, but better enable them to move on and forget the stress and its associations more quickly than females once it has passed. Situations or conditions in which recovery after stress exposure is prolonged may be more relevant than the magnitude of response in mediating a negative health outcome (Linden et al. 1997; Sapolsky et al. 2000), and thus the female's enhanced emotional memory and resistance to stress-induced memory impairment may convey greater susceptibility to developing depression or anxiety in response to a significant negative stress.

Conclusions

The ovarian steroid hormones exert a profound and dynamic effect on CNS development and function throughout the life cycle, modulating many structures and systems which are implicated in affective and psychotic disorders. Regulation occurs through many processes, including both genomic and non-genomic effects, resulting in altered neuronal sensitivity and responsivity to various stimuli.

The greater degree of fluctuation of a female's hormonal milieu across the lifespan may, in at least some, thus enhance the potential for aberrant neurotransmission and stress response. Though much research has been carried out on sex-specific differences in the healthy brain, future adequately-powered studies are needed whose primary aim should be to investigate these differences in patients with psychiatric disorders, especially those which are known to have significant prevalence or course differences between the sexes.

References

Allen J *et al.* (2003). Sexual dimorphism and asymmetries in the gray-white composition of the human cerebrum. *Neuroimage*, **18**, 880–94.

Allen LS *et al.* (1989). Two sexually dimorphic cell groups in the human brain. *Journal of Neuroscience*, **9**, 497–506.

Altemus M (2006). Sex differences in depression and anxiety disorders: Potential biological determinants. *Hormones and Behavior*, **50**, 534–8.

Arato M *et al.* (2004). Digit length pattern in schizophrenia suggests disturbed prenatal hemispheric lateralization. *Progress in Neuro-psychopharmacology & Biological Psychiatry*, **28**, 191–4.

Baxter L *et al.* (1987). Cerebral glucose metabolic rates in normal human females versus normal males. *Psychiatry Research*, **21**, 237–45.

Bethea CL *et al.* (2000). Steroid regulation of tryptophan hydroxylase protein in the dorsal raphe of macaques. *Biological Psychiatry*, **47**, 562–76.

Bethea CL *et al.* (2002). Diverse actions of ovarian steroids in the serotonin neural system. *Frontiers in Neuroendocrinology*, **23**, 41–100.

Bethea CL *et al.* (2006). Nuclear factor kappa B in the dorsal raphe of macaques: an anatomical link for steroids, cytokines and serotonin. *Journal of Psychiatry & Neuroscience*, **31**(2), 105–14.

Bingaman EW *et al.* (1994). Androgen inhibits the increases in hypothalamic corticotropin releasing hormone (CRH) and CRH immunoreactivity following gonadectomy. *Neuroendocrinology*, **59**, 228–34.

Blier P (2001). Crosstalk between the norepinephrine and serotonin systems and its role in the antidepressant response. *Journal of Psychiatry & Neuroscience*, **26**(Suppl), S3–S10.

Burgess LH and Handa RJ (1992). Estrogen alters adrenocorticotropic hormone and corticosterone secretion and glucocorticoid receptor mediated function. *Endocrinology*, **131**, 1261–9.

Cahill L *et al.* (2001). Sex-related difference in amygdala activity during emotionally influenced memory storage. *Neurobiology of Learning and Memory*, **75**, 1–9.

Cahill L *et al.* (2004). Sex-related hemispheric lateralization of amygdala function in emotionally influenced memory: an FMRI investigation. *Learn & Memory*, **11**, 261–6.

Calizo LH and Flanagan-Cato LM (2000). Estrogen selectively regulates spine density within the dendritic arbour of rat ventromedial hypothalamic neurons. *Journal of Neuroscience*, **20**, 1589–1596.

Canli T *et al.* (1999). Sex differences in the neural basis of emotional memories. *Proceedings of the National Academy of Sciences*, **99**, 10789–94.

Choi DC *et al.* (2007). Bed nucleus of the stria terminalis subregions differentially regulate hypothalamic-pituitary-adrenal axis activity: implications for the integration of limbic inputs. *Journal of Neuroscience*, **27**(8), 2025–34.

Clark AS *et al.* (1988). Androgen binding and metabolism in the cerebral cortex of the developing rhesus monkey. *Endocrinology*, **123**, 932–940.

Conrad CD *et al.* (2004). Acute stress impairs spatial memory in male but not female rats: influence of estrous cycle. *Pharmacology, Biochemistry, and Behavior*, **78**, 569–79.

Cyr M *et al.* (2002). Estrogenic modulation of brain activity: implications for schizophrenia and Parkinson's disease. *Journal of Psychiatry and Neuroscience*, **27**, 12–27.

Davidson RJ *et al.* (2002). Depression: perspectives from affective neuroscience. *Annual Review of Psychology*, **53**, 545–74.

Dickerson SS and Kemeny ME (2004). Acute stressors and cortisol responses: a theoretical integration and synthesis of laboratory research. *Psychological Bulletin*, **130**, 355–91.

Etgen AM *et al.* (2001). Mechanisms of ovarian steroid regulation of norepinephrine receptor-mediated signal transduction in the hypothalamus: implications for female reproductive physiology. *Hormones and Behavior*, **40**, 169–77.

Figueiredo HF *et al.* (2007). Estrogen potentiates adrenocortical responses to stress in female rats. *American Journal of Physiology, Endocrinology and Metabolism*, **292**(4), E1173–E1182.

Filipek PA *et al.* (1994). The young adult human brain: an MRI-based morphometric analysis. *Cerebral Cortex*, **4**, 344–360.

Finegan J *et al.* (1988). A window for the study of prenatal sex hormone influences on postnatal development. *Journal of Genetic Psychology*, **150**, 101–12.

Fink G *et al.* (1996). Estrogen control of central neurotransmission: effect on mood, mental state, and memory. *Cellular and Molecular Neurobiology*, **16**, 325–44.

Galea LM *et al.* (1997). Sex differences in dendritic atrophy of CA3 pyramidal neurons in response to chronic restraint stress. *Neuroscience*, **81**, 689–97.

Gallucci WT *et al.* (1993). Sex differences in sensitivity of the hypothalamic–pituitary–adrenal axis. *Health Psychology*, **12**, 420–5.

Giedd JN *et al.* (1997). Sexual dimorphism of the developing human brain. *Progress in Neuro-psychopharmacology & Biological Psychiatry*, **21**, 1185–201.

Goldstein J *et al.* (2001). Normal sexual dimorphism of the adult human brain assessed by in vivo magnetic resonance imaging. *Cerebral Cortex*, **11**, 490–7.

Goldstein JM *et al.* (2002). Impact of normal sexual dimorphisms on sex differences in structural brain abnormalities in schizophrenia assessed by magnetic resonance imaging. *Archives of General Psychiatry*, **59**, 154–64.

Gorski RA *et al.* (1978). Evidence for a morphological sex difference within the medial preoptic area of the rat brain. *Brain Research*, **148**, 333–46.

Gundlah C *et al.* (2002). Ovarian steroid regulation of monoamine oxidase-A and –B mRNAs in the macaque dorsal raphe and hypothalamic nuclei. *Psychopharmacology (Berl)*, **160**, 271–82.

Gur RE *et al.* (2004). A sexually dimorphic ratio of orbitofrontal to amygdala volume is altered in schizophrenia. *Biological Psychiatry*, **55**, 512–17.

Haier R *et al.* (2005). The neuroanatomy of general intelligence: sex matters. *Neurimage*, **25**, 320–327.

Hamann S (2005). Sex differences in the responses of the human amygdala. *Neuroscientist*, **11**, 288–93.

Harasty J *et al.* (1997). Language-associated cortical regions are proportionally larger in the female brain. *Archives of Neurology*, **54**, 171–6.

Heinsbroek RPW *et al.* (1991). Sex differences in the behavioral consequences of inescapable footshocks depend on time since shock. *Physiology & Behavior*, **49**, 1257–63.

Hermel EES *et al.* (2006). Influence of sex and estrous cycle, but not laterality, on neuronal somatic volume of the posterodorsal medial amygdala of rats. *Neuroscience Letters*, **405**, 153–8.

Heuser IJ *et al.* (1994). Age-associated changes of pituitary–adrenocortical hormone regulation in humans: importance of gender. *Neurobiology of Aging*, **15**, 227–31.

Hines M *et al.* (1992). Sex differences in subregions of the medial nucleus of the amygdala and the bed nucleus of the stria terminalis of the rat. *Brain Research*, **579**, 321–6.

Jones MT *et al.* (1972). Characteristics of fast feedback control of corticotrophin release by corticosteroids. *Journal of Endocrinology*, **55**, 489.

Kaasinen V *et al.* (2001). Sex differences in extrastriatal dopamine D2-like receptors in the human brain. *American Journal of Psychiatry*, **158**, 308–11.

Kant GJ *et al.* (1983). Comparison of stress response in male and female rats: pituitary cyclic AMP and plasma prolactin, growth hormone and corticosterone. *Psychoneuroendocrinology*, **8**, 421–8.

Karkanias GB *et al.* (1997). Estradiol reduction of alpha 2-adrenoceptor binding in female rat cortex is correlated with decreases in alpha 2A/D-adrenoceptor messenger RNA. *Neuroscience*, **81**, 593–7.

Kirschbaum C *et al.* (1993). The 'Trier Social Stress Test' – a tool for investigating psychobiological stress responses in a laboratory setting. *Neuropsychobiology*, **28**, 76–81.

Kirschbaum C *et al.* (1996). Short-term estradiol treatment enhances pituitary-adrenal axis and sympathetic responses to psychological stress in healthy young men. *Journal of Clinical Endocrinology and Metabolism*, **81**, 39–43.

Kirschbaum C *et al.* (1999). Impact of gender, menstrual cycle phase, and oral contraceptives on the activity of the hypothalamic-pituitary-adrenal axis. *Psychosomatic Medicine*, **61**, 154–62.

Koopman P *et al.* (1991). Male development of chromosomally female mice transgenic for SRY. *Nature*, **351**, 117–21.

Kornstein SG *et al.* (2000). Gender differences in treatment response to sertraline versus imipramine in chronic depression. *American Journal of Psychiatry*, **157**, 1445–52.

Kudielka BM *et al.* (2004). HPA axis responses to laboratory psychosocial stress in healthy elderly adults, younger adults, and children: impact of age and gender. *Psychoneuroendocrinology*, **29**, 83–98.

Kudielka BM and Kirschbaum C (2005). Sex differences in HPA axis responses to stress: a review. *Biological Psychology*, **69**, 113–32.

Kugaya A *et al.* (2003). Increase in prefrontal cortex serotonin 2A receptors following estrogen treatment in postmenopausal women. *American Journal of Psychiatry*, **160**, 1522–4.

Laakso A *et al.* (2002). Sex differences in striatal presynaptic dopamine synthesis capacity in healthy subjects. *Biological Psychiatry*, **52**, 759–63.

Le Saux M *et al.* (2006). ERbeta mediates the estradiol increase of D2 receptors in the rat striatum and nucleus accumbens. *Neuropharmacology*, **50**, 451–7.

Le Saux M and Di Paolo T (2005). Changes in 5-HT1A receptor binding and G-protein activation in the rat brain after estrogen treatment: comparison with tamoxifen and raloxifene. *Journal of Psychiatry & Neuroscience*, **30**, 110–17.

Le Saux M and Di Paolo T (2006). Influence of oestrogenic compounds on monoamine transporters in rat striatum. *Journal of Neuroendocrinology*, **18**, 25–32.

Linden W *et al.* (1997). Physiological stress reactivity and recovery: conceptual siblings separated at birth? *Journal of Psychosomatic Research*, **42**, 117–35.

Lindholm J and Schultz-Moller N (1973). Plasma and urinary cortisol in pregnancy and during estrogen treatment. *Scandinavian Journal of Clinical and Laboratory Investigation*, **31**, 119–22.

Lu NZ and Beathea CL (2002). Ovarian steroid regulation of 5-HT1A receptor binding and G protein activation in female monkeys. *Neuropsyhcopharmacology*, **27**, 12–24.

Luine V (2002). Sex differences in chronic stress effects on memory in rats. *Stress*, **5**, 205–16.

McCormick CM *et al.* (2002). Peripheral and central sex steroids have differential effects on the HPA axis of male and female rats. *Stress*, **5**, 235–24.

McCarthy MM (2008). Estradiol and the developing brain. *Physiological Reviews*, **88**, 91–134.

Mendrek A *et al.* (2005). An fMRI study of sex differences in emotion processing in schizophrenia. *Schizophrenia Bulletin*, **31**, 427.

Mendrek A *et al.* (2007). Sex differences in the cerebral function associated with processing of aversive stimuli by schizophrenia patients. *Australian and New Zealand Journal of Psychiatry*, **41**, 136–41.

Mendrek A (2007). Reversal of normal cerebral sexual dimorphism in schizophrenia: evidence and speculations. *Medical Hypotheses*, **69**, 896–902.

Mizoguchi K *et al.* (1992). Stress induces neuronal death in the hippocampus of castrated rats. *Neuroscience Letters*, **138**, 157–60.

Mizukami S *et al.* (1983). Sexual difference in nuclear volume and it ontogeny in the rat amygdala. *Experimental Neurology*, **79**, 569–75.

Moses-Kolko EL *et al.* (2003). Widespread increases of cortical serotonin type 2A receptor availability after hormone therapy in euthymic post menopausal women. *Fertility and Sterility*, **80**, 554–9.

Mozley L *et al.* (2001). Striatal dopamine transporters and cognitive functioning in healthy men and women. *American Journal of Psychiatry*, **158**, 1492–9.

Naftolin F *et al.* (1975). The formation of estrogens by central neuroendocrine tissues. *Recent Progress in Hormone Research*, **31**, 295–319.

Patchev VK *et al.* (1995). Implications of estrogen-dependent brain organization for gender differences in hypothalamo-pituitary-adrenal regulation. *FASEB Journal*, **9**, 419–23.

Pau KY *et al.* (2000). Oestrogen upregulates noradrenaline release in the mediobasal hypothalamus and tyrosine hydroxylase gene expression in the brainstem of ovariectomized rhesus macaques. *Journal of Neuroendocrinology*, **12**, 899–909.

Pecins-Thompson M *et al.* (1996). Ovarian steroid regulation of tryptophan hydroxylase mRNA expression in rhesus macaques. *Journal of Neuroscience*, **16**, 7021–9.

Pecins-Thompson M *et al.* (1998). Regulation of serotonin re-uptake transporter mRNA expression by ovarian steroids in rhesus macaques. *Brain Research. Molecular Brain Research*, **53**, 120–9.

Pfaff DW (1966). Morphological changes in the brains of adult rats after neonatal castration. *Journal of Endocrinology*, **36**, 415–16.

Pheonix CH *et al.* (1959). Organizing action of prenatally administered testosterone propionate on the tissues mediating mating behaviour in the female guinea pig. *Endocrinology*, **65**, 369–82.

Pohjalainen T *et al.* (1998). Sex differences in the striatal dopamine D2 receptor binding characteristics in vivo. *American Journal of Psychiatry*, **155**, 768–73.

Procopio M *et al.* (2006). The hormonal environment in utero as a potential aetiological agent for schizophrenia. *European Archives of Psychiatry and Clinical Neuroscience*, **256**, 77–81.

Putnam K *et al.* (2005). Sex-related differences in stimulated hypothalamic pituitary-adrenal axis during induced gonadal suppression. *Journal of Clinical Endocrinology and Metabolism*, **90**, 4224–31.

Raisman G and Field PM (1971). Sexual dimorphism in the preoptic area of the rat. *Science*, **173**, 731–3.

Raps D *et al.* (1971). Plasma and adrenal corticosterone levels during the different phases of the sexual cycle in normal female rats. *Experientia*, **27**, 339–40.

Reiman E *et al.* (1996). The application of positron emission tomography to the study of the normal menstrual cycle. *Human Reproduction*, **11**, 2799–805.

Roca CA *et al.* (2005). Sex-related differences in stimulated hypothalamic-pituitary-adrenal axis during induced gonadal suppression. *Journal of Clinical Endocrinology and Metabolism*, **90**, 4224–31.

Roelfsema F *et al.* (1993). Sex-dependent alteration in cortisol response to endogenous adrenocorticotropin. *Journal of Clinical Endocrinology and Metabolism*, **77**, 234–40.

Rohleder N *et al.* (2001). Sex differences in glucocorticoid sensitivity of proinflammatory cytokine production after psychosocial stress. *Psychosomatic Medicine*, **63**, 966–72.

Rubinow DR *et al.*(2002). Gonadal hormones and behaviour in women: concentrations versus context. In: DW Pfaff *et al.* (eds) *Hormones, Brain and Behaviour*, pp. 37–73. Academic Press, New York.

Sapolsky RM *et al.* (2000). How do glucocorticoids influence stress responses? Integrating permissive, suppressive, stimulatory, and preparative actions. *Endocrine Reviews*, **21**, 55–89.

Sapolsky RM (2003). Stress and plasticity in the limbic system. *Neurochemical Research*, **28**, 1735–1742.

Schlinger BA and Arnold AP (1991). Androgen effects on the development of the zebra finch song system. *Brain Research*, **561**, 99–105.

Seeman MV (1995). Sex differences in predicting neuroleptic response. In: W Gaebel and AG Awad (eds) *The Prediction of Neuroleptic Response*, pp. 51–64. Springer-Verlag, Vienna.

Seidlitz YI and Diener E (1998). Sex differences in the recall of affective experiences. *Journal of Personality and Social Psychology*, **74**, 262–71.

Sholl SA and Kim KL (1989). Estrogen receptors in the rhesus monkey brain during fetal development. *Brain Research. Developmental Brain Research*, **50**, 189–96.

Simerly RB *et al.* (1990). Distribution of androgen and estrogen receptor mRNA-containing cells in the rat brain: an in situ hybridization study. *Journal of Comparative Neurology*, **294**, 76–95.

Smith LJ *et al.* (2004). Effects of ovarian steroids and raloxifene on proteins that synthesize, transport, and degrade serotonin in the raphe region of macaques. *Neuropsychopharmacology*, **29**, 2035–45.

Steenbergen HI *et al.* (1990). Sex-dependent effects of inescapable shock administration on shuttlebox-escape performance and elevated plus-maze behavior. *Physiology & Behavior*, **48**, 571–6.

Stroud LR *et al.* (2002). Sex differences in stress responses: social rejection versus achievement stress. *Biological Psychiatry*, **52**, 318–27.

Svec F (1988). Differences in the interaction of RU 486 and ketoconazole with the second binding site of the glucocorticoid receptor. *Endocrinology*, **123**, 1902–6.

Swaab DF and Hofman MA (1995). Sexual differentiation of the human hypothalamus in relation to gender and sexual orientation. *Trends in Neurosciences*, **18**, 264–70.

Uhart M *et al.* (2006). Gender differences in hypothalamic-pituitary-adrenal (HPA) axis reactivity. *Psychoneuroendocrinology*, **31**(5), 642–52.

Uno H *et al.* (1989). Hippocampal damage associated with prolonged and fatal stress in primates. *Journal of Neuroscience*, **9**, 1705–11.

Vamvakopoulos NC and Chrousos GP (1993). Evidence of direct estrogenic regulation of human corticotrophin-releasing hormone gene expression. *Journal of Clinical Investigation*, **92**, 1896–902.

Van de Kar LD *et al.* (1991). Amygdaloid lesions: differential effect on conditioned stress and immobilization-induced increases in corticosterone and rennin secretion. *Neuroendocrinology*, **54**, 89–95.

Viau V and Meaney MJ (1991). Basal and stress hypothalamic-pituitary-adrenal activity in cycling and ovariectomized-steroid treated rats. *Endocrinology*, **129**, 2503–11.

Warren SG *et al.* (1995). LTP varies across the estrous cycle: enhanced synaptic plasticity in proestrus rats. *Brain Research*, **703**, 26–30.

Wilkinson M *et al.* (1983). Prolonged estrogen treatment induces changes in opiate, benzodiazepine and beta-adrenergic binding sites in female rat hypothalamus. *Brain Research Bulletin*, **11**, 279–81.

Wolf OT *et al.* (2001). The relationship between stress induced cortisol levels and memory differs between men and women. *Psychoneuroendocrinology*, **26**, 711–20.

Wong D *et al.* (1988). In vivo measurement of dopamine receptors in human brain by positron emission tomography. Age and sex differences. *Annals of the New York Academy of Sciences*, **515**, 203–14.

Woolley CS and McEwen BS (1992). Estradiol mediates fluctuation in hippocampal synapse density during the estrous cycle in the adult rat. *Journal of Neuroscience*, **12**, 2549–54.

Woolley CS *et al.* (1997). Estradiol increases the sensitivity of hippocampal CA1 pyramidal cell to NMDA receptor-mediated synaptic input: correlation with dendritic spine density. *Journal of Neuroscience*, **17**, 1848–59.

Yoshimura S *et al.* (2003). Sex-differences in adrenocortical responsiveness during development in rats. *Steroids*, **68**, 439–45.

Young EA (1996). Sex differences in response to exogenous corticosterone. *Molecular Psychiatry*, **1**, 313–19.

Zhou JN *et al.* (1995). A sex difference in the human brain and its relation to transexuality. *Nature*, **378**, 68–70.

CHAPTER 6

Lesbianism and mental health

Kristian Aleman and Ronald Doctor

Etymology, definition, prevalence, and art

Etymologically the adjective 'lesbian' is traced back to 1591 from 'Lesbius', emanating from the Greek conception 'lesbios of Lesbos'. Lesbos is an island in the north-eastern Aegean Sea in Greece and was the great lyric poet Sappho's home (born sometime between 630 and 612 BC). Sappho is famous for her erotic and romantic verses and is associated with homosexual relationships between women.

Adrienne Rich (1980), a feminist poet in the late 20th century, outlined a continuum of lesbian intimacy ranging from sexual to platonic relationships. In the broadest definition of lesbianism, Rich proposed that the female who sidestepped traditional married life in order to combat male tyranny might be seen at one end of the continuum, usually connected with feminism. In the 1970s the radical lesbians declared, 'A lesbian is the rage of all women condensed to the point of explosion' (McCoy and Hicks 1979).

Henri de Toulouse-Lautrec, the prominent 19th century French post-impressionist painter, injured as a young boy, became short, midget-like, and suffered from a sense of being an outsider. He empathized with prostitutes and represented them in his art. He became acquainted with lesbians and noted that these women often protectively turned to each other for love. His artistic inspiration emerged from their intense intimacy. When Toulouse-Lautrec observed two women sleeping entwined on a couch, he pronounced: 'This is superior to everything. Nothing can compare to something so simple.'

Being a lesbian most often involves both romantic feelings and sexual attraction toward other women. Today the prevalence of female and male homosexuals plus bisexuals is estimated by the Stonewall organization to be between 5–7% among people in the United Kingdom. One crucial research observation of homosexual people relating to mental health seems to be whether they can openly stand for their homosexual identity or not. The identity process of 'coming out' is associated with healthier self-acceptance and self-esteem.

Theory of homosexuality

Richard von Krafft-Ebing considered homosexuality as pathological. In his book *Psychopathia Sexualis* (Krafft-Ebing 1886) homosexuality was registered as one of over 200 other sexual deviances. He postulated that this pathological phenomenon either emanated from birth or was acquired from the environment.

Sigmund Freud (1905) in a controversial book postulated that humans at birth are 'polymorphous perverse'. Freud adopted a more accepting stance of diverse sexuality and did not regard this as immoral; on the contrary, he considered the infant was naturally open to all kinds of sexual orientations before her actual sexual orientation was formed by the resolution of the Oedipal complex occurring around the age of three to five years. In the 'negative' Oedipal complex (Freud 1924), where the child becomes homosexual, the child does not identify herself with the mother. The girl first tries to identify with her mother but abandons her search and turns towards her father. During this frustrating loss of female identification she experiences a 'penis envy' and incorporates the father's gender identity and later turns her 'masculine' identity and love to the mother or other women.

Freud thought homosexuality should not be assessed as a form of pathology. In 1935 Freud wrote a letter to an American mother (Jones 1957, pp. 208–9):

> Homosexuality is assuredly no advantage, but it is nothing to be ashamed of, no vice, no degradation, it cannot be classified as an illness; we consider it to be a

variation of the sexual function produced by a certain arrest of sexual development. Many highly respectable individuals of ancient and modern times have been homosexuals, several of the greatest men among them (Plato, Michelangelo, Leonardo da Vinci, etceteras). It is a great injustice to persecute homosexuality as a crime, and cruelty too . . .

If [your son] is unhappy, neurotic, torn by conflicts, inhibited in his social life, analysis may bring him harmony, peace of mind, full efficiency whether he remains a homosexual or not . . .

Although Freud was open-minded in efforts to investigate homosexuality, his theory has been criticized (Burch 1993) to be too one-dimensional, with an emphasis on masculinity, a unitary form of gender identity. It is not solely an over-identification with the 'masculinity' for the little girl, although many lesbians are considered as 'tomboys'. Burch (1993) discusses that gender identity in human beings (both males and females, heterosexual and homosexual) might be fluid, more multifaceted, on a continuum from more or less masculinity to more or less femininity. Over time an individual may develop various dominating gender identity role patterns either in fantasy or in reality. According to Winnicott's (1971) 'potential space' this fluidity might be understood as a psychological predicament for creativity and psychic expansiveness. This psychic play and reality within the lesbian personalities and between their relationships might turn to an enlarged sense of what is feminine.

Outcome from empirical research

Outcome from recent research (American Psychiatric Association 2000) has opposed earlier findings that sexual orientation would be innate and fixed. It suggests a maturational process across an individual's lifetime. By 1973, empirical research had accumulated unmistakably that the American Psychiatric Association removed the diagnosis of homosexuality as a mental disorder from the *Diagnostic and Statistical Manual of Mental Disorders* (DSM). However, homosexuals are still a focus of mental health research because they tend to be more vulnerable as compared to heterosexuals. One crucial parameter seems to be antigay attitudes, which undoubtedly affects homosexuals' regulation of self-esteem. Even though research on lesbians started intensely in the late 1980s, there are still limitations in most of the studies. Outcome studies from empirical research have carefully investigated certain mental phenomena and accumulated a database supported by

several studies in each phenomenon. The different phenomena are summarized in the following sections.

Depression

The essential research of lesbianism and mental health is the prevalence of depression. It is up to several times higher in lesbians compared to women in general (Cochran 2001; Matthews *et al.* 2002). Lesbians have a higher prevalence of depression as compared to gay men and bisexual people. On the other hand, the two latter groups have other significant mental problems (e.g. anxiety) that lesbians do not experience as much.

Except for the uni- or bipolar manic–depressive mood disorders, which are partly genetic, depression exists on a psychological continuum, from mild to moderate depression, ultimately to severe melancholia. Important parameters are often seen in clinical work. For instance, a woman thinks: 'people will welcome my lesbianism and I will try to come out', in combination with not having worked through her gender identity enough. This constellation might lead to depression; firstly there is frustration, which to a certain degree results in aggression. Aggression that has no adequate channels might escalate to 'intro-aggression', i.e. the aggression turns inwards, which is typical for depression.

Gilman *et al.* (2001) investigated the probability of mental disorders in homosexuals. They used the representative household survey data from the National Comorbidity Survey. A total of 2.1% of men were homosexuals and 1.5% of women were lesbians. The DSM-III-R (American Psychiatric Association 1987) was applied to assess criteria for psychiatric disorders. The homosexuals experienced more prevalence of anxiety, mood difficulties, different substance use disorders, and suicidal thoughts, than compared to heterosexuals.

Cochran *et al.* (2007) found evidence that homosexuals experience elevated risk of mental health; the percentage of persons interviewed and assessed as homosexuals was about 4.8%. Lesbians and bisexual females had an increase of depressive disorders as compared to heterosexual females. This correlation was not found between gay men and heterosexual men.

Drug, alcohol, and tobacco abuse

There are several empirical studies showing that lesbians abuse drugs, like marijuana, tobacco, inhalants, cocaine, and analgesics more than the comparison groups of heterosexual women (Gilman *et al.* 2001; Cochran *et al.* 2004, 2007). A greater amount of studies show an increased significance of lesbians suffering from alcohol abuse or dependency in comparison to females in general. Female drug abusers report themselves more often as lesbians compared to women in general. Drug abuse and lesbianism constitute a phenomenon that ought to be more researched, while studies in problematic drinking are more prevalent.

In 1994, one national study in the United Kingdom, called the 'Project of LSD' (cited in Mullen 1998), embraced a sample of 287 persons at a Gay Pride festival. Fifty-six per cent were homosexual men and females and 8% were bisexual. Interesting results were documented as shown in Table 6.1.

It is clear in this study that lesbians suffer from using a broad range of substances, especially alcohol, tobacco, cannabis, and tranquilizers, as shown in many other research studies (e.g. Bux 1996). Fifty-two per cent of these substance users utilized two or more drugs during the same period.

In the United States, Cochran and coworkers (2004) investigated whether there were any differences in drug abuse or drug dependency between homosexuals and heterosexuals. From a sample of 194 homosexuals (98 men and 96 females) and 9714 heterosexuals (3922 men, 5792 women) they applied a cross-sectional national household interview investigation. The results showed consistent elevated drug abuse in homosexuals compared to the control group. Lesbians fulfilled criteria for both dysfunctional use and dependency of marijuana and analgesics.

In a Swedish study, Bergmark (1999) investigated the drinking patterns among Swedish homosexual men and lesbians (n=1720) as compared to two nationally representative survey groups. She documented that alcohol constituted an important 'core' in the community of lesbians and gays. Furthermore it was shown that lesbians had higher-risk behaviour of alcohol level and addiction consequences. Lesbians were seldom abstainers and unfortunately the alcohol consumption did not decrease with aging, as it does in the general population.

Eating disorder as related to obesity

Boehmer and colleagues conducted a recently published study (2007) examining whether lesbians suffer from a higher weight or obesity than women with other sexual orientations. Population estimates, from The National Survey of Family Growth (2002), of obesity across different groups of sexual orientation in 6000 women were compared. The statistical analysis resulted in lesbians having double the risk of both overweight and obesity compared to heterosexual women. Interestingly, bisexual women and those who were assessed as 'something else', i.e. besides heterosexual, lesbian, or bisexual women, did not show any risks of either being overweight or obese.

This up-to-date study confirms what previous research (e.g. Aaron *et al.* 2001) has indicated, i.e. lesbians do have higher risks of eating disorders that affect mental health. The consequences lead to morbidity—coronary heart disease, stroke, diabetes and certain forms of cancers. Ultimately mortality increases in lesbians as a secondary phenomenon to obesity.

Experiencing violence

The mental phenomenon of violence in lesbian relationships challenges stereotypes of traditional women as related to non-domestic violence. Fortunata and Kohn (2003) investigated psychosocial characteristics and personality traits of lesbian batterers and factors connected with domestic violence in lesbian relationships. The subjects in this study consisted of 100 lesbians in current relationships, where 33 were assessed as batterers and 67 non-batterers. The lesbian batterers reported experiences of sexual abuse, childhood physical abuse, and greater risks of alcohol abuse. Batterers were assessed as having personality traits of being aggressive, antisocial, borderline, and paranoid. They also showed more alcohol-dependency, drug-dependency, and delusional clinical symptoms compared to non-batterers.

Table 6.1 Prevalence of substance use in male and female homosexuals

Substance	Homosexual men	Lesbians
Alcohol	81%	86%
Tobacco	48%	52%
Cannabis	41%	38%
Ecstasy	19%	9%
Speed	13%	9%
Poppers	32%	9%
Cocaine	5%	3%
LSD (lysergic acid diethylamide)	8%	4%
Tranquilizers	18%	14%
Prozac®	8%	3%

To comprehend the various forms of violence in lesbian relationships, especially the batterers, Coleman (1994) emphasized an understanding from a multidimensional theory of partner abuse; crucially, it must build upon individual personality dynamics. The psychodynamics in this article were related to the borderline and narcissistic personality disorders. In relation to drugs and alcohol these disorders and also similar traits as Fortunata and Kohn (2003) discovered, irrespective of lesbianism, homosexuality, or heterosexuality, are always connected to difficulties in handling aggressive affects (Aleman 2007). However, in the empirical research field of lesbianism and mental health, there should be several more such studies conducted before pointing to the prevalence of borderline and narcissistic personality disorders in lesbians and particularly the batterers.

Another form of experiencing violence is witnessing violence and perpetrating violence against others. Russell et al. (2001) examined hate crimes committed against lesbians, gay, and bisexual youths compared to heterosexual youths. They applied representative data from the National Longitudinal Study of Adolescent Health. Lesbian (and gay men plus bisexual) youths did experience extreme forms of violence compared to heterosexual youths. The same groups of youths also reported experiences of witnessing violence. These findings provide strong evidence that lesbian youths have to handle very complex situations and affects that certainly influence their mental states of mind.

Suicide

During adolescence, lesbians (and gay men plus bisexual persons) attempt suicide up to six times more than heterosexuals. Lesbians' vulnerability to depression, substance abuse, and experience of violence are known risk factors for attempted and completed suicide. Historically, research about gay men and suicide has been far more studied than in lesbians. Still, it seems probable that there are greater attempts of suicide among young lesbians, because young gay men, who 'come out' with their gender identity are consistently more prevalent, as compared to young lesbians, who tend to come out later or never. Therefore, it is most possible that a major proportion of young lesbians who attempt suicide are disguised within the general numbers of young females who attempt suicide.

The highest prevalence of suicide is among lesbians who are isolated from help or support. Those who identify their sexuality early on, run a particularly high risk of attempted suicidal. Even young lesbians (and gays) who identify themselves as 'tomboys' (and 'sissies'), i.e. developing an atypical gender stereotype, are more at suicidal risk.

Lesbians suffer far more from suicidal attempts, depression, and also from dependency on substances than heterosexual women and heterosexual men or homosexual men (Saghir and Robins 1973; Bell and Weinberg 1978; Lewis et al. 1982; Blume 1985; McKirnan and Peterson 1989; Schilit et al. 1990). In a recent published study (Silenzio et al. 2007), the authors analysed current data from the National Longitudinal Study of Adolescent Health. Again, results showed that lesbians (and gay men plus bisexuals) suffered from more suicidal ideation and suicide attempts as compared to heterosexual respondents.

Lesbians (and gay men plus bisexuals) have greater prevalence of deliberate self-harm and say that physical harm gives them a sense of relief. Lesbians and gay men are more likely than bisexuals to refer to their gender identity as a reason for harming themselves. Empirical research suggests that self-harm might be connected to difficulties in being out in society (King and McKeown 2003) or having experienced rejection from other people. Self-harm is associated with low self-esteem and high anxiety. A greater number of homophobic incidents are reported among self-harming lesbians as compared to those without a history of self-harm. Bisexual people are reported having higher prevalence of self-harm than either lesbians or gay men (Bennett 2004).

In general, among people who are homosexual or bisexual, being the victim of a homophobic incident is commonly reported. Female homosexuals more commonly report verbal abuse, while male homosexuals more likely report experience of physical assault. Hate crimes have a serious effect on the quality of life of victims—many of them alter their behaviour in public spaces by not openly displaying affection. One study in the United Kingdom conducted by Wake et al. (1999) found that 82% of all incidents are not reported.

Discussion

Empirical studies use many different definitions of lesbianism as lesbianism, i.e. from people who solely fantasize about it to those who act it out, making it difficult to make meaningful comparisons. Lesbianism is often assessed as both behavioural, i.e. desire or attraction, and cognitive, i.e. sense of identity. Lesbians therefore constitute subgroups of females whose mental health and risk behaviours have not been well researched.

Interestingly, lesbians are found among all subpopulations of females and are represented in all socioeconomic strata, and all ages in ethnic and racial groups. There is no clear assessment of demographic category characteristics and neither a clear lesbian single type of family, community, or culture. Since the view of sexual identity and sexual behaviour varies with culture, race and ethnicity, assessment of lesbianism must take these factors into account.

Generally, the majority of lesbian, gay, and bisexual people together do not experience mental health problems, although research suggests that lesbians are at higher risk of mental disorder (particularly depression), suicidal behaviour, substance abuse, eating disorders, and experiencing violence. Returning to the concept of the borderline syndrome (and narcissism) that is not yet documented in lesbians from several empirical studies, in fact, all aforementioned psychological phenomena usually occur in one or other way in the borderline syndrome. Within this syndrome one might say that individuals do not solely abuse substances but also food or intimate emotions because of their primary identity diffusion (Kernberg 1975). However, evidence indicates that the increased risk of mental disorder in lesbians is linked to experiences of discrimination (Mays and Cochran 2001). They are more likely to report both daily and lifetime discrimination than heterosexual people. Lesbians more commonly experience verbal and physical intimidation than heterosexual women (King and McKeown 2003). Antigay stigma has been linked to an increase in deliberate self-harm in lesbians.

It should be recognized that mental distress can be caused by many factors unconnected with sexuality. Homosexual people do face particular psychological pressures living in a discriminatory and heterosexist society. Furthermore internalized homophobia, with associated feelings of low self-esteem and self-hatred, can lead to emotional distress. Being homosexual is not in itself a mental health problem, but coping with the consequences of discrimination can be highly detrimental to lesbian mental health. A Health Education Authority mental health promotion on 'sexual identity' states that: 'some studies have suggested that internalized homophobia is a risk factor for alcohol and drug dependency. Anxiety, depression, self-harm, suicide and attempted suicide have all been linked with the combined effects of the experience of prejudice and discrimination and internalized negative feelings'. A Department of Health leaflet states that those at increased risk of suicide include people 'whose sexual orientation brings them into conflict with their family or others'.

There is a real problem of awareness of alcohol and drug misuse in lesbians. The following description of the United States in the 1970s (O'Donnell *et al.* 1978) could be written of the United Kingdom in 2002:

> One in every three gay persons abuses alcohol and is either an alcoholic or is rapidly heading towards that destination. This is more than three times the estimate of problem drinkers in the general population. Alcoholism is not talked about very much in the lesbian community. Some of us think we don't know anyone who drinks heavily. But most of us do know women who drink heavily—we just do not recognize the extent of the problem.

The difference between the United States and the United Kingdom is that the former has been discussing and debating alcohol use and recovery for several decades to the extent where now there are many lesbian and gay Alcoholics Anonymous (AA) groups and 'clean and sober' social events, which provide some of the social functions previously provided by the lesbian/gay bar subculture. This is not the case in the United Kingdom. Reasons suggested for this include the problems of dealing with societal oppression, using alcohol and drugs as a means of coping with depression, and the pivotal role of 'bar culture' in homosexual social networks.

Lesbians (gay men and bisexuals) use mental health services more frequently than their heterosexual counterparts. Over 40% of lesbians reported negative or mixed reactions from mental health professionals when they disclosed their sexual orientation. One in five lesbians and gay men and a third of bisexual men stated that a mental health professional made a causal link between their sexual orientation and their mental health problem (King and McKeown 2003). Lesbians reported not being confident about accessing mental health services (Mitchell *et al.* 2001). Reports of problems are observed in their encounters with mental health professionals, ranging from lack of empathy about sexual orientation to incidents of homophobia. There are acknowledged difficulties for mental health professionals in getting the balance right.

Morris *et al.* (2001) documented that 'coming out' with gender identity is evidently beneficial to mental health. Self-esteem is associated with good mental health. Lesbians (and gay men) were more confident with their sexual identity and more likely to have parents and siblings to whom they had disclosed their sexual identity than their bisexual counterparts. Lesbians were more likely to communicate that their sexual orientation was important to their identity than heterosexual women (Bennett 2004).

It seems that lesbians (gay men and bisexuals) are overlooked in mental health policy making. Lesbians are at increased risk of both attempted and completed suicide. Despite this, their needs have not been addressed in the series of Annual Reports from National Suicide Prevention Strategy for England. Current government policy focuses on the importance of choice in mental health services. However, there is not much available information on appropriate service provision which could give lesbians' choice. A report documented by the mental health charity of homosexuals and bisexuals, PACE, listed several recommendations for including these people in the National Service Framework for Mental Health (McFarlane 1998). These involved promoting mental health for homosexuals and bisexuals in public exposures and positive imagery, preventing suicide, improvements of contact with services, and ensuring needs are addressed within the Care Programme Approach.

References

Aaron DJ et al. (2001). Behavioral risk factors for disease and preventive health practices among lesbians. *American Journal of Public Health*, **91**, 972–5.

Aleman K (2007). 'Psychoanalytic Conceptions of the Mind in Drug Abusers. Methods Exploring Personality Disorders, Traits, and Defense Mechanisms.' Doctoral thesis, Lund University, Lund, Sweden.

American Psychiatric Association (1987). *Diagnostic and Statistical Manual of Mental Disorders, Third Edition Revised*, American Psychiatric Association, Washington, DC.

American Psychiatric Association (2000). *Lesbian and Bisexual Issues*. Council on minority mental health and mental disparities; American Psychiatric Association, Washington DC.

Bell AP and Weinberg MS (1978). *Homosexualities: A Study of Diversity Among Men and Women*. Mitchell Beazley, London.

Bennett J (2004). *Emotional well-being and social support study: An overview*. University of Strathclyde, Glasgow.

Bergmark KH (1999). Drinking in the Swedish gay and lesbian community. *Drug & Alcohol Dependence*, **56**, 133–43.

Blume ES (1985). Substance abuse (of being queer, magic pills and social lubricants). In: H Hidalgo et al. (eds) *Lesbian and Gay Issues: Resource Manual for Social Workers*, pp. 79–87. National Association of Social Workers, Silver Springs, MD.

Boehmer U et al. (2007). Overweight and obesity in sexual-minority women: evidence from population-based data. *American Journal of Public Health*, **97**, 1134–40.

Burch B (1993). Gender identities, lesbianism, and potential space. *Psychoanalytic Psychology*, **10**, 359–75.

Bux D (1996). The epidemiology of problem drinking in gay men and lesbians: a critical review. *Clinical Psychological Review*, **16**, 277–98.

Cochran SD (2001). Emerging issues in research on lesbians' and gay men's mental health: Does sexual orientation really matter? *American Psychologist*, **56**(11), 929–47.

Cochran SD et al. (2004). Prevalence of non-medical drug use and dependence among homosexually active men and women in the US population. *Addiction*, **99**, 989–98.

Cochran SD et al. (2007). Mental health and substance use disorders among Latino and Asian American lesbian, gay, and bisexual adults. *Journal of Consulting and Clinical Psychology*, **75**, 785–94.

Coleman VE (1994). Lesbian battering: the relationship between personality and the perpetration of violence. *Violence and Victims*, **9**, 139–52.

Fortuna B and Kohn CS (2003). Demographic, psychosocial, and personality characteristics of lesbian batterers. *Violence and Victims*, **18**, 557–68.

Freud S (1905). Three essays on the theory of sexuality. In: *The Standard Edition of the Complete Psychological Works of Sigmund Freud, 7 (1901–1905): A Case of Hysteria. Three Essays on Sexuality and Other Works*, pp. 123–246. Hogarth Press and the Institute of Psychoanalysis, 1953, London.

Freud S (1924). The dissolution of the Oedipus complex. In: *The Standard Edition of the Complete Psychological Works of Sigmund Freud, 19 (1923–1925): The Ego and the Id and Other Works*, pp. 171–80. Hogarth Press and the Institute of Psychoanalysis, 1961, London.

Gilman SE et al. (2001). Risk of psychiatric disorders among individuals reporting same-sex sexual partners in the National Comorbidity Survey. *American Journal of Public Health*, **91**, 933–9.

Jones E (1957). *Sigmund Freud: Life and work, Vol. 3*. Hogarth, London.

Kernberg OF (1975). *Borderline conditions and pathological narcissism*. Jason Aronson Inc, New York.

King M and McKeown E (2003). *Mental health and social wellbeing of gay men, lesbians and bisexuals in England and Wales: A summary of findings*. Mind, London.

Krafft-Ebing R (1886). *Psychopathia sexualis*. Reprinted by Bloat Books, Burbank, CA (1999).

Lewis CE et al. (1982). Drinking patterns in homosexual and heterosexual women. *Journal of Clinical Psychiatry*, **43**, 277–9.

Matthews AK et al. (2002). Prediction of depressive distress in a community sample of women: the role of sexual orientation. *American Journal of Public Health*, **92**, 1131–9.

Mays VM and Cochran SD (2001). Mental health correlates of perceived discrimination among lesbian, gay, and bisexual adults in the United States. *American Journal of Public Health*, **91**(11), 1869–76.

McCoy S and Hicks M (1979). A psychological retrospective on power in the contemporary lesbian-feminist community. *Frontiers: A Journal of Women Studies*, **4**, 65–9.

McFarlane L (1998). *Diagnosis homophobic: The experiences of lesbians, gay men and bisexuals in mental health services*. PACE, London.

McKirnan DJ and Peterson PL (1989). Alcohol and drug use among homosexual men and women: Epidemiology and population characteristics. *Addictive Behaviors*, **14**, 545–53.

Mitchell M *et al.* (2001). *"What are you like?" Understanding the health needs and improving services for lesbians, gay men and bisexuals in Buckinghamshire and Milton Keynes: Report of the Lesbian, Gay and Bisexual 'Lifestyle' and Health Needs Assessment.* Institute for Health Services Research, University of Luton, Luton.

Morris JF, Waldo CR, and Rothblum ED (2001). A model for predictors and outcomes of outness among lesbian and bisexual women. *American Journal of Orthopsychiatry*, **71**, 61–71.

Mullen A (1999). Social inclusion: reaching out to bisexual, gay and lesbian youth. *Research Briefing Paper* **1** in The Lesbian Information Service (www.lesbinform.fsnet. co.uk).

O'Donnell M *et al.* (1978). *Lesbian Health Matters.* Santa Cruz, Up Press.

Rich A (1980). Compulsory heterosexuality and lesbian existence. *Signs*, **5**, 631–60.

Russell ST *et al.* (2001). Same-sex romantic attraction and experiences of violence in adolescence. *American Journal of Public Health*, **91**, 903–6.

Saghir MT and Robins E (1973). *Male and Female Homosexuality: A Comprehensive Investigation.* Willliams & Wilkins, Baltimore, MD.

Schilit R *et al.* (1990). Substance use as a correlate of violence in intimate lesbian relationships. *Journal of Homosexuality*, **19**, 51–65.

Silenzio VMB *et al.* (2007). Sexual orientation and risk factors for suicidal ideation and suicide attempts among adolescents and young adults. *American Journal of Public Health*, **97**, 2017–19.

Wake I *et al.* (1999). *Breaking the Chain of Hate: A National Survey Examining Levels of Homophobic Crime and Community Confidence towards the Police Service.* National Advisory Group/Policing Lesbian and Gay Communities, Manchester.

Winnicott DW (1971). *Playing and Reality.* Tavistock, London.

CHAPTER 7

Attachment and women's mental health

Daniel McQueen and Ronald Doctor

Introduction

In this chapter we will present a brief account of attachment theory and its evolution, then describe the contribution of attachment theory to the understanding of some key disorders that are more frequently seen in women.

Attachment

Attachment theory is identified with John Bowlby, a child psychiatrist and psychoanalyst and Mary Ainsworth (née Salter), a research psychologist, amongst others. Before completing his medical degree Bowlby had worked in a school for maladjusted children. This introduced him to the lasting effects on personality development of deficient early family relationships (Bretherton 1992). Bowlby's first published study was of the characteristics and family backgrounds of juvenile thieves. In this study he drew attention to the most prolific thieves, clinically described as affectionless characters, who uniformly had backgrounds characterized by combinations of complete or prolonged separation from the mother between 12 months and 4 years, anxious or ambivalent mothers or foster mothers, fathers who hated them, a family history of mental illness or had experienced recent trauma. (Bowlby 1944a, 1944b).

Attachment and ethology

Bowlby used the perspective of ethology (the scientific study of animal behaviour) to see attachment to caregivers as a *primary instinctual behavioural system*. Bowlby hypothesized that evolutionary pressure had led to the development of an instinctual system of attachment to caregivers, and a complementary system of caregiving by parents or kin to infants, to ensure the survival of infants and hence of the clan and species. Bowlby argued that the evolutionary environment in which attachment developed was that of nomadic hunter-gatherer tribes and that the specific evolutionary pressure driving attachment was protection from predation. The goal of the attachment system is then to maintain proximity to caregivers who would provide safety from danger. As such, attachment is of equal biological importance to feeding and mating for survival of the species (Bowlby 1957, 1969).

Bowlby also took from ethology the idea of *critical periods* in development during which a specific behavioural system is particularly sensitive to the environment. Bowlby demonstrated that the attachment system is particularly sensitive to the environment during the first three or four years of life. Appropriate interactions with a caregiver during this period will allow the development of normal attachment behaviour. Outside of the critical period the attachment behaviour system will not be so responsive to the environment. If appropriate interactions do not occur sufficiently during the critical period, or development is disturbed for some other reason, then the attachment system will not develop normally. Later experiences have less impact than experiences during the critical period (Bowlby 1969).

In three seminal papers Bowlby argued that the infant's attachment behaviour is made up of a number of component instinctual responses, clinging, sucking, and following, plus smiling and crying which had the purpose of eliciting care from caregivers. These appear in the first year of life and become increasingly focused on the mother during the second six months of life (Bowlby 1958). He argued that the intensity of attachment and the degree of distress aroused by separation from the mother could not be explained by previous theories (Bowlby 1960a). In his third paper he argued that grief and mourning are present in children whenever attachment behaviour is activated in the child and the attachment figure is not available, and that repeated disruption of attachment relationships during the critical period of the early years may result in the individual being unable to develop the capacity for relationships in depth (Bowlby 1960b). Bowlby theorized that attachment behaviours are encoded in mental representations of the individual in relation to others; he called these *internal working models* (Bowlby 1969).

Attachment classification

Ainsworth conducted longitudinal naturalistic studies of mothers and infants less than two years of age observed at home in rural Uganda and of mothers with newborn babies in Baltimore, United States. These observations were complemented by observations in a laboratory procedure know as the *strange situation*. The strange situation was designed to measure levels of exploratory behaviour in infants of 12 months of age under circumstances of high and low stress. In the strange situation mother and baby are observed in a laboratory playroom, then an unfamiliar woman joins them. After three minutes the mother leaves the baby with the stranger for three minutes before she returns and the stranger leaves the mother and baby together. The mother then leaves again and the baby is alone for a further three minutes. Finally mother returns to the baby.

An unexpected observation made in the strange situation experiment was the range of infant behaviour on reunion with the mother. The majority of infants displayed attachment behaviour, sought proximity, interaction, or contact with their mother on reunion, and thus reassured returned to playing. These were described as *secure* (B). A second group of infants appeared to suppress attachment behaviour and ignored their mother on her return, even though they had searched for her in her absence. These were described as *insecure-avoidant* (A). A third group were surprisingly angry with their mothers and showed high levels of attachment behaviour that didn't terminate—they wouldn't settle even after she returned. These were described as *insecure-ambivalent* (C) (also called *insecure-resistant*). Just over half the infants were classified as secure with the remainder divided between the two insecure categories (Ainsworth *et al.* 1978).

It was shown that the reunion behaviour in the strange situation correlated with the quality of the mother–infant interaction at home. The infants with more harmonious relationships with their mothers showed secure attachment in the strange situation, while those with less harmonious relationships showed insecure-avoidant or insecure-ambivalent behaviour (Ainsworth *et al.* 1978).

In addition to describing the infants' behaviour the attachment classification is also related to the infants' perception of the availability of the caregiver. Securely attached infants have internalized the expectation of an adult who will respond to their distress, when they feel threatened they are able to direct attachment behaviours (crying, approaching, seeking contact) towards the caregiver, and they are able to take comfort from their caregivers' reassurances. In this way the parents of securely attached infants promote their infants' exploration of the world. This is not the case with infants who are insecurely attached. Insecurely attached infants do not expect a caregiver to be reliably responsive.

Insecure attachments develop when the infants do not have a mental representation of a responsive caregiver in times of need, such as when they feel fearful or helpless. These infants develop different strategies to gain access to their caregiver in order to survive.

In Ainsworth's original study, the mothers of insecure-avoidant infants showed aversion to physical contact when the infants sought it and expressed little emotion in interaction with their infants. Insecure-avoidant attachment is therefore an adaptive strategy on the part of the infants of defensively turning away from their distress and minimizing their attachment behaviour in order to maintain proximity to a caregiver who is aversive to contact and is rejecting. These infants therefore have less access to their own feelings and have lower expectations of help being available.

The mothers of infants later classified as insecure-ambivalent were found to be less sensitive to their babies and more interfering with their children's behaviour. Thus insecure-ambivalent attachment is a strategy of maximizing attachment behaviour to gain the attention of a caregiver who is inconsistently available to the infant. Because these infants are so enmeshed in issues of caretaker availability they are unable to make accurate appraisals of the level of threat and the availability of help (Ainsworth 1978). Insecure attachments are therefore considered to be adaptive in that they offer an organized strategy for gaining protection from the caregiver.

Disorganized attachment

Subsequent researchers reported difficulty classifying some infants' strange situation behaviour in samples where the children had been maltreated. The behaviour of infants from maltreated samples was often found to be contradictory or disorganized, they seemed to lack an organized strategy for dealing with reunion with their parent in the strange situation and did not fit neatly into any of the secure/insecure categories. This led to the addition of a fourth attachment category, *disorganized* (D). Behaviour during reunion that is described as disorganized includes contradictory, misdirected, or fragmented behaviour patterns, e.g. approaching and moving away from the parent, crying against the wall, stereotypies, freezing or slowing, or disoriented behaviour (Main and Solomon 1990).

Disorganized attachment behaviour arises when infants are overwhelmed by separation and can be induced when toddlers are given conflicting signals, confusing signals, or exposed to inescapable situations. Conceptually, disorganization is explained by the coexistence of two contradictory urges: the urge to seek safety from the attachment figure and the wish to flee from the attachment figure because the attachment figure is the source of distress or fear.

In addition to the strange situation, which assesses attachment behaviour, a number of tools have been devised to measure and classify attachment representations in older children, adolescents, and adults. For a review see Prior and Glaser (2006). The *Adult Attachment Interview* is widely used to assess the state of mind of adults with regard to attachment. It consists of an hour-long interview in which adults are asked to describe early attachment relationships and experiences and to evaluate the effects of these on their personality and functioning (Main *et al.* 1985) The transcripts of the interviews are then classified on the basis of form and content into Secure/autonomous (F), Dismissing (Ds), Preoccupied (E); subsequently a fourth category has been added, Unresolved/disorganized (U/d). The categories use similar constructs to the classification of infant behaviour in the strange situation.

About 50–80% of maltreated infants show disorganized attachment, and 15–25% of children in low-risk non-maltreated samples also demonstrate disorganized attachment (van IJsendoorn *et al.* 1999).

Dissociation

Dissociative phenomena in adults are of particular interest for several reasons. Unresolved/disorganized attachment on the Adult Attachment Interview is conceptually linked to dissociative phenomena arising whilst discussing loss and trauma themes. Unresolved/disorganized attachment in caregivers in the Adult Attachment Interview predicts disorganized attachment in their offspring in the strange situation. Dissociative phenomena in the strange situation support disorganized attachment classification. Disorganized infants have been shown to go on to display and report raised levels of dissociative behaviour and symptoms at 16 and 19 years (Ogawa *et al.* 1997; Weinfield *et al.* 1999).

Once dissociation is established as a defence then it tends to occur at lower thresholds in the future. During the pre-school period, children who have been maltreated show increasing levels of dissociation compared to non-maltreated peers who show decreasing levels of dissociation (Macfie *et al.* 2001).

Unresolved attachment and frightening/frightened behaviour

A number of explanations exist for disorganized attachment in low-risk samples. A number of the children in low-risk samples will have experienced maltreatment. A proportion of infants may be more sensitive to maternal insensitivity due to genetic variation, specifically variations in a dopamine receptor subtype (Gervai 2007).

A hypothesis that has generated much research is that mothers who show frightening or frightened behaviour unknowingly place their infants in situations of inescapable fear, the infant is frightened by the parent's behaviour and thus wants to flee, and yet the infant also wants to approach the parent as the person with whom the infant wishes to seek safety.

Main and Hesse (1990) found a strong association between parents being in the unresolved/disorganized category on the Adult Attachment Interview (ie unresolved or disorganized when discussing *their own* experiences of loss or abuse), and their infants demonstrating disorganized attachment in the strange situation. Over 90% of unresolved/disorganized mothers had disorganized infants. Only 16% of mothers who had experienced loss, but did not show unresolved/disorganized attachment, had disorganized infants. This finding has been replicated in a number of studies (Fonagy *et al.* 1991; van IJzendoorn 1995).

Based on behaviours shown in the Adult Attachment Interview that suggested that the parent was experiencing some degree of dissociation while recounting traumatic events, Main and Hesse have described a scale of frightening (FR) behaviours shown by parents. These include direct indices of dissociation, anomalous and inexplicable threatening behaviour, timid/deferential (role inverting) behaviour, sexualized behaviour towards the infant, and disorganized/disoriented behaviour compatible with disorganized infant behaviours.

They hypothesize that unresolved, partially dissociated traumatic experiences intrude into the parent's mind and are manifest in degrees of dissociated behaviour, and that it is these states of dissociation in the parent that the infant finds frightening, and which lead to disorganization of their infant's attachment. Further evidence supporting the link between frightening (FR) parental behaviour and disorganization of infant attachment has been reported in high-risk samples. For a review see Hesse and Main (1999).

Reflective function

The ability to think about or reflect on one's own mental states (intentions, wishes, feelings, and beliefs) or on the mental states of others is known as reflective function or mentalization. It is a largely preconscious activity. The social biofeedback theory of parental affect-mirroring suggests that the infant learns to recognize its own affects through seeing them contingently mirrored in its parent and over time is thus able to internalize the representation of its own affect states, which leads to the sense of having a mind. This requires a caregiver who is sensitively attuned to their child's mental states. In this way the acquisition of mentalization is intimately linked to the quality of attachment relationships, and the development of a coherent or integrated sense of self and others.

Infants who have caregivers who are insensitive or poorly attuned to their mental states will have less opportunity to learn about their own mental states through contingent affect mirroring. Infants who experience their caregivers as frightened or frightening will avoid contemplating the contents of their caregivers' minds. Infants whose attachment is disorganized do not develop an integrated image of themselves or their caregiver. A dissociated and unintegrated sense of self and other disrupts the acquisition of reflective function and leads to emotional disability. In this way, attachment disorganization limits mentalization. It is beyond the scope of this chapter to describe in detail the development of mentalization. For a detailed account see Fonagy *et al.* (2004).

Intergenerational transmission of attachment

There is evidence that attachment patterns are transmitted from mothers and fathers to children. The attachment status of adults prior to the birth of their children is highly predictive of their unborn children's future attachment classification in the strange situation at one year (Fonagy *et al.* 1991).

Role reversal is one aspect of disorganized attachment that has been studied in depth. In role reversal, parents and children swap roles; a parent looks to their child to fulfil their own emotional needs, and a child may attempt to meet the parent's unmet emotional needs in order to sooth the parent's distress and thus achieve a greater feeling of security in that relationship. Mothers who reported role reversal with their mothers during the Adult Attachment Interview engaged in higher levels of role reversal with their toddler-aged daughters. Furthermore, when fathers reported role reversal with their mothers during the Adult Attachment Interview, then their female partners tended to engage in higher levels of role reversal with their toddler-aged sons, indicating that assertive mating allows the transmission of mother–son role reversal through the son's choice of partner (Macfie 2005).

Attachment, adaptation, and psychopathology

Bowlby argued that early attachment experiences are critical for developing a sense of mastery, emotional self-regulation, and interpersonal effectiveness. He argued that the internal working models of relationships that determine behaviour are adaptable to changing environments, but that they can become defensively distorted and that this will lead to rigidity and a failure of adaptation to the changing environment. The principal cause of defensive distortions and splits is the need to keep an internal working model of a good helpful parent separate from an internal working model of a frightening parent.

Infants whose caregivers are sensitive and responsive learn that they can get their needs met and be effective in the world. Infants whose caregivers are insensitive or inconsistent do not develop this sense of autonomy (Bowlby 1973).

A number of large longitudinal studies of attachment have been running for many years. The largest and longest running study of attachment is the Minnesota Longitudinal Study of Parents and Children (Sroufe *et al.* 2005), which began in 1975 with 267 pregnant first-time mothers; they were below the official poverty line and as such it is a high-risk sample. It studied the mothers before and after the birth, and the children throughout their lives and into (at the time of writing) their 28th year. It has demonstrated a number of important continuities between infant attachment and subsequent behaviour, as discussed in the following sections.

Attachment, adaptation, and psychopathology in childhood

Children who were securely attached in infancy show greater social competence. They were shown to be more cooperative with adults, more appropriate in their help-seeking behaviour from teachers, and more confident in their play when compared to insecurely attached children. Securely attached children were better able to modulate their negative feelings, expressed less anger and aggression during play with their peers, and were not found to be either bullies or bullied. Children with insecure-avoidant attachment showed more bullying behaviour towards their peers during play, and insecure-resistant children were more likely to be the victims of insecure-avoidant children. Children with secure attachment histories were rated as more socially competent by teachers throughout school and adolescence. Secure children were better at adhering to group norms and showed more leadership ability. Girls with a history of secure attachment were rated as having relationships that were more intimate. For a review of the findings of the Minnesota Longitudinal Study see Weinfield *et al.* (1999).

Insecure-avoidant attachment sequelae

The Minnesota Study found that early insecure-avoidant attachment was significantly associated with aggression in boys, and in adolescence with childhood-onset antisocial behaviour (Egeland and Carlson 2004). Insecure-avoidant five-year-olds were more likely to bully insecure-ambivalent peers (Weinfield *et al.* 1999).

Insecure-ambivalent attachment sequelae

Warren *et al.* (1997) found in the Minnesota sample that after controlling for other key variables, anxious-ambivalent attachment was significantly associated with anxiety disorders among teenagers.

Disorganized attachment sequelae

Disorganized attachment appears to be most important in terms of predicting later poor functioning and disturbance. Disorganized attachment is related to increased cortisol secretion in response to stress, indicating the infants' lack of an effective strategy for dealing with stress. It is associated with mild delay on the Bayley Scales of Infant Development. Disorganized attachment is strongly associated with later controlling and role reversal behaviour of children with their parents (Main and Cassidy 1988). Disorganized children perform less well in tests of reasoning and delay-of-gratification task, even after controlling for self-esteem and intelligence quotient. Disorganized children are less competent in their play with peers, have higher rates of peer hostility and aggression, and are at greater risk of developing behaviour problems and oppositional defiant disorder (Greenberg 1999). Disorganized children and adolescents display and report raised levels of dissociative behaviour and symptoms at 16 and 19 years (Ogawa *et al.* 1997; Weinfield *et al.* 1999). For detailed review of disorganized attachment in childhood the reader is directed to Lyons-Ruth and Jacobvitz (1999) and Hesse and Main (2000).

Attachment, adaptation, and psychopathology in adulthood

Research on the relationship between attachment and mental health in adulthood largely depends on two strategies: assessing the concurrent attachment status of the adult using the Adult Attachment Interview, or using recall of parental behaviour and recall of adverse childhood experiences that can allow suppositions about the likely nature of the early attachment relationship.

The Adult Attachment Interview has been used in a wide number of different clinical and non-clinical groups. Generally, secure/autonomous attachment is underrepresented in clinical groups and appears to act as a protective factor. This is in line with Bowlby's hypothesis that individuals with secure attachment view themselves as competent and have an expectation that help will be available when required, and that they will be able to use it.

Depression

The central thesis of attachment theory is the primary organizing influence of attachment to caregivers. It is to be expected, therefore, that the loss through death of the primary caregiver in childhood should have far reaching consequences. Brown and Harris (Brown *et al.* 1977; Brown and Harris 1978) demonstrated in a series of studies of women with depression, in both a community and hospital setting, that the death of the mother before the age of 11 years was the major factor determining vulnerability to depression in response to further losses in later life. Death of the mother before 11 years also determined the severity and symptomatology of the depression. Women whose mothers had died before they were 11 had much higher rates of melancholic depression (characterized by retardation and other somatic features). Drawing on the ideas of learned helplessness (Seligman 1975) and hopelessness in depression (Beck 1967) the authors showed that depressed women who had lost their mother before the age of 11 years were also less likely to seek treatment for their depression than other depressed women. They hypothesized that the early loss of the mother permanently lowered the women's self-esteem and sense of mastery, and increased the chance that the women would passively endure future trauma, rather than expecting and seeking a solution.

Parkes (1991) studied an outpatient sample of adults with complicated bereavement. He used *basic trust in self or others* as a proxy measure for good early attachment experiences. He found that people without basic trust were more vulnerable to developing complicated bereavement. In his sample the patients with basic trust and complicated bereavement had all experienced particularly difficult bereavements that were either multiple or unexpected. Among the patients low in basic trust, only a minority had experienced multiple or unexpected bereavements; 58% had experienced a single, expected death. This indicates that people with basic trust only developed complicated bereavement after multiple or unexpected bereavements, whereas people lacking in basic trust were vulnerable to developing complicated bereavements even after a single death which they had had time to prepare for. Grief reactions complicated by feelings of ambivalence towards the dead person were significantly more likely to arise following the death of a parent.

The direct research evidence on attachment styles among depressed adults is inconsistent. In part this arises from samples being drawn from different populations—out patients, inpatients, or patients in tertiary referral centres. Furthermore, inclusion and exclusion criteria vary between the different studies; some control for comorbid personality disorder, others do not. Some research reports only the three-way classification (Secure/autonomous, Dismissing, Preoccupied), others also use the four-way classification (Secure/autonomous, Dismissing, Preoccupied, Unresolved/disorganized). Finally, the diagnostic category of depression is in itself probably heterogeneous with regard to attachment behaviours, including depressed individuals with insecure-dismissive (externalizing) strategies and depressed individuals with insecure-ambivalent (internalizing) strategies. Generally among depressed patients there are lower levels of Secure/autonomous attachment and higher rates of Preoccupied and Unresolved/disorganized attachment (Dozier *et al.* 1999).

Postnatal depression

Postnatal depression is more common in mothers who have insecure attachment, specifically insecure-anxious (enmeshed and fearful) attachment styles (Bifulco *et al.* 2004). Toddler offspring of depressed mothers have significantly more insecure attachments and behavioural problems than do toddlers with non-depressed mothers (Cicchetti *et al.* 1998).

Parental, and particularly maternal, depression is associated with an increased risk of childhood emotional and behavioural disorders in their children. As the children of depressed parents grow up, there is a two- to threefold increase in rates of depression, anxiety, substance misuse, and physical illness when their children reach adolescence and adulthood. Effective treatment of maternal depression leads to a reduction in emotional and behavioural disturbance in their children (Weissman *et al.* 2005, 2006a, 2006b).

Anxiety

Anxiety disorders are also heterogeneous and often comorbid with other disorders, particularly depression. Focusing on generalized anxiety disorder, the prospective studies of Warren *et al.* (1997) showing that insecure-ambivalent attachment in the strange situation at one year was associated with anxiety disorders at 17 years. Fonagy *et al.* (1996), in a sample of psychiatric inpatients at the Cassel Hospital (Richmond, UK), a tertiary referral centre for people with particularly severe and complex difficulties, found that using the four-way classification, unresolved/disorganized attachment status was present in 7% of controls, 75% of patients, and 86% of patients with a diagnosis of anxiety. Due to their severity these patients are unlikely to be representative of all those with anxiety.

Dissociative disorders

Adults who experience clinically significant dissociation are most likely to be diagnosed as having chronic post-traumatic stress disorder, dissociative disorders (multiple personality disorder, dissociative identity disorder, depersonalization), or borderline personality disorder.

Dissociative identity disorder is, by definition, a disorganized state of the self. Ninety per cent of people with dissociative identity disorder have been found to have a history of childhood sexual abuse (Fonagy and Target 1995).

Post-traumatic stress disorder, by definition, is a state of being unresolved with respect to trauma, and therefore of unresolved/disorganized attachment (de Zulueta 2006). Diagnostic criteria for post-traumatic stress disorder emphasize the experiences of people who have experienced circumscribed traumatic events. However, it is recognized in DSM IV that children exposed to repeated, protracted interpersonal trauma such as childhood sexual or physical abuse or neglect, exhibit characteristic symptoms, including impaired affect modulation, dissociative symptoms, somatic complaints, feelings of ineffectiveness, shame, guilt, despair, hopelessness, feeling permanently damaged, hostility, social withdrawal, feeling constantly threatened, and impaired relationships with others (American Psychiatric Association 1997). This constellation of symptoms has been referred to as complex post-traumatic stress disorder (Herman 1992, van der Kolk et al. 2005). It is very likely that children exposed to this early environment would have disorganized attachment.

Borderline personality disorder

Borderline personality disorder is a disorder of personality development characterized by: instability in affects, identity, and relationships; feelings of emptiness; strenuous efforts to avoid feelings of abandonment that lead to feelings of psychic disintegration. It is used to describe a wide range of difficulties and behaviours. The backgrounds of people diagnosed with borderline personality disorder are characterized by reports of neglect, abuse, and early separations (Gabbard 2005). As a consequence, people with borderline personality disorder show high rates of unresolved/disorganized attachment. In the Cassel Hospital sample, 89% of inpatients with borderline personality disorder had unresolved attachment status (Fonagy et al. 1996).

Eating disorders

An argument has been made to link some eating disorders with dissociation on the basis that the serious distortions of body image are related to dissociation (Liotti 1999). In the case of a woman with anorexia and a severe distortion of her body image, the dissociation might occur between two internal working models of herself, one of a little girl who is starving hungry for love and approval from an emotionally unavailable mother, and an incompatible internal working model of a good kind mother with a very bad greedy little girl, who must control her greediness. However, eating disorders and dissociation are considered separately here.

Attachment research in people with eating disorders shows that insecure attachment is the norm with a mixture of insecure-ambivalent/preoccupied attachment and insecure-avoidant/dismissive attachment; among more disturbed populations unresolved classifications predominate.

Ringer et al. (2007) using the Adult Attachment Interview found that all of their patients with eating disorders were insecurely attached with half being preoccupied and the rest mainly using a combination of preoccupied and dismissing strategies. Using a self-report questionnaire (the Reciprocal Attachment Questionnaire), Ward et al. (2000) in a mixed inpatient and outpatient sample of women at a tertiary referral centre found that patients scored higher than controls on most scales but particularly Compulsive Care-Seeking and Compulsive Self-Reliance, creating a 'push–pull' dilemma in their attachment relationships. Troisi et al. (2005) using the Attachment Style Questionnaire found that eating disorder patients had higher rates of insecure-anxious attachment but no elevation in insecure-avoidant scales. Later Troisi et al. (2006) found that childhood separation anxiety and preoccupied attachment best predicted negative body image. Latzer et al. (2002) using the Adult Attachment Scale found that eating disorder patients had higher scores on both insecure-avoidant and insecure-ambivalent attachment than controls.

In the Cassel inpatient sample Fonagy et al. (1996) using the Adult Attachment Interview found that patients with eating disorders on the three-way classification had high rates of insecure-preoccupied attachment (64%) and on the four-way classification all but one (93%, 13/14) were unresolved. Interestingly, the eating disorder patients differed from the other patient groups in having significantly elevated scores for idealization of parents; this sample is probably more severely disturbed than the other groups, coming from an exclusively inpatient sample with high levels of comorbidity at a national centre.

Conclusion

The attachment system is an instinctual behavioural system that evolved to reduce predation of the young. The early years are a critical period for the development of attachment. Attachment is patterned by parental sensitivity, responsiveness, and availability. It is disrupted by trauma, separation, or loss. Attachment styles tend to endure in the absence of marked social environmental change. Attachment styles are mediated by the subject's internal working models—these are mental representations of how relationships work. Internal working models determine how individuals perceive and act in their social environment. Internal working models can become defensively structured in which case they become less adaptive to later environmental change.

Secure attachment is associated with a sense of competence and a belief that help will be available if needed; it is associated with emotional resilience under stress. Insecure attachment is associated with vulnerability to emotional trauma. Insecure dismissive attachment is associated with reduced help seeking behaviour. Disorganized attachment arises when caregivers are frightened or frightening or show dissociative behaviour. Individuals with disorganized attachment lack an organized strategy for obtaining security from an attachment figure, who is seen as both a source of fear and of safety. Individuals with disorganized attachment display a lack of integration of self and other, they are most vulnerable to develop later psychiatric illness. Attachment styles are transmitted between generations, directly through parenting behaviour and indirectly by assortive mating.

References

Ainsworth MDS *et al.* (eds) (1978). *Patterns of Attachment: A Psychological Study of the Strange Situation.* Erlbaum, Hillsdale, NJ.

Ainsworth MDS and Eichberg CG (1991). Effects on infant-mother attachment of mother's unresolved loss of an attachment figure or other traumatic experience. In: CM Parkes *et al.* (eds) *Attachment Across the Life Cycle*, pp. 160–83. Routledge, New York.

American Psychiatric Association (1997). *Diagnostic and Statistical Manual of Mental Disorders. Fourth edition, text re*vision. American Psychiatric Association, Washington, DC.

Beck AT (1967). *Depression: Clinical, Experimental and Theoretical Aspects.* Harper and Row Inc, New York.

Bifulco A *et al.* (2004). Maternal attachment style and depression associated with childbirth: preliminary results from a European and US cross-cultural study. *British Journal of Psychiatry*, **184**(suppl. 46), s31–s37.

Bowlby J (1944a). Forty-four juvenile thieves: their characters and home-life. *International Journal of Psycho-Analysis*, **25**, 19–53.

Bowlby J (1944b). Forty-four juvenile thieves: their characters and home-life (II). *International Journal of Psycho-Analysis*, **25**, 107–28.

Bowlby J (1951). *Maternal Care and Mental Health.* WHO Monograph Series 2, Geneva.

Bowlby J (1957). An ethological approach to research in child development. *British Journal of Medical Psychology*, **30**, 230–40. Reprinted in: J Bowlby (1997) (ed) *The Making and Breaking of Affectional Bonds*, Tavistock Publications and Routledge, London and New York.

Bowlby J (1958). The nature of the child's tie to his mother. *International Journal of Psycho-Analysis*, **39**, 350–73.

Bowlby J (1960a). Separation anxiety. *International Journal of Psycho-Analysis*, **41**, 89–113.

Bowlby J (1960b). Grief and mourning in infancy and early childhood. *Psychoanalytic Study of the Child*, **15**, 9–52.

Bowlby J (1969). *Attachment and Loss (Vol. 1), Attachment.* Hogarth Press and the Institute of Psycho-Analysis, London.

Bowlby J (1973). *Attachment and Loss (Vol. 2), Separation: Anxiety and Anger.* Hogarth Press and the Institute of Psycho-Analysis, London.

Bowlby J (1980). *Attachment and Loss (Vol. 3), Loss: Sadness and depression.* Hogarth Press and the Institute of Psycho-Analysis, London.

Bowlby J (1997). *The Making and Breaking of Affectional Bonds.* Tavistock Publications and Routledge, London and New York.

Bretherton I (1991). The roots and growing points of attachment theory. In: CM Parkes *et al.* (eds), *Attachment Across the Life Cycle*, pp. 9–32. Routledge, London and New York.

Bretherton I (1992). The origins of attachment theory: John Bowlby and Mary Ainsworth. *Developmental Psychology*, **28**, 759–75.

Broberg AG *et al.* (2001). Eating disorders, attachment and interpersonal difficulties: A comparison between 18- to 24-year-old patients and normal controls. *European Eating Disorders Review*, **9**(6), 381–96.

Brown GW *et al.* (1977). Depression and loss. *British Journal of Psychiatry*, **130**, 1–18.

Brown GW and Harris T (1978). *The Social Origins of Depression: A Study of Psychiatric Disorder in Women.* Tavistock, London.

Cicchetti D *et al.* (1998). Maternal depressive disorder and contextual risk: contributions to the development of attachment insecurity and behavior problems in toddlerhood. *Development and Psychopathology*, **10**, 283–300.

Dozier M *et al.* (1999). Attachment and Psychopathology in Adulthood. In: J Cassidy and PR Shaver (eds) *Handbook of attachment theory and research*, pp. 497–519. Guilford, New York.

Egeland B and Carlson E (2004). Clinical applications of attachment. In: L Atkinson (ed) *Attachment and Psychopathology*, pp. 27–48. Lawrence Erlbaum Associates, Inc, Mahwah, NJ.

Egeland B *et al.* (1988). Breaking the cycle of abuse. *Child Development*, **59**, 1080–8.

Fonagy P and Target M (1995). Dissociation and trauma. *Current Opinion in Psychiatry*, **8**, 161–6.

Fonagy P and Target M (1997). Attachment and reflective function: their role in self organisation. *Development and Psychopathology*, **9**, 679–700.

Fonagy P *et al.* (1991). Maternal representations of attachment during pregnancy predict the organization of infant-mother attachment at one year of age. *Child Development*, **62**, 891–905.

Fonagy P *et al.* (1996). The relation of attachment status, psychiatric classification, and response to psychotherapy.

Journal of Consulting and Clinical Psychology, **64**(1), 22–31.

Fonagy P *et al.* (2004). *Affect Regulation, Mentalisation, and the Development of the Self*. Karnac Books, London.

Gabbard GO (2005). *Psychodynamic Psychiatry in Clinical Practice*. American Psychiatric Publishing, Washington, DC and London.

Gervai J *et al.* (2007). Infant genotype may moderate sensitivity to maternal affective communications: attachment disorganization, quality of care, and the DRD4 polymorphism. *Social Neuroscience*, **2**(3–4), 307–19.

Greenberg MT (1999). Attachment and psychopathology in childhood. In: J Cassidy and PR Shaver (eds) *Handbook of Attachment: Theory, Research, and Clinical Applications*, pp. 469–96. Guilford, New York.

Grossmann KE *et al.* (eds) (2005). *Attachment from Infancy to Adulthood. The Major Longitudinal Studies*. Guilford Press, New York.

Herman JL (1992). Complex PTSD: a syndrome in survivors of prolonged and repeated trauma. *Journal of Traumatic Stress*, **5**, 377–91.

Hesse E and Main M (1999). Second-generation effects of unresolved trauma in nonmaltreating parents. *Psychoanalytic Inquiry*, **19**, 481–540.

Hesse E and Main M (2000). Disorganized infant, child, and adult attachment. *Journal of the American Psychoanalytic Association*, **48**, 1097–127.

Latzer Y *et al.* (2002). Attachment style and family functioning as discriminating factors in eating disorders. *Contemporary Family Therapy: An International Journal*, **24**(4), 581–99.

Liotti G (1999). Understanding the dissociative processes. *Psychoanalytic Inquiry*, **19**, 757–83.

Lorenz K (1935). Der kumpan in der umvelt des vogels [Companionship in bird life]. In: CH Schiller (ed and trans) *Instinctive behaviour*, pp. 83–128. International Universities Press, New York.

Lyons-Ruth K and Jacobvitz D (1999). Attachment disorganization: Unresolved loss, relational violence, and lapses in behavioral and attentional strategies. In: J Cassidy and PR Shaver (eds) *Handbook of Attachment: Theory, Research, and Clinical Applications*, pp. 520–54. Guilford, New York.

Macfie J *et al.* (2001). The development of dissociation in maltreated preschool children. *Development and Psychopathology*, **13**, 223–254.

Macfie J *et al.* (2005). Intergenerational transmission of role reversal between parent and child: dyadic and family systems internal working models. *Attachment & Human Development*, **7**(1), 51–65.

Madigan S *et al.* (2006). Unresolved states of mind, anomalous parental behavior, and disorganized attachment: a review and meta-analysis of a transmission gap. *Attachment & Human Development*, **82**, 89–111.

Main M and Cassidy J (1988). Categories of response to reunion with the parent at age six: Predictable from attachment classifications and stable over a one-month period. *Developmental Psychology*, **24**, 415–26.

Main M and Hesse E (1990). Parents' unresolved traumatic experiences are related to infant disorganized attachment status: Is frightened and/or frightening parental behavior the linking mechanism? In: MT Greenberg *et al.* (eds) *Attachment in the Preschool Years: Theory, Research, and Intervention*, pp. 161–82. University of Chicago Press, Chicago, IL.

Main M and Solomon J (1990). Attachment in the preschool years: Theory, research and intervention. In: MT Greenberg *et al.* (eds) *Procedures for Identifying Infants as Disorganized/disorientated during the Ainsworth Strange Situation*. University of Chicago Press, Chicago, IL.

Main M *et al.* (1985). Security in infancy, childhood and adulthood: a move to the level of representations. Growing points of attachment theory. In: I Bretherton and E Waters (eds) *Monographs of the Society for Research in Child Development*, **50**, 66–104.

Ogawa J *et al.* (1997). Development and the fragmented self: A longitudinal study of dissociative symptomatology in a non-clinical sample. *Development and Psychopathology*, **4**, 855–879.

Oliver J (1988). Successive generations of child maltreatment. *British Journal of Psychiatry*, **153**, 543–53.

Parkes CM (1991). Attachment, bonding and psychiatric problems after bereavement in adult life. In: CM Parkes *et al.* (eds). *Attachment Across the Life Cycle*, pp. 160–83. Routledge, New York.

Prior V *et al.* (2006). *Understanding Attachment and Attachment Disorders. Theory, Evidence and Practice*. Jessica Kingsley Publishers, London and Philadelphia, PA.

Ringer F and Crittenden PM (2007). Eating disorders and attachment: the effects of hidden family processes on eating disorders. *European Eating Disorders Review*, **15**, 119–30.

Seligman MEP (1975). *Helplessness: On Depression, Development and Death*. WH Freeman, San Francisco, CA.

Sroufe LA *et al.* (2005). *The Development of the Person: The Minnesota Study of Risk and Adaptation from Birth to Adulthood*. Guilford Press, New York.

Troisi A *et al.* (2005). Early separation anxiety and adult attachment style in women with eating disorders. *British Journal of Clinical Psychology*, **44**, 89–97.

Troisi A *et al.* (2006). Body dissatisfaction in women with eating disorders: relationship to early separation anxiety and insecure attachment. *Psychosomatic Medicine*, **68**, 449–53.

van der Kolk BA *et al.* (2005). Editorial: Disorders of extreme stress: The empirical foundation of a complex adaptation to trauma. *Journal of Traumatic Stress*, **18**(5), 389.

van IJzendoorn MH (1995). Adult attachment representations, parental responsiveness and infant attachment: A meta-analysis on the predictive validity of the Adult Attachment Interview. *Psychological Bulletin*, **117**, 387–403.

van IJzendoorn M *et al.* (1999). Disorganised attachment in early childhood: meta-analysis of precursors, concomitants, and sequelae. *Development and Psychopathology*, **11**, 225–49.

Ward A *et al.* (2000). Attachment patterns in eating disorders: past in the present. *International Journal of Eating Disorders*, **28**(4), 370–6.

Warren SL *et al.* (1997). Child and adolescent anxiety disorders and early attachment. *Journal of the American Academy of Child and Adolescent Psychiatry*, **36**, 637–44.

Weinfield NS *et al.* (1999). The Nature of Individual Differences in Infant–Caregiver Attachment. In: J Cassidy and P Shaver (eds) *Handbook of Attachment: Theory, Research, and Clinical Applications*, pp. 68–88. Guilford Press, New York.

Weissman MM *et al.* (2005). Families at high and low risk for depression: a 3-generation study. *Archives of General Psychiatry*, **62**, 29–36.

Weissman MM *et al.* (2006a). Remissions in maternal depression and child psychopathology: a STAR*D child report. *Journal of the American Medical Association*, **295**, 1389–98.

Weissman MM *et al.* (2006b). Offspring of depressed parents: 20 years later. *American Journal of Psychiatry*, **163**, 1001–8.

World Health Organization (1992). *The International Classification of Diseases, (ICD-10): Classification of Mental and Behavioural Disorders: Clinical Descriptions and Diagnostic Guidelines. Tenth revision.* WHO, Geneva.

Zulueta F de (1999). Borderline personality disorder as seen from an attachment perspective: a revue. *Criminal Behaviour and Mental Health*, **9**, 237–53.

Zulueta F de (2006). The treatment of psychological trauma from the perspective of attachment research. *Journal of Family Therapy*, **28**, 334–51.

CHAPTER 8

Maternal mental health: an ethical base for good practice

Michael Göpfert, Nora McClelland, and James Wilson

Introduction

In this chapter we argue that the four principles of medical ethics, beneficence, non-maleficence, respect for autonomy, and justice (Gillon 1985; Beauchamp and Childress 2001), a new Family Interest Principle (introduced later in the chapter), and a consideration of 'capacity' provide a reasoned practice guide for work with mothers experiencing health problems, focusing here on mental health when a parent is a patient. Our concern is the relationship of the clinician with a parent and through the parent their child. Ethics of service provision or services planning (e.g. Culyer 2001; McLachlan 2005; see also Chapter 35, this volume), or the provision of other services (e.g. education, child protection) although intensely relevant to this area are not addressed in this chapter nor will we deal with the complex aspects of medical ethics relating to the treatment of children (Baines 2008). We use the term 'parent' to refer to any adult person who fulfils a substantive parental role with a child. Defining what counts as a family will in certain circumstances be contentious. There are diverse patterns of family arrangements that may be influenced by cultural, political, economic, and temporal factors. For the purposes of our discussion, we define a family in terms of its role in child-rearing, as a group of at least one adult and at least one child, living together in long-term relationships on an ongoing basis, with vested interest in the well-being of each of the family members.

Ethical principles of good practice

Mental health practice is particularly sensitive to prejudice and political influence. Parental mental health practice is even more ethically complex because of the central role of the parent–child relationship. Good mental health practice with parents requires us not just to think about the parent as a person, or about the child in isolation from the parent, but in addition to think about the quality of the parent–child relationship within which both parent and child(ren) define themselves. Our argument is based on four assumptions about the parent–child relationship which we propose are fundamental to the ethics of parental mental health practice.

Four basic assumptions regarding the parent–child relationship and parental mental health

Where the family is viable, the best interests of the child are held within the parent–child relationship

The welfare of the child is held to be paramount in law in all decisions made on the behalf of the child (Children Act 1989). This principle, enshrined in family law, has assumed influence in informing generic decision-making when children's welfare may be affected (see Jackson 2002). Commonly, this is referred to as the principle of 'paramountcy' of 'the best interest of the child' (e.g. Paul 2004). There is an extensive literature on the idea of the best interests of children (e.g. Elliston 2007), consideration of which lies beyond the scope of this chapter. What is important for our purposes is the assumption that, whichever account of the best interests of the child is settled on, the best interests of the child are primarily held within the parent–child relationship, supported through the 'community', i.e. formal and informal institutions for and cultural patterns of childcare. There will of course be cases where the parent–child relationship is not viable, and hence the best interests of the child are best pursued outside the parent–child relationship.

• The notion of a viable relationship requires some further consideration here. A judgement about the viability of the parent–child relationship is complex and is, in essence, central to child protection. A determination of non-viable parent–child relationships will often result in enforced regulation or even dissolution of a family by the State through the available legal frameworks (primarily the Children Act 1989 and related Human Rights law). Within English law, interference in family is justified by the State through the need to protect children from harm, where harm is defined as ill treatment or impairment of health or development and/or impairment suffered from seeing or hearing the ill-treatment of another. The degree and nature of such interference in family life must be proportionate to the need to protect the interests of children: the removal of children from their parents care is to be regarded as a 'draconian' and 'extremely harsh' measure, requiring 'exceptional justification' and 'extraordinarily compelling reasons' (Mumby, X Council v B (Emergency Protection Orders) [2005] 1 FLR 341)

• Article 8 of the European Convention on Human Rights provides both adults and children with the qualified right to respect for private and family life. State interference in this right is limited; it must be proportionate and in accord with law and justified as necessary in a democratic society in the interests of national security, public safety or the economic well-being of the country, for the prevention of disorder or crime, for the protection of health or morals, or for the protection of the rights and freedoms of others

• Article 8 confers a positive obligation on the state to provide opportunities for family life to develop and be maintained (X v Iceland 1976), for example, through supporting parent–child contact arrangements when a parent is in hospital and/or family reunification at a parent's discharge from hospital. For the State not to do so could constitute a violation of Article 8 (B v UK 1987)

• Case law emerging from the European Court of Human Rights (ECtHR) defines family life, as pertaining to Article 8, broadly in terms of the existence of close personal ties of some permanence (Marckx v Belgium 1979) not necessarily determined solely by biological ties (X, Y and Z v UK 1997) or determined by marital status, (Keegan v Ireland 1994).

Cases before the ECtHR in relation to family life are often characterized by clashes of interest, between parents, children, and the Nation State. The ECtHR upholds the view that the interests of any child will be of paramount concern in any matters before it. Circumstances found to justify State interference in family life are primarily those that concern the physical health, welfare, and safety of a child including the child's need for protection from serious psychological impairment, lack of care and guidance, and any serious risks to the child's future development. The discussion of human rights for people diagnosed with mental ill health has traditionally centred on: Article 3, the right to be protected from torture or degrading treatment or punishment; Article 5, the right to liberty and security of the person; and Article 6, the right to a fair hearing. However, as legal commentators note, there is opportunity for parents who experience mental ill health and whose contact with their children has been restricted or denied by legal intervention to appeal against an interference to human rights protected by Article 8 to the ECtHR (Gostin 2000; Hale 2007). This opportunity is increasingly being taken up and judgments are highlighting that whilst the interventions by the State may be justified, the State is often found to be in violation of Article 8 by failing in its duty to support family relationships (Prior 2003).

The social role dimension

Being a child and becoming and being a parent—while representing basic biological facts—are social roles fundamental to individual and social identity (Bowlby 1988). For women, becoming or being a mother may be a particularly significant aspect of identity that may be conflicted when women experience mental illness, by negative social and professional attitudes towards gender, mental health, and/or parenting (Krumm *et al.* 2006). The parent–child relationship is only one social role relationship; there are many others that people engage in during their lifetime, for example, as partner, worker, or patient. Any social interaction can at the same time be construed as a social role relationship. A parent is necessarily involved in a number of major social role relationships supporting the viability of their role as parent. Without this network of relationships the child for whom the role of child is an essential basic necessity, may be affected adversely.

The attachment relationship dimension

Within a parent–child relationship a parent's contribution is quintessentially their capacity for preoccupation with the child, both in terms of instrumental and emotional care (Bowlby 1969/1999; Hill 2004). The attachment relationship is an asymmetrical one, and children are primary partners in parenting as a cooperative process (James and Prout 1990). They contribute through both their responsiveness to, and the demands they make on, their parent. This means the parent has the capacity to be preoccupied with the child but does not always have to be, and the child will contribute to triggering the parent into a state of preoccupation as needed. This facet of relationship is often seen as critical in mediating effects of parental mental ill health on children. For example, severe postnatal depression may prevent a mother from being appropriately triggered into this state of preoccupation. Hence, apart from generic issues of abuse (a reversal of needs and roles by means of power) this parental availability within the parent–child relationship needs to be of concern to the professional working with issues of parental mental health.

Mental ill health does not automatically result in impaired parenting capacity

Recovery from ill health implies resumption of social roles including that of parent, but parental ill health—including mental ill health—does not automatically imply that parenting capacity is impaired (Adshead *et al.* 2004; Göpfert *et al.* 2004b). Conceptually, recovery is complex. Recovery may be partial, the level of previous function may not always be restored, and as a dynamic process recovery may create change and support changing. It is not permissible to assume that parenting capacity will be automatically impaired as a result of parental mental ill health. However, parenting might be impaired and acknowledging the social role of parenting and the dynamic nature of parenting in the recovery process, this must be considered when working with a parent with mental health issues.

The implication of these assumptions is that instead of thinking simply about the mother, or the child, practitioners need to think about the parent–child(ren) relationship. This will often require acknowledging a complex system of variously interlinked and interdependent relationships that are likely to exist in a family situation. Parent–child relationships may be complicated further not solely by number (children as opposed to child) but also by the nature of the particular relationship (e.g. age, stage, developmental needs), culture, and by the number of adults involved in parenting roles.

The four principles of medical ethics applied to parental mental health

Medical ethics is located within a range of force fields mainly between the poles of 'autonomy' and 'paternalism/welfarism' which is reflected in the following discussion of the four principles. This is because sometimes the health professional must act in the best interests of a patient without the patient's explicit consent (paternalism—usually in a clinical crisis) while at other times a patient may make a decision that by medical standards and values might be considered not to be in his/her best interests (e.g. refusing a blood transfusion or rejecting psychotropic medication). With the introduction of the parenting dimension and the 'best interests of the child' matters can become more complex, but the four principles of medical ethics can provide some guidance.

1 Beneficence

The principle of beneficence concerns the 'moral obligation to act for the benefit of others, helping them to further their important and legitimate interests, often by preventing or removing possible harms' (Beauchamp 2008). It is important when thinking of the principle of beneficence to realise that we must also reflect on the appropriate scope of the principle: for instance, who is it that healthcare professionals have a duty to benefit—is it solely the parent-patient, or does it also include their children (Gillon 1994)? Should healthcare professionals be thinking even more widely so that they also think about what benefits society more broadly? And how should healthcare professionals take into account the relationships between patients and their families when thinking about benefiting them: should they view each person as an isolated individual, or should we give some intrinsic weight to the relationships through which patients define themselves?

If we take it that our focus should be on benefiting each person as an isolated individual, and that the healthcare professional's duty of beneficence extends at least as far as the best interests of the child(ren) of the parent-patient, then it has been argued that acting in accord with beneficence for the parent-patient creates potential for professional conflict with the child's best interest (see Weir and Douglas 1999). Some practitioners argue that in order to manage or avoid this conflict, they should not get involved with the other side of the pair and should either attend to the needs of the child, or the parent only and not overextend themselves by thinking about their relationship.

However, we argue that it is a mistake to start from the assumption that the child's best interests and the best interests of the parent-patient are separate and in conflict. This greatly underestimates the degree to which both the parent's and the child's best interests are held within and constituted by the best interests of the family unit that their individual interests are invested in. The mutual investment in the family unit provides a subsidy for family relationships and roles which in turn subsidize individual interests. This claim for the primacy of the relationship is based on a view of the parent role as a basic aspect of adult life (assumption 2, 'The social role dimension') and that the needs of the adult are met, at least in a substantive part, when the needs of their children are met. Consequently the needs of the adult have to be met in such a way that enables them to meet their obligations to the child in fulfilment of their parental role. From the perspective of the child, their primary need is for someone to be appropriately preoccupied with them; and it is reasonable to think that, apart from circumstances where the parent–child relationship is clearly nonviable (see earlier), this role will be best provided by the parent.

It follows that rather than thinking simply about what would be to the benefit of the parent-patient, and then separately about what would benefit the parent-patient's children, it is not only legitimate but in fact ethically required to consider the best interests of the family as a unit. (We call this the Family Interest Principle, and discuss its implications in more detail later.)

2 Nonmaleficence

The principle of nonmaleficence relates to obligations not to harm others, and in an extended sense also covers obligations not to allow others to come to harm. There will remain some cases where even with the best support that can be provided, the parent–child relationship may not be able to be made viable, and in such cases the principle of nonmaleficence comes to the fore, i.e. a principle that no harm should come to either the mother or the child.

Clearly, children can be harmed through their parent's mental ill health (d'Orban 1979; Falkov 1996; Reder and Duncan 1999). Moreover, a mothers' role, identity, and adult integrity (and in some instances her life), may be seriously harmed by any adversity she may cause her children. It is therefore of paramount importance that mental health professionals do not underestimate these possibilities, and act to prevent any harm to children and their mothers resulting directly or indirectly from parental mental ill health through child abuse or neglect, including consideration of treatment effects.

3 Respect for autonomy

Respect for individual autonomy is a central principle of medical ethics and links with the legal construct of 'capacity' (see later). The freedom to orchestrate one's own life is commonly considered an important part of what makes life valuable. Autonomy provides the basis for personal responsibility. What is necessary for action to be judged autonomous is that an individual can respond adequately to the requirements of a given situation; having understood, weighed up, and considered the various alternative courses of action, the person chooses to act and has responsibility for their choice, if freely made. Professional judgement made in the best interest of another person must take account of claims for autonomy (McClelland 2006).

Autonomy and beneficence are at times positioned in conflict, for example, loss of rationality is often seen as a feature of mental ill health, particularly when this is associated with distorted perceptions of reality or values as a result of a psychotic disorder. Yet social stereotypes, based upon race and gender, pervade and influence diagnostic process and perceptions of rationality. For instance, borderline personality disorder is predominantly diagnosed in women (DSM-IV). So diagnosed, women may be deemed unable to tolerate or control emotions. On that basis, women may be treated as less than fully rational autonomous human beings. This conflict may be particularly evident for parent-patients. Safeguards for 'autonomy' are reflected in various legal considerations, e.g. adult decision-making capacity (Mental Capacity Act [England and Wales] 2005) or independent representation of the child (Article 12, United Nations Convention on the Rights of the Child (1989)). The literature also reflects the dominant ethics discourse regarding parental duty, and children's rights and autonomous interests (e.g. Clayton 1997; Green 1997; Jackman *et al.* 2007) resonating with a wider debate about autonomy and its associated conceptual dilemmas (Ruddick 2001; O'Neill 2003; Wilson 2007).

When we are thinking of the ethics of maternal mental health, the traditional debate about autonomy needs to be reconstructed. Traditional debates around autonomy often fail to take account of the importance of relationships, and view autonomy primarily in terms of independence. However, as many feminist and communitarian writers have pointed out, when a mother is invested in her parental role, her attachment to the social role of being a parent and to her children are at the core of what she reflectively values in her life. Her autonomy is thus not primarily constituted by her ability to separate herself from her children, but rather in the security of the relationship she has with them. It follows that respect for her autonomy requires supporting her role as a parent (Mackenzie and Stoljar 2000). However, it is important to recognize that a mother may not wish (or be able) to assume parental responsibilities because of illness (Thomas and Kalucy 2003), personality, or preferences. This can be particularly problematic if a mother attributes responsibility for any problem to others, including a child or professional, and this may be difficult to acknowledge, especially if the parental role is caught up in power battles with professionals. Where parental commitment is limited or absent, mediation on behalf of the child's best interests and adult autonomy is required and legal process may be inevitable. 'Help' under such circumstances may be perceived by the parent-patient and/or the child as an imposition and adult claims for autonomy may conflict directly with the child's best interests. The professional duty through beneficence is to recognize and support the parental role if viable. The emerging legal framework of 'capacity' deals with many aspects of autonomy (see later).

4 Justice

Health professionals have a dual obligation to recognize the needs of children and parents when dealing with either child or parent as patient. Adverse effects of parental ill health may be experienced disproportionately by children, for example, if children assume age-inappropriate caring roles in order to help (Bleuler 1974; Aldridge and Becker 2003). Justice can be found in the recognition of need, validation of experiences, and the provision of practical support to both mother and child within, and additional to, the family relationship. There is a political dimension to the ethical debate of justice, involving consideration of equity and equality, reflecting the tension between paternalism and autonomy (Culyer 2001; McLachlan 2005). This is an issue of policy well beyond the ethics of the individual professional relationship with patients. However, it is important to acknowledge that the political dimension seriously impacts on what the individual professional's options may be (see Honneth 2008).

For instance, the State has devolved the power to suspend parent-child relationships to Courts and agencies with responsibility for safeguarding children. When parenting is judged inadequate and a child is permanently removed from their parent's care there is no continuing duty of care owed to that parent by children's services. This may reflect an unethical position taken by the State towards women whose personal identity is bound to their parental role as mothers but have lost the care of their child.

5 The Family Interest Principle

When we are thinking about mental health practice with parents, it is helpful to supplement the four

principles with a fifth, which we call the Family Interest Principle: as long as the family unit including any parent-child relationship is viable, any individual's needs and best interests are to a significant degree constituted by the interests of the family as a whole, and so individual welfare needs will mainly be met by supporting the viability of the family as a whole. We believe that this is a principle that many practitioners use in their thinking and day-to-day practice, but which has not so far received a name. It recognizes the fact that the whole of the family (like any cohesive group) is more than the sum of its constituent parts.

The Family Interest Principle is a useful addition to the four principles because it allows us to integrate perspectives which would otherwise be in irreconcilable conflict. It does so in two chief ways. First, as we saw in the discussion of beneficence, by focusing on benefiting the family as a whole, it allows us to appropriately consider both interests of the parent-patient and their child(ren). This avoids the difficulties caused by an exclusive focus on either the interests of the parent-patient, or on the child: if professionals focus on a 'patient's' best interests alone (without consideration of her role, e.g. as mother) they may deny a mother's obligations to her child(ren), undermining her adult status, roles, and responsibilities. A similar argument can be made that any exclusive focus on the 'best interests of the child' without detailed consideration of the parent-child relationship may not be in the best interest of anyone (McClelland and Göpfert 2005). Hence, if we redirect our attention to that of the best interest of the parent-child(ren) relationship we will tend to better serve the interests of all provided that family relationships are in principle viable and both parent and child(ren) place value on, and are invested in, maintaining their relationship (assumption 1, 'Where the family is viable, the best interests of the child are held within the parent-child relationship').

Second, the Family Interest Principle allows us to find a way of valuing the perspective of the child which escapes the traditional polarization between autonomy and beneficence/paternalism where the child is either considered as a separate being or as dependent on other's wisdom. Lee (2005) has argued that the child should not just be considered as a separate being with their own sets of rights and interests. As the child is embedded in a network of relationships and social interaction, the child can be considered as separable from the parents but not separate. Separateness can only be achieved through the child's development. This development is dependent on the child's togetherness with the parent who is a critical part of their social world. A parent enables their child to explore and learn about the world because they are there for the child to come back to. As the relationship between parent and child is reciprocal in a complementary manner, the parent is also required to be able to be separable without being separate; the parental capacity for preoccupation with the child can be triggered any time when needed. The Family Interest Principle thus provides an ethically effective way of taking account of the child's need to be separable and accommodates the need to consider the child's own needs in isolation from the parent but never as completely separated from their parent. Seeing the child as 'separable' enables us to consider the needs of the child as distinct from others while also considering their dependency without conceptual conflict. The matrix of mutual family roles enables fairness and justice through recognition (see also Honneth 2008).

It is important to note, however, that the Family Interest Principle will provide appropriate guidance only where the family relationship is viable. Dealing with a non-viable family as if it were viable may be damaging for individual family members. It may be difficult in some situations to conclude that a family unit is no longer viable: this might be particularly the case where family secrets such as abuse or incest exist. However, consideration of the Family Interest Principle is dependent on the existence of a family unit that is invested in the welfare, safety, and well-being of all its members. When the protection of a child from harm cannot be sustained by the family, and additional support from services to the family is rejected by the family or cannot be sufficient to protect family members from harm, then the family relationship is no longer viable (see discussion earlier). However, even in this case it is important to some degree to keep the family as a whole in mind in order to address the needs of individual family members. For instance, a child might be feeling anxious and troubled about the fate of their parent(s) but the knowledge that they are given appropriate help and support can make an essential contribution to the child's psychological welfare by alleviating guilt. Similarly a mother who has failed in her parental role may find it easier to deal with the consequences if she knows that her child is well looked after. Family members continue to carry the family they belong to in their minds, even if it does not exist as a living group anymore.

Using these principles

The four principles, when combined with the Family Interest Principle are a helpful guide to identifying and

categorizing the kind of ethical issues which arise in maternal mental health (and probably generally in parental health), but it is important to recognize that they represent a framework for moral thinking, rather than an algorithm (Beauchamp and Childress 2001, p.15). These principles on their own will not tell us what to do when we are faced with a moral dilemma; but they will at least enable us to see clearly what the source of the dilemma is, and to think more reasonably and defensibly in deciding which option to take. Further guidance comes from consideration of the legal position on mental capacity.

Mental capacity

It is important for professionals dealing with mothers and their children to understand the issues of mental capacity and competence as these concepts influence our work. There are unresolved issues in terminology (e.g. Bielby 2005) which can be particularly pertinent in clinical practice in situations involving mothers with mental health issues. Competence may be defined as either task-specific or agent-related, and capacity as defined in the Mental Capacity Act refers to the person's capacity to make specific decisions (overlapping with task-specific competence), as well as to the transferable 'capacity' in the strict legal sense where, for example, legal capacity can be exercised through 'Lasting Power of Attorney'.

When we are thinking about the ethics of mental health practice with parents, issues of competence and capacity arise in at least three different directions simultaneously. First, there is the question of the mental capacity of the parent to consent to decisions about their own treatment; second, there is the question of the parenting capacity of the parent; and third, there is the question of the capacity of the child. In addition, it is easy for issues of capacity and competence to get confused, to contaminate one another and lead to pseudo-legal solutions of relationship conflicts when it would clearly be most appropriate for parent and child to work out a joint decision (Paul 2004). Legally, 'parenting capacity' falls under the framework of the Children Act 1989 only, therefore the more legal arguments about issues of capacity and competence—while conceptually relevant to issues of parenting—are not dealt with here in any detail but the conceptual issues will be referred to in outline.

The mental capacity of the parent

In England and Wales the Mental Capacity Act 2005 provides a legal framework through which proxy decision-making on behalf of people over 16 years who do not have capacity to make those decisions for themselves is authorized. The Act provides some legal safeguards for both those making decisions and those on whose behalf the decisions are made. The jurisdiction of the Mental Capacity Act can encompass children under the age of 16 years if they lack capacity and are likely to continue to lack capacity beyond the age of 18 in relation to their property and affairs. With regard to young people aged 16–17 there are specific considerations in the Mental Capacity Act; for example, a person under 18 years may not make a legally binding advance decision. Professionals will need to continue to be mindful of the range of legislative powers that may apply in their work with young people and may need to consider the Children Act 1989 and the Mental Health Act 1983 (particularly relevant following the amendments in 2007) in their practice.

The Mental Capacity Act 2005 imposes a decision-specific and functional approach to capacity. The following principles apply regarding capacity:

1. Mental capacity should always be assumed

2. A person's ability to make decisions must be optimized before concluding that capacity is absent

3. It should be remembered that mental capacity is not static and assessment of capacity is decision specific. Any judgment must take into account the nature of the decisions to be made

4. Patients are entitled to make unwise decisions. It is not the decision but the process which determines if capacity is absent

5. Decisions made for people lacking mental capacity must be made in their best interest

6. Such decisions must be the least restrictive options(s) and respectful of basic rights and freedoms.

The Act takes capacity to be decision specific. Before any adult can be declared to lack capacity to make a particular decision, it must be established that the person 'is unable to make a decision for himself in relation to the matter because of an impairment of, or a disturbance in the functioning of, the mind or brain'. More specifically, capacity is tested by whether the person can understand information given to them, retain that information long enough to be able to make a decision, weigh up the information available to make a decision, and communicate their decision.

The Mental Capacity Act has specifically refrained from extending powers under this Act for proxy

decision-making related to particular family relationships. The particular decisions excluded in the Mental Capacity Act include:

- Consent to marriage, civil partnership

- Consent to divorce (after two-year separation) or dissolution of civil partnership

- Consent to sexual relationships

- Consent to placing a child for adoption or the making of an adoption order

- Discharging parental responsibilities in matters not relating to a child's property

- Giving consent under the Human Fertilisation and Embryology Act 1990.

The exclusions acknowledge the particular nature of these decisions, which are distinct from care treatment and property decisions and that other jurisdictions can provide better safeguards.

In clinical practice the assessment whether a parent-patient has mental capacity to consent to matters relating to their children's care may present particular complexity. For example, a mother who is a single parent with no extended family support who experiences a severe mental health crisis that necessitates admission to hospital is inevitably placed in a dilemma in relation to her children's care. The mental health crisis may not impair mental capacity for parental decision-making. Her options are:

- Accept informal admission (Section 131, Mental Health Act 1983) and seek support from the Local Authority for her children's care (Sections 17, 20, Children Act 1989)

- To refuse admission to hospital (neglect own needs) to continue to care for her children (parent's prioritization of children) and consequently risk compulsory detention (Sections 2, 3, Mental Health Act 1983)

- If her mental health crisis does not meet the legal criteria to justify compelling her admission, the presence or nature of any risk to her children will need to be considered. This may involve the local authority children's services undertaking an assessment of the children's needs, either with a view to their welfare (Section 17, Children Act 1989) or their protection (Section 47, Children Act 1989)

- If her admission to hospital is legally compelled, and over-rides her autonomy, her children will require accommodating by the local authority. This may be negotiated on a voluntary basis (Sections 17, 20,

Children Act 1989) unless the mother's capacity to consent to an agreement with the local authority is challenged (see later).

In this example as the mother has parental responsibility and if her mental capacity for decision-making in relation to her children is unchallenged she can enter into an arrangement with the local authority to provide temporary care for her children (Statutory Instrument 1991/890, reg 3). Whilst she may fear this may result in the permanent loss of her children, and research would indicate these fears are not without some evidential justification (see Barn 1993; Howard *et al.* 2001; Stanley *et al.* 2003; Park *et al.* 2006), she retains the legal power to remove her children from local authority care at any time (Section 20(8), Children Act 1989). In clinical practice, as we argued earlier, mental health professionals have an ethical obligation through beneficence and respect for autonomy to incorporate a commitment to the patient's parental role. In this scenario this would apply to all the potential options outlined earlier. This obligation would also apply if this scenario included some consideration of Community Treatment Orders introduced by the recent amendments to Section 17, Mental Health Act 1983. The Family Interest Principle applied in this instance would enable professionals to ensure consideration of, and support for, the parent–child relationship in planning and delivering services to the family.

In clinical practice, parent-patients may at times lack capacity to make some decisions or consent to the provision of any services considered (by professionals) necessary for their own care or treatment or the welfare of their children. This adds a further dimension of ethical complexity. For example, consider a mother who has a learning disability and a diagnosis of borderline personality disorder. She experiences fluctuating changes in her state of mind that influence her decision-making and she does not always sufficiently comprehend and retain information to weigh it up and make a decision. She also has difficulty in communicating and sticking to her decisions in a reliable manner over a period of time. Her capacity for decision-making is clearly an issue. For professionals the task in working with the mother is to balance competing ethical claims of autonomy (which depends on capacity) and beneficence when we act in our patient's best interests. In working with the parent-patient the Mental Capacity Act (2005) excludes proxy decision-making on behalf of her children's interests (i.e. her parental role and responsibility) from its applications and therefore the main legal framework for decision-making remains the Children Act.

If in this scenario, as a consequence of some mental health crisis, the mother's admission to hospital is thought necessary, the consideration of mental capacity creates a potential for different options and outcomes from those outlined earlier. In this instance she may also refuse admission to hospital, wishing to care for her children (prioritizing her children and neglecting her own needs). Similarly she may risk compulsory detention through the provisions of the Mental Health Act 1983 but there will be an additional option for professionals provided through the Mental Capacity Act (from April 2009). If her mental health crisis does not warrant over-riding autonomy through a compulsory admission (Section 2, 3, Mental Health Act 1983), but she is judged not to have the capacity to make a decision about admission that professionals believe to be in her best interest, she may be deprived of liberty and admitted to hospital through Section 4, Mental Capacity Act 2005. In this instance the judgement of capacity to make decisions about her own care and treatment is likely to remove the option of an informal admission too. The law compels practitioners to act in accord with beneficence.

However, mental capacity is decision specific: if she has mental capacity to make decisions about her own care and treatment and does not meet the legal criteria to justify compelling her admission she is free to refuse this (or agree to informal admission). But consideration of any risk to her children will still be required as part of a mental health service responsibility. As in the scenario described, the local authority children's services are likely to become involved to assess the children's needs. Here the differences in the scenarios may begin to emerge more clearly in relation to parental responsibility. Assessments of mental capacity may be required here in relation to the mother's mental capacity in her parental role to make decisions on behalf of her children. At each decision the test of mental capacity applies. In the context of parenting decisions the assessment of mental capacity is highly complex.

Parenting capacity

The principle of 'parental responsibility', whilst undefined in English law by the Children Act 1989, is implicitly rooted in a model of human development where the assumption is of a requirement for parental care and substitute decision-making (care-taking) whilst capacity for autonomy and independence develops in the child (Baines 2008). The Children (Scotland) Act 1995 has made an attempt to define parental responsibility and sets out the intended scope for parental responsibility recognizing the changing balance of this as the child matures. Parental responsibility creates a moral and legal duty for the 'best interests' or 'welfare' of the child to be of paramount concern for the parent until such time when the child is judged a fully autonomous agent and then no longer has an entitlement to parental action on their behalf. At this time, parental responsibility as a legal obligation ends although parents are likely to feel a moral duty for much longer.

In the case of the child, 'best interest' is variously and sometimes idealistically defined (Elliston 2007), but a common working assumption is that a parent will make decisions about a child's best interest based on what that child would decide for themselves if they had adult capacity. For example, the mother who compels her child to comply with a feared dental examination acts in their child's future interest in having teeth in adulthood to justify over-riding the wishes of the child in the present.

Parental responsibility then, is based on the assumption of a child's inherent lack of mental capacity. However, this is modified by the principle of children's rights, and notions of 'Gillick competence' that apply to children who have reached sufficient understanding to make up their own mind in relation to a particular issue, usually regarding medical treatment or intervention. Gillick competence requires the child to have sufficient understanding and intelligence to enable him or her to understand fully what is proposed, and the consequences of refusing. There are a number of issues and potential discrepancies with the question of Gillick competence. For instance, Elliston (2007) points out that in England (differently from Scotland) there is a difference in practice between the right to refuse any treatment (e.g. life-saving blood transfusion) and the right to consent to treatment (e.g. contraception). This seems to hold for parents' refusal of treatment of their child as well in the case of the refusal of treatment by a child against the parents' wishes, e.g. in the case of life-threatening anorexia. The details of the argument are beyond the scope of this chapter but it is clear that the reasoning may vary across a range of considerations of capacity. For example, for children it has also been argued that they may lack the capacity to make decisions with long-term consequences in the here-and-now because they may not have developed sufficient wisdom, or sufficient stability of opinion/values. This introduces the wisdom of decision-making and maturity as requirements for a child to have capacity which in effect sets a different and inequitable standard to the test of mental capacity for decision-making for adults

where the wisdom of a decision is not at issue. These issues await further clarification (Elliston 2007).

At the start of this discussion of mental capacity we referred to a problem in misunderstanding terminology between competence and mental capacity. In working with parent-patients there is potential for further confusion through the use of the term 'parenting capacity'. The framework for the assessment of children in need (Department of Health 2000) incorporates an assessment of parenting capacity. This focuses specifically on a parent's ability to respond to and meet their children's needs. Critical dimensions of capacity include a parent's ability to provide basic care, warmth, stimulation, stability, guidance, and boundaries. Although in principle outside the scope of this chapter, some fundamental differences between concepts of mental capacity and parenting capacity need to be highlighted. In the Mental Capacity Act 2005 a person lacks mental capacity in relation to a matter if, at that time, the person is unable to make a decision in relation to the particular matter because of an impairment of, or disturbance in, the functioning of the mind or brain. It does not matter if the impairment or disturbance is permanent or temporary. There is a diagnostic threshold for mental capacity judgements. Judgements of parenting capacity do not overtly incorporate any diagnostic criteria. However myth and stigma associated with mental health diagnosis are pervasive and are likely to influence judgements. It might also be argued that whilst assessments of mental capacity are not based on the perceived wisdom of a decision, assessments of parenting capacity demand that parents act wisely in regard to the decisions they make about their children. In making judgements about mental capacity there is a need to optimize opportunity and capacity for decision-making, this may involve taking time. In making judgements about children's needs the focus may relate to speed, as a child's needs related to their development cannot wait for their parent's recovery.

It is important in such situations that adult mental health and disability services become active and engaged in supporting parent-patients and local authority children's workers in assessing mental and parenting capacity. The local authority requires parental consent in order to provide services to the children. If, as a consequence of mental health and/or disability, a mother experiences difficulty in understanding or retaining information or her affective state influences decisions, tensions are likely to emerge between the mother and services as her mental capacity related to specific parenting decisions will also be changeable. This is likely to influence judgements about her parenting capacity. In this situation the likelihood that formal legal proceedings will be taken by the local authority to assume parental responsibility is increased. Acting in accord with beneficence and adopting a Family Interest Principle through assessment and practice may provide a framework for mental health practitioners to use as a guide to the ethical dilemmas they will inevitably face in such situations.

Other and contextual issues

The Family Interest Principle is important to consider in practice with mothers with mental health problems in a number of issues:

- When dealing with complex mental health problems a more detailed understanding of women's experiences as patients and how this affects their maternal role is required

- Mental health legislation stipulates that psychiatric hospitals have written policies on the arrangements for children visiting patients stating that a child's visit should be permitted only if this would be in the child's best interests and such decisions should be regularly reviewed (Mental Health Act Code of Practice 1999). Prescriptive guidance may be unhelpful. A visit to the parent in hospital decided upon in a child's best interest may not always contribute to the recovery of the parent. A visit whilst causing no detriment to the child may at times be of great benefit for the patient. Suitable visiting facilities and balanced consideration of the needs of both child and parent may be more helpful; by acting in the parent's best interests professionals may support the parental role, consequently acting in the interest of the child and of the family as a whole

- It is incorrect to automatically assume prioritizing a mother's needs is not in the child's best interest (Göpfert *et al.* 2004a, 2004b). Sometimes supporting and enabling a child to contribute to the care of the mother and considering with a mother how this is done rather than whether or not it happens (Byng Hall 2002, 2008) may be in everyone's best interest

- Detention under mental health legislation may signal that the child's best interests cannot be sufficiently held within the mother–child relationship. It may be the responsibility of the detaining adult mental health professional in consultation with the mother maintaining her parental role to ensure her children's needs are adequately met. This is likely to include

a consideration of support for ongoing contact when appropriate in order to sustain the family relationship

- Many factors, such as poverty, domestic violence, torture, persecution, and stigma, may affect a mother's parenting capacity. Such factors interact with, and may be exacerbated by, mental ill health and vice versa but they usually are beyond amelioration by mental health intervention only. It might be important to consider the needs of the family as a whole

- Many children have been harmed by State intervention aimed at their protection. The final arbiter of any intervention will be the long-term outcome and there is limited evidence which allows us to be mindful of this. Yet there are ample illustrations in the public domain where the judgements of professionals and the judiciary were wanting (see also Göpfert *et al.* 1996 for a more detailed consideration of risk from risk assessment and 'help'). In a difficult situation where it is not clear whether a family may be viable, especially when involving issues of psychological harm, the balance has to be a best estimate of the long-term outcome of supporting the family as a whole against the best interests of any family member but especially the child in a family that is judged nonviable because of the significant harm to the child. It is important to recognize that family relationships are from time to time harmful and hurtful, that life itself is a risk, and that we cannot nor should protect children from all risks because that in itself may be more harmful than beneficial

- There is a question whose responsibility it should be to be concerned as a professional or service about the parental role if a parent is a patient, about the safety of the child, and about the needs of the family. There is no clarity in the literature but an emerging understanding that maybe it should be equally the concern of all (e.g. the 'Think Family' policy of the UK Government). Some publications also acknowledge that maybe this should especially be the adult mental health services' task as they are looking after the patient who is the parent (e.g. Howard 2000; Howard *et al.* 2008; Chao and Kuti 2009). In keeping with the Family Interest Principle it might be most appropriate that any professional who is involved with one member of a family has a duty and a right to consider the welfare of the family as a whole, take appropriate action, and reasonably expect other services or professionals to be responsive. By implication this means that adult mental health services will have to consider the family and the welfare and interests of children as a matter of routine. This, in turn, has consequences for skill mix and training requirements for adult mental health staff.

Family care plans have been found to be an ethically-based means for managing complexity and ensuring adequate mental health and social care of parent and child (Reupert and Mayberry 2007; Reupert *et al.* 2008). An adapted version of the 'best interest checklist' required by the Mental Capacity Act could be integrated into this and be very helpful to professionals and families alike. In the United Kingdom we also have guidelines on considering the parental role of patients for use with the revised care programme approach (Department of Health 2008).

Concluding comment

We know that many women with mental health issues are mothers (Jenkins *et al.* 2003; Singleton *et al.* 2003; Skapinakis *et al.* 2003) but our understanding of the relationship between gender, mental health, and parenting remains limited (Reupert and Mayberry 2009). Collectively we often regard women and men as both different, when they may not be, e.g. legal position of infanticide (Dobson and Sales 2000), and similar, when there may be fundamental gender differences, e.g. formation of attachment patterns (Minnis *et al.* 2007). Therefore mental health practice has a limited although expanding evidence base (see Chapter 3, this volume) and traditionally has largely ignored the parenting role. We hold that this is ethically unacceptable and have proposed principles of good practice when dealing with mothers with mental health issues. Becoming a father is a very different process from becoming a mother. The process of how something comes about partially determines the outcome hence the relationship between mother and child is intrinsically different from that of father and child. We do not yet know how this should be considered in mental health practice but we do know that we are currently most commonly dealing with mothers when parental mental health issues need to be considered. Gendered service provision remains a complex issue (see Chapter 35, this volume) and difficult to address. Attending to the mother–child relationship as a central concern in adult mental health will not only assist in gender-appropriate service provision but also in improving family life and child mental health. We outlined an argument for the abandonment of individual claims for primacy of best interests in favour of developing an alternative claim for the family's best interest, a Family Interest Principle. This acknowledges

that best may well not be 'the best' but as good as it can be within the parameters of finding the best balance between benefit and harm. Principles of medical ethics can be helpfully extended to the parent–child relationship. This has implications for theory of medical ethics, requiring greater inclusion in training and policy development, to inform ethical practice. Much of this is in keeping with recent United Kingdom and Australian government policies (Department for Children, Schools and Families 2003; Australian Government 2004; Social Exclusion Task Force 2007).

Acknowledgments

The following have made substantial contributions by way of comments to the content of this chapter: Paul Baines, Alder Hey Hospital, Liverpool; Anne Morris, University of Liverpool; Julia Nelki, Alder Hey Hospital, Liverpool; David Pilgrim, University of Central Lancashire. James Wilson's contribution to this work was undertaken at UCLH/UCL who received a proportion of funding from the Department of Health's NIHR Biomedical Research Centres funding scheme.

References

Adshead G *et al.* (2004). Personality disorder in parents: developmental perspectives. In: M Göpfert *et al.* (eds), *Parental Psychiatric Disorder*, 2nd edition, pp. 271–309. Cambridge University Press, Cambridge.

Aldridge J and Becker S (2003). *Children Caring for Parents with Mental Illness: Perspectives of Young Carers, Parents and Professionals*. Policy Press, Bristol.

Australian Government; Department of Health and Ageing (2004). *Principles and actions for services and people working with children of parents with a mental illness*. Commonwealth of Australia, Canberra.

Baines P (2008). Medical ethics for children: applying the four principles to paediatrics. *Journal of Medical Ethics*, **34**, 141–5.

Barn R (1993). *Black children in the Public Care System*. British Agency for Adoption and Fostering, London.

Beauchamp T (2008). The principle of beneficence in applied ethics. In: EN Zalta (ed) *The Stanford Encyclopedia of Philosophy*. http://plato.stanford.edu/archives/spr2008/entries/principle-beneficence.

Beauchamp T and Childress JF (2001). *Principles of Biomedical Ethics*, 5th edition. Oxford University Press, Oxford.

Bielby P (2005). The conflation of competence and capacity in English medical law: A philosophical critique. *Medicine, Health Care and Philosophy*, **8**, 357–69.

Bleuler M (1974). The offspring of schizophrenics. *Schizophrenia Bulletin*, **8**, 93–107.

Bornstein MH and Cote LR (2006). *Acculturation and Parent-Child Relationships: Measurement and Development*. Lawrence Erlbaum Associates, Philadelphia, PA.

Bowlby J (1969/1999). *Attachment and Loss (vol. 1), Attachment*, second edition. Basic Books, New York.

Bowlby J (1988). *A Secure Base: Parent-Child Attachment and Healthy Human Development*. Basic Books, New York.

Byng Hall J (2002). Relieving parentified children's burdens in families with insecure attachment patterns. *Family Process*, **41**(3), 375–88.

Byng Hall J (2008). The significance of children fulfilling parental roles: implications for family therapy. *Journal of Family Therapy*, **30**, 147–62.

Chao O and Kuti G (2009). Supporting children of forensic in-patients: whose role is it? *Psychiatric Bulletin*, **33**, 55–7.

Children Act (1989). *The Stationery Office*, London.

Clayton EW (1997). Legal and ethical commentary: the dangers of reading duty too broadly. *Journal of Law Medicine and Ethics*, **25**, 19–21.

Culyer AJ (2001). Equity – some theory and its policy implications. *Journal of Medical Ethics*, **27**, 275–83.

D'Orban PT (1979). Women who kill their children. *British Journal of Psychiatry*, **134**, 560–71.

Dawson A and Garrard E (2006). In defence of moral imperialism: four equal and universal prima facie principles. *Journal of Medical Ethics*, **32**, 200–4.

Dent JR (2006). Motherhood versus patienthood: a conflict of identities. *Medical Humanities*, **32**, 20–4.

Department for Children, Schools and Families (2003). *Every Child Matters*. The Stationery Office, Norwich.

Department of Health (2000). *Framework for the Assessment of Children in Need and their Families*. The Stationery Office, London. http://www.dh.gov.uk/prod_consum_dh/groups/dh_digitalassets/@dh/@en/documents/digitalasset/dh_4014430.pdf (accessed 28.12.09).

Department of Health (2008). *Care Programme Approach (CPA) Briefing: Parents with mental health problems and their children*. http://www.cpaa.org.uk/files/cpa-briefing-parents-with-m-h-probs.pdf (accessed 28.12.09).

Department of Health and Welsh Office (1999). *Code of Practice (Mental Health Act 1983)*. The Stationery Office, London.

Dobson V and Sales B (2000). The science of infanticide and mental illness. *Psychology, Public Policy and Law*, 6(4) 1098–112.

Elliston S (2007). *Best Interests of the Child in Healthcare*. Routledge, Abingdon.

Falkov A (1996). *Study of Working Together 'Part 8' Reports: Fatal Child Abuse and Parental Psychiatric Disorder*. Department of Health, London.

Gillon R (1985). *Philosophical Medical Ethics*. Wiley, London.

Gillon R (1994). Medical ethics: four principles plus attention to scope. *British Medical Journal*, **309**, 184.

Göpfert M *et al.* (1996). The assessment and prediction of parenting capacity. In: M Göpfert *et al.* (eds), *Parental Psychiatric Disorder*, first edition, pp. 271–309. Cambridge University Press, Cambridge.

Göpfert M *et al.* (2004a). The construction of parenting and its context. In: M Göpfert, J Webster, and M Seeman (eds) *Parental Psychiatric Disorder*, second edition, pp. 62–84. Cambridge University Press, Cambridge.

Göpfert M *et al.* (2004b). Formulation and assessment of parenting. In: M Göpfert, J Webster, and M Seeman (eds) *Parental Psychiatric Disorder*, second edition, pp. 93–111. Cambridge University Press, Cambridge.

Gostin L (2000). Human rights of persons with mental disabilities: European Convention of Human Rights. *International Journal of Law and Psychiatry*, **23**(2), 125–59.

Green RM (1997). Parental autonomy and the obligation not to harm one's child genetically. *Journal of Law, Medicine & Ethics*, **25**, 5–15.

Hale B (2007). Justice and equality in mental health law: the European experience. *International Journal of Law and Psychiatry*, **30**, 18–28.

Harbour A (2006). The Mental Capacity Act and young people. *Child and Adolescent Mental Health*, **11**(1), 53–4.

Hill J (2004). Parental psychiatric disorder and the attachment relationship. In: M Göpfert *et al.* (eds) *Parental Psychiatric Disorder*, second edition, pp. 50–61.Cambridge University Press, Cambridge.

Honneth A (2008). *Reification: A New Look at an Old Idea (Berkeley Tanner Lectures)*. Open University Press, Maidenhead.

Howard LM (2000). Psychotic disorders and parenting – the relevance of patient's children for general psychiatry services. *Psychiatric Bulletin*, **24**, 324–6.

Howard LM, Kumar C, Thornicroft G (2001). The psychosocial characteristics of mothers with psychotic disorders. *British Journal of Psychiatry*, **178**, 427–32.

Howard L *et al.* (2008). *CAN-M: Camberwell Assessment of Need for Mothers*. RCPsych Publications, London.

Jackman L *et al.* (2007). Ethical decision-making in paediatric intensive care: whose "best interests" are we serving? *Archives of Disease in Childhood*, **2**(suppl 1), A34–A36.

Jackson E *et al.* (2002). Conception and the irrelevance of the Welfare Principle. *Modern Law Review*, **65**, 176–203.

James A and Prout A (eds) (1990). *Constructing and Reconstructing Childhood: Contemporary Issues in the Sociological Study of Childhood*. Routledge Falmer, London.

Jenkins R *et al.* (2003). British Psychiatric Morbidity Survey. *International Review of Psychiatry*, **15**(1), 14–18.

Kopelman LM (2007). The best interest standard for incompetent or incapacitated persons of all ages. *Journal of Law, Medicine & Ethics*, **35**, 187–96.

Krumm S and Becker T (2006). Subjective views of motherhood in women with mental illness – a sociological perspective. *Journal of Mental Health*, **15**(4), 449–60.

Lee N (2005). *Childhood and Human Value*. Open University Press, Maidenhead.

Mackenzie C and Stoljar N (eds) (2000). *Relational Autonomy: Feminist Perspectives on Autonomy, Agency and the Social Self*. Oxford University Press, New York.

Maitra B (1995). Assessment of parenting. In: P Reder and C Lucey (eds) *Giving Due Consideration to the Family's Racial and Cultural Background*. Routledge, London.

McClelland N (2006). Beneficence in ethical practice in diagnosis and treatment of personality disorder. *Therapeutic Communities*, **27**(4), 477–93.

McClelland N and Göpfert M (2005). 'The needs of parents with mental health issues and the best interests of the child: What do we need to work together?' Paper presented at BASPCAN Conference, Leeds, 4 October 2005.

McLachlan HV (2005) Justice and the NHS: a comment on Culyer. *Journal of Medical Ethics*, **31**, 379–82.

Mental Capacity Act (2005). The Stationery Office, London.

Mental Health Act (1983). The Stationery Office, London.

Minnis H *et al.* (2007). Genetic, environmental and gender influences on attachment disorder behaviours. *British Journal of Psychiatry*, **190**, 490–5.

Mumby J in *X Council v B (Emergency Protection Orders)* [2004] EWHC 2015 (Fam); [2005] 1 FLR 341, para 57.

O'Neill O (2003). Some limits of informed consents. *Journal of Medical Ethics*, **29**, 4–7.

Park JM *et al.* (2006). Involvement in the child welfare system among mothers with serious mental illness. *Psychiatric Services*, **57**, 493–7.

Paul M (2004). Decision-making about children's mental health care: ethical challenges. *Advances in Psychiatric Treatment*, **10**, 301–11.

Prior P (2003). Removing children from the care of adults diagnosed with mental illnesses: a clash of human rights? *European Journal of Social Work*, **6**(2), 179–90.

Reder P and Duncan S (1999). *Lost Innocents: A follow-up study of fatal child abuse.* Routledge, London.

Reupert AE and Mayberry DJ (2007). Families affected by parental mental illness: Issues and intervention points for stakeholders. *American Journal of Orthopsychiatry*, **77**(3), 362–9.

Reupert A and Mayberry D (2009). Fathers' experience of parenting with a mental illness. *Families in Society*, **90**(1), 61–8.

Reupert AE *et al.* (2008). Care plans for families affected by parental mental illness. *Families in Society*, **89**(1), 39–43.

Rogers WA (2006). Feminism and public health ethics. *Journal of Medical Ethics*, **32**, 351–4.

Ruddick W (2001). Medical Ethics. In: L Becker and C Becker (eds) *Encyclopedia of Ethics*, 2nd edition. Garland, New York.

Singleton N *et al.* (2003). Psychiatric morbidity among adults living in private households 2000. *International Review of Psychiatry*, **15**(1), 65–73.

Skapinakis P *et al.* (2003). Clarifying the relationship between unexplained chronic fatigue and psychiatric morbidity: results from a community survey in Great Britain. *International Review of Psychiatry*, **15**(1), 57–64.

Social Exclusion Task Force (2007). *Reaching Out: Think Families.* The Cabinet Office, London. http://www.cabinetoffice.gov.uk/media/cabinetoffice/social_exclusion_task_force/assets/think_families/think_families_full_report.pdf (accessed 28.12.09).

Stanley N *et al.* (2003). *Child Protection and Mental Health Services: Inter-professional Responses to the Needs of Mothers.* Policy Press, Bristol.

Statutory Instrument No 890 (1991). Children and Young Persons: Arrangements for Placement of Children (General) Regulations. London, The Stationery Office. http://www.opsi.gov.uk/si/si1991/Uksi_19910890_en_1.htm (accessed 28.12.09).

Tallis R (2004). *Hippocratic Oaths: Medicine and its Discontents.* Atlantis, London.

Thomas L and Kalucy R (2003). Parents with mental illness: lacking motivation to parent. *International Journal of Mental Health Nursing*, **12**(2), 153–7.

Weir A and Douglas A (1999). *Child Protection and Adult Mental Health – Conflict of Interest?* Butterworth-Heinemann, Oxford.

Wilson J (2007). Is respect for autonomy defensible? *Journal of Medical Ethics*, **33**, 353–6.

United Nations Convention on the Rights of the Child (1989). *United Nations Convention on the Rights of the Child U.N. Doc. A/Res/44/25 (1989). Version 7.* United Nations, New York.

CHAPTER 9

Women as carers

Irene Cormac

Introduction

A carer is a non-professional person who provides help and support to people who are sick, infirm, or disabled (Singleton *et al.* 2002). The person receiving care (care recipient) may need assistance with several aspects of their life including personal care, nursing care, housekeeping, emotional support, and finances (Levine 2004).

In the United Kingdom (UK), carers contribute about £57 million to society. The 2001 UK census found that there were 5.7 million carers of whom 3.3 million were women, and about 1.25 million carers provide over 50 hours of caring per week (Office of National Statistics 2003). Mostly carers are aged 45–64 years old and two-thirds are married (Singleton *et al.* 2002).

Social trends affect the availability of carers, for example, the number of women in paid employment, patterns of marriage, and numbers of lone parents (Department of Heath 1999). Many topics in this chapter are relevant to carers of both genders, caring for those with physical or mental disorders, or a combination of these.

Often women become carers on the basis of family, cultural, or religious expectations. The role of carer may be additional to family roles as a daughter, sister, mother, aunt, grandmother, partner, spouse, or as a relative by marriage. A woman may choose the caring role, or it may be assigned to her or she accepts the role because no one else is available. There may be cultural or practical reasons for women to be carers, for example, if their income is less important, if they have caring experience, or the role of carer is an extension of a pre-existing role as parent, spouse, or partner.

Carers are affected by the duration and timing in their life of their caring duties. They are also affected by other roles and responsibilities, within and outside their family lives, by the extent of their previous social integration, and by their previous level of emotional well-being (Moen *et al.* 1995).

The experience of being a carer can be positive and rewarding for both carer and care recipient. Benefits can include receiving love and affection, a sense of achievement from developing and using skills in caring, the development of personal attributes such as tolerance and patience, as well as the carer experiencing less guilt and enjoying the satisfaction of meeting religious and social expectations (Cassells *et al.* 2003).

In the United States, a study of adult daughters caring for elderly parents suggested that women's satisfaction with life was related to an accumulation of mastery (perceived competence and control) across their roles as mother, wife, employee, and carer (Christensen *et al.* 1998).

Burden of care

Caring can be difficult physically and mentally, and thus affects the health and well-being of a carer. The burden of care experienced by women in midlife was found to be greater when there was coresidence, lower satisfaction with social support, and poorer health in the carer (Knight *et al.* 1998).

A survey by the Office of National Statistics found that 18% of carers felt worried most of the time, 33% of carers said that caring made them feel depressed, and 21% of female carers had neurotic symptoms (Singleton *et al.* 2002). This survey also reported that in care recipients, 67% had physical problems, 19% had physical and mental health problems, 7% had mental health problems, and the remainder had problems of old age. Carers who had more than eight family members to whom they felt close were less likely to have health problems (13%) compared with of carers in smaller social groups (26%) (Singleton *et al.* 2002).

Trajectory of the illness or disability

Demands on a carer vary during the trajectory of the illness or disability of the care recipient, whether these conditions are physical, mental, or a combination of both. For example, the trajectory of a brief episode of psychosis is significantly different from the trajectory of a chronic physical illness, such as multiple sclerosis.

Early phase

In the early stages of diagnosis and treatment of an illness or disability, it is common for carers and family members to grieve for the loss of health of the care recipient or for what the future might have been. The care recipient may experience similar feelings. A common reaction is to search for causes for the care recipient's illness, attribute self-blame for failure to recognize the condition earlier, and to attribute blame to others for perceived or actual discrepancies in care. Some carers respond by becoming closer to the care recipient and take steps to make the best of the remaining time together.

Adjustment and continuum phases

The phase of adjustment varies in timing, extent, and duration. Carers find it easier to cope if they accept the changes in their situation and if they previously enjoyed a good relationship with the care recipient. Previously established patterns of behaviour within families and relationships are likely to be reactivated and are sometimes maladaptive. With increasing frustration and tiredness, the benign intentions of a carer can be overcome, leading to a range of possible outcomes from malevolent thoughts about the care recipient, to rebuking the care recipient, responding slowly to care needs, to rough physical handling.

Terminal phase of illness and bereavement

The end stages of an illness or disability can be sudden or gradual; short or prolonged. Caring for a dying person is highly stressful and can be overwhelming with or without support (Walsh *et al.* 2007). Some carers and care recipients have been shown to benefit from more tailored services and more palliative care (Kristjanson *et al.* 2005). During the transition from caring to bereavement, wife and daughter carers have been found to experience depressive symptoms (Li 2005). Elderly carers experience more depression after the unexpected death of their spouse and highly stressed

carers show increased social isolation following bereavement (Burton *et al.* 2006).

Challenges in caring

Carers coping with a person with mental health problems have most difficulty dealing with fluctuations in the mental illness or disorder, unpredictable behaviour, restlessness, disturbance at night, pacing, and suicide threats (Perring *et al.* 1992). A study of mostly female carers (80%) providing care for relatives with dementia found that 52% of care recipients needed assistance with bathing and dressing, 40% with walking, 36% with toileting, 28% with feeding, along with physical comorbidities (92%) (Bridges-Webb *et al.* 2007).

Carers tend to modify their behaviour to the demands of caring and can become constantly watchful, whilst trying to prevent adverse events such as wandering and falls. Sleep disturbance is a common problem for carers. Role changes may take place. For example, the role of a mother that formerly existed with her daughter may be reversed when the mother develops care needs, following the onset of dementia. For sexual partners, sexual intimacy may cease which may be much missed (Box 9.1).

A carer may have difficulty working and have periods of absence due to caring duties. The financial burden of caring may increase when a care recipient needs more complex care. Emotional responses such as embarrassment (perhaps from episodes of incontinence or socially inappropriate behaviour) can lead to carers withdrawing from social contact and becoming isolated (Kristjanson and Aoun 2004). Mothers caring for children with learning disabilities with severe behaviour problems (mostly physical aggression) were emotionally stressed by 'secondary stressors' arising from social isolation, limitations on lifestyle, and self-blame (Johnson *et al.* 2006).

Coping with caring

Carers tend to maintain their sense of well-being if they enjoy the caring role and if time is available for other activities which maintain subjective well-being (Pinquart and Sorensen 2004). In a Swedish study of carers aged over 75 years, the most commonly used coping strategies by women and men were keeping emotions tightly under control, taking one day at a time, remembering the good times, establishing priorities and keeping them in focus, and reminding themselves that others could be in a worse situation (Ekwall *et al.* 2007).

Box 9.1 Effect of changes on the carer	
Changes due to care needs	**Effect on the carer**
Household routine changes	Disruption to family life
Demand for care increases	Less time for work/ relaxing
Prolonged illness or disability	Carer role persists or extends
Risk of adverse events, e.g. falls	Watchfulness and constant vigilance
Adverse events and practical difficulties	Problem-solving skills used more by carer
Unable to undertake usual tasks	Develops new skills, e.g. gardening
Personal care needed	Change in balance of relationship
Financial burden increases	Financial difficulties and debt
Physical changes in care recipient	Sexual intimacy decreases
Sleeping difficulties	Sleep deprivation and exhaustion
Embarrassment, guilt, and shame	Withdrawal from friends/ colleagues
Less support from others	Social isolation and loneliness
Adapted from Cassells *et al.* (2003).	

Although parents normally provide care for their children, this role takes on another dimension if a child has physical or mental disabilities. In Iceland, mothers of children with mental disorders were found to a higher prevalence of psychiatric disorders (55%) than fathers (26%), leading to recommendations that psychiatric services for children should ensure that mothers receive support as well as the child (Guethmundsson and Tomasson 2002).

In the USA, a study of the mothers of young children receiving critical care found that mothers who received a specially designed educational and behavioural programme had better maternal coping outcomes, with fewer subsequent child adjustment problems (Melynk *et al.* 2004). The intervention comprised education about the behaviour and emotions that young children display during and after hospital admission, with parent participation in the child's care, guided play using puppets, medical and nursing role play, and reading a story about a child in hospital (ibid.).

In a Canadian study, the physical health and psychological well-being of carers of children with cerebral palsy (mainly mothers) was directly related to the child's behaviour and the demands of caring (Raina *et al.* 2005). This study highlighted the benefits and importance of the immediate family working closely together and of parents receiving cognitive and behavioural strategies to assist with the management of their child's care.

In caregivers of stroke victims, severe cognitive decline, and emotional and behavioural changes in the care recipient were found to be the main precipitants for carer 'burnout', with the greatest risk of burnout in women and young caregivers who had poor health (van den Heuvel *et al.* 2000).

Relinquishing caring

The decision to transfer a care recipient from home to institutional care may be triggered by the ill health of the carer, lack of support for the carer, an increase in the burden of care for the care recipient, or the development an unacceptable level of risk at home. Carers who feel overwhelmed are more likely to place a care recipient in institutional care (Grant *et al.* 2000). Carers may have great difficulty in relinquishing caring at home, with feelings of guilt, shame, and anxiety. They may continue to provide long-term emotional and financial support to the care recipient.

Needs of carers

Key priorities for carers are to receive a satisfactory standard of care from health professionals, to have the information they need, sufficient support, and help for the care recipients and themselves (Department of Health 1999). Carers also want flexible employment, adequate state benefits, and for their own health needs to be met (ibid.). A survey by Carers UK (2008) recommended improvements in state benefits for carers, before and after retirement, and for carer's health to be improved by regular health checks, for carers to have training for their role, regular breaks, and a system to help carers during crises.

Resources for carers

Information for carers and care recipients

A wealth of information for carers is available on the Internet and from books and leaflets published by the voluntary sector, government, social services, and by

> **Box 9.2** Information for carers
>
> Department of Work and Pensions: http://www.dwp.gov.uk
>
> NHS Direct: http://www.nhsdirect.nhs.uk
>
> NHS Choices (the official website of the NHS): http://www.nhs.uk
>
> Princess Royal Trust for Carers: http://www.carers.org
>
> Rethink: http://www.rethink.org
>
> Royal College of Psychiatrists: http://www.rcpsych.ac.uk/mentalhealthinformation.aspx
>
> UK Government website: http://www.direct.gov.uk
>
> *The Essential Carer's Guide* by Mary Jordan (2006). Hammersmith Press, London.

professional organizations such as the Royal College of Psychiatrists (Box 9.2). Information and resources are also available from a national network of carers' centres and from some GP practices. Carers may want different information depending on the phase of caring; maybe information about a physical or mental condition, how to deal with problems that have arisen, or what the services are available and how to gain access to them.

Services for carers

Many carers are keen to receive help from outside agencies but others prefer family and friends to help. As care needs vary over time, it is best if services can be tailored to the level of need. As young care recipients move into adulthood, 'parent' carers may have to accept being less involved in their son's or daughter's care, negotiate 'new terms' of engagement with their adult 'child', and accept the influence of other carers.

Carers and care recipients may need financial assistance and advice; for example, on how to obtain tax breaks, Carers' Allowance, and other state benefits. Legal advice and services may be required for preparing a will, registration of an Advanced Directive, or for property matters. Care recipients may have to stop driving and relinquish their driving licence.

Older women carers may find that they have to take over responsibilities previously undertaken by their partners. Carers may need training in lifting and handling or other aspects of caring. They may need to use equipment such as a wheelchair or hoist. Carers living at a distance may only be able to visit at weekends, and need to arrange help for the care recipient from local carers' organizations and statutory services.

Many carers want to work, attend college, social events, and to continue with their hobbies. They may require assistance to arrange help with caring duties, transport, and mobility. Carers may prefer to have a few hours of help with nursing care, or instead chose help with the gardening. When it all gets to be too much, carers and families may require advice and support to arrange funding and a suitable placement in institutional care.

Throughout the UK, there are carers' centres and telephone advice lines run by the voluntary sector and others, providing a range of emotional and practical support from individual support, help to arrange day care services, and access to respite care. Many carers find this kind of support invaluable.

Barriers to obtaining care

Steps must be taken to overcome barriers to communication, perhaps due to language or educational differences, and to avoid discrimination. It is best to arrange for a professional interpreter rather than a member of the family for privacy. Health professionals must be sensitive to the needs of women who want to see only female staff, for whatever reason, including cultural or religious reasons.

Women who are socially excluded (such as the homeless, refugees, women with addictions, and mentally disordered offenders) are less likely to be aware of the support and services available to them.

Lesbian and gay carers need the same level of support as other carers, and may feel that they have to 'come out' to health professionals so that they can receive the care normally afforded to other couples (Carers UK 2003). Lesbian and gay carers can have difficulty arranging residential care if their partner is not recognized as the next of kin, and fear discrimination by professional carers (ibid.).

Information sharing and confidentiality

Carers want information about the care recipient's condition and treatment. Yet they often feel ignored and 'starved of information' in healthcare settings (Hervey and Ramsay 2004). Doctors tend to make two types of errors with carers; excluding the carer while talking to the patient and visa versa (Levine 2004). Healthcare professionals and doctors have a duty to abide by their professional codes of conduct about confidentiality. The General Medical Council (2004) and the Royal College of Psychiatrists (2006) have produced useful information for doctors on confidentiality.

The understandable reluctance of health professionals to breach patients' confidentiality can be seen by carers as unhelpful or even obstructive. In order to address this, the Royal College of Psychiatrists produced a leaflet on 'Confidentiality and Carers' to facilitate sharing information between patients, carers and mental health professionals (Royal College of Psychiatrists 2005a). Care recipients can be asked if they are willing to share some information with carers and may be less reluctant to do so, if it is clear that that sensitive information will be kept confidential (ibid.).

Health professionals need training to improve attitudes towards carers and knowledge of carers' issues. The Royal College of Psychiatrists (2005b) has produced a training resource for psychiatrists, for delivery by mental health professionals and carers, containing copies of information leaflets for patients and carers on mental health conditions and services, together with a list of contact details of voluntary sector organizations.

Health and well-being of carers

Carers who are most vulnerable to health problems are women and those with pre-existing health problems (Cormac *et al.* 2006). In 2006, the 'Carer's Week' survey (http://www.carers.org.uk) found that carers aged 18–35 years old had the highest rates of depression (61%), anxiety (82%), and isolation (78%), and fewer friends (70%), whereas carers aged over 65 had received support from their GPs (60%) and 40% of these had received health checks.

In mothers of adults with learning disabilities, the responsibility for caring may last for decades, yet the mother's physical health may not necessarily be affected by the caring role (Chen *et al.* 2001). Caregivers who report experiencing mental or physical strain were found to have a 63% increase in the risk of dying than non-carers (relative risk: 1.63) (Schulz and Beach 1999). High burdens of care experienced by female carers may increase the risk of coronary heart disease in women (Lee *et al.* 2003).

Being a carer of an elderly person is not a risk factor per se for a psychiatric disorder. However, depression has been found to be more common in women carers (47%) of elderly people with dementia (Livingston *et al.* 1996). Loneliness has been found to be a factor in the development of depression in women carers of spouses with dementia (Beeson 2003). In comparison with non-carers, moderate cognitive impairment has been found in women carers aged 70–79 years old who provided care to their disabled or ill husbands (Lee *et al.* 2004).

Support programmes should focus on self-efficacy, social support, and coping strategies (van den Heuvel *et al.* 2001). Support from family and friends, respite care, hobbies, and employment are important factors in maintaining carer well-being.

Healthcare professionals should identify carers, especially in primary care settings which are usually the first services contacted by carers. Carers should be offered an assessment of their emotional and physical health, advice on their rights, and information on how to obtain an assessment of their carer recipient's needs (Hare 2004). Screening programmes should be set up to identify 'hidden carers'.

Legislation and policies for carers

In the UK, legislation and government policies have been designed to assist carers. Some voluntary sector organizations are keen to lobby for further improvements in legislation and services for carers (Box 9.3).

In England and Wales, the Mental Capacity Act 2005 has been designed to prevent carers from being overly restrictive and gives rights to those who lack capacity. A person can nominate someone else to act on their behalf, by creating a Lasting Power of Attorney, with

---

Box 9.3   Legislation and policies

In England and Wales, three Acts have been passed relating to carers

Carers Recognition and Services Act 1995 gives rights to carers to have an assessment of their needs from the local authority when their care recipient has a needs assessment.

Carers and Disabled Children's Act 2000 gives the right to anyone who has regular and substantial caring commitments to have an assessment and to have help to continue caring. Local authorities can also provide services at their discretion to carers.

Carers (Equal Opportunities) Act 2004 places a duty on local authorities to inform carers of their rights to an assessment of their own needs including opportunities for employment and lifelong learning. Social services are given powers to request help from other statutory bodies to assist in the provision of services for carers, for example, housing.

Other relevant legislation and government documents

The Delayed Discharge Act 2003 and the National Service Frameworks: Mental Health NSF 1999, Older Peoples NSF 2001, Valuing People 2001, and Supporting People with Long-term Conditions 2005.

registration at the Office of Public Protection. Advance Statements of wishes can be prepared and Advance Decisions can be made about life-sustaining treatment. Useful information for care recipients, carers, and health professionals is available in the Code of Practice (Mental Capacity Act 2005). Similar legislation has been enacted in Scotland, the Adults with Incapacity (Scotland) Act 2000, also with a code of practice.

Whenever possible, care recipients should make their own decisions about personal, financial, and property matters. Mental capacity in adults should be assumed be present until it is found to be lacking. Health professionals should assess and record mental capacity, and provide help to a person to overcome any hindrance to communication and understanding.

Conclusions

In the UK, women are responsible for providing the most care, often at a cost to their own health and well-being. Care packages for women as carers should take account of their own needs, life course, other roles and responsibilities, together with the specific needs of the care recipient; so women as carers can continue to provide care for their care recipients for as long as they wish to do so, or until events overtake them.

References

Adults with Incapacity (Scotland) Act (2000). www.opsi.gov. uk/legislation/scotland/acts2000/asp_20000004_en_1

Beeson RA (2003). Loneliness and depression in spousal caregivers of those with Alzheimer's disease versus non-caregiving spouses. *Archives of Psychiatric Nursing*, **17**, 135–43.

Bridges-Webb C *et al.* (2007). Patients with dementia and their carers. *Annals of New York Academy of Sciences*, **1114**, 130–6.

Burton AW *et al.* (2006). Bereavement after caregiving or unexpected death: effects on elderly spouses. *Aging and Mental Health*, **10**(3), 319–26.

Carers UK (2003). *Policy briefing on Lesbian and Gay Carers.* Carers UK, London. http://www.carersuk.org

Carers UK (2008) *Carers Voices: Shaping the 2008 National Strategy for Carers.* Carers UK, London. http//:www. carersuk.org

Cassell C *et al.* (2003). The impact of incontinence on older spousal caregivers. *Journal of Advanced Nursing*, **42**, 607–16.

Chen SC *et al.* (2001). Health status of mothers of adults with intellectual disability. *Journal of Intellectual Disability Research*, **45**, 439–99.

Christensen KA *et al.* (1998). Mastery in women's multiple roles and well-being: adult daughters providing care to impaired parents. *Health Psychology*, **17**(2), 163–71.

Cormac I and Tihanyi P (2006). Meeting the mental and physical healthcare needs of carers. *Advances in Psychiatric Treatment*, **12**, 162–72.

Department of Health (1999). *Caring about Carers: a National Strategy for Carers.* Department of Health, London.

Ekwall AK *et al.* (2007). Older caregiver's coping strategies and sense of coherence in relation to quality of life. *Journal of Advanced Nursing*, **57**, 584–96.

General Medical Council (2004). *Confidentiality: Protecting and Providing Information.* http://www.gmc-uk.org/guidance/ library/confidential.asp.

Grant JS *et al.* (2000). Sociodemographic, physical, and psychosocial characteristics of depressed and non-depressed family caregivers of stroke survivors. *Brain Injury*, **14**, 1089–100.

Guethmundsson OO and Tomasson K (2002). Quality of life and mental health of parents of children with mental health problems. *Nordic Journal of Psychiatry*, **56**, 413–17.

Hare P (2004). Keeping carers healthy: the role of community nurses and colleagues. *British Journal of Nursing*, **9**, 155–9.

Hervey N and Ramsay R (2004). Carers as partners in care. *Advances in Psychiatric Treatment*, **10**, 81–4.

Johnson RF *et al.* (2006). Caring for children with learning disabilities who present problem behaviours: a maternal perspective. *Journal Child Health Care*, **10**(93), 188–98.

Knight RG *et al.* (1998). Caregiving and well-being in a sample of women in midlife. *Australian and New Zealand Journal of Public Health*, **22**, 616–20.

Kristjanson LJ and Aoun S (2004). Palliative care for families: remembering the hidden patients. *Canadian Journal of Psychiatry*, **49**(6), 359–65.

Kristjanson LJ *et al.* (2005). Palliative care and support for people with neurodegenerative conditions and their carers. *International Journal of Palliative Nursing*, **12**(8) 368–77.

Lee S *et al.* (2003). Caregiving and risk of coronary heart disease in US women. *A prospective study. American Journal of Preventative Medicine*, **24**(2), 113–19.

Lee S *et al.* (2004). Does caregiving stress affect cognitive function in older women? *Journal of Nervous and Mental Disease*, **192**, 51–7.

Levine C (2004). The good doctor: the carer's perspective. *Clinical Medicine*, **4**, 244–5.

Li LW (2005). From caregiving to bereavement: trajectories of depressive symptoms among wife and daughter caregivers. *Journal Gerontology British Psychological Sciences Society*, **60**(4), 190–8.

Livingston G *et al.* (1996). Depression and other psychiatric morbidity in carers of elderly people living at home. *British Medical Journal*, **312**, 153–6.

Mental Capacity Act (2005) *Code of Practice.* Public Guardianship Office. London. http://www.dca.gov.uk/ menincap/legis.htm

Melynk BM *et al.* (2004). Creating opportunities for parent empowerment: program effects on the mental health/

coping outcomes of critically ill young children and their mothers. *Pediatrics*, 113(6), e597–607.

Moen P *et al.* (1995). Caregiving and women's well-being: a life course approach. *Journal of Health Society and Behaviour*, **36**(3), 259–73.

Office of National Statistics (2003). *Census 2001: National report for England and Wales*. HMSO, London.

Perring C *et al.* (1992). *Families caring for people diagnosed as mentally ill: the literature re-examined*. HMSO, London.

Pinquart M and Sorensen S (2004). Associations of caregiver stressors and uplifts with subjective well-being and depressive mood: a meta-analytic comparison. *Ageing and Mental Health*, **8**, 438–49.

Raina P *et al.* (2005). The health and well-being of caregivers of children with cerebral palsy. *Pediatrics*, **115**(6), e626–36.

Robinson KM and Steele D (1995). The relationship between health and social support in caregiving wives as perceived by others. *Journal of Advanced Nursing*, 21, 88–94.

Royal College of Psychiatrists (2005a). *Carers and Confidentiality in Mental Health. Issues Involved in Information-sharing*. Royal College of Psychiatrists, London.

Royal College of Psychiatrists (2005b). *Partners in Care Training Resource*. Royal College of Psychiatrists, London.

Royal College of Psychiatrists (2006). *Council Report CR133*. Royal College of Psychiatrists, London.

Schulz R and Beach SR (1999). Caregiving as a risk factor for mortality: the caregiver health effects study. *Journal of American Medical Association*, **282**(23), 2215–19.

Singleton N *et al.* (2002). *Mental health of Carers*. Office for National Statistics, London.

Walsh K *et al.* (2007). Reducing emotional distress in people caring from patients receiving palliative care. *British Journal of Psychiatry*, **190**, 142–7.

van den Heuvel *et al.* (2001). Risk factors for burn-out in caregivers of stroke patients, and possibilities for intervention. *Clinical Rehabilitation*, **15**, 669–7.

PART 2

Clinical Aspects: Women and Mental Health

PART 2A

Clinical Aspects of Mental Illness in Women

CHAPTER 10

Anxiety disorders in women

Heather A. Church and James V. Lucey

Introduction

Anxiety disorders are common in women and although often disabling they are eminently treatable (Kessler *et al.* 2005, 2007; NCS-R 2007). Nevertheless for many reasons they are frequently under diagnosed and/or inadequately managed (Wang *et al.* 2005; Wittchen and Jacobi 2005). Sufferers may not seek professional help, may receive incorrect diagnoses, or have symptoms of anxiety confused with medical complaints, especially cardiac complaints (Leon *et al.* 1995; Wang *et al.* 2005). While both men and women with anxiety disorders often receive suboptimal treatment, this is especially true for women. Women are more likely to receive benzodiazepines and are less likely to avail themselves of other effective pharmacological or psychological treatments (van der Waals *et al.* 1993). Moreover, women are more likely than men to suffer with anxiety disorders (NCS-R 2007). In this chapter we will present epidemiological data on specific anxiety disorders in women. We will review management, as well as consider hormonal and perinatal issues in relation to anxiety disorders in women.

Epidemiology

Anxiety disorders are the most prevalent of all psychiatric conditions, occurring in approximately one-third (31.2%) of the population throughout their lifetime. This was supported in two significant and recent epidemiological studies, the National Comorbidity Survey Replication (NCS-R) and the World Health Organization's World Mental Health Survey Initiative (Kessler *et al.* 2005, 2007). Anxiety disorders occur more frequently in women than men, as demonstrated by the data presented in Table 10.1 modified from the NCS-R (2007). The most prevalent lifetime psychiatric disorders, respectively, were major depressive disorder, alcohol abuse, specific phobia, social phobia, and conduct disorder (Kessler *et al.* 2005).

Presentation

The median age of onset for anxiety disorders is 11 years, with 75% developing the conditions between six and 21 years (Kessler *et al.* 2005). Separation anxiety disorder and specific phobia have an early age of onset (median range 7–14), whereas generalized anxiety disorder (GAD), panic disorder (PD), and post-traumatic stress disorder (PTSD) occur during later ages (median range 24–50) (Kessler *et al.* 2007).

It is estimated that fewer than 40% of people with a lifetime psychiatric disorder receive professional treatment (Kessler *et al.* 1994). For those who do seek treatment for anxiety disorders, there is a delay in presentation ranging from nine to 23 years. Delay in presenting for treatment is particularly associated with those with an early age of onset of the disorder, who are married, have poor educational attainment, or are members of racial or ethnic minorities (Wang *et al.* 2005). Patients with anxiety disorders present to general practitioners more often than to psychiatrists (Lepine 2002), so that the vast majority of anxiety disorders are treated in the community, by primary care providers. Of those presenting with anxiety disorders, approximately one-third receive medication treatment only, one-fifth receive psychological treatment only, one-quarter receive both medication and psychological treatment, while one-quarter receive no treatment (Wittchen and Jacobi 2005).

Confounders

In a recent review, Bekker *et al.* (2007) explored potential confounders contributing to the apparently increased prevalence of anxiety disorders in women. They concluded that men may find it difficult to report anxiety symptoms because of societal pressures and traditional roles. Moreover men are more likely to abuse alcohol in certain anxiety disorders so that their symptoms may be underreported. In addition, different diagnostic criteria may be a source of bias. Peters *et al.*

Table 10.1 Lifetime prevalence of anxiety disorders in women and gender ratio

Anxiety disorder	Percentage of lifetime prevalence in women	Ratio female:male
Panic disorder	6.2	2:1
Agoraphobia without panic	1.6	1.5:1
Specific phobia	15.8	1.8:1
Social phobia	13	1.2:1
Generalized anxiety disorder	7.1	1.7:1
Post-traumatic stress disorder	9.7	2.7:1
Obsessive–compulsive disorder	3.1	2:1
Separation anxiety disorder	10.8	1.5:1
Any anxiety disorder	36.4	1.5:1

(2006) reported that women with PTSD were twice as likely to meet ICD-10 criteria; however, there was no gender difference when DSM-IV criteria were used.

Economic and social cost

Anxiety disorders confer several significant burdens. The economic burden relates to both the direct costs to the healthcare system, such as treatment and hospitalization, and to the indirect costs such as unemployment, decreased work attendance, and suicide (Greenburg et al. 1999). Around 85% of the economic burden is due to loss of productivity, which highlights the importance of employers in the prevention and the promotion of mental health (Smit et al. 2006).

Although there is little available data on caregiver burden in anxiety disorders, a recent review article concluded that caregiver burden in obsessive–compulsive disorder (OCD) is equivalent to that in schizophrenia and that relatives of those with PTSD experience a significant burden. Obviously this burden falls disproportionately on women. However, other anxiety disorders have not been studied in relation to caregiver burden (Kalra et al. 2008).

Specific disorders

Panic disorder (PD)

PD is a common condition and with a reported lifetime prevalence of 4.7% (NCS-R 2007). PD is approximately twice as common in women as in men (Alonso et al. 2004; NCS-R 2007). The age of onset is typically in the early to middle twenties (Weissman et al. 1997). Approximately one-third of those with PD seek help from a mental health professional, while one-quarter avail themselves of general medical services in a primary care setting, possibly because of the similarity of physiological symptoms of panic to cardiac symptoms (Leon et al. 1995).

Clinical features of panic differ according to gender. Women are more likely to experience breathing difficulties and faintness with panic attacks (Sheikh 2002) and overall report more symptoms of PD than men (Dick et al. 1994). A worrying statistic is that women are three times more likely to relapse in the long term than men (Yonkers et al. 2003).

PD confers an 83% chance of comorbidity with one or more other psychiatric disorders (anxiety disorder, mood disorder, substance use disorders, and impulse control disorders) (Kessler et al. 2006). With regard to comorbid Axis II disorders, men are more likely to have borderline and schizoid personality disorder, whereas histrionic and cluster C (especially dependent) personality disorders are found more commonly in women (Barzega et al. 2001a). Women have also been known to have higher rates of bulimia nervosa at the onset of PD (Barzega et al. 2001b).

The aetiology of PD is multifactorial. Childhood trauma is a significant risk factor (Zlotnick et al. 2008). Women with PD (60%) were more likely to have been sexually abused than women with other anxiety disorders (30.8%) (Stein et al.1996). There is debate about gender specific genetic risk factors for PD (Kendler et al. 2001). There is evidence of an excess of high monoamine oxidase A (MAO-A) gene promoter alleles in women with PD. MAO-inhibitors (MAO-Is) are considered effective treatment in PD, which suggests that an increase in MAO-A activity is a risk factor for PD in females (Deckert et al. 1999). There is some support for catechol-O-methyltransferase (COMT) Val158met polymorphism as a possible specific risk factor in women. This polymorphism has been implicated in amygdala and prefrontal cortical activation in PD (Domschke et al. 2007, 2008).

Panic disorder with agoraphobia (PDA)

Agoraphobia is 20 times more common among individuals with PD than among those without it. The comorbidity of PD and agoraphobia ranges from 22.5–58.2% (Weissman et al. 1997). Interestingly, the comorbidity of PDA with drug dependence, bipolar I disorder, social phobia, specific phobia, generalized anxiety, and personality disorders is greater than in PD without agoraphobia (Grant *et al.* 2006). Yonkers *et al.* (1998) reported men suffer more from isolated PD whereas women more likely have PDA. However, the NCS-R (2007) reported both PD and PDA were more common in women. In addition, alcohol misuse is more common in men with PDA than in women (Cox *et al.* 1993).

In patients with PDA, women reported a greater subjective perception of agoraphobic avoidance while males were significantly more likely than females to anticipate the serious physical consequences of panic attacks (Latas *et al.* 2006). A recent three-year longitudinal study compared primary care patients with PD and PDA. Seventy-five per cent of patients with PD had experienced a recovery from their panic symptoms as opposed to 25% in patients with PDA. This indicates a more chronic course of PDA with fewer episodes of recovery and supports a pathway towards agoraphobia with increasing severity of PD (Francis *et al.* 2007).

Phobias

Specific phobia

In the NCS-R study, specific phobia was the third most common psychiatric condition with a lifetime prevalence of 12.5%. Women are approximately twice as likely to develop a specific phobia as men (Magee *et al.* 1996; NCS-R 2007). Specific phobia has the earliest age of onset of all anxiety disorders, with a mean age of presentation of seven years (Kessler *et al.* 2005). There is some evidence for different ages of presentation depending on subtype. Animal and environmental phobias begin early in life, whereas situational phobias present later (Becker *et al.* 2007). In relation to gender, women report more animal phobias, whereas men report fear of heights (acrophobia) (Curtis *et al.* 1998; Becker *et al.* 2007). Comorbid anxiety disorders are common, but less so than with most other anxiety disorders (Michael and Margraf 2004). This is understandable, given how circumscribed specific phobia is and its limited interaction with the lifestyle and psychosocial circumstances of the patient. Becker *et al.* (2007) reported that women with specific phobia experienced a lifetime prevalence of 28.3% for other anxiety disorders, 13.7% for affective disorders, 3.2% for somatoform disorders, 2.2% for substance related disorders, and 4% for eating disorders.

In the aetiology of simple phobias, genetic factors may contribute as well as traumatic childhood events (Kendler *et al.* 1992a). An association with a COMT gene polymorphism in simple phobia has been observed, which suggests that genetic predisposition may increase the risk of simple phobia developing after suitable anxiogenic events (Hajduk 2004).

Social phobia

Social phobia has a lifetime prevalence of 12.1% and occurs almost equally between men and women (NCS-R 2007). The mean age of onset is mid teens to early twenties (Magee *et al.* 1996; Kessler *et al.* 2005).

Women with social phobia report greater difficulty in speaking to authority figures, performing in front of an audience, entering a room, being the centre of attention, expressing disagreement to others they know, and giving a party. Men reported greater fears of urinating in public bathrooms and returning goods to a store (Turk *et al.* 1998).

Social phobia is associated with significant psychiatric comorbidity as well as treatment seeking and functional impairment. Around 83% of people with social phobia have another lifetime psychiatric disorder (Magee *et al.* 1996). Women with social phobia were more likely to have agoraphobia and men with social phobia were more likely to have substance misuse disorders (Yonkers *et al.* 2001). The degree of impairment in social phobia is related to the number of fears (Ruscio *et al.* 2008). Data from the Harvard/Brown Anxiety Disorders Research Program study (HARP) has shown that of all sufferers from anxiety disorders, people with social phobia were those least likely to recover (Bruce *et al.* 2005). In an eight-year longitudinal study, only 38% of women and 32% of men experienced complete remission during the study (Yonkers *et al.* 2001). Approximately one third of people with social phobia reported severe functional impairment at some point in their life. Predictably social phobia is also associated with relatively poorer educational attainment and an unmarried social circumstance (Magee *et al.* 1996).

There is now evidence for a genetic predisposition with a chromosome 16 risk locus in social phobia (Gelernter *et al.* 2004). Polymorphisms within the COMT gene locus in women are associated with low extroversion and high neuroticism, which are traits associated with social phobia (Stein *et al.* 2005). However, Rapee and Spence (2004) concluded that while genetic factors play a role in a range of emotional disorders only a few such factors are specific for social phobia.

Generalized anxiety disorder (GAD)

The lifetime prevalence of GAD is 5.7%, with GAD occurring almost twice as often in women than in men (Kessler *et al.* 2001; NCS-R 2007). GAD typically presents in the late teens to late twenties (Kessler *et al.* 2001). It is the most common anxiety disorder in older adults, being relatively persistent compared to other disorders in this age group (55–85 years) (Beekman *et al.* 1998). Unfortunately, GAD tends to follow a chronic course with few remissions. Due to the high prevalence rate in primary care (8%), a significant burden on the primary care service has been reported (Wittchen 2002).

The lifetime comorbidity with other Axis I psychiatric disorders is approximately 90%, with major depression (62.4%), dysthymia (39.5%), alcohol dependence (37.9%), simple phobia (35.1%), social phobia (34.4%), and drug abuse (27.6%) being most likely. GAD is associated with being separated/widowed/divorced, age over 24 years, unemployment, or being in a low paying job (Wittchen *et al.* 1994). There is a high rate of comorbid depression among the anxiety disorders, especially GAD, leading to questions about the primacy of anxiety or depression in women (Parker and Hadzi-Pavlovic 2001, 2004). Genetic risk factors for GAD and major depression are more strongly correlated in women. Major depression and GAD share a heritable personality component—neuroticism—about which many theories have been expounded, not the least of which is the idea of a dimensional relationship between anxiety and depression (Kendler *et al.* 2007).

Twin studies have shown that genetic factors account for approximately a 30% risk of GAD development (Kendler *et al.* 1992b). Abnormalities in adrenaline and serotonin have been implicated in GAD, as well as depression (Gorman *et al.* 2002).

Obsessive–compulsive disorder (OCD)

The lifetime prevalence of OCD is 2.3%, with twice as many female sufferers as male (NCS-R 2007). Men present earlier than women (21.1 vs. 24.3 years mean age at presentation) (Lensi *et al.* 1996). OCD is considered to be among the 10 most disabling of all medical and psychiatric conditions in the world, according to the World Health Organization, yet it takes on average 10 years from the appearance of symptoms to appropriate intervention (Pinto *et al.* 2006). Women with OCD are more likely to be married with children and to have a past history of an eating disorder or depression, while men are more likely to have a history of anxious personality traits (Castle *et al.* 1995; Bogetto *et al.* 1999). Also, women were more likely to have anxiety, eating, and impulse-control disorders (de Mathis *et al.* 2008), emphasizing the proposed link, and suggested classification in DSM-V that would see OCD reclassified on an impulsive–compulsive spectrum.

People with OCD tend to have a chronic course with persistent disabling symptoms (Alonso *et al.* 2001). In turn, the quality of life reported by those with OCD is impaired and is directly related to the severity of the OCD, particularly obsessional symptoms (Eisen *et al.* 2006). Women were found to experience more contamination/cleaning symptoms whereas men were found to report sexual/religious themes. Gender differences have not been found regarding aggressive/checking, symmetry/ordering, or hoarding dimensions (Labad 2008). Women were found to report a stressful event prior to symptoms as well as present more acutely and have a more difficult disease course and a worse outcome than men (Bogetto *et al.* 1999; Lochner *et al.* 2004).

Comorbid psychiatric and neuropsychiatric conditions are common in OCD. The age of onset is associated with specific comorbidities. A younger age of onset is associated with tic, anxiety, somatoform, eating, and impulse-control disorders. Lengthy illness duration is associated with fewer tics and with comorbid depressive disorder (Diniz *et al.* 2004; de Mathis *et al.* 2008).

Women with OCD more commonly report personal histories of child sexual abuse (Lochner *et al.* 2004). There is also evidence for genetic susceptibility in OCD and synergistic gender-gene effects. Variants of the COMT gene and the MAO-A gene, which are linked to high MAO-A activity, have been found to contribute to OCD susceptibility with a sexually dimorphic pattern, suggesting differences in genetic susceptibility to OCD between the sexes (Karayiorgou *et al.* 1999). In a study where patients were given the tricyclic serotonin reuptake inhibitor clomipramine (by an intravenous route), women showed a better antiobsessional response to the infusion than men, with the authors suggesting that serotonergic mechanisms may be more important in women than in men (Mundo *et al.* 1999).

Post-traumatic stress disorder (PTSD)

The lifetime prevalence of developing PTSD is 6.8%. Twice as many women develop the disorder than men (NCS-R 2007). In the NCS, 51.2% of women and 60.7% of men reported at least one traumatic event in their lives, yet the estimated risk of developing PTSD was

20.4% for women and 8.1% for men (Kessler *et al.* 1995).

Although women have a slightly lower average lifetime exposure to trauma, developing PTSD may depend on the type of trauma and its meaning. Rape and sexual abuse occur more commonly in women. Women have higher PTSD rates after childhood trauma than men, which suggests that trauma exposure in women at a young age can be a risk factor (Breslau *et al.* 1997). Women are also at greater risk of developing PTSD later on in life as a result of a minor traumatic event, if they have experienced a prior violent assault (Breslau *et al.* 2007). The effect of previous trauma suggests a kindling effect, with initial insults causing damage at early developmental stages and influencing the perception of later trauma, thus increasing the likelihood of PTSD.

People with PTSD score higher on 'neuroticism' scales and lower on 'agreeableness', suggesting there are predisposing personality traits in the development of the disorder (Chung *et al.* 2007). There is some evidence for lower cortisol levels being associated with the development of PTSD; however, there are conflicting studies which may indicate more complex neuroendocrine aetiology (Resnick *et al.* 1995; McFarlane *et al.* 1997; Yehuda 2002; Meewisse *et al.* 2007). The results of studies of catecholamine levels have been varied, with notably raised catecholamine levels in those with symptomatic PTSD in some studies, suggesting that increased sympathetic arousal is linked to PTSD symptoms (Kosten *et al.* 1987; Yehuda *et al.* 1992). In another study, however, no differences were found between PTSD and control groups (Mellman *et al.* 1995).

Women are more likely to meet avoidance/numbing and arousal criteria, to avoid thoughts and situations associated with the event. They tend to lose interest in significant activities, have a sense of a foreshortened future, trouble sleeping, difficulty concentrating, and an exaggerated startle response (Fullerton *et al.* 2001).

PTSD in women has been linked to major depression, substance use disorders, other anxiety disorders, somatoform disorders, dissociative disorder, eating disorders, and borderline personality disorder (Kessler *et al.* 1995; Brady *et al.* 2000). Many women with PTSD (44%) meet the criteria for three or more other psychiatric diagnoses over their lifetime (Kessler *et al.* 1995). This data would suggest an underlying neurobiological diathesis inducible in youth given adverse environments, and a feedback effect on development, causing greater susceptibility to the harmful effects of future trauma.

Treatment

There has been little research on specific treatments aimed at women with anxiety disorders. If there are biological and psychological determinants of gender differences in anxiety disorder, specific treatment should be beneficial. Van der Waals' research (1993) showed females were twice as likely as men to be prescribed benzodiazepines in general practice without the benefit of a specific diagnosis. Patients with anxiety disorders often present such disorders to their general practitioner, but some do not receive a specific diagnosis for years (Kessler *et al.* 1995; Lepine 2002; Wang *et al.* 2005). This suggests women with anxiety disorders are being treated primarily with benzodiazepines and that other treatments such as antidepressants and psychotherapy are dismissed as potential treatments.

Some specific treatment considerations for women are worth considering. In GAD, women appear to have a poorer response to the specific serotonin reuptake inhibitor (SSRI) fluoxetine than men, particularly if they are older at the age of presentation (Simon *et al.* 2006). The SSRI sertraline was found to be effective in treating GAD with no identifiable gender differences (Steiner *et al.* 2005). In PD, there is some evidence that the noradrenaline reuptake inhibitor desipramine may be more effective in women than men (Kalus *et al.* 1991). Women achieved greater improvement than men in terms of panic frequency, when treated with the SSRI sertraline (Clayton *et al.* 2006).

There is no data on gender-specific treatment of social phobia; however, Ruscio (2008) reported an inverse relationship between the number of symptoms and those receiving treatment for the disorder. Yonkers *et al.* (2001) studied a group of patients for eight years, observing that there was no significant difference in relapse rates between men and women; however, women with poor baseline functioning and a history of suicide attempts were found to have a more chronic course. The type of treatment was not controlled but approximately 80% of the women had received benzodiazepines.

In PTSD, sertraline appears to be beneficial to both men and women, with better results in men in terms of relapse prevention and acute exacerbation of PTSD symptoms (Davidson *et al.* 2001). In OCD treated with intensive residential care, females with less severe symptoms at discharge had lower initial OCD severity and better initial psychosocial functioning (Stewert *et al.* 2006). Although behavioural and cognitive therapies play a role in the treatment of anxiety disorders, gender differences have not been studied in any significant way.

Menstruation/menopause—women's hormonal cycle

Two conditions occurring in the week prior to menstruation have anxiety as a clinical feature: premenstrual tension syndrome (PMT), which is classified in the ICD-10 diagnosis, and premenstrual dysphoric disorder (PMDD), which is classified as a DSM-IV disorder. Symptoms of PMDD include depressed or labile mood, anxiety, irritability, anhedonia, difficulty concentrating, lethargy, hyper/insomnia, cravings for certain foods, physical symptoms, and a feeling of being out of control. In the DSM-IV (American Psychiatric Association 2000) PMDD disorder, five or more symptoms must be present during the last week of the luteal phase and one of these symptoms must be of a mood disturbance to fulfil criteria. The ICD-10 (World Health Organization 1992) requires only one distressing physical or mood symptom to have PMT. There appears to be associations with these conditions and anxiety disorders, specifically GAD and PD which are considered differential diagnoses of PMT (Freeman 2003).

Hsiao et al. (2004) reported 78% and 68% of patients with GAD and PD respectively had premenstrual syndrome, with 52% and 36% respectively experiencing premenstrual exacerbation (PME), which suggests that women's hormonal cycles play a role in anxiety symptoms. McLeod (1993) found that women with GAD and premenstrual syndrome reported a worsening of symptoms in the premenstrual and follicular phase of the menstrual cycle, while those with GAD alone did not report these findings. There is some evidence of worsening of anxiety symptoms in the premenstrual phase of PD (Cameron et al. 1988; Stein et al. 1989; Cook et al. 1990).

Women with OCD reported a worsening of their symptoms at menarche, during the premenstrual phase and at menopause (Williams et al. 1997; Labad et al. 2005; Vulink et al. 2006). In PTSD, exogenous corticotrophin-releasing-factor (CRP) and adrenocorticotropic hormone (ACTH) leads to pituitary and adrenal hyperactivity in premenopausal women, suggesting that cortisol hyperactivity may have a role in the pathogenesis of PTSD (Rasmusson et al. 2001). There are no available data on social phobia or simple phobia and the female reproductive cycle.

SSRIs are first-line pharmacological treatment of PMDD. Other antidepressants can be used if SSRIs are unsuccessful. Hormones that suppress ovulation are of limited use because of their adverse effects. Anxiolytics, spironolactone, and non-steroidal anti-inflammatory drugs can be used as supportive care to relieve PMDD symptoms (Jarvis et al. 2008).

Pregnancy/postpartum

Pregnancy and the postpartum period can be a cause of exacerbation in pre-existing conditions such as depression, schizophrenia, and bipolar affective disorder. However, anxiety disorders in the perinatal period have been much neglected. In a study of mothers living in a residential mother/infant programme, one-third met the criteria for an anxiety disorder. Among those women with an anxiety disorder, two-thirds had experienced mild to moderate depression in their pregnancy (Phillips et al. 2007). Sutter-Dallay (2004) reported that one-quarter of women experience an anxiety disorder in pregnancy and found those women to be three times as likely to develop postnatal depression. In a recent review, Ross and McLean (2006) concluded that there is evidence that both GAD and OCD are more prevalent amongst prenatal and postpartum women than in the general population. It appears that anxiety disorders in the perinatal period are common and can be associated with comorbid illness.

Most anxiety disorders commence around the childbearing years. Anxiety disorders in pregnancy and postpartum can occur de novo or be pre-existing. In a study examining anxiety through pregnancy into postpartum, most cases of postnatal anxiety were preceded by antenatal anxiety; however, there was a mean decrease in anxiety across this period (Heron et al. 2004). This supports prevalence data in GAD which shows higher rates of anxiety during pregnancy than in the postpartum period (8.5% vs. 4.4–8.2%) (Sutter-Dallay et al. 2004; Wenzel et al. 2003, 2005). This understudied area could have implications in furthering our knowledge of the aetiology of anxiety disorders in women and in recognizing the importance of proper diagnosis and treatment. Data on specific anxiety disorders are limited but will be discussed.

There is a 2.5% prevalence rate of PD in the perinatal period (Guler et al. 2008a) but there are conflicting data on the severity of symptoms across the perinatal period. It was reported in another study by Guler et al. (2008b) that those women who suffered from PD during pregnancy experienced a marked improvement in panic symptoms during the first six weeks postpartum. However, in women with pre-existing PD, Cohen et al.

(1994) reported a worsening of symptoms over their postpartum course in 35% of cases, while 55% remained the same and 10% improved. Northcott and Stein (1994) reported a worsening of symptoms in about 63% of cases over the postnatal period.

In OCD, over half (54%) of women reported symptoms related to the baby during the perinatal period, with obsessive thoughts of harm towards their child occurring more frequently postpartum (Labad *et al.* 2005). In a review by Pigott (2003), it was concluded that in about 20–30% of cases, symptoms are worse in the postpartum period. The exacerbation of OCD symptoms in some women may put these women at an increased risk of developing postpartum depression (Williams *et al.* 1997).

Perinatal PTSD has been studied in relation to the mode of infant delivery. In a recent review, Ross and McLean (2006) found that studies revealed conflicting evidence. It appears the childbirth experience rather than the type of delivery is more associated with developing PTSD. Termination of pregnancy has been linked by some to PTSD and social anxiety. There is an increased risk of both PTSD and social anxiety; depending upon the number of terminations a woman has undergone (Steinberg *et al.* 2008). There are no available data on specific phobia in the perinatal period.

References

Alonso J *et al.* (2004). Prevalence of mental disorders in Europe: results from the European Study of the Epidemiology of Mental Disorders (ESEMeD) project. *Acta Psychiatrica Scandinavica Supplement*, **420**, 21–7.

Alonso P *et al.* (2001). Long-term follow-up and predictors of clinical outcome in obsessive-compulsive patients treated with serotonin reuptake inhibitors and behavioral therapy. *Journal of Clinical Psychiatry*, **62**, 535–40.

American Psychiatric Association (2000). *Diagnostic and Statistical Manual of Mental Disorders, fourth edition*. American Psychiatric Association, Washington, DC.

Barzega G *et al.* (2001a). Gender-related distribution of personality disorders in a sample of patients with panic disorder. *European Psychiatry*, **16**, 173–9.

Barzega G *et al.* (2001b). Gender-related differences in the onset of panic disorder. *Acta Psychiatrica Scandinavica*, **103**, 189–95.

Becker ES *et al.* (2007). Epidemiology of specific phobia subtypes: findings from the Dresden Mental Health Study. *European Psychiatry*, **22**, 69–74.

Beekman AT *et al.* (1998). Anxiety disorders in later life: a report from the Longitudinal Aging Study Amsterdam. *International Journal of Geriatric Psychiatry*, **13**, 717–26.

Bekker MHJ *et al.* (2007). Anxiety Disorders: Sex differences in prevalence, degree, and background, but gender-neutral treatment. *Gender Medicine*, **4**, Supplement B, 178–93.

Bogetto F *et al.* (1999). Gender-related clinical differences in obsessive-compulsive disorder. *European Psychiatry*, **14**, 434–41.

Brady KT *et al.* (2000). Comorbidity of psychiatric disorders and posttraumatic stress disorder. *Journal of Clinical Psychiatry*, **61**, 22–32.

Breslau N and Anthony JC (2007). Gender differences in the sensitivity to posttraumatic stress disorder: An epidemiological study of urban young adults. *Journal of Abnormal Psychology*, **116**, 607–11.

Breslau N *et al.* (1997). Sex differences in posttraumatic stress disorder. *Archives of General Psychiatry*, **54**, 1044–8.

Bruce SE *et al.* (2005). Influence of psychiatric comorbidity on recovery and recurrence in generalized anxiety disorder, social phobia, and panic disorder: a 12-year prospective study. *American Journal of Psychiatry*, **162**, 1179–87.

Cameron OG *et al.* (1988). Menstrual fluctuation in the symptoms of panic anxiety. *Journal of Affective Disorders*, **15**, 169–74.

Castle DJ *et al.* (1995). Gender differences in obsessive compulsive disorder. *Australian and New Zealand Journal of Psychiatry*, **29**, 114–17.

Chung MC *et al.* (2007). Comorbidity and personality traits in patients with different levels of posttraumatic stress disorder following myocardial infarction. *Psychiatry Research*, **152**, 243–52.

Clayton AH *et al.* (2006). Sex differences in clinical presentation and response in panic disorder: pooled data from sertraline treatment studies. *Archives of Women's Mental Health*, **9**, 151–7.

Cohen LS *et al.* (1994). Postpartum course in women with preexisting panic disorder. *Journal of Clinical Psychiatry*, **55**, 289–92.

Cook BL *et al.* (1990). Anxiety and the menstrual cycle in panic disorder. *Journal of Affective Disorders*, **19**, 221–6.

Cox BJ *et al.* (1993). Gender effects and alcohol use in panic disorder with agoraphobia. *Behaviour Research and Therapy* **31**, 413–416.

Curtis GC *et al.* (1998). Specific fears and phobias. Epidemiology and classification. *British Journal of Psychiatry*, **173**, 212–17.

Davidson J *et al.* (2001). Efficacy of sertraline in preventing relapse of posttraumatic stress disorder: results of a 28-week double-blind, placebo-controlled study. *American Journal of Psychiatry*, **158**, 1974–81.

de Mathis MA *et al.* (2008). Obsessive-compulsive disorder: influence of age at onset on comorbidity patterns. *European Psychiatry*, **23**, 187–94.

Deckert J *et al.* (1999). Excess of high activity monoamine oxidase A gene promoter alleles in female patients with panic disorder. *Human Molecular Genetics*, **8**, 621–4.

Dick CL *et al.* (1994). Epidemiology of psychiatric disorders in Edmonton. *Panic disorder. Acta Psychiatrica Scandinavica Supplement*, **376**, 45–53.

Diniz JB *et al.* (2004). Impact of age at onset and duration of illness on the expression of comorbidities in obsessive-compulsive disorder. *Journal of Clinical Psychiatry*, **65**, 22–7.

Domschke K *et al.* (2007). Meta-analysis of COMT val158met in panic disorder: ethnic heterogeneity and gender specificity. *American Journal of Medical Genetics B: Neuropsychiatric Genetics*, **144B**, 667–3.

Domschke K *et al.* (2008). Influence of the catechol-O-methyltransferase val158met genotype on amygdala and prefrontal cortex emotional processing in panic disorder. *Psychiatry Research*, **163**, 13–20.

Eisen JL *et al.* (2006). Impact of obsessive-compulsive disorder on quality of life. *Comprehensive Psychiatry*, **47**, 270–5.

Francis JL *et al.* (2007). Characteristics and course of panic disorder and panic disorder with agoraphobia in primary care patients. *Primary Care Companion to the Journal of Clinical Psychiatry*, **9**, 173–9.

Freeman EW (2003). Premenstrual syndrome and premenstrual dysphoric disorder: definitions and diagnosis. *Psychoneuroendocrinology*, **28**(Suppl 3), 25–37.

Fullerton CS *et al.* (2001). Gender differences in posttraumatic stress disorder after motor vehicle accidents. *American Journal of Psychiatry*, **158**, 1486–91.

Gelernter J *et al.* (2004). Genome-wide linkage scan for loci predisposing to social phobia: evidence for a chromosome 16 risk locus. *American Journal of Psychiatry*, **161**, 59–66.

Gorman JM *et al.* (2002). New developments in the neurobiological basis of anxiety disorders. *Psychopharmacological Bulletin*, **36**(Suppl 2), 49–67.

Grant BF *et al.* (2006). The epidemiology of DSM-IV panic disorder and agoraphobia in the United States: results from the National Epidemiologic Survey on Alcohol and Related Conditions. *Journal of Clinical Psychiatry*, **67**, 363–74.

Greenberg PE *et al.* (1999). The economic burden of anxiety disorders in the 1990s. *Journal of Clinical Psychiatry*, **60**, 427–35.

Guler O *et al.* (2008a). The prevalence of panic disorder in pregnant women during the third trimester of pregnancy. *Comprehensive Psychiatry*, **49**, 154–8.

Guler O *et al.* (2008b). Course of panic disorder during the early postpartum period: a prospective analysis. *Comprehensive Psychiatry*, **49**, 30–4.

Hajduk A (2004). A search for psychobiological determinants of anxiety disorders. Annales Academiae Medicae Stetinensis **50**, 65–75.

Heron J *et al.* (2004). The course of anxiety and depression through pregnancy and the postpartum in a community sample. *Journal of Affective Disorders*, **80**, 65–73.

Hsiao MC *et al.* (2004). Premenstrual symptoms and premenstrual exacerbation in patients with psychiatric disorders. *Psychiatry and Clinical Neurosciences*, **58**, 186–90.

Jarvis CI *et al.* (2008). Management strategies for premenstrual syndrome/premenstrual dysphoric disorder. *Annals of Pharmacotherapy*, **42**, 967–78.

Kalra H *et al.* (2008). Caregiver burden in anxiety disorders. *Current Opinion in Psychiatry*, **21**, 70–3.

Kalus O *et al.* (1991). Desipramine treatment in panic disorder. *Journal of Affective Disorders*, **21**, 239–44.

Karayiorgou M *et al.* (1999). Family-based association studies support a sexually dimorphic effect of COMT and MAOA on genetic susceptibility to obsessive-compulsive disorder. *Biological Psychiatry*, **45**, 1178–89.

Kendler KS *et al.* (1992a). The genetic epidemiology of phobias in women. The interrelationship of agoraphobia, social phobia, situational phobia, and simple phobia. *Archives of General Psychiatry*, **49**, 273–81.

Kendler KS *et al.* (1992b). Generalized anxiety disorder in women. A population-based twin study. *Archives of General Psychiatry*, **49**, 267–72.

Kendler KS *et al.* (2001). Panic syndromes in a population-based sample of male and female twins. *Psychological Medicine*, **31**, 989–1000.

Kendler KS *et al.* (2007). The sources of co-morbidity between major depression and generalized anxiety disorder in a Swedish national twin sample. *Psychological Medicine*, **37**, 453–62.

Kessler RC *et al.* (1994). Lifetime and 12-month prevalence of DSM-III-R psychiatric disorders in the United States. Results from the National Comorbidity Survey. *Archives of General Psychiatry*, **51**, 8–19.

Kessler RC *et al.* (1995). Posttraumatic stress disorder in the National Comorbidity Survey. *Archives of General Psychiatry*, **52**, 1048–60.

Kessler RC *et al.* (2001). The epidemiology of generalized anxiety disorder. *Psychiatric Clinics of North America*, **24**, 19–39.

Kessler RC *et al.* (2005). Prevalence, severity, and comorbidity of 12-month DSM-IV disorders in the National Comorbidity Survey Replication. *Archives of General Psychiatry*, **62**, 617–27.

Kessler RC *et al.* (2006). The epidemiology of panic attacks, panic disorder, and agoraphobia in the National Comorbidity Survey Replication. *Archives of General Psychiatry*, **63**, 415–24.

Kessler RC *et al.* (2007). Lifetime prevalence and age-of-onset distributions of mental disorders in the World Health Organization's World Mental Health Survey Initiative. *World Psychiatry*, **6**, 168–76.

Kosten TR *et al.* (1987). Sustained urinary norepinephrine and epinephrine elevation in post-traumatic stress disorder. *Psychoneuroendocrinology*, **12**(1), 13–20.

Labad J *et al.* (2005). Female reproductive cycle and obsessive-compulsive disorder. *Journal of Clinical Psychiatry*, **66**, 428–35.

Labad J *et al.* (2008). Gender differences in obsessive-compulsive symptom dimensions. *Depression and Anxiety*, **25**(10), 832–8.

Latas M *et al.* (2006). Gender differences in psychopathologic features of agoraphobia with panic disorder. *Vojnosanitetski Pregled*, **63**, 569–74.

Lensi P *et al.* (1996). Obsessive-compulsive disorder. Familial-developmental history, symptomatology, comorbidity and course with special reference to gender-related differences. *British Journal of Psychiatry*, **169**, 101–7.

Leon AC *et al.* (1995). The social costs of anxiety disorders. *British Journal of Psychiatr*, **27**(Suppl), 19–22.

Lepine JP (2002). The epidemiology of anxiety disorders: prevalence and societal costs. *Journal of Clinical Psychiatry*, **63**(Suppl 14), 4–8.

Lochner C *et al.* (2004). Gender in obsessive-compulsive disorder: clinical and genetic findings. *European Neuropsychopharmacology*, **14**, 105–13.

Magee WJ *et al.* (1996). Agoraphobia, simple phobia, and social phobia in the National Comorbidity Survey. *Archives of General Psychiatry*, **53**, 159–68.

McFarlane AC *et al.* (1997). The acute stress response following motor vehicle accidents and its relation to PTSD. *Annals of the New York Academy of Sciences*, **821**, 437–41.

McLeod DR *et al.* (1993). The influence of premenstrual syndrome on ratings of anxiety in women with generalized anxiety disorder. *Acta Psychiatrica Scandinavica*, **88**, 248–51.

Meewisse ML *et al.* (2007). Cortisol and post-traumatic stress disorder in adults: systematic review and meta-analysis. *British Journal of Psychiatry*, **191**, 387–92.

Mellman TA *et al.* (1995). Nocturnal/daytime urine noradrenergic measures and sleep in combat-related PTSD. *Biological Psychiatry*, **38**, 174–9.

Michael T and Margraf J (2004). Epidemiology of anxiety disorders. *Psychiatry*, **3**, 2–6.

Mundo E *et al.* (1999). Effect of acute intravenous clomipramine and antiobsessional response to proserotonergic drugs: is gender a predictive variable? *Biological Psychiatry*, **45**, 290–4.

NCS-R (2007) *NCS-R Update Jun 17 2007: Lifetime prevalence of DSM-IV/WMH-CIDI disorders by sex and cohort.* http://www.hcp.med.harvard.edu/ncs/ftpdir/table_ncsr_LTprevgenderxage.pdf.

Northcott CJ and Stein MB (1994). Panic disorder in pregnancy. *Journal of Clinical Psychiatry*, **55**, 539–42.

Parker G and Hadzi-Pavlovic D (2001). Is any female preponderance in depression secondary to a primary female preponderance in anxiety disorders? *Acta Psychiatrica Scandinavica* **103**, 252–6.

Parker G and Hadzi-Pavlovic D (2004). Is the female preponderance in major depression secondary to a gender difference in specific anxiety disorders? *Psychological Medicine*, **34**, 461–70.

Peters L *et al.* (2006). Gender differences in the prevalence of DSM-IV and ICD-10 PTSD. *Psychological Medicine*, **36**, 81–9.

Phillips J *et al.* (2007). Rates of depressive and anxiety disorders in a residential mother-infant unit for unsettled infants. *Australian and New Zealand Journal of Psychiatry*, **41**, 836–42.

Pigott TA (2003). Anxiety disorders in women. *Psychiatric Clinics of North America*, **26**, 621–72.

Pinto A *et al.* (2006). The Brown Longitudinal Obsessive Compulsive Study: clinical features and symptoms of the sample at intake. *Journal of Clinical Psychiatry*, **67**, 703–11.

Rapee RM and Spence SH (2004). The etiology of social phobia: empirical evidence and an initial model. *Clinical Psychology Review*, **24**, 737–67.

Rasmusson AM *et al.* (2001). Increased pituitary and adrenal reactivity in premenopausal women with posttraumatic stress disorder. *Biological Psychiatry*, **50**, 965–77.

Resnick HS *et al.* (1995). Effect of previous trauma on acute plasma cortisol level following rape. *American Journal of Psychiatry*, **152**, 1675–7.

Ross LE and McLean LM (2006). Anxiety disorders during pregnancy and the postpartum period: A systematic review. *Journal of Clinical Psychiatry*, **67**, 1285–98.

Ruscio AM *et al.* (2008). Social fears and social phobia in the USA: results from the National Comorbidity Survey Replication. *Psychological Medicine*, **38**, 15–28.

Sheikh JI *et al.* (2002). Gender differences in panic disorder: findings from the National Comorbidity Survey. *American Journal of Psychiatry*, **159**, 55–8.

Simon NM *et al.* (2006). Preliminary support for gender differences in response to fluoxetine for generalized anxiety disorder. *Depression and Anxiety*, **23**, 373–6.

Smit F *et al.* (2006). Costs of nine common mental disorders: implications for curative and preventive psychiatry. *Journal of Mental Health Policy Economics*, **9**, 193–200.

Stein MB *et al.* (1989). Panic disorder and the menstrual cycle: panic disorder patients, healthy control subjects, and patients with premenstrual syndrome. *American Journal of Psychiatry*, **146**, 1299–303.

Stein MB *et al.* (1996). Childhood physical and sexual abuse in patients with anxiety disorders and in a community sample. *American Journal of Psychiatry*, **153**, 275–7.

Stein MB *et al.* (2005). COMT polymorphisms and anxiety-related personality traits. *Neuropsychopharmacology*, **30**, 2092–102.

Steinberg JR and Russo NF (2008). Abortion and anxiety: what's the relationship? *Social Science & Medicine*, **67**, 238–52.

Steiner M *et al.* (2005). Gender differences in clinical presentation and response to sertraline treatment of generalized anxiety disorder. *Human Psychopharmacology*, **20**, 3–13.

Stewart SE *et al.* (2006). Outcome predictors for severe obsessive-compulsive patients in intensive residential treatment. *Journal of Psychiatric Research*, **40**, 511–19.

Sutter-Dallay AL *et al.* (2004). Women with anxiety disorders during pregnancy are at increased risk of intense postnatal depressive symptoms: a prospective survey of the MATQUID cohort. *European Psychiatry*, **19**, 459–63.

Turk CL *et al.* (1998). An investigation of gender differences in social phobia. *Journal Anxiety Disorders*, **12**, 209–23.

van der Waals FW *et al.* (1993). Sex differences among recipients of benzodiazepines in Dutch general practice. *British Medical Journal*, **307**, 363–6.

Vulink NC *et al.* (2006). Female hormones affect symptom severity in obsessive-compulsive disorder. *International Clinical Psychopharmacology.*, **21**, 171–5.

Wang PS *et al.* (2005). Failure and delay in initial treatment contact after first onset of mental disorders in the National Comorbidity Survey Replication. *Archives of General Psychiatry*, **62**, 603–13.

Weissman MM *et al.* (1997). The cross-national epidemiology of panic disorder. *Archives of General Psychiatry*, **54**, 305–9.

Wenzel A *et al.* (2003). Prevalence of generalized anxiety at eight weeks postpartum. *Archives of Women's Mental Health*, **6**, 43–9.

Wenzel A *et al.* (2005). Anxiety symptoms and disorders at eight weeks postpartum. *Journal of Anxiety Disorders*, **19**, 295–311.

Williams KE and Koran LM (1997). Obsessive-compulsive disorder in pregnancy, the puerperium, and the premenstruum. *Journal of Clinical Psychiatry*, **58**, 330–4.

Wittchen HU *et al.* (1994). DSM-III-R generalized anxiety disorder in the National Comorbidity Survey. *Archives of General Psychiatry*, **51**, 355–64.

Wittchen HU (2002). Generalized anxiety disorder: prevalence, burden, and cost to society. *Depression and Anxiety*, **16**, 162–71.

Wittchen HU and Jacobi F (2005). Size and burden of mental disorders in Europe–a critical review and appraisal of 27 studies. *European Neuropsychopharmacology*, **15**, 357–76.

World Health Organization (1992). *Clinical Descriptions and Diagnostic Guidelines (ICD-10)*. World Health Organization, Geneva.

Yehuda R *et al.* (1992). Urinary catecholamine excretion and severity of PTSD symptoms in Vietnam combat veterans. *Journal of Nervous Mental Disease*, **180**, 321–5.

Yehuda R (2002). Current status of cortisol findings in post-traumatic stress disorder. *Psychiatric Clinics of North America*, **25**, 341–68.

Yonkers KA *et al.* (1998). Is the course of panic disorder the same in women and men? *American Journal of Psychiatry*, **155**, 596–602.

Yonkers KA *et al.* (2001). An eight-year longitudinal comparison of clinical course and characteristics of social phobia among men and women. *Psychiatric Services*, **52**, 637–43.

Yonkers KA *et al.* (2003). Chronicity, relapse, and illness–course of panic disorder, social phobia, and generalized anxiety disorder: findings in men and women from 8 years of follow-up. *Depression and Anxiety*, **17**, 173–9.

Zlotnick C *et al.* (2008). Childhood trauma, trauma in adulthood, and psychiatric diagnoses: results from a community sample. *Comprehensive Psychiatry*, **49**, 163–9.

CHAPTER 11

Depression in women

Jona Lewin

Introduction

Depression in women is common and has attracted increasing interest. It affects women disproportionately and besides the emotional suffering, it has a major impact on their ability to function in their various roles.

An analysis of the effect of depression on disability adjusted life years (DALYs) by Murray and Lopez (1996) showed that depression was the second leading cause of disease burden after ischaemic heart disease. However, depression proved to be the leading cause of disability for women worldwide. The most likely reasons are the disproportionate prevalence of depression and the severity of its impact on a woman's life course.

Possible reasons for the gender difference in depression prevalence could include a greater number of first-onset episodes, longer duration of depressive episodes, a greater recurrence of depression in women than in men, or a combination of these factors.

This question was addressed by three large epidemiological studies conducted in the United States, which showed that the greater number of first-onset depressive episodes in women and not gender differences in the duration or recurrence of depression is responsible for the gender difference (Eaton *et al.* 1997; Keller and Shapiro 1981; Kessler *et al.* 1993). It can therefore be concluded that women have greater rates of first-onset depression than men, but once they are depressed, both have episodes of similar duration and are equally likely to have recurrent depressive episodes.

The subsequent question arises why do women have greater rates of first-onset depression than men? This is most likely based on the fact that there are significant biological- and socialization-related differences between women and men. Women experience certain stressors more frequently than men and women may also react differently to these stressors, either due to different biological or socialization factors.

In the rest of this chapter I will describe epidemiological evidence about the difference in prevalence of depression, examine the phases in the life cycle of a woman, and consider social, psychological, and biological aetiological factors.

Epidemiology—size of problem

The lifetime prevalence of depression in women has been found to be consistently greater than in men in a number of countries and cultures, including the United States, Puerto Rico, New Zealand, France, Iceland, Taiwan, Korea, and Germany (Weissman *et al.* 1996).

The Office of Population Census and Surveys (OPCS) survey of 10 000 adults living in private households in the United Kingdom found that women were more likely than men to suffer from a neurotic health problem (Meltzer *et al.* 1995).

These findings were confirmed by Jenkins *et al.* (1997), who carried out a National Psychiatric Morbidity Survey of Great Britain; 10 108 of 13 000 selected adults were interviewed. The overall one-week prevalence of neurotic disorder was 12.3% in males and 19.5% in females. Unmarried and postmarital groups had a high rate of disorder, as did single parents and people living on their own. Unemployment was strongly associated with neurotic disorder. Individual neurotic disorders were all significantly commoner in women, with the exception of panic disorder.

The National Comorbidity Survey (NCS) in the United States (Kessler *et al.* 1993) showed that the lifetime prevalence of a major depressive disorder was 21.3% for women and 12.7% for men. These findings were confirmed in the NCS Replication (NCS-R) study, which showed similar findings (Kessler *et al.* 2003).

The very large, six-nation European study DEPRES (Depressive Research in European Society) (Angst *et al.* 2002) establishes the sex difference at the level of both major depressive disorder (female:male = 1.7) and of the various depressive symptoms. Very few studies have shown ratios close to unity, and they have usually been in restricted populations.

The largest study, which found minimal gender differences, was the North-Trondelag Health Study (HUNT), which was carried out in Norway on 92 100 individuals. They found minimal gender differences in dimensional depression scores and in prevalence rates of depression. Both these measures were found to increase continuously with age in both genders (Stordal *et al.* 2001).

Life cycle of women and depression

A number of studies have shown that at certain periods during the life cycle of a woman the prevalence of depression is increased. These periods have been identified as the postpubertal, perimenstrual, perinatal, and perimenopausal phases.

Postpubertal phase

Some studies of depression in children have shown that prepubertal boys and girls have similar levels of depressive disorder, while other studies have shown that prepubertal boys had greater rates of depression than prepubertal girls (Nolen-Hoeksema and Girgus 1994; Twenge and Nolen-Hoeksema 2002). Studies of postpubertal children showed that from age 12 onwards the rate of depression in girls increased substantially whereas the rates of depression in boys increased slightly or not at all (Angold *et al.* 1998; Twenge and Nolen-Hoeksema 2002). However, the rates of substance abuse and criminal behaviour increased in boys from the age of 12 onwards to a much greater degree than in girls (Angold *et al.* 1998).

Angold *et al.* (1999) investigated whether the morphological changes associated with puberty or the hormonal changes were more strongly associated with increased rates of depression in adolescent girls. The results showed that the increased rate of depression in adolescent girls was not related to the morphological changes which occurred during puberty and the authors therefore concluded that the causal factors of the increase in depression in females during the postpubertal phase are most likely associated with changes in androgen and oestrogen levels.

Perimenstrual phase

Henshaw (2007) defined perimenstrual syndrome as any constellation of psychological and physical symptoms that recur regularly in the luteal phase of the menstrual cycle, remit for at least one week in the follicular phase, and cause distress and functional impairment. The characteristics of functional impairment have been reported in various studies (Hylan *et al.* 1999; Pearlstein *et al.* 2000). However, the precise relationship between premenstrual syndrome/premenstrual dysphoric disorder and mood disorder has remained unclear (Henshaw 2007). Although premenstrual syndrome responds well to selective serotonin reuptake inhibitors (SSRIs), the onset of depression is more rapid than that of major depression (Kim *et al.* 2004).

The close temporal relationship between the symptoms of the perimenstrual syndrome and the menstrual cycle suggests a strong biological aetiological factor. The hypothalamic–pituitary–adrenal (HPA) axis, the gamma-aminobutyric acid (GABA) system, the serotonergic system, and the endogenous opioids have been implicated in the aetiology of the perimenstrual syndrome (Halbreich 2003). Craig *et al.* (2004) have established that oestrogens can affect the cholinergic, serotonergic, dopaminergic, and noradrenergic systems (Craig *et al.* 2004). I will discuss biological factors of depression in women in more detail later in this chapter.

Perinatal phase

About 50–80% of woman experience 'postpartum blues' within the first few days of giving birth. This condition is characterized by no more than two weeks of mild depressive symptoms of mood instability, tearful anxiety, and insomnia (Ahokas *et al.* 2001).

Perinatal depression encompasses depressive episodes, which occur either during pregnancy or during the first 12 months after delivery. A population study (Andersson *et al.* 2006) found that depression was more prevalent during mid-gestation than postpartum. In a population-based sample of 1555 women in Sweden, anxiety and depression were more prevalent during mid-trimester (~30%) than postpartum (16%). A history of psychiatric disorder, being single, and obesity were risk factors for new-onset postpartum psychiatric disorder.

A systematic review published in 2004 (Bennett *et al.* 2004) showed the prevalence at first, second, and third trimesters to be 7.5%, 12.8%, and 12%, respectively. A more recent systematic review and meta-analysis of perinatal depression found the prevalence of depression in the first trimester at 11.0%, which dropped to 8.5% in the second and third trimester. After delivery, the prevalence of depression rose to its highest level in the third month at 12.9%. In the fourth through seventh months postpartum the prevalence of depression declined slightly, staying in the range of 9.9–10.6%, after which it declined to 6.5% (Gavin *et al.* 2005).

Apart from the effects on psychological health, antenatal depressive symptoms have been associated with increased risk of obstetric interventions such as epidural analgesia, operative deliveries, and admissions to neonatal units (Chung *et al.* 2001).

Postnatal depression has been associated with lower quality interaction between mothers and their infant (Stein *et al.* 1991), with subsequent greater child insecurity in attachment relationships (Marmorstein *et al.* 2004) and higher levels of psychiatric disturbances amongst their children (Murray and Stein 1989).

Perimenopause and menopause

The perimenopause has been described as a 'tumultuous and distressing endocrine event' (Taylor 2002) with oscillations between episodes of hypo-oestrogenism and hyperoestrogenism (Shideler *et al.* 1989). Pior (1998) demonstrated that oestrogen variability is significantly higher in the perimenopause than in any other natural reproductive phase in women, including puberty.

Epidemiological studies found an increase in depressive symptoms in perimenopausal women compared with premenopausal women (Bromberger *et al.* 2001, 2003).

The results of these studies were confirmed in findings from the following prospective studies. Harlow *et al.* (2003) reported an association between menopausal transition and increased risk for clinical depression, particularly in women with a history of depression. Another longitudinal study found a significantly greater risk for episodes of clinical depression around menopause than when the women were premenopausal (Schmidt *et al.* 2004). Freeman *et al.* (2004) found that women in the menopausal transition were up to three times more likely to report depressive symptoms than premenopausal women.

In a longitudinal eight-year prospective cohort study of 231 women with no history of depression at the beginning of the study, Freeman *et al.* (2004) found the transition to menopause and its changing hormonal milieu were strongly associated with new onset of depressed mood.

Cohen *et al.* (2006) examined the association between the menopausal transition and onset of first lifetime episode of depression among women with no history of previous depressive episodes. In a longitudinal, prospective study of 460 subjects, after adjusting for age at study enrolment and history of negative life events, they found that premenopausal women with no lifetime

history of major depression who entered the menopause were twice as likely to develop significant depressive symptoms as women who remained premenopausal. The increased risk for depression was somewhat greater in women with self-reported vasomotor symptoms.

Bebbington *et al.* (1998) carried out a prospective study on 9792 subjects. Social variables, which were likely to contribute to a postmenopausal decline in depressive disorders, were controlled in logistic regression analysis. The results showed that there was a clear reversal of the sex difference in prevalence of depression in those over the age of 55. This could not be explained for in terms of differential effects of marital status, child care, or employment status. This study adds to the view that sex difference in prevalence of depression is less apparent in later middle age. This could largely be due to biological causes or due to a combination of biological factors and social factors other than those controlled for in this study.

Aetiological factors

The interpretation of the evidence for specific biological or social vulnerabilities to depression in women can be ideologically driven, as the choice between social, psychological, and biological causes can be represented as the choice between seeing women either as socially disadvantaged, or as inherently vulnerable with all the associated implications of inferiority.

However, there is likely to be interplay between these two groups. Biological factors may influence psychological and social factors and vice versa. For instance, in the perinatal phase a woman is more likely to react with depressed mood to psychological and social stressors than at other times in her life. There is considerable research evidence of biological, psychological, and social aetiological factors, and the interaction of these factors.

Biological factors

The strong association between mood disturbance and the transitions in women's lives, which is characterized by hormonal shifts, suggests a causal link. It is well established that oestradiol and progesterone modulate the neurotransmitter and neuroendocrine systems, including those involving monoamines.

A number of studies have examined the relationship between changing hormone levels in women and mood disorder. In this context oestrogen has been investigated most extensively. Oestrogen is a term used to include the three major hormones oestradiol, oestriol, and oestrone. Oestradiol is the most potent oestrogen and the predominant form circulating in the body from menarche to menopause (Shervin 1997). Premenopausally, 95% of oestradiol is produced by the ovaries and 5% from fat cells.

After menopause, oestrone is partly converted to oestradiol, but this amounts to much less oestradiol than was available premenopausally (Lobo 1997; Steiner et al. 2003). Oestriol is produced by the placenta. The most significant source of oestrogen after the menopause when ovarian function fails is the weaker oestrogen oestrone, which is produced in fat cells. The menopause has been described as 'a period of low effective oestrogen' (Douma et al. 2005).

Oestrogen affects more than 400 bodily functions. Among other brain functions oestrogen increases the rate of degradation of monoamine oxidase and intraneural serotonin transport, both of which serve to increase serotonin availability in the synapse, and as a result enhance mood (Carretti et al. 2005).

Some studies on the relationship of gonadal hormones and depression in women have shown that some women develop depression or experience an exacerbation of an existing depression during periods when hormone levels change substantially. These periods include the premenstrual phase of the menstrual cycle, during the postpartum period, and periods of unpredictable ovulation, which include puberty and perimenopause. (Lobo 1997; Shervin 1997; McEwen 1999; Carretti et al. 2005).

Kumar and Robson (1984) and Rubinow et al. (1998) have suggested that oestrogen may provide protection against depression. They reported an increased incidence of depressive symptoms during periods associated with low oestrogen concentrations, e.g. premenstrual and postpartum. However it has also been reported that depression may be equally high at times of high oestrogen concentration, such as the antenatal period (Evans et al. 2001). Furthermore, there is some evidence that the prevalence of depression decreases postmenopausally, at a time when oestrogen levels are significantly reduced (Kessler et al. 1993; Bebbington et al. 1998).

It has been proposed that the precipitous drop in oestrogen following delivery triggers depression (Deakin 1989; Gregoire et al. 1996; Ahokas et al. 2001). It has also been suggested that women with a history of depression are at increased risk for the mood destabilizing effects of gonadal steroids and therefore postnatal depression (Bloch et al. 2000).

Studies on women with polycystic ovary syndrome have been carried out in order to investigate the role of oestrogen in depression. Polycystic ovary syndrome is a common and pervasive endocrine disorder with varied presentation and usually reduced oestrogen production. The common clinical features include hirsuitism, infertility, menstrual disturbance, and obesity. Several studies have established that women with polycystic ovary syndrome are more likely to experience symptoms of depression than comparison healthy groups. (Elsenbruch et al. 2003; Weiner et al. 2004; Hollinrake et al. 2005; Lane 2006).

Studies, which tried to identify specific features of polycystic ovary syndrome, which might be the cause of depression, have found mixed results. Neither high androgen levels (Rasgon et al. 2003; Hollinrake et al. 2005), hirsuitism (Keegan et al. 2003), or infertility (McCook 2002; Himelein and Thatcher 2006) were found to significantly correlate with depression among women with polycystic ovary syndrome. In one study, higher free testosterone levels were associated with more positive mood states (Weiner et al. 2004). Higher body mass was associated with greater depression in one study (Rasgon et al. 2003), but unrelated to depression in another (McCook 2002).

It has also been suggested that oestrogen may have a role as an antidepressant. However, methodological difficulties have affected the few studies in this area. These include small number of subjects and the lack of control groups. In postpartum depression, oestrogen therapy may be useful both as prophylaxis in vulnerable individuals (Sichel et al. 1995) and as treatment (Klaiber et al. 1979; Gregoire et al. 1996). There is also some evidence that women taking oestrogen replacement therapy may respond better to fluoxetine (Schneider et al. 1997).

In the perimenopause, oestrogen replacement therapy has been found to be effective in reducing mild depressive symptoms (Epperson et al. 1999) and it has been reported to be an effective treatment for depression (Schmidt et al. 2000; Soares et al. 2001). However, it is difficult to determine from these studies whether the oestrogen is treating menopausal symptoms, such as sleep deprivation and anergia, or the depression per se.

According to Cutter et al. (2003) there is currently little evidence to suggest that oestrogen is a useful treatment for depression during the menopause or at any other time.

Social and psychological factors

Social adversity and chronic stress

During the last 30 years there have been significant changes in family structures across Western Europe with divorce and remarriage rates increasing. Findings from the 1998 General Household Survey in the United Kingdom show that 38% of births were outside marriage compared with 26% 10 years earlier. Nevertheless, 61% of the 1998 births were registered jointly by parents living in the same address.

Between 1971 and 1990, the number of divorced and separated women with children rose from 290 000 to 650 000, and the number of lone mothers from 90 000 to 390 000. In the late 1980s, European figures showed that the United Kingdom had a lone parent rate of 17%, which was amongst the highest in Europe (Millar 1997).

Targosz et al. (2003) carried out a study on 5281 women and found that lone mothers had prevalence rates of depressive episode of 7%, about three times higher than any other group. The milder condition, mixed anxiety/depression, was also increased in frequency. These increased rates of depressive conditions were no longer apparent after controlling for measures of social disadvantage, stress, and isolation.

Lone mothers tend to suffer higher rates of material disadvantage than mothers who are in a relationship (Targosz et al. 2003). Poverty has been associated with a number of chronic uncontrollable negative life conditions, including inadequate housing, dangerous neighbourhoods, and financial uncertainties. The stresses of poverty can undermine parenting skills, increase relationship conflicts, reduce self-esteem, and undermine coping strategies. There is also an increased risk of a number of acute stressors, including exposure to crime and violence and physical and sexual assault (Belle and Doucet 2003). One study of low-income women in the United States showed that 83% of these women had a history of physical or sexual abuse (Bassuk et al. 1998). Heneghan et al. (1998) confirmed these findings in a study of inner-city mothers. They reported that poor financial status, poor health status, or activity limitation due to illness were associated with higher levels of depressive symptoms.

Belle and Doucet (2003) showed that poverty is the one stressor most consistently correlated with depression in women. Depressive symptoms were more common among people with low incomes, particularly mothers with young children.

Weich et al. (2001) investigated gender difference in rates of the most common mental disorders, anxiety and depression, on 9947 subjects in a seven-year, population-based cohort study. The odds ratio for the gender difference in the future prevalence of common mental disorders was 1.92 (95% confidence interval: 1.75–210).

They also found that gender differences in common mental disorders were not explained by differences in the number or type of social roles occupied by men and women, or by reverse causality. They suggested that further studies should consider characteristics of social roles, such as demand, control, and reward.

Other studies have pointed to the importance of social factors, as the sex ratio for depression is not universally maintained across all sociodemographic categories. It is, for instance, much more marked in married than in never-married women (Bebbington et al. 1981; Weissman and Klerman 1977; Lindeman et al. 2000,) and young married women looking after small children appear to be particularly at risk, at least in some societies (Brown and Harris 1978, Ensel 1982).

However, marital status has different associations with affective disorders in different cultures. Married women are at low risk of depressive disorder in Mediterranean countries (Mavreas et al. 1986; Vazquez-Barquero et al. 1987), in rural New Zealand (Romans-Clarkson et al. 1988), and among British Orthodox Jews (Lowenthal et al. 1995). These societies all accord a high value to the home-making role of women. However, irrespective of cultural background, unsupported mothers appear to be at particular risk of depression (Targosz et al. 2003).

It is therefore important to take into account that not only are social variables important in influencing the sex ratio for depression, but the association with sociodemographic factors is itself affected by more subtle sociocultural influences. The pervasiveness of the sex ratio can be seen as a reflection of the all-pervading feature of social disadvantage experienced by women worldwide in different communities.

Life events

A number of studies have shown a clear relationship between the experience of stressful life events and onset of depression (Brown and Harris 1978; Mazure 1998). Several studies have tried to establish whether women experience more frequent or more severe life events or are more sensitive to the depressive effects of life events. Some studies found that women experience more negative life events than men (Brown and Birley 1968; Bebbington et al. 1991), others found no gender difference in life events occurrence (Uhlenhuth and Paykel 1973; Perris 1984), while some found that the risk for depression following life events is greater for women than for men (Uhlenhuth and Paykell 1973; Kessler and McLeod 1984; Nazroo et al. 1997; Maciejewski et al. 2001). Other studies found that women experience certain kind of negative life events more often than men (Wagner and Compas 1990; Weiss *et al.* 1999).

A study by Maciejewski *et al.* (2001), who analysed data from a nationwide community-based sample of 1024 men and 1800 women, found no gender differences in exposure to a number of stressful life events. However, women were approximately three times more likely than men to experience major depression in the wake of a stressful life event. It has been suggested that certain cognitive characteristics in women may contribute to this increased stress reactivity in women (Abramson *et al.* 2002).

The difference in reactivity to life events could be based on gender-related biological predisposing factors. However, there is also evidence that women are more likely than men to have had previous adverse experiences, which can act as vulnerability factors to depression.

A Finnish population study (Veijola *et al.* 1998) showed that a disturbed mother–child relationship and neurotic symptoms in childhood are stronger predisposing factors to depression in women than in men.

Women are at greater risk of suffering sexual and physical abuse, which includes child sexual abuse, rape, and male partner violence (Koss *et al.* 2003). Sexual and physical abuse tends to occur at various points across the lifespan. Prior victimization increases the risk of repeat victimization and adolescent victimization is the strongest risk factor of continued victimization (Koss *et al.* 2003).

Abuse is a potent risk factor for depression both immediately after the abuse and throughout the survivors' lifetime (Weiss *et al.* 1999). The National Women's Study (Saunders *et al.* 1999) found that women who had been the victim of completed rape in childhood had a lifetime prevalence of depression of 52%, compared to 27% in non-victimized women. A meta-analyses of 18 studies of depression and intimate violence found that mean prevalence rates of depression among abused women was 48% (Golding 1999). It has been concluded that childhood physical abuse is the strongest predictor of adult depression in all ethnic groups after controlling for background characteristics that are risk factors for both abuse and depression (Dube *et al.* 2001; Oddone-Paolucci *et al.* 2001).

Another vulnerability factor for women is the affiliative style of relationships, as women tend to have a stronger affiliative style in their social relationships than men. This style of social relationships includes close emotional communication and intimate personal relationships. This has been attributed to biological factors as well as gender role socialization (Feingold 1994). Although gender differences in affiliative style are apparent before puberty, they tend to intensify during pubertal transition (Maccoby 1990). Adolescent girls tend to spend more time talking than their male peers and with increasing age their conversations reflect an increasing interpersonal focus (Raffaelli and Duckett 1989).

It has been suggested that this process of gender role socialization may prepare adolescent girls for caregiving roles, but at the same time the pubertal intensification in affiliative orientation may sensitize postpubertal girls to the depressogenic effect of certain negative life events, and in particular events that represent conflicts, breaches, or losses within interpersonal relationships (Cyranowski *et al.* 2000).

Conclusions

The increased prevalence of depression amongst women compared to men and the heightened risk at various phases in the life cycle of women has been well documented. A number of studies have tried to establish the responsible aetiological factors for the increased rates of depression. No definite factor has been identified and it is likely that a combination of biological, social, and psychological factors interact to contribute to the increased rates of depression. Attempts to prevent and treat depressive episodes in women need to focus on a wide range of biological, social, and psychological risk factors.

References

Abramson LY *et al.* (2002). Cognitive vulnerability-stress models of depression in a self-regulatory and psychological context. In: IH Gotlib and CL Hammen (eds) *Handbook of Depression*, 268–94. Guilford Press, New York.

Ahokas A *et al.* (2001). Estrogen deficiency in severe postpartum depression: successful treatment with sublingual physiological 17beta-estradiol: a preliminary study. *Journal of Clinical Psychiatry*, **62**, 332–6.

Andersson L *et al.* (2006). Depression and anxiety during pregnancy and six months postpartum: a follow-up study. *Acta Obstatrica Gynecologica Scandivanvica*, **85**, 937–44.

Angold A *et al.* (1998). Puberty and depression: the roles of age, pubertal status, and pubertal timing. *Psychological Medicine*, **28**, 51–61.

Angold A *et al.* (1999). Pubertal changes in hormone levels and depression in girls. *Psychological Medicine*, **29**, 1043–53.

Angst J *et al.* (2002). Gender differences in depression: epidemiological findings from the European Depression I and II Studies. *European Archives of Psychiatry and Clinical Neuroscience*, **252**, 201–9.

Bassuk E *et al.* (1998). Prevalence of mental health and substance use disorders among homeless and low-income housed mothers. *American Journal of Psychiatry*, **155**, 1561–4.

Bebbington P *et al.* (1981). The epidemiology of mental disorders in Camberwell. *Psychological Medicine*, **11**, 561–80.

Bebbington PE *et al.* (1991). Adversity in groups with an increased risk of minor affective disorder. *British Journal of Psychiatry*, **158**, 33–48.

Bebbington PE *et al.* (1998). The influence of age and sex on the prevalence of depressive conditions: report from the National Survey of Psychiatric Morbidity. *Psychological Medicine*, **28**, 9–19.

Belle D and Doucet J (2003). Poverty, inequality, and discrimination as sources of depression among U.S. women. *Psychology of Women Quarterly*, **27**, 101–13.

Bennett HA *et al.* (2004). Prevalence of depression during pregnancy: a systematic review. *Obstetrics and Gynecology*, **103**, 698–709.

Bloch M *et al.* (2000). Effects of gonadal steroids in women with a history of postpartum depression. *American Journal of Psychiatry*, **157**, 924–30.

Bromberger JT *et al.* (2001). Psychological distress and natural menopause: a multiethnic community study. *American Journal of Public Health*, **91**, 1435–42.

Bromberger JT *et al.* (2003). Persistent mood symptoms in a multiethnic community cohort of pre- and peri-menopausal women. *American Journal of Epidemiology*, **158**, 347–56.

Brown GW and Birley J (1968). Crises and life changes and the onset of schizophrenia. *Journal of Health and Social Behaviour*, **9**, 203–14.

Brown GW and Harris T (1978). *Social Origins of Depression*. Tavistock, London.

Carretti N *et al.* (2005). Serum fluctuations of total and free tryptophan levels during the menstrual cycle are related to gonadotrophins and reflect brain serotonin utilization. *Human Reproduction*, **20**, 1548–53.

Chung TK *et al.* (2001). Antepartum depressive symptomatology is associated with adverse obstetric and neonatal outcomes. *Psychosomatic Medicine*, **63**, 830–4.

Cohen LS *et al.* (2006). Risk for new onset of depression during the menopausal transition: The Harvard study of moods and cycles. *Archives of General Psychiatry*, **63**, 385–90.

Craig M *et al.* (2004). Oestrogens, brain function and neuropsychiatric disorders. *Current Opinion in Psychiatry*, **17**, 209–14.

Cutter WJ *et al.* (2003). Oestrogen, brain function, and neuropsychiatric disorders. *Journal of Neurology, Neurosurgery and Psychiatry*, **74**, 837–40.

Cyranowski JM *et al.* (2000). Adolescent onset of the gender difference in life time rates of major depression: A theoretical model. *Archives of General Psychiatry*, **57**, 21–7.

Deakin JFW (1989). Relevance of hormone CNS interactions to psychological changes in the puerperium. In: R Kuma and IF Brockington (eds) *Motherhood and Mental Illness 2: Causes and Consequences*, pp. 113–32. Butterworth, London.

Douma SL *et al.* (2005). Estrogen-related mood disorders. Reproductive life cycle factors. *Advances in Nursing Science*, **28**, 364–75.

Dube SR *et al.* (2001). Child abuse, household dysfunction, and the risk of attempted suicide throughout the life span: findings form the adverse childhood experience study. *Journal of the American Medical Association*, **286**, 3089–96.

Eaton W *et al.* (1997). Natural history of Diagnostic Interview Schedule/DSM-IV Major Depression. *Archives of General Psychiatry*, **54**, 993–9.

Elsenbruch S *et al.* (2003). Quality of life, psychosocial wellbeing, and sexual satisfaction in women with polycystic ovary syndrome. *Journal of Clinical Endocrinology and Matabolism*, **88**, 5801–7.

Ensel WM (1982). The role of age in the relationship of gender and marital status to depression. *Journal of Nervous and Mental Disease*, **170**, 536–43.

Epperson CN *et al.* (1999). Gonadal steroids in the treatment of mood disorders. *Psychosomatic Medicine*, **61**, 676–97.

Evans J *et al.* (2001). Cohort study of depressed mood during pregnancy and after childbirth. *British Medical Journal*, **343**, 257–60.

Feingold A (1994). Gender differences in personality: a meta-analysis. *Psychological Bulletin*, **116**, 429–56.

Freeman EW *et al.* (2004). hormones and menopausal status as predictors of depression in women in transition to menopause. *Archives of General Psychiatry*, **61**, 62–70.

Gavin NI *et al.* (2005). Perinatal depression: a systematic review of prevalence and incidence. *Obstetrics and Gynecology*, **106**, 1071–83.

Golding J (1999). Intimate partner violence as a risk factor for mental disorders: a meta-analysis. *Journal of Family Violence*, **14**, 99–132.

Gregoire AJP *et al.* (1996). Transdermal oestrogen for treatment of severe postnatal depression. *Lancet*, **347**, 930–3.

Halbreich U (2003). The etiology, biology, and evolving pathology of premenstrual syndromes. *Psychoneuroendocrinology*, **28**, 1–99.

Harlow BL *et al.* (2003). Depression and its influence on reproductive endocrine and menstrual cycle markers associated with perimenopause. *Archives of General Psychiatry*, **20**, 29–36.

Heneghan AM *et al.* (1998). Depressive symptoms in inner-city mothers of young children; who is at risk? *Pediatrics*, **102**, 1394–400.

Henshaw CA (2007). PMS: diagnosis, aetiology, assessment and management. *Advances in Psychiatric Treatment*, **13**, 139–46.

Himelein MJ and Thatcher SS (2006). Polycystic ovary syndrome: a review. *Obstetrical and Gynecological Review*, **61**, 723–32.

Hollinrake EM *et al.* (2005). Increased risk of depression in women with polycystic ovary syndrome. In: *Proceedings of the 61st Annual Meeting of the American Society for Reproductive Medicine, 15–19 October, 2005.* Montreal, Canada.

Hylan TR *et al.* (1999). The impact of premenstrual symptomatology on functioning and treatment-seeking behaviour: experience form the United States, United Kingdom, and France. *Journal of Women's Health and Gender-Based Medicine*, **8**, 1043–52.

Jenkins R *et al.* (1997). The National Psychiatric Morbidity Surveys of Great Britain – initial findings from the Household Survey. *Psychological Medicine*, **27**, 775–89.

Keegan A *et al.* (2003). 'Hirsuitism': a psychological analysis. *Journal of Health Psychology*, **8**, 327–45.

Keller M and Shapiro R (1981). Major depressive disorder: Initial results from a one year prospective naturalistic follow-up study. *Journal of Nervous Mental Disorders*, **169**, 761–8.

Kessler R and McLeod J (1984). Sex differences in vulnerability to undesirable life events. *American Sociological Review*, **49**, 620–31.

Kessler RC *et al.* (1993). Sex and depression in the National Comorbidity Survey I: Lifetime prevalence, chronicity, and recurrence. *Journal of Affective Disorders*, **29**, 85–96.

Kessler RC, Berglund P, Demler O *et al.* (2003). The epidemiology of major depressive disorder. Results from the National Comorbidity Survey Replication (NCS-R). *JAMA*, **289**, 3095–105.

Kim DR *et al.* (2004). Premenstrual dysphoric disorder and psychiatric co-morbidity. *Archives of Women's Mental Health*, **7**, 37–47.

Klaiber EL *et al.* (1979). Estrogen therapy for sever persistent depressions in women. *Archive of General Psychiatry*, **36**, 550–4.

Koss MP *et al.* (2003). Depression and PTSD in survivors of male violence: Research and training initiatives to facilitate recovery. *Psychology of Women Quarterly*, **27**, 130–42.

Kumar R and Robson KM (1984). A prospective study of emotional disorders in childbearing women. *British Journal of Psychiatry*, **144**, 35–47.

Lane DE (2006). Polycystic ovary syndrome and its differential diagnosis. *Obstetric and Gynecology Survey*, **61**, 125–35.

Lindeman S *et al.* (2000). The 12-month prevalence and risk factors for major depressive episode in Finland: representative sample of 5993 adults. *Acta Psychiatrica Scandinavica*, **102**, 178–84.

Lobo RA (1997). The postmenopausal state and estrogen deficiency. In: R Lindsay et al. (eds) *Estrogens and Antiestrogens*. Lippincott-Raven, Philadelphia, PA.

Lowenthal K *et al.* (1995). Gender and depression in Anglo-Jewry. *Psychological Medicine*, **25**, 1051–64.

Maccoby E (1990). Gender and relationships: a developmental account. *American Psychologist*, **45**, 513–20.

Maciejewski PK *et al.* (2001). Sex differences in event-related risk for major depression. *Psychological Medicine*, **31**, 593–604.

Marmorstein NR *et al.* (2004). Psychiatric disorders among offspring of depressed mothers: associations with paternal psychopathology. *American Journal of Psychiatry*, **161**, 1588–94.

Mavreas VG *et al.* (1986). Prevalence of psychiatric disorder in Athens: a community study. *Social Psychiatry*, **21**, 172–81.

Mazure CM (1998). Life stressors as risk factors in depression. *Clinical Psychology: Science and Practice*, **5**, 291–313.

McCook JG (2002). 'The influence of hyperandrogenism, obesity and infertility on the psychosocial health and well-being of women with polycystic ovary syndrome.' Dissertation. University of Michigan, Ann Arbor, MI.

McEwen BS and Alves SE (1999). Estrogen actions in the central nervous system. *Endocrinology Review*, **20**, 279–307.

Meltzer H *et al.* (1995). *OPCS Survey of Psychiatric Morbidity in Great Britain, Report 1.* HMSO, London.

Millar J (1997). State, family and personal responsibility: the changing balance for the lone mothers in the UK. In: C Ungerson and M Kember (eds) *Women and Social Policy*, 2nd edition. pp. 146–62. Macmillan, Basingstoke.

Murray L and Stein A (1989). The effects of postnatal depression on the infant. *Baillieres Clinical Obstetrics and Gynaecology*, **3**, 921–33.

Murray CJ and Lopez AD (1996). *The global burden of disease: a comprehensive assessment of mortality and disability from diseases, injuries, and risk factors in 1990 and projected to 2020.* Harvard University Press, Boston, MA.

Nazroo JY *et al.* (1997). Gender differences in the onset of depression following a shared life event: a study of couples. *Psychological Medicine*, **27**, 9–19.

Nolen-Hoeksema S and Girgus JS (1994). The emergence of gender differences in depression in adolescence. *Psychological Bulletin*, **115**, 424–43.

Oddone-Paolucci E *et al.* (2001). A meta-analysis of the published research on the effects of child sexual abuse. *Journal of Psychology*, **135**, 17–36.

Pearlstein TB *et al.* (2000). Psycho-social functioning in women with premenstrual dysphoric disorder before and after treatment with sertraline or placebo. *Journal of Clinical Psychiatry*, **61**, 101–9.

Perris H (1984). Life events and depression, part 1: effect of sex, age, and civil status. *Journal of Affective Disorders*, **7**, 11–24.

Prior JC (1998). Perimenopause: the complex endocrinology of the menopausal transition. *Endocrinology Review*, **19**, 397–428.

Raffaelli M and Duckett E (1989). "We were just talking...": conversations in early adolescence. *Journal of Youth and Adolescence*, **18**, 567–82.

Rasgon NL *et al.* (2003). Depression in women with polycystic ovary syndrome: clinical and biochemical correlates. *Journal of Affective Disorders*, **74**, 299–304.

Romans-Clarkson SE *et al.* (1988). Marriage, motherhood and psychiatric morbidity inNew Zealand. *Psychological Medicine*, **18**, 983–90.

Rubinow DR *et al.* (1998). Estrogen-serotonin interactions: implications for affective regulation. *Biological Psychiatry*, **44**, 839–50.

Saunders B *et al.* (1999). Prevalence, case characteristics, and long-term psychological correlates of child rape among women: A national survey. *Child Maltreatment*, **4**, 187–200.

Schmidt PJ *et al.* (2000). Estrogen replacement in perimenopause related depression: a preliminary report. *American Journal of Obstetrics and Gynecology*, **183**, 414–20.

Schmidt PJ *et al.* (2004). A longitudinal evaluation of the relationship between reproductive status and mood in perimenopausal women. *American Journal of Psychiatry*, **161**, 2238–44.

Schneider LS *et al.* (1997). Estrogen replacement and response to fluoxetine in a multicentre geriatric depression trial. Fluoxetine Collaborative study Group. *American Journal of Geriatric Psychiatry*, **5**, 97–106.

Shervin BB (1997). Estrogenic effects on the central nervous system: clinical aspects. In: R Lindsey *et al.* (eds) *Estrogens and Antiestrogens*, pp. 75–87. Lippincott-Raven, Philadelphia, PA.

Shideler SE *et al.* (1989). Ovarian-pituitary hormone interactions during the menopause. *Maturitas*, **11**, 331–9.

Sichel DA *et al.* (1995). Prophylactic estrogen in recurrent postpartum affective disorder. *Biological Psychiatry*, **38**, 814–18.

Soares CN *et al.* (2001). Efficacy for the treatment of depressive disorders in perimenopausal women: a double-blind, randomized, placebo-controlled trial. *Archives of General Psychiatry*, **58**, 529–34.

Stein A *et al.* (1991). The relationship between post-natal depression and mother-child interaction. *British Journal of Psychiatry*, **158**, 46–52.

Steiner M *et al.* (2003). Hormones and mood: from menarche to menopause and beyond. *Journal of Affective Disorders*, **74**, 67–83.

Stordal E *et al.* (2001). Depression in relation to age and gender in the general population: the Nord-Trondelag Health Study (HUNT). *Acta Psychiatrica Scandinavica*, **104**, 210–16.

Targosz S *et al.* (2003). Lone mothers, social exclusion and depression. *Psychological Medicine*, **33**, 715–22.

Taylor M (2002). Alternative medicine and the peri-menopause, an evidence based review. *Obstetric Gynecological Clinical Journal of North America*, **29**, 555–73.

Twenge J and Nolen-Hoeksema S (2002). Age, gender, race, SES, and birth cohort differences on the Children's Depression Inventory: a meta-analysis. *Journal of Abnormal Psychology*, **111**, 578–88.

Uhlenhuth EH and Paykel ES (1973). Symptom intensity and life events. *Archives of General Psychiatry*, **28**, 473–7.

Vazques-Barquero J *et al.* (1987). A community mental health survey in Cantabria; a general description of morbidity. *Psychological Medicine*, **17**, 227–42.

Veijola J *et al.* (1998). Sex differences in the association between childhood experiences and adult depression. *Psychological Medicine*, **28**, 21–7.

Wagner BM and Compas BE (1990). Gender, instrumentality and expressivity: moderators of the relation between stress and psychological symptoms during adolescence. *American Journal of Community Psychology*, **18**, 383–406.

Weich S *et al.* (2001). Social roles and the gender difference in rates of common mental disorders in Britain: a 7-year, population based cohort study. *Psychological Medicine*, **31**, 1055–64.

Weiner CL *et al.* (2004). Androgens and mood dysfunction in women; comparison of women with polycystic ovarian syndrome to healthy controls. *Psychosomatic Medicine*, **66**, 356–62.

Weiss EL *et al.* (1999). Childhood sexual abuse as a risk factor for depression in women: Psychosocial and neurobiological correlates. *American Journal of Psychiatry*, **156**, 816–28.

Weissman MM and Klerman GL (1977). Sex differences and the epidemiology of depression. *Archives of General Psychiatry*, **34**, 98–111.

Weissman MM *et al.* (1996). Cross-national epidemiology of major depression and bipolar disorder. *Journal of the America Medical Association*, **276**, 292–9.

CHAPTER 12

Schizophrenia in women

Anita Riecher-Rössler, Marlon Pflüger, and Stefan Borgwardt

Introduction

Sex and gender differences in schizophrenic disorders are one of the most exciting areas of psychiatry, both for clinicians and researchers. For researchers, these differences could be a window to explore the aetiology or at least some pathogenetic mechanisms of these disorders as sex differences—especially regarding age of onset—are one of the most stable and well-established findings in schizophrenic psychoses. Not only biological differences but also differences regarding psychosocial factors influencing the outbreak and the course of these disorders are certainly of great importance in this context.

More knowledge about these mechanisms could also be helpful for developing new therapeutic strategies. For clinicians such new therapeutic strategies would be most welcome. A better understanding of the differences between men and women and their specific needs would also allow to provide specific services tailored to their different life circumstances.

Gender differences

Epidemiological and clinical gender differences

Gender differences in schizophrenia have been described for a long time. In particular, differences in age at onset have been found in many studies (Häfner et al. 1989, 1993a, b; Jablensky et al. 1992). Less consistent are the findings concerning differences in symptomatology and the course of the disease.

Inconsistencies might be partly due to methodological problems in earlier studies (Riecher-Rössler and Rössler 1998). Thus, populations examined were frequently neither representative nor restricted to first-contact patients or first admissions. Often the studies did not rely on direct investigation or standardized assessment.

Few studies on this topic fulfil the essential methodological standards. One which does is the DOSMD Study (Determinants of Outcome of Severe Mental Disorders) by the World Health Organization (WHO), in which 1379 first-contact patients in 12 centres all over the world were examined (Jablensky et al. 1992). Another one is the Finnish First Contact Study by Salokangas and Stengard (1990), who examined 227 first-contact patients. In our own studies on gender differences (Häfner et al. 1989, 1993a, b; Riecher-Rössler et al. 1992) we examined a representative population of 267 first-time hospitalized patients directly and with standardized instruments retrospectively. We also examined 1169 first-time hospitalized patients using data from the Danish Case Register. In these studies many of the mentioned gender differences could be confirmed.

Age of onset

Concerning the difference in age of onset observed in many centres of the WHO studies (Jablensky et al. 1992) as well as in the Danish and the Mannheim Case Register (Häfner et al. 1989), the age of women at first contact or first admission was higher than that of men. The difference was on average between three and a half and nearly six years. In our direct investigation of the first onset of the disease we could demonstrate that this gender difference is genuine and is already evident at the first onset of signs and symptoms of the disease; there is not just a delay in help-seeking or hospital admission among women (Häfner et al. 1993a, b).

Searching for the explanation to this gender difference, a number of psychosocial factors have been suggested. However, none of them has so far been empirically proven (for a review see Riecher-Rössler and Häfner 2000).

The DOSMD study by the WHO shows that the observed sex difference in the age of onset is a phenomenon found in almost all cultures investigated all over the world (Jablensky et al. 1992). This finding probably also speaks against psychosocial causes of the gender difference.

At the same time we were able to show that the cumulative lifetime risk for men and women is identical (Häfner *et al.* 1989, 1993a, b). Men just fall ill earlier than women. This shows that gender has no stable influence on the outbreak of the disease, but that this influence is modulated by age. Men show their peak of first admissions in their early twenties, women only in their late twenties. Furthermore, there is a second, smaller peak of onsets in women after the age of 45 (Häfner *et al.* 1989, 1993a, b).

This distribution, together with the lack of psychosocial explanations for the gender difference in age of onset, directed our attention towards the oestrogen hypothesis (Riecher-Rössler and Häfner 1993a, b). According to this hypothesis, women are protected against schizophrenia between puberty and menopause to some extent by their relatively high physiological oestrogen production during this phase. Then, around age 45, several years before menopause sets in, oestrogen production begins to fall. Women lose the protection oestrogens potentially offer, and this may account for the second peak of illness onset in women after age 45.

The oestrogen hypothesis is not only based on epidemiological data, but also on increasing evidence from clinical and basic research, which shows that oestrogens have significant effects on the mental state of women, including women suffering from schizophrenia (see later).

Symptomatology

As to the symptom-related gender differences noted in symptoms, it has often been reported that negative symptoms occur more frequently in men and affective symptoms more often in women. More recent studies have not consistently confirmed these findings. Addington *et al.* (1996) have shown that gender differences in negative and affective symptoms disappear when the sample is restricted to narrowly defined schizophrenia. Also, in our own direct investigation we did not find many gender differences, especially with respect to psychotic symptoms. The differences we found were more related to illness behaviour. For example, men showed more self-neglect or drug abuse, while women tended to be overadaptive (Häfner *et al.* 1993a, b).

Comorbidity, especially the greater prevalence of substance abuse in men, might have contributed to the gender differences found in the studies, which did not control for this. It may also be that negative symptoms have been reported more often in men, since men on average are prescribed higher doses of neuroleptics, and negative symptom rating scales do not always adequately distinguish between negative symptomatology and the neuroleptic side effects (Seeman 1996a).

Course

Women have often been reported to have a more favourable course and a better psychosocial 'outcome' than men (Riecher-Rössler and Rössler 1998). They were said to have fewer and shorter hospital stays, better social adjustment, and a better living situation than men, whereas the *symptom-related* course seems to be similar for both genders. Women's mortality also seems to be lower, mainly due to their lower suicide rate.

However, looking at more recent and more reliable studies, it seems important to differentiate carefully, i.e. between narrowly or broadly defined schizophrenia, young or older women, etc.

Thus, e.g. in our study based on the Danish Case Register cohort, the frequency and duration of hospitalizations over a 10-year period were the same for both genders when the analyses were restricted to narrowly defined schizophrenia (Maurer 1995). Similar results were found in the Nottingham subsample of the DOSMD study (Harrison *et al.* 1996).

Retterstøl (1991) showed that a more favourable course of disease is only observed in women up to menopause where after this the course deteriorates. Also Ciompi and Müller (1976) found that the symptoms in schizophrenic women are relatively mild at a young age, but become worse as age advances. In men, this pattern was reversed. Seeman (1983) demonstrated that only young women show a better response to neuroleptics as compared to men of the same age group.

There are several reasons for these contradictory results. Firstly, gender differences might be partly due to artefacts, e.g. results of gender-specific diagnostic habits. As a consequence of this, some differences disappear if one looks only at narrowly defined core-schizophrenia.

Secondly, the remaining 'true' effects of gender are—at least in part—age-dependent: on the one hand there is obviously a direct influence of actual age on the symptom-related course of disease. In view of the aforementioned results, this could be due to with the protective effect of oestrogens in younger women up to menopause.

The better overall social course of women on the other hand might also be a consequence of the higher age of *onset* and the accordingly better social integration of the female patients to start with. The first symptoms in men usually occur around the age of 20, but in women not until the mid 20s; thus, at illness onset women have usually already achieved much more stability in their various social roles as compared to men. Very often, women have already completed education, have a stable job and partnership, might be married, and so on. This better social integration significantly improves the prognosis—at least for the *social* course of the illness.

Finally, there are indications that women receive different and potentially better treatment than men do. Salokangas and Stengard (1990) were able to show that psychiatric teams primarily recommend psychotherapy for women, but rehabilitation concentrating on working capacity and basic social skills for men. Moreover, women actually used psychotherapy more often than men did.

A further reason for the better course in women is probably their better compliance and possibly also a lower susceptibility to expressed emotions. Other potentially contributing psychosocial factors have not yet been sufficiently examined (Riecher-Rössler and Rössler 1998; Riecher-Rössler 2000).

Summing up the findings on *epidemiological and clinical gender differences*, the lifetime risk for schizophrenia seems to be the same in men as in women. Women fall ill later and tend to have a better course of illness despite only few differences in symptoms to begin with. This applies especially to young women. After age 40, women not only fall ill twice as frequently as men, their symptoms and the course of their disease also seem to be worse.

The explanations for these gender differences are probably biological as well as psychosocial. It seems that the female sex hormone estradiol has a certain protective effect in young women (see later). The tendency for the course to be better in women certainly also has to do with the later age of onset, which is associated with better social integration. Other contributing factors could be better care offered to women and women's better compliance.

Gender differences in neuroimaging

Male and female patients with schizophrenia have the same pattern of structural brain abnormalities, but male patients appear to manifest greater severity, especially with regard to ventricular enlargement (Nopoulos *et al.* 1997). Sex as well as schizophrenic psychosis might also influence structural lateralization of the brain. Results remain relatively mixed, particularly at the regional level (Beaton 1997; Shapleske *et al.* 1999). Nonetheless, empirical evidence supporting the presence of greater structural asymmetries in men compared to women are

well replicated in perisylvian, temporal, and orbital brain regions (Wada *et al.* 1975; Witelson and Kigar 1992; Bryant *et al.* 1999; Good *et al.* 2001; Knaus *et al.* 2004). Other structural imaging findings, however, fail to support the presence of sex differences in right-frontal and left-occipital width asymmetries or in hemispheric length asymmetries (Chui and Damasio 1980; Narr *et al.* 2007). Recent structural and functional magnetic resonance imaging (MRI) findings suggest disrupted sexual brain dimorphisms in schizophrenia are associated with sex-specific language deficits (Sommer *et al.* 2003) and left hippocampal abnormalities (Bühlmann *et al.* 2009), in particular, contribute to language dysfunction among men (Walder *et al.* 2007). In functional MRI studies, sex differences in cerebral activations in schizophrenia patients deviate from what has been observed in the general population. In men, exposure to and experience of negative affect evoked significantly greater activations in the thalamus, cerebellum, temporal, occipital, and posterior cingulate cortex, while women exhibited greater activations in the left middle frontal gyrus (Mendrek *et al.* 2007). Advances in neuroimaging techniques allow for a detailed investigation of morphometric and functional variability in the brain. It should be emphasized that sex differences in brain structure and function refer to average differences between men and women and that differences between individuals within each sex are much greater than the average difference between sexes (Resnick and Driscoll 2008).

Gender differences in neuropsychology

The presence of neuropsychological impairment in patients suffering from schizophrenia is well established matter of fact. Deficits affect the areas of memory, attentional processes, and executive functions. Language, motor, and visuospatial abilities are less consistently impaired (for a review see Gopal and Variend 2005). However, gender differences with regard to neuropsychological capabilities in schizophrenia are an issue of controversy. Some research groups underscore inferior neuropsychological performance in men (e.g. Goldstein *et al.* 1998), others in women (e.g. Perlick *et al.* 1992), and finally there is a substantial number of reports which cannot provide evidence for gender differences at all (e.g. Goldberg *et al.* 1995).

In this context it is important to note that the impairment of neuropsychological functions depends on a wide variety of conditions, which might differ between men and women; i.e. the age of onset (Hoff *et al.* 1996), the severity of negative symptoms (O'Leary *et al.* 2000), or the overall symptom severity. Neuropsychological performance in women may fluctuate with their monthly cycling oestrogen levels, complicating the isolation of gender effects even more (Hoff *et al.* 2001). Contrary to women, strong laterality effects have been reported for male patients indicating a more pronounced impairment in language skills as compared to visuospatial capabilities (Ragland *et al.* 1999).

More recent reports emphasize conceptual differences of gender and sex in terms of a more psychosocially founded and multidimensional term of gender on the one hand versus a biologically reduced and dichotomous term of sex on the other hand. Lewine *et al.* (2006) report results that clearly indicate stronger gender than sex effects. While sex yielded two main effects in the domains of language and visual perception in favour of men, gender was associated with five main effects (language, verbal and spatial memory, visual perception, and motor speed) favouring the 'feminine' over the 'masculine' individuals. In this study gender was defined as 'gender role', i.e. the overt behaviour displayed in society to establish a position associated with the evaluation of one's gender.

The same controversy holds true considering the course of the illness as a determining factor for gender differences in neurocognitive functions. There is only scarce evidence for gender differences in the first episode of psychosis. One of the few studies shows that men outperform women in tests tackling visuospatial abilities while women perform superior in verbal learning and memory (Albus *et al.* 1997). However, Hoff *et al.* (1998) could not find any gender differences in first-episode patients of psychosis after controlling for symptom severity.

There is hardly any evidence concerning individuals at-risk for or in a prodromal state of psychosis. Weiser *et al.* (2000) retrospectively analysed military draft board data and reported on individuals who later developed schizophrenia. In these prodromal individuals women performed poorer than men in a small set of verbal as well as non-verbal tests. Currently, there is no prospective study regarding individuals in a clinically defined prodromal state of psychosis.

Specific needs and treatment options

These findings on gender differences clearly indicate that we need a more gender-sensitive attitude in our diagnostic and therapeutic approaches.

As regards biological aspects, consideration needs to be given to the large field of gender-specific pharmacotherapy in general and especially in pregnancy and during nursing. This broad topic, however, exceeds the scope of this chapter. Other important biological influences are those of gonadal dysfunction and oestrogens, which will be discussed in the next section. And just as important as considering these gender-specific biological influences is a gender-sensitive approach in the psychosocial treatment of schizophrenia, which means taking into account the influence of gender roles, sexuality, or motherhood.

Gonadal function and oestrogens

Recent research increasingly points to the importance of oestrogens and the hypothalamic–pituitary–gonadal axis in schizophrenic psychoses.

On the one hand there are reports of gonadal dysfunction and states of oestrogen deficiency in women with schizophrenia; on the other hand there is mounting evidence from clinical as well as from epidemiological and basic research that estradiol, the main component of oestrogens, exerts protective effects in schizophrenia.

Research findings
Basic research findings and oestrogens
Important findings from basic research were the identification of oestrogen receptors in the limbic system of the brain, and the observation that the effects of oestrogens in rodents are, in some respects, similar to those of neuroleptics. Furthermore, it was shown that oestrogens can modulate the sensitivity and number of dopamine receptors. It was therefore hypothesized that oestrogens exert their antipsychotic effects in a manner similar to that of traditional neuroleptics, at least partly by blockade of dopaminergic transmission (for review see Riecher-Rössler and Häfner 1993a, b).

We now know that oestrogens, and especially 17-beta-estradiol (the natural oestrogen that is most active in the brain), produce many other neuroprotective and psychoprotective effects. For example, they appear to improve cerebral blood flow and glucose metabolism, promote neuronal sprouting and myelination, enhance synaptic density and plasticity, facilitate neuronal connectivity, act as antioxidants, and inhibit neuronal cell death. They have also been shown to exert profound effects on brain differentiation during development, particularly during late gestation and during the early postnatal period, and are important in normal maintenance of brain function during ageing (for reviews see Cyr *et al.* 2002; Goldstein *et al.* 2002; Oesterlund 2002; Vedder and Behl 2005).

In a well-controlled MRI study, Goldstein *et al.* (2002) showed that normal patterns of sexual brain dimorphism (brain regions found to be structurally different between normal men and women) are disrupted in schizophrenia, especially in the cortex. Apart from later 'activational' effects of circulating hormones (e.g. during puberty), those investigators suggested that these early 'organizational' effects of gonadal hormones that occur during the developmental period (which is probably critical for at least some forms of schizophrenia) could be partly responsible for that finding.

The mechanisms of action of oestrogens are now known not only to depend on the classical genomic pathway but also to involve non-genomic, rapid interactions, which explains the differing latency of effects. They clearly modulate the dopaminergic and other neurotransmitter systems that are believed to be relevant to schizophrenia, such as the serotonergic and glutamatergic system, but also the noradrenergic and cholinergic system (for reviews see Garcia-Segura *et al.* 2001; Stahl 2001a, 2001b; Cyr *et al.* 2002; McEwen 2002; Oesterlund 2002;). Recently it has even been suggested that 17-beta-estradiol in the brain might rather be regarded as a neurotransmitter itself than as a hormone (Balthazart and Ball 2006).

There are at least two subtypes of oestrogen receptors, namely oestrogen receptor-a and oestrogen receptor-b, which are transcribed from two distinct genes (Oesterlund 2002). Autopsy studies showed that oestrogen receptor-a messenger RNA is expressed in discrete areas of the human brain such as amygdala, hypothalamus, cerebral cortex, and hippocampus; these areas are associated with neuroendocrine function, as well as with emotion, memory, and cognition (Oesterlund *et al.* 2000).

Epidemiological findings and oestrogens

Epidemiological studies into sex differences in schizophrenic disorders suggest that the physiologically high estradiol production in young fertile women contributes to the later age of onset of schizophrenia in women as compared with men, to the second peak of onset in women around the menopause, and to the better course of the disease in young women (Häfner *et al.* 1993a, b; Riecher-Rössler *et al.* 1997). A number of risk factors appear to counteract the protective effect of oestrogens. Thus, the sex difference in age of onset diminishes in the subgroup of cases with a genetic risk and in patients with perinatal complications (Könneke *et al.* 2000; Häfner 2005).

Recent results regarding age of menarche further support the hypothesis that physiological oestrogens play a protective role against development of the disease. We could demonstrate a significantly later age of menarche in a representative group of first admitted women with schizophrenia as compared with a healthy control group (Riecher-Rössler 2002). Seeman and coworkers (Cohen *et al.* 1999; Hayeems and Seeman 2005) found that later menarche was associated with an earlier onset of the illness, an association that was independent of factors such as family history and obstetric complications.

Clinical findings and oestrogens

Clinically, psychotic symptomatology has often been found to correlate with the oestrogenic state of women (for reviews see Riecher-Rössler and Häfner 1993a, b; Seeman 1996a). For example, during high oestrogen phases such as pregnancy, chronic psychoses appear to improve, whereas there is an excess of psychoses after delivery.

Psychosis associated with oestrogen withdrawal due to conditions other than the puerperium was recently reviewed by Mahé and Dumaine (2001). Those investigators reported cases of premenstrual psychosis; postabortion psychosis; and psychoses associated with removal of hydatiform mole, cessation of oral contraceptives, clomiphene and tamoxifen administration (both oestrogen receptor antagonists), and gonadorelin agonist administration (which blocks pituitary stimulation of endogenous oestrogen secretion). Psychotic episodes were acute, short, and with a wide range of psychotic, but also affective, symptomatology. Recurrences were often reported when oestrogen withdrawal recurred, and puerperal psychosis was frequent in the history of the patients who were affected.

Psychotic symptoms in schizophrenic patients have also often been shown to deteriorate premenstrually or perimenstrually (i.e. in the low oestrogen phase of the cycle; for review see Riecher-Rössler and Häfner 1993a, b; Seeman 1996b; Riecher-Rössler 2002). Most studies, however, did not correlate symptomatology with estradiol serum levels directly. This was also true for a more recent study (Choi *et al.* 2001), which found only behavioural, affective, and somatic symptoms in schizophrenia (not psychotic ones) to be associated with menstrual cycle phase. In fact, an elevated number of admissions during the perimenstrual period has also been identified in other disorders (Althaus *et al.* 2000), and exacerbation of many psychiatric symptoms (not only psychotic ones) during the perimenstrual period was observed in schizophrenia patients (Riecher-Rössler *et al.* 1994; Harris 1997). In theory, this lack of specificity is to be expected because of the multiple effects of oestrogens on mental functioning.

Rather than examining cyclic fluctuations, Hoff *et al.* (2001) assessed the relation between average oestrogen levels from four consecutive weeks on the one hand and psychopathology and cognitive function on the other hand in 22 female inpatients with chronic schizophrenia, aged 22–63 years. There was no significant association between oestrogen levels and psychopathology, but higher average oestrogen levels were strongly associated with better cognitive abilities. However, this finding may partly be due to the effects of ageing.

Studies conducted in cases of late-onset schizophrenia demonstrated the importance of age. We showed not only that there are twice as many women as men with onset of schizophrenia beyond the age of 40 years, but also that they suffered from unexpectedly severe disease in terms of symptomatology and course (Riecher-Rössler *et al.* 1997; Riecher-Rössler 2002). One explanation for this could again be the loss of oestrogens just before and during menopause. In accordance with those findings are the results of long-term studies in schizophrenia, which have shown that the course of schizophrenia in women tends to deteriorate during the menopause and thereafter (for review see Riecher-Rössler and Häfner 1993a, b; Riecher-Rössler and Rössler 1998).

Intervention studies with oestrogens

Intervention studies have also been conducted over long periods, mainly with positive results (Korhonen *et al.* 1995; Lindamer *et al.* 1997) (for a review see Riecher-Rössler and Häfner 1993a, b). In a systematic trial conducted in 1996, Kulkarni *et al.* (1996) found that schizophrenic women receiving estradiol as an adjunct to neuroleptic treatment exhibited more rapid improvement in psychotic symptoms than did women receiving neuroleptics only. In a double-blind, 28-day, placebo-controlled study (Kulkarni *et al.* 2001), 12 women were administered transdermal 17-beta-estradiol (patches) 50 mg/24 hours, another 12 women received 100 mg/24 hours, and the third group received placebo. The 100-mg group experienced greater improvement than either the 50-mg or the placebo groups; striking improvements were observed with respect to key psychotic symptoms. Louza *et al.* (2004) could not find a respective effect, which they themselves discuss to be possibly due to then having used conjugated oestrogens rather than 17-beta-estradiol, which is known to be active in the brain.

Hormone replacement therapy in postmenopausal women also appears to exert a positive effect. Lindamer *et al.* (2001) reported on a community sample of peri-menopausal and postmenopausal women with schizophrenia. Of the women studied, 24 were on hormone replacement therapy for gynaecological reasons and 28 had never received such therapy. The users of hormone replacement therapy needed a relatively lower average dose of antipsychotic medication and suffered from less severe negative symptomatology.

Ahokas *et al.* (2000) demonstrated positive effects of oestrogen substitution in women with postpartum psychosis. In those women who exhibited sustained oestrogen deficiency states, the substitution of 17-beta-estradiol, without any further medication, yielded a dramatic antipsychotic effect within one week. However, the proportion of schizophrenia-like psychoses in the sample was not given.

Regarding the therapeutic effect of oestrogens, it must be noted that both, the numerous direct effects on the brain as well as indirect effects may play a role. For example, oestrogens may also increase blood levels of antipsychotic drugs via their actions on liver metabolism (Yonkers *et al.* 1992).

Hypo-oestrogenism in women with schizophrenia

Several studies have recently confirmed earlier findings of disturbed gonadal function and hypo-oestrogenism in schizophrenic women (Riecher-Rössler and Häfner 1993a, b; Riecher-Rössler *et al.* 1994; Kulkarni *et al.* 1996; Riecher-Rössler *et al.* 1998; Choi *et al.* 2001; Hoff *et al.* 2001; Huber *et al.* 2001; Bergemann *et al.* 2002; Canuso *et al.* 2002; Smith *et al.* 2002; Zhang-Wong and Seeman 2002). They describe menstrual irregularities and reduced blood levels of estradiol, progesterone, and gonadotropins (follicle-stimulating hormone, luteinizing hormone) throughout the menstrual cycle, as well as an ovulation in the majority of women with schizophrenia. Reduced fertility was also reported.

There appear to be multiple reasons for these disturbances. Partly, they are probably a consequence of stress and/or neuroleptic-induced hyperprolactinaemia, which is known to suppress gonadal function (Maguire 2002). However, these are probably not the only causes, because other psychiatric disorders accompanied by similar 'stress' do not show the same disturbances or at least not to the same degree (Riecher-Rössler *et al.* 1998; Huber *et al.* 2001), and hypo-oestrogenism was observed long before the introduction of neuroleptics. Furthermore, recent findings are not unequivocal. Smith *et al.* (2002) found the dose of typical neuroleptics to correlate with prolactin levels especially in women and prolactin to correlate inversely with estradiol serum levels. In contrast to these findings, Huber *et al.* (2001) were unable to identify a significant association of prolactin and estradiol in 43 women with acute psychosis, 14 women with other diagnoses, and nine healthy control women. Nevertheless, women with schizophrenia had significantly lower estradiol serum levels than did the control women. Women with other psychiatric diagnoses fell in between the psychotic and the healthy group with regard to estradiol and prolactin levels. Also, in 16 premenopausal women with schizophrenia and schizoaffective disorders, Canuso *et al.* (2002) found a high rate of ovarian dysfunction and estradiol levels below normal, irrespective of medication type or prolactin status. Interestingly, Warner *et al.* (2001) found prolactin levels in unmedicated schizophrenic patients to be even lower than in control individuals. Those investigators suggested that this was due to a disordered dopaminergic system because dopamine tonically inhibits prolactin.

Taken together, these results imply that the hypothalamic–pituitary–gonadal axis is disturbed in many women with schizophrenia, and that the reasons for this are far from clear, yet. An interesting research question in this context is whether gonadal dysfunction with oestrogen deficiency could even be part of the underlying pathogenetic process, at least in a subgroup of women (Riecher-Rössler 2002).

Implications for clinicians and researchers

Further research into the impact of gonadal function and oestrogens on schizophrenia is warranted because new diagnostic and therapeutic strategies could emerge that would benefit the many women worldwide who suffer from this disorder.

Assessment and therapy of gonadal dysfunction

Because there is growing evidence that many even younger women with schizophrenia are in a state of oestrogen deficiency, in the future oestrogens and the gonadal axis should be considered more seriously in the treatment of women with schizophrenia. Psychiatric history taking should always include questions regarding menstrual irregularities, amenorrhoea, and galactorrhoea. Also, prolactin and oestrogen serum levels should be tested, if necessary. Gonadal dysfunction and hypo-oestrogenic states can often be found even in menstruating women (Riecher-Rössler *et al.* 1994; Riecher-Rössler *et al.* 1998; Smith *et al.* 2002). In addition, hyperprolactinaemia is clearly underdiagnosed (Maguire 2002). Some authors have therefore suggested routine laboratory tests (Smith *et al.* 2002).

Most neuroleptics can cause hyperprolactinaemia and can—especially if they are taken over a number of years—theoretically induce 'iatrogenic early menopause' via suppression of physiological estradiol production. The attendant risks include both short-term effects, such as hot flushes and sexual dysfunction, and long-term consequences, including osteoporosis and potentially cardiovascular disease or cognitive deterioration (Maguire 2002; Oesterlund 2002). In schizophrenic patients, these risks are further increased by additional risk factors such as smoking, poor diet, and reduced exercise (Smith *et al.* 2002).

Furthermore, menopausal complaints may lead to compliance problems. In the case of hyperprolactinaemia with secondary oestrogen deficiency, prolactin-sparing neuroleptics, e.g. clozapine, quetiapine, aripiprazol, or maybe olanzapine (Maguire 2002), should therefore be preferred. If a switch to these neuroleptics is not possible for clinical reasons or if hypo-oestrogenism persists despite switching, then oestrogens should be substituted. Issues regarding contraception must be taken into account in such cases because, when switching to prolactin-sparing neuroleptics, the menstrual cycle often normalizes and fertility is regained, with high risk for unplanned pregnancy (Neumann and Frasch 2001).

Estradiol as a therapeutic agent?

First trials of oestrogens in schizophrenia indicate that estradiol could be used as an adjunct to neuroleptic medication. However, further replication of these findings in larger controlled studies by different groups are needed before recommendations for broad clinical application can be made.

In women who suffer from frequent perimenstrual psychotic relapses, 'cycle modulated' neuroleptic therapy or, if contraception is needed at the same time, continuous use of oral contraceptives without hormone-free intervals may be strategies worthy of research (Braendle *et al.* 2001; Riecher-Rössler 2002).

Even more promising could be hormonal replacement with oestrogens in women with schizophrenia in peri- and postmenopause, since oestrogens in other disorders such as depression have proven to be especially helpful when they are used to restore hormonal balance.

In any case, oestrogen replacement therapy ameliorates perimenopausal complaints, which can act as stressors and theoretically provoke relapses. Hormone replacement therapy has also been recommended for other reasons, such as for prophylaxis of osteoporosis, for a delay of the age-dependent cognitive decline, and possibly also for Alzheimer's disease (for a review see Riecher-Rössler and de Geyter 2007). Schizophrenia may be an additional indication to be studied.

Research should also be conducted concerning the best mode of hormone replacement therapy for psychiatric patients. Progestogens are usually added to oestrogens in order to prevent endometrial cancer, but they can antagonize the positive effects of oestrogens with respect to mental state (Braendle *et al.* 2001; Cyr *et al.* 2002). Furthermore, other risks associated with hormone therapy, such as breast cancer and cardiovascular disease for certain combinations, must be considered (Writing Group for the Women's Health Initiative Investigators 2002), although these risks have been overestimated lately due to uncritical interpretations of studies such as the Women's Health Initiative Study (Pines *et al.* 2007; Riecher-Rössler and de Geyter 2007; Rossouw *et al.* 2007).

Nevertheless, alternatives to conventional hormone replacement therapy, compounds with more specific and potent oestrogenic activity in the brain as opposed to other tissues, should be sought (Halbreich 2002; Riecher-Rössler 2002). Such compounds would both minimize the side effects of hormonal therapy and permit new therapeutic strategies in men. Possible candidates are the selective oestrogen receptor modulators, which have agonist or antagonist properties that depend on the target tissue. However, the effects of the available selective oestrogen receptor modulators on the brain remain to be clarified. Raloxifene, for example, appears to exert its main effects on the bone, although recent data suggest that it also acts on different brain receptors (Cyr *et al.* 2002). Also, the synthetic steroid tibolone appears to cause less endometrial proliferation, but its effects on the central nervous system are still not clear, apart from the fact that it appears to have an androgenic effect and increases beta-endorphin levels, with improvement in mood and libido (Davis 2002). Further studies on the brain-specific effects of selective oestrogen receptor modulators and other oestrogenic compounds (e.g. phyto-oestrogens, xeno-oestrogens, and dihydroepiandrosterone) are urgently needed.

In summary, hopes are emerging that oestrogens, as neuroprotective and psychoprotective adjunctive therapies, may complement the traditional drug therapies in schizophrenia in the future. However, it must be emphasized that most strategies are still being researched. In particular, results from larger controlled clinical trials are needed before oestrogens may be recommended as adjunct therapy in younger women

without proven oestrogen deficiency. In contrast, other strategies should already be part of standard clinical care (Grigoriadis and Seeman 2002). These include examination of the gonadal axis, with therapeutic consequences, if indicated. Regarding oestrogen replacement therapy, it must be stressed that the decision must always be made on the basis of an individual risk–benefit assessment (NAMS 2000; Writing Group for the Women's Health Initiative Investigators 2002) and in close cooperation with a gynaecologist.

For future research, many questions remain unresolved, not only regarding new therapeutic strategies and compounds but also regarding the poorly understood disturbances of oestrogens and the hypothalamic–pituitary–gonadal axis in women with schizophrenia. Further research in this area may even contribute to our understanding of the pathogenesis of this disease, at least in a subgroup of women.

Gender role and sexuality

Gender role

Gender-sensitive therapy also means being sensitive to gender differences in symptom perception and illness concept, in coping, illness, and help-seeking behaviour (Riecher-Rössler 2000). The influence of current social roles (partnership, motherhood, professional roles, etc.), social status, social stress, and social support has to be taken into account just as much as the influence of gender-specific socialization and 'gendered' role behaviour.

It also means that we should be more aware of the practical needs of our patients. Thus, day-treatment or weekend home-leaves during a hospital stay for a housewife and mother may be a much greater stress than for a man, who may be free of any duties at home.

Also, significantly more women than men with schizophrenia have children, which is often associated with specific burdens and stressors (see later).

Also the later age of onset in women means that the disease has different effects on them than on men. As a consequence of this, women frequently have to cope with losses in many forms, such as in relationships with partners or children, or in the professional sphere. Thus, whereas for men the goal is often to attain certain roles for the very first time, for women, the focus in therapy often has to be the maintenance or re-establishment of certain roles.

Sexuality

Most women with schizophrenia are sexually active (Miller 1997), although sexual desire and orgasmic function can be impaired not only by the illness itself, but also by side effects of medication, especially anti-psychotic-induced hyper-prolactinaemia (see earlier).

Women with schizophrenia often suffer from sexual victimization, experience sexual abuse, or feel pressured to sexual activities which place them at risk for sexually transmitted diseases (for a review see Seeman and Fitzgerald 2000). When hospitalized, women often feel threatened by the aggressive or sexually assaultive behaviour of male patients. Doctors should be aware of these problems, ask their female patients actively regarding problems in this area, and offer specific help in form of counselling and arranging practical help. Cooperation with gynaecologists, social workers, specialized institutions for women such as women's shelters and counselling agencies is often required. Establishing special 'women's areas' in hospitals can be helpful.

Motherhood

In recent times, more women with schizophrenia are married and more often they have children. In a review, Mary Seeman (2004) concludes that over 50% of all female patients with schizophrenia become mothers, a percentage close to the general population. But pregnancy and motherhood can be difficult for women with schizophrenia.

Infertility and desiring motherhood

Many women with schizophrenia desiring motherhood can not fulfil this wish without difficulties. Due to the disease or neuroleptics they can be infertile, often they do not have a suitable and reliable partner. These aspects should always be inquired when caring for women with schizophrenia and they should receive the necessary counselling. If a child is desired, the woman's general situation should be considered, if possible together with her partner. What is the expected course of the disease? What would the effect of the additional burden of caring for a child be? What psychosocial support is there for mother and child? How much support can be offered? What are the father's wishes and his situation? How is his psychosocial stability? If, after carefully considering these aspects, motherhood seems possible, the question of whether the course of the disease permits a temporary pause from the neuroleptic medication needs to be addressed, the patient should have been stable and without relapse for at least one to two years. It is advisable to taper out the medication slowly and the contraception should not be stopped before the patient is medication free. Otherwise a teratogenic effect of the neuroleptics during the first three months of pregnancy cannot be definitely excluded.

Unwanted pregnancy

Unwanted or at least unplanned pregnancies are not rare. In these cases the pregnancy is often noticed very late and a doctor is consulted to discuss a termination, or confronted with the question whether the medication could have led to deformations of the child. These women need to be advised very carefully and their own wishes, possible ambivalence, and their capacity of judgement should be taken into account. Medication during the first trimester alone is not a reason for interrupting a pregnancy, as on the whole the risk of teratogenicity is low. However, the patient should have access to good prenatal care with specialized ultrasound monitoring etc. if she wants to bring the pregnancy to term.

Motherhood

For a woman affected with schizophrenia, motherhood can be a considerable strain, not only because of the care the child needs. The fear that the child could be taken away if she cannot cope has also to be taken into consideration. Partners who may be able to give support usually do not live with the mothers or are unknown (for a review see Seeman 2004). So, some of these fears are well founded, they can be very stressful for these women, and can maintain pathological processes of the disease as well as delaying remission. Because of these fears, many women do not seek help, which causes a vicious circle. Here psychiatric institutions which offer low threshold, specialized care are urgently needed. Parents with psychiatric diseases, especially single mothers, often do not accept the usual offers of care, such as day centres for patients with psychiatric diseases, as they do not want to be separated from their children and these can not be cared for in such institutions. Also most of the institutions are not suited for the care of young children. Here a specialized setting and specific experience with the cooperation of the various professions such as psychiatrists, psychiatric nurses, social workers, midwives, pedagogues, etc., is necessary. Specialized parent/child programmes can specifically train those skills which individuals with a psychiatric disease often do not have spontaneously or sufficiently, the so called 'parenting skills' (Hofecker Fallahpour and Riecher-Rössler 2002).

Specialized institutions with these specific settings and experience are being founded, especially in Anglo-American countries (for reviews see Oyserman et al. 1994; Seeman 2004). One of their main aims besides treatment and rehabilitation is the training of parenting. The parents' skills are trained and improved in a special 'parenting rehabilitation' which includes an initial assessment followed by a long-term programme with parenting classes, support groups for parents and children, therapeutic kindergartens, etc. (Oyserman *et al.* 1994; Mowbray *et al.* 2001; Seeman 2004).

Summary and conclusions

Schizophrenic disorders show a later age of onset in women and a slightly better course especially in young women. As to pathogenesis there is some evidence that the age difference might be at least partly due to the female sex hormone estradiol being a protective factor. Differences in course might also have to do with this biological factor, but at the same time with the psychosocial advantages of a higher age of onset and other psychosocial factors. Thus, gender differences in schizophrenia are obviously determined by biological as well as psychosocial factors and the complex interplay of both.

For the clinician this means that therapy has to be based on a multilevel approach that integrates biological, psychological, and social factors and takes into account the specific needs of women, including their needs in specific life circumstances such as motherhood.

For research, gender differences in schizophrenic psychoses could be a valuable paradigm regarding the interplay between biological and psychosocial factors. Understanding gender differences could help understanding the complex pathogenetic mechanisms of these disorders and give valuable clues to new therapies.

References

Addington D *et al.* (1996). Gender and affect in schizophrenia. *Canadian Journal of Psychiatry*, **41**, 265–8.

Ahokas A *et al.* (2000). Positive treatment effect of estradiol in postpartum psychosis: a pilot study. *Journal of Clinical Psychiatry*, **61**, 166–9.

Albus M *et al.* (1997). Are there gender differences in neuropsychological performance in patients with first-episode schizophrenia? *Schizophrenia Research*, **28**, 39–50.

Althaus G *et al.* (2000). [The effect of the menstruation cycle on manifestations of psychiatric diseases]. *Fortschritte der Neurologie-Psychiatrie*, **68**, 357–62.

Balthazart J and Ball GF (2006). Is brain estradiol a hormone or a neurotransmitter? *Trends in Neurosciences*, **29**, 241–9.

Beaton AA (1997). The relation of planum temporale asymmetry and morphology of the corpus callosum to handedness, gender, and dyslexia: a review of the evidence. *Brain and Language*, **60**, 255–322.

Bergemann N *et al.* (2002). Acute psychiatric admission and menstrual cycle phase in women with schizophrenia. *Archives of Women's Mental Health*, **5**, 119–26.

Braendle W *et al.* (2001). Sexualhormone und psyche – ergebnisse des 2. Interdisziplinären Frankfurter Gesprächs zur Kontrazeption. *Frauenarzt*, **42**, 154–60.

Bryant NL *et al.* (1999). Gender differences in temporal lobe structures of patients with schizophrenia: a volumetric MRI study. *American Journal of Psychiatry*, **156**, 603–9.

Bühlmann E *et al.* (2009). Hippocampus abnormalities in at risk mental states for psychosis? — A cross-sectional high resolution region of interest magnetic resonance imaging study. *Journal Psychiatric Research* (article in press).

Canuso CM *et al.* (2002). Antipsychotic medication, prolactin elevation, and ovarian function in women with schizophrenia and schizoaffective disorder. *Psychiatry Research*, **111**, 11–20.

Choi SH *et al.* (2001). Changes in premenstrual symptoms in women with schizophrenia: a prospective study. *Psychosomatic Medicine*, **6**, 822–9.

Chua WL *et al.* (2005). Estrogen for schizophrenia. *Cochrane Database of Systematic Reviews*, **4**, CD004753.

Chui HD and Damasio AR (1980). Human cerebral asymmetries evaluated by computerized tomography. *Journal of Neurology, Neurosurgery, and Psychiatry*, **43**, 873–8.

Ciompi L and Müller C (1976). *Lebensweg und Alter der Schizophrenen*. Springer, Berlin.

Cohen RZ *et al.* (1999). Earlier puberty as a predictor of later onset of schizophrenia in women. *American Journal of Psychiatry*, **156**, 1059–64.

Cyr M *et al.* (2002). Estrogenic modulation of brain activity: implications for schizophrenia and Parkinson's disease. *Journal of Psychiatry & Neuroscience*, **27**, 12–27.

Davis SR (2002). The effects of tibolone on mood and libido. *Menopause*, **9**, 162–70.

Garcia-Segura LM *et al.* (2001). Neuroprotection by estradiol. *Progress in Neurobiology*, **63**, 29–60.

Goldberg TE *et al.* (1995). Lack of sex differences in the neuropsychological performance of patients with schizophrenia. *American Journal of Psychiatry*, **152**, 883–8.

Goldstein JM *et al.* (1998). Are there sex differences in neuropsychological functions among patients with schizophrenia? *American Journal of Psychiatry*, **155**, 1358–64.

Goldstein JM *et al.* (2002). Impact of normal sexual dimorphisms on sex differences in structural brain abnormalities in schizophrenia assessed by magnetic resonance imaging. *Archives of General Psychiatry*, **59**, 154–64.

Good CD *et al.* (2001). A voxel-based morphometric study of ageing in 465 normal adult human brains. *Neuroimage*, **14**, 21–36.

Gopal YV and Variend H (2005). First-episode schizophrenia: a review of cognitive deficits and cognitive remediation. *Advances in Psychiatric Treatment*, **11**, 38–44.

Grigoriadis S and Seeman MV (2002). The role of estrogen in schizophrenia: implications for schizophrenia practice guidelines for women. *Canadian Journal of Psychiatry*, **47**, 437–42.

Häfner H (2005). Gender differences in schizophrenia. In: N Bergemann and A Riecher-Rössler (eds) *Estrogen Effects in Psychiatric Disorders*, pp. 53–94. Springer, Wien.

Häfner H *et al.* (1989). How does gender influence age at first hospitalization for schizophrenia? *Psychological Medicine*, **19**, 903–18.

Häfner H *et al.* (1993a). The influence of age and sex on the onset and early course of schizophrenia. *British Journal of Psychiatry*, **162**, 80–6.

Häfner H *et al.* (1993b). Generating and testing a causal explanation of the gender difference in age at first onset of schizophrenia 3. *Psychological Medicine*, **23**, 925–40.

Halbreich U (2002). The spectrum of estrogens, estrogen agonists and SERMS. *International Journal of Neuropsychopharmacology*, **5**(Suppl 1), S12.

Harris AH (1997). Menstrually related symptom changes in women with schizophrenia. *Schizophrenia Research*, **27**, 93–9.

Harrison G *et al.* (1996). Predicting long-term outcome of schizophrenia: an overview. *Psychological Medicine*, **26**, 697–705.

Hayeems R and Seeman MV (2005). Puberty and schizophrenia onset. In: N Bergemann and A Riecher-Rössler (eds) *Estrogen Effects in Psychiatric Disorders*, pp. 95–106. Springer, Wien.

Hofecker Fallahpour M and Riecher-Rössler A (2002). Ein treffpunkt für psychisch kranke eltern und ihre kinder. *Pro Mente Sana Aktuell*, **2**, 22–3.

Hoff AL *et al.* (1996). A neuropsychological study of early onset schizophrenia. *Schizophrenia Research*, **20**, 21–8.

Hoff AL *et al.* (2001). Association of estrogen levels with neuropsychological performance in women with schizophrenia. *American Journal of Psychiatry*, **158**, 1134–9.

Hoff AL *et al.* (1998). Sex differences in neuropsychological functioning of first-episode and chronically ill schizophrenic patients. *American Journal of Psychiatry*, **155**, 1437–9.

Huber TJ *et al.* (2001). Estradiol levels in psychotic disorders. *Psychoneuroendocrinology*, **26**, 27–35.

Jablensky A *et al.* (1992). Schizophrenia: manifestations, incidence and course in different cultures. *a World Health Organization ten-country study. Psychological Medicine*, **20**(Suppl 20), 1–97.

Knaus TA *et al.* (2004). Sex-linked differences in the anatomy of the perisylvian language cortex: a volumetric MRI study of gray matter volumes. *Neuropsychology*, **18**, 738–47.

Könneke R *et al.* (2000). Main risk factors for schizophrenia: increased familial loading and pre- and peri-natal complications antagonize the protective effect of oestrogen in women. *Schizophrenia Research*, **44**, 81–93.

Korhonen S *et al.* (1995). Successful estradiol treatment of psychotic symptoms in the premenstrual phase: a case report. *Acta Psychiatrica Scandinavica*, **92**, 237–8.

Kulkarni J *et al.* (1996). A clinical trial of the effects of estrogen in acutely psychotic women. *Schizophrenia Research*, **20**, 247–52.

Kulkarni J *et al.* (2001). Estrogen – a potential treatment for schizophrenia. *Schizophrenia Research*, **48**, 137–44.

Lewine RR *et al.* (2006). Sex, gender, and neuropsychological functioning in schizophrenia. *Journal of Clinical and Experimental Neuropsychology*, **28**, 1362–72.

Lindamer LA *et al.* (2001). Hormone replacement therapy in postmenopausal women with schizophrenia: positive effect on negative symptoms? *Biological Psychiatry*, **49**, 47–51.

Lindamer LA *et al.* (1997). Gender, estrogen, and schizophrenia. *Psychopharmacology Bulletin*, **33**, 221–8.

Louza MR *et al.* (2004). Conjugated estrogens as adjuvant therapy in the treatment of acute schizophrenia: a double-blind study. *Schizophrenia Research*, **66**, 97–100.

Maguire GA (2002). Prolactin elevation with antipsychotic medications: mechanisms of action and clinical consequences. *Journal of Clinical Psychiatry*, **63**(Suppl 4), 56–62.

Mahé V and Dumaine A (2001). Oestrogen withdrawal associated psychoses. *Acta Psychiatrica Scandinavica*, **104**, 323–31.

Maurer K (1995). Der geschlechtsspezifische Verlauf der Schizophrenie über 10 Jahre. Kovac, Hamburg.

McEwen B (2002). Interplay between membrane and genomic actions of estrogens. *International Journal of Neuropsychopharmacology*, **5**, 12.

Mendrek A *et al.* (2007). Sex differences in the cerebral function associated with processing of aversive stimuli by schizophrenia patients. *Australian and New Zealand Journal of Psychiatry*, **41**, 136–41.

Miller LJ (1997). Sexuality, reproduction, and family planning in women with schizophrenia. *Schizophrenia Bulletin*, **23**, 623–35.

Mowbray CT *et al.* (2001). Life circumstances of mothers with serious mental illnesses. *Psychiatric Rehabilitation Journal*, **25**, 114–23.

NAMS (2000). A decision tree for the use of estrogen replacement therapy or hormone replacement therapy in postmenopausal women: consensus opinion of the North American Menopause Society. *Menopause*, **7**, 76–86.

Narr KL *et al.* (2007). Asymmetries of cortical shape: effects of handedness, sex and schizophrenia. *Neuroimage*, **34**, 939–48.

Neumann NU and Frasch K (2001). Olanzapin und schwangerschaft – zwei kasuistiken. *Nervenarzt*, **72**, 876–8.

Nopoulos P *et al.* (1997). Sex differences in brain morphology in schizophrenia. *American Journal of Psychiatry*, **154**, 1648–54.

O'Leary DS *et al.* (2000). Cognitive correlates of the negative, disorganized, and psychotic symptom dimensions of schizophrenia. *Journal of Neuropsychiatry and Clinical Neuroscience*, **12**, 4–15.

Oesterlund MK (2002). The role of estrogens in neuropsychiatric disorders. *Current Opinion in Psychiatry*, **15**, 307–12.

Oesterlund MK *et al.* (2000). The human forebrain has discrete estrogen receptor messenger RNA expression: high levels in the amygdaloid complex. *Neuroscience*, **95**, 333–42.

Oyserman D *et al.* (1994). Resources and supports for mothers with severe mental illness. *Health & Social Work*, **19**, 132–42.

Perlick D *et al.* (1992). Gender differences in cognition in schizophrenia. *Schizophrenia Research*, **8**, 69–73.

Pines A *et al.* (2007). IMS updated recommendations on postmenopausal hormone therapy. *Climacteric*, **10**, 181–94.

Ragland JD *et al.* (1999). Neuropsychological laterality indices of schizophrenia: interactions with gender. *Schizophrenia Research*, **25**, 79–89.

Resnick SM *et al.* (2008). Sex differences in brain aging and Alzheimer's disease. In: J Becker *et al.* (eds) *Sex Differences in the Brain: From Genes to Behavior*, pp. 427–54. Oxford University Press, Oxford.

Retterstøl N (1991). Course and outcome in paranoid disorders. *Psychopathology*, **24**, 277–86.

Riecher-Rössler A (2000). Psychische erkrankungen bei frauen – einige argumente für eine geschlechtersensible psychiatrie und psychotherapie. *Psychosomatische Medizin und Psychotherapie*, **46**, 129–39.

Riecher-Rössler A (2002). Estrogen effects in schizophrenia and their potential therapeutic implications - review. *Archives of Women's Mental Health*, **5**, 111–18.

Riecher-Rössler A and De Geyter C (2007). The forthcoming role of treatment with oestrogens in mental health. *Swiss Medical Weekly*, **137**, 565–72.

Riecher-Rössler A and Häfner H (1993). Schizophrenia and oestrogens - is there an association? *European Archives of Psychiatry and Clinical Neuroscience*, **242**, 323–8.

Riecher-Rössler A and Häfner H (2000). Gender aspects in schizophrenia: bridging the border between social and biological psychiatry. *Acta Psychiatrica Scandinavica. Supplementum*, **407**, 58–62.

Riecher-Rössler A and Rössler W (1998). The course of schizophrenic psychoses: what do we really know? a selective review from an epidemiological perspective. *European Archives of Psychiatry and Clinical Neuroscience*, **248**, 189–202.

Riecher-Rössler A *et al.* (1992). Is age of onset in schizophrenia influenced by marital status? Some remarks on the difficulties and pitfalls in the systematic testing of a 'simple' question. *Social Psychiatry and Psychiatric Epidemiology*, **27**, 122–8.

Riecher-Rössler A *et al.* (1994). Can estradiol modulate schizophrenic symptomatology? *Schizophrenia Research*, **20**, 203–14.

Riecher-Rössler A *et al.* (1997). What do we really know about late-onset schizophrenia? *European Archives of Psychiatry and Clinical Neuroscience*, **247**, 195–208.

Riecher-Rössler A *et al.* (1998). Gonadal function and its influence on psychopathology. A comparison of schizophrenic and non-schizophrenic female inpatients. *Archives of Women's Mental Health*, **1**, 15–26.

Rossouw JE *et al.* (2007). Postmenopausal hormone therapy and risk of cardiovascular disease by age and years since menopause. *Journal of the American Medical Association*, **297**, 1465–77.

Salokangas RK and Stengard E (1990). Gender and short-term outcome in schizophrenia. *Schizophrenia Research*, **3**, 333–45.

Seeman MV (1983). Interaction of sex, age and neuroleptic dose. *Comprehensive Psychiatry*, **24**, 125–8.

Seeman MV (1996a). Schizophrenia, gender and affect. *Canadian Journal of Psychiatry*, **41**, 263–4.

Seeman MV (1996b). The role of estrogen in schizophrenia. *Journal of Psychiatry & Neuroscience*, **21**, 123–7.

Seeman MV (2004). Schizophrenia and motherhood. In: M Göpfert *et al.* (eds) *Parental Psychiatric disorder. Distressed Parents and their Families*, 2nd edition, pp. 161–71. Cambridge University Press, Cambridge.

Seeman MV and Fitzgerald P (2000). Women and schizophrenia: clinical aspects. In: D Castle *et al.* (eds) *Women and Schizophrenia*, pp. 35–50. Cambridge University Press, Cambridge.

Shapleske J *et al.* (1999). The planum temporale: a systematic, quantitative review of its structural, functional and clinical significance. *Brain Research: Brain Research Reviews*, **29**, 26–49.

Smith S *et al.* (2002). The effects of antipsychotic-induced hyperprolactinaemia on the hypothalamic-pituitary-gonadal axis. *Journal of Clinical Psychopharmacology*, **22**, 109–14.

Sommer IE *et al.* (2003). Language lateralization in female patients with schizophrenia: an FMRI study. *Schizophrenia Research*, **60**, 183–90.

Stahl SM (2001a). Effects of estrogen on the central nervous system. *Journal of Clinical Psychiatry*, **62**, 317–18.

Stahl SM (2001b). Why drugs and hormones may interact in psychiatric disorders. *Journal of Clinical Psychiatry*, **62**, 225–6.

Vedder H and Behl C (2005). Estrogens in neuropsychiatric disorders: from physiology to pathophysiology. In: Bergemann N and Riecher-Rössler A (eds) Estrogen Effects in Psychiatric Disorders, pp. 1–30. Springer, New York.

Wada JA *et al.* (1975). Cerebral hemispheric asymmetry in humans. Cortical speech zones in 100 adults and 100 infant brains. *Archives of Neurology*, **32**, 239–46.

Walder DJ *et al.* (2007). Neuroanatomic substrates of sex differences in language dysfunction in schizophrenia: a pilot study. *Schizophrenia Research*, **90**, 295–301.

Warner MD *et al.* (2001). Lower prolactin bioactivity in unmedicated schizophrenic patients. *Psychiatry Research*, **102**, 249–54.

Weiser M *et al.* (2000). Gender differences in premorbid cognitive performance in a national cohort of schizophrenic patients. *Schizophrenia Research*, **45**, 185–90.

Witelson SF and Kigar DL (1992). Sylvian fissure morphology and asymmetry in men and women: bilateral differences in relation to handedness in men. *Journal of Comparative Neurology*, **323**, 326–40.

Writing Group for The Women's Health Initiative
  Investigators (2002). Risks and benefits of estrogen plus
  progestin in healthy postmenopausal women. *Journal of
  the American Medical Association*, **288**, 321–33.

Yonkers KA *et al.* (1992). Gender differences in
  pharmacokinetics and pharmacodynamics of
psychotropic medication. *American Journal of Psychiatry*,
  149, 587–95.

Zhang-Wong J and Seeman MV (2002). Antipsychotic drugs,
  menstrual regularity, and osteoporosis risk. *Archives of
  Women's Mental Health*, **5**, 93–8.

CHAPTER 13

Women with borderline personality disorder: aetiology, assessment, and prognosis

Sarah Majid

Introduction

Personality disorders are developmental conditions appearing in childhood or adolescence and continuing into adulthood. They are characterized by deeply ingrained and enduring patterns of behaving, feeling, and relating that deviate significantly from the average individual in a culture. They are usually associated with subjective distress and problems in social functioning and performance across multiple social and occupational domains. Borderline personality disorder (BPD) is characterized by emotional instability, unstable relationships, and impulsive, often dangerous, behaviour. It has been typically regarded as an untreatable condition, with patients often disliked and avoided by professionals and understandably alienated and angry with services. BPD patients are commonly but not exclusively women, and often present with associated difficulties such as eating disorders and self-harm. They are significant utilizers of mental health services, have high rates of unemployment, and 10% commit suicide. As women, many patients are parents themselves with important implications for treatment and risk assessment.

In this chapter I review aetiological theories, including neurobiological and psychosocial and attachment-based models, and more current work focusing on mentalization. I go on to consider the assessment and diagnosis of BPD in women in particular, and the natural history of the disorder, bearing in mind findings from recent research.

In Chapter 14 I review the treatment approaches with a focus on recent developments in therapy.

Epidemiology

Borderline personality disorder is a common condition with prevalence estimates in the community of 0.2–1.8%, and a recent study finding of 0.7% in a sample of 626 British householders (Coid *et al.* 2006). The majority of patients are women—around 70% of most samples, so that most of the research data describes women (Widiger and Weissman 1991) They are more likely to visit their general practitioner, accounting for 4–6% of attenders, though are often underdiagnosed (Moran *et al.* 2000) Rates are higher in psychiatric outpatients (8–11%) and inpatients (14–20%) and over 50% in services dealing with eating disorder, drug and alcohol dependency, or chronic self-harm. The highest rates are in forensic services (60–80%) (Blackburn *et al.* 1990; Zanarini 1998).

Sociodemographic data highlights significant impairment in interpersonal and occupational function and women with BPD are commonly separated, divorced, or never married with high rates of unemployment or occupational instability (Skodol *et al.* 2002a). Black and minority ethnic groups appear to be under-represented in samples, and it is unclear whether this reflects actual reduced prevalence or bias in diagnosis and referral.

Suicidality is frequent with parasuicidal acts in 84% (Black 2006) and increased risk of actual suicide (Cheng *et al.* 1997). Sixty to 70% attempt suicide at some point in their life, and 10% complete suicide (Oldham 2006). This risk is compounded by comorbid depression.

Clinical features

BPD is characterized by a pervasive pattern of instability of mood, interpersonal relationships, affect and self-image, with intolerance of being alone. Patients also have chronic feelings of emptiness or boredom and impulsive behaviour including self-harm, binging, and drug abuse. Disturbed behaviours such as self-mutilation frequently occur in the context of intense abandonment/engulfment/annihilation anxieties, typically in the context of intense and problematic interpersonal relationships. Patients with BPD may develop paranoid symptoms under stress becoming suspicious with magical thinking or ideas of reference. These transient psychotic episodes are typically precipitated by interpersonal crises that leave the patient feeling abandoned, and are not usually prolonged. Assessment may be complicated by drug or alcohol abuse which commonly makes patients more paranoid—although it may also be resorted to as self-medication for disturbing transient psychotic symptoms. These features are reflected in the ICD-10 and DSM IV definitions (see Table 13.1) and supported by research looking at descriptive discriminating. The characteristic intense attachments and abandonment anxieties mean patients often regress in therapeutic relationships. Clinicians are prone to typical countertransference difficulties including rescue fantasies, guilt feelings, boundary transgressions, rage and hatred, anxiety and terror, and profound feelings of helplessness, and teams often become split in their responses to patients and views on appropriate management. This can make women with BPD a challenging group to work with.

Table 13.1 ICD-10 (World Health Organization 1992) and DSM-IV (American Psychiatric Association 2000) definitions of BPD

ICD-10
F60.3: Emotionally unstable personality disorder
Marked tendency to impulsive action with emotional instability. Minimal ability to plan ahead and outbursts of intense anger may often lead to violence or behavioural explosions. These are easily precipitated when impulsive acts are criticized or threatened by others
F 60.30 Impulsive type with predominant emotional instability and lack of impulse control
Outbursts of violence or threatening behaviour are common, particularly in response to criticism
F 60.31 Borderline type
Several characteristics of emotional instability. In addition, the patients own self-image, aims and internal preferences (including sexual) often unclear or disturbed. Usually chronic feelings of emptiness. A liability to involvement in intense and unstable relationships may cause repeated emotional crises and be associated with excessive efforts to avoid abandonment and a series of suicidal threats or acts of self-harm
DSM-IV: criteria for borderline personality disorder
A pervasive pattern of instability of interpersonal relationships, self-image and affects and marked impulsivity beginning in early adulthood and present in a variety of contexts, as indicated by at least 5 of the following:
1. Frantic efforts to avoid real or imagined abandonment
2. A pattern of unstable and intense interpersonal relationships characterized by alternating between extremes of idealization and devaluation
3. Identity disturbance: markedly and persistently unstable self-image or sense of self
4. Impulsivity in at least two areas that are potentially self-damaging (e.g. spending, sex, substance abuse, reckless driving, binge eating)
5. Recurrent suicidal behaviour, gestures, or threats, or self-mutilating behaviour
6. Affective instability due to a marked reactivity of mood (e.g. intense episodic dysphoria, irritability or anxiety lasting a few hours and only rarely more than a few days)
7. Chronic feelings of emptiness
8. Inappropriate intense anger or difficulty controlling anger (e.g. frequent displays of temper, constant anger, recurrent physical fights)
9. Transient, stress-related paranoid ideation or severe dissociative symptoms

Historically, clinicians were attempting to understand patients who seemed too disturbed for classical psychoanalysis as neurotics, but not as unwell as schizophrenics. Hoch and Polatin (1949) referred to them as having 'pseudoneurotic schizophrenia', and further studies delineated the syndrome showing that patients did not deteriorate into schizophrenia over time. More recent descriptive studies have identified quasi-psychotic thought, abandonment/engulfment/annihilation concerns as differentiating BPD from other personality disorders. (Zanarini *et al.* 1990), though there remains considerable overlap in clinical samples.

Psychoanalytic clinicians have understood BPD symptoms as arising from core intrapsychic features with impaired ego functioning including inability to plan, difficulty managing primitive impulses, and predominance of primary (irrational) over secondary process (logical) thinking (Stern 1938; Knight 1953). These were further systematized by Kernberg who conceptualized borderline personality organization as underlying a number of personality disorders including borderline, narcissistic, antisocial, histrionic (characterized in DSM as cluster B disorders) and paranoid personality disorder, all located between neurotic and psychotic conditions. His model highlights ego weakness with low anxiety tolerance and poor impulse control and emphasizes core features of identity diffusion, partially intact reality testing, pathological internalized object relations, and the use of primitive defences (splitting, primitive idealization, projection, projective identification, denial and omnipotence, and devaluation) (Kernberg 1975).

The splitting process of separating contradictory aspects of others (along with the associated feelings) means that others or self tend to be seen as all bad or all good, though there may be rapid oscillations between. This contributes to the instability of self-identity and affect in relationships with others, and is a familiar aspect of the clinical experience of working with borderline patients. These features have been supported by empirical research showing BPD patients to use more splitting, projection, and acting out, with this discriminating from other personality disorders (Zanarini *et al.* 1990). Splitting is also a key feature in cognitive formulations of BPD that emphasize dichotomous thinking alongside typical cognitions such as 'the world is dangerous and malevolent', 'I am powerless and vulnerable', 'I am inherently unacceptable', and 'I am uncared for' (Beck and Freeman 1990).

Intense anxieties about separation and abandonment (with conflict about the expression of anger and emotional need) are greater in patients with BPD compared with antisocial personality disorder (ASPD) or bipolar disorder (Perry and Cooper 1986). They tend to become deeply attached and rely on transitional objects (Cardasis *et al.* 1997). This has been linked with failed early attachment experiences with a number of studies demonstrating insecure attachment characterized by alternating fear of involvement and intense neediness (Bartholomew *et al.* 2001).

BPD patients have also been shown to have characteristic temperament dimensions A seven-year follow-up study identified impulsiveness-related traits (such as novelty seeking and low cooperativeness) as predicting BPD compared with other personality disorder and non-clinical controls independent of attachment style and parental bonding reports (Links *et al.* 1999; Fossati *et al.* 2001).

Bateman and Fonagy (2004) conceptualize BPD in terms of a core unstable or reduced capacity to mentalize, i.e. make sense of oneself and others on the basis of intentional mental states (desires, beliefs, feelings) understood as distinct from events in the world. In the absence of this capacity, individuals revert to more primitive modes of thinking characterized by psychic equivalence, teleological thinking, and pretend mode. This leads to difficulties making sense of and managing intense feelings in interpersonal interactions. This is compounded by a hypersensitive attachment system and an internalized 'alien self' representation that profoundly disturbs any sense of self-coherence leading to impulsive disturbed behaviours. This is understood as explaining the observed characteristic clinical picture.

Comorbidity

Women with BPD have high rates of comorbid psychiatric diagnoses, often three or more, particularly mood disorders. In a study of 409 outpatients, of 59 diagnosed with BPD, 61% had comorbid major depressive disorder, 29% panic disorder with agoraphobia, and 13% substance misuse (Zimmerman and Mattia 1999; Skodol 2002b). Women with BPD with impulsive behaviour have increased rates of comorbid eating disorder compared with men who show higher rates of substance abuse and antisocial personality (Zlotnick 2002).

Course and prognosis of borderline personality disorder

Longitudinal studies of the course of BPD show a stability of diagnosis over time, and suggest that long-term outcomes are better than for most serious psychiatric disorders, with most patients improving symptomatically over time—although the risk of actual suicide remains significant at 10% (Oldham, 2006). Increased suicide risk has been associated with severity of psychopathology, previous attempts, affective instability, comorbid mood disorder, dual diagnosis, history of abuse, negative life events, and younger age (Links 2007). One 27-year follow-up study showed that patients continued to improve into late middle age with only 8% of BPD sample still meeting criteria for diagnosis (Paris and Zweig-Frank 2001).

A substantial prospective follow-up study by Zanarini *et al.* (2003, 2006) followed 362 adult inpatients with PD over six years. Two hundred and ninety met criteria for BPD and 94% were reassessed at two, four, and six years by interviewers blind to previous information. Of these, one-third showed remission at two years, half at four years, and two-thirds at six years. Overall, 73.5% had met criteria for remission at some stage, and only 6% of these experienced recurrences. Despite the decline in symptoms, the BPD group remained symptomatically distinct from the axis II comparison group. The impulsive symptoms, self-mutilation, suicide attempts, quasi psychotic thought, and treatment regressions seemed to improve most quickly. The affective and enduring temperament-based symptoms such as anger and emptiness, difficulty tolerating aloneness, and concerns about abandonment appear to be more chronic and persisted at six years. However, the available evidence suggests that BPD patients tend to remain functionally seriously impaired, even if they no longer meet criteria for diagnosis (Skodol *et al.* 2002b).

It is advisable not to diagnose personality disorder before the age of 18; however, borderline characteristics and symptoms are often identifiable at an earlier age (Bradley *et al.* 2005). Studies looking at childhood and adolescent precursors suggest that antisocial behaviour in adolescent girls is associated with BPD in adulthood. An interesting longitudinal study of 407 adolescents from a community sample showed a stability of cluster B symptoms aged 12–20 (Crawford *et al.* 2001a, 2001b). In girls (n = 199) internalizing symptoms (anxiety and depression) age 10–14 years predicted cluster B symptoms in adolescence, but externalizing symptoms in adolescence (12–17 years) predicted cluster B symptoms at age 17–24 (independent of earlier cluster B symptoms). The stability of abnormal personality constellations, supports a link with biologically predetermined disposition.

Aetiology

Most theoreticians propose a multifactorial aetiology of BPD with evidence for the importance of genetic, neurobiological, and psychosocial factors that supports a model of constitutional vulnerability influencing resilience to early environment and subsequent life events (Zanarini and Frankenberg 1997). Studies of the impact of trauma and attachment on the developing brain increasingly integrate neurobiological observations and psychosocial attachment-based models.

Genetic factors

Family studies support the heritability of BPD and its independence from schizophrenia, schizotypal PD, and depression. The role of genetic factors is supported by a large twin study (Torgersen *et al.* 2000) of 92 monozygotic (MZ) and 129 dizygotic (DZ) twin pairs which found 35% concordance in MZ and 7% in DZ twins

Table 13.2 Factors associated with good and poor prognosis in BPD (Links *et al.* 1998)

Poor prognosis
History of childhood sexual abuse in childhood, incest or parental brutality
Family history of mental illness, maternal psychopathology
Early age of first psychiatric contact with chronic symptoms
Phenomenological predictors: higher affective instability, magical thinking and aggression in relationships, impulsivity and substance abuse and overall greater severity of disorder. Comorbid antisocial, paranoid or paranoid features
Good prognosis
High IQ
Absence of narcissistic entitlement
Absence of parental divorce

meeting criteria for narrow definition of BPD using SCID-II. Heritability for personality disorder generally was 0.6, and for BPD specifically 0.69. The pattern of personality traits that describes BPD (including tendency to unstable affect, unstable cognitive functioning, unstable sense of self, and unstable interpersonal relationships) has also been shown to be highly heritable by phenotypic factor analysis, as are specific traits such as self-control.(Livesley et al. 1998).

Neurobiological abnormalities

A number of structural and functional neurobiological abnormalities have been demonstrated in subjects with BPD compared with healthy controls. The evidence has been extensively reviewed in Bateman and Fonagy (2004).

Neurotransmitter abnormalities

The impulsivity characteristic of BPD patients has been linked to dysfunctions of the serotonergic system. Studies link abnormal levels of serotonin metabolites with attempted suicide and externally directed aggression, with low 5-hydroxyindoleacetic acid levels in lumbar cerebrospinal fluid (CSF) and blunted neuroendocrine responses to fenfluramine. There is some evidence localizing these abnormalities to areas involved in inhibiting limbic aggression in the orbital-frontal cortex, ventral-medial cortex and cingulated cortex (Soloff et al. 2003). This is consistent with the reduction of impulsive aggression clinically by selective serotonin re-uptake inhibitors (SSRIs) independent of depression when used in high doses or for longer duration (Coccaro 1998). Reduced 5-HT (serotonin) synthetic capacity in medication free BPD subjects has also been demonstrated in corticostriatal sites by functional positron emission tomography scanning. Studies of potential candidate genes have associated the serotonin transporter 'S' allele and the tryptophan hydroxylase (TPH) 'L' allele with impulsivity and neuroticism (Lesch et al. 1996). The 5-HT 1b receptor gene has been linked to suicide attempts (New et al. 2001).

Noradrenergic abnormalities have also been noted in BPD patients and associated with risk taking and sensation seeking. Increased CSF dopamine concentrations have been shown in BPD patients with comorbid schizotypal presentations. These may signal vulnerabilities to childhood and adult environmental stressors which themselves impact on catecholamine and cortisol levels (Caspi et al. 2002, 2003).

Enhanced amygdala activation

Enhanced amygdala activation has been shown in BPD subjects shown affectively stimulating images (mutilated bodies, crying children, scenes of violence and danger) compared with healthy female controls (Herpetz et al. 2001). Enhanced activation to facial expressions of emotion, with a tendency to attribute negative attributes (threatening, untrustworthy possibly plotting) to neutral faces has also been shown (Donegan et al. 2003). A hypersensitive amygdala may predispose subjects to be hypervigilant and overreactive to benign emotional expressions, contributing to the extreme sensitivity that typically complicates BPD subjects' relationships.

This may be part of a pattern of hypothalamic–pituitary–adrenal (HPA) hypersensitivity resulting from trauma. Hyper-responsiveness of the HPA axis has been demonstrated in women with BPD with a history of sexual abuse, with enhanced adrenocorticotropic hormone (ACTH), and cortisol responses to the dexamethasone/ corticotropin-releasing hormone (CRH) challenge compared with non-abused BPD and healthy controls (Rinne et al. 2002). A number of magnetic resonance imaging (MRI) studies have shown reduced hippocampal and amygdala volumes in women with BPD, a finding also associated with trauma (see later).

Greater amygdala neuronal activity in response to fearful stimuli has also been linked with the short allele of the serotonin transporter (5HTT) promoter gene in normal individuals (Hariri et al. 2002).

Reduced prefrontal controls

Reduced frontal and prefrontal inhibitory controls may contribute to amygdala hyperactivity and a difficulty extinguishing a fear response and shutting down the generation of negative affect in women with BPD.

There is evidence for reduced medial and orbital frontal lobe volumes in BPD patients (Lyoo et al. 1998). Frontal lobe abnormalities have been consistently associated with aggressive behaviour in a variety of PD subjects, and in personality change following orbitofrontal cortex lesions and prefrontal injury. The frontal lobe is thought to play a role in a variety of executive brain functions involved in affective responsiveness, social and personality development, self-awareness, and consciousness. There may be a range of prefrontal and subcortical-frontal connecting systems that account for alterations in frontal lobe functioning in subjects with BPD and other personality disorders.

As noted earlier, reduced prefrontal metabolic and serotonergic activity have been associated with impulsive aggression in patients with BPD and ASPD (Soloff et al. 2003). This area is also connected with structures involved in rewards, drives, and motivation, and delayed gratification associated with increased serotonergic activity which may be relevant to the capacity to direct attention, suppress irrelevant stimuli, and make non-impulsive choices based on likelihood of reward. This seems highly relevant to borderline pathology and comorbid conditions such as eating disorders, addiction problems, ASPD, and conduct disorder.

The medial prefrontal region is also importantly activated in mentalization tasks, which involves several different brain structures working together, and is thought to be relevant to the specific difficulties BPD patients struggle with.

Psychosocial factors

A number of psychosocial factors have been associated with BPD through their increased prevalence in the histories of patients. High rates of parental psychopathology, parental loss and separation, conflictual relationships, childhood trauma, abuse, and neglect all contribute to a disturbed, unstable, and non-nurturing family environment and interfere with intrapsychic and interpersonal development (Zanarini 2000).

Family history of psychopathology

Women with BPD have increased rates of psychiatric disorder in one or both biological parents compared with psychiatric controls, and controlling for childhood abuse and comorbidity. One study found 71% outpatients with BPD had at least one parent with axis 1 disorder compared with 30% non-BPD (Goldman, 1993). In a study of female inpatients, in 82% both parents met criteria for parental psychopathology, with severity associated with BPD severity (Schacknow *et al.* 1997). Though studies have shown increased rates of mood disorders and substance abuse, overall parental pathology appears heterogeneous, contributing to an unstable family environment.

Parental loss or separation

Women with BPD have high rates of parental loss and separation through divorce, parental illness, or death—80% in an early study by Walsh (1977). This has been supported by subsequent research and the level of disruption appears to be greater than for psychotic, depressed, or other PD controls. Prolonged early separation of at least one to three months appears to be significant.

Disturbed relationship with parents

Studies show most families to have a high degree of discord. The Walsh study (1977) reported two-thirds of patients' relationships with parents as highly conflictual including hostility, devaluation or abuse, with 57% of patients perceiving themselves as overinvolved with one parent—and most reporting at least one parent remote and lacking attachment feelings. Problems with both parents are likely to be the common pathogenic influence (Frank and Paris, 1981). Zanarini emphasizes an invalidating family environment where emotional distress is denied, undermining self-perceptions of internal states and failure to discriminate feelings of self and other (Zanarini 2000; Fruzzetti 2005).

Neglect

A number of studies have associated neglect and childhood abuse with personality disorder. A retrospective study comparing 358 inpatients with BPD with 109 axis II controls showed that 91% reported sexual abuse, 62% in childhood compared with 32% controls, and 92% some kind of neglect. Eighty-four per cent showed biparental failure with females with BPD characteristically reporting female caretaker neglect and male caretaker abuse. Fifty per cent reported biparental denial of the validity of their thoughts and feelings (Zanarini, 2000). The prospective New York Children in the Community Study (Johnson *et al.* 1999, 2000) followed-up 738 youths from 1975–1993. This showed that childhood abuse substantially increased the risk of Cluster B personality disorders, and BPD in particular. Emotional, physical, and supervision neglect were all associated with increased risk for personality disorder. Supervision neglect includes allowing a child to go out as she pleases, being tolerant of drug abuse including cannabis, with prevalence of 30% supervision neglect amongst Cluster B diagnoses (including BPD). This remained significant after controlling for abuse.

Childhood trauma and maltreatment

Women with BPD frequently have a history of trauma, with a substantial percentage reporting sexual abuse with increased prevalence than psychiatric comparison groups. Studies also show increased rates of physical abuse, though this does not always discriminate from other axis II (personality disorder) patients. In a review by Zanarini (2000) 40–70% BPD reported sexual abuse in childhood or adolescence compared with 19–46% controls. Across the studies, 40–50% of this abuse was by non-relatives, about 25% by fathers and 25% by siblings. A study comparing women with BPD with axis II female controls highlighted sexual abuse as the only significant multivariate predictor in the diagnosis of BPD—with the reported rate of 71% compared with 46%. Abuse more commonly involved penetration (fivefold), non-relatives (threefold), and multiple perpetrators (Paris *et al.* 1994). The impact of abuse is importantly mediated by caregiver response and the family environment (Bradley *et al.* 2005).

Neurobiological impact of stress

Maltreatment is known to disrupt psychological development causing delays and deficits across a range of cognitive, emotional, and behavioural achievements including IQ, symbolic function, and emotional regulation skills. This is supported by findings from neurobiological research on the developing brain and the impact of trauma. There is evidence that cortical and subcortical brain structures continue developing into late adolescence—and maltreated children show reduced intracranial and cerebral volumes that may account for pervasive areas of difficulty. There is evidence for the impact of stress on the serotonergic system, with 5-HT1A and B receptor alterations in the hippocampus and cortex and reduced serotonin levels. It has been suggested that trauma has long-term affects on the hypothalamic–pituitary axis with lower resting levels of ACTH and cortisol secretion but a hyper-responsiveness during acute stress. Fifty per cent of women with BPD appear to show non-suppression on dexamethasone suppression test. Elevated glucocorticoids may themselves have neurotoxic effects accounting for smaller hippocampal volumes (found in studies of women with histories of childhood sexual abuse, adult PTSD, and BPD) and may affect the developing brain. There has been particular interest in the functioning of the anterior cingulated region of the medial prefrontal cortex. Studies have shown reduced N-acteylaspartate levels in maltreated children, and reduced blood flow in women with PTSD during traumatic imagery or recounting memories of sexual abuse (Shin *et al.* 1999; Bremner *et al.* 1999; see Gabbard *et al.* 2006 for a review).

Attachment

Early theorists linked the problems of BPD patients with early developmental difficulties, with excessive splitting (Kernberg 1975) or mothering deficits leading to failure of object constancy (Adler and Buie 1979) and of separation-individuation (Mahler 1971; Masterson and Rinsley1975). The emphasis on early mothering experiences is supported by more recent findings from attachment research that show an association between diagnosis of BPD with insecure preoccupied classifications on the Adult Attachment Interview. Increased attachment insecurity persists after comparison with normative, psychiatric and other personality disorder controls and after controlling for physical and sexual abuse (Fossati 2001; Nickell *et al.* 2002) Gunderson (1996) emphasizes the intolerance of

aloneness and the inability to evoke a soothing introject, and understands patterns of borderline experience and behaviour in terms of the insecurely attached infant—with clinging, fearfulness about dependency needs, terror of abandonment, and constant monitoring of caregiver proximity—linking this to disorganized attachment in infancy as a predisposing condition. This is supported by two longitudinal studies following infants into early adulthood that report an association between insecure attachment and BPD symptoms (Lyons-Ruth *et al.* 2005). Schore (2001) proposes that secure attachment is important for brain development, and it has been linked with the development of symbolic function and metacognitive capacities in memory, comprehension, communication, and reasoning capacity (Fonagy 2006).

Mentalization model

Bateman and Fonagy (2004) have integrated both neurobiological findings and attachment research in the development of their model which places deficits in mentalizing at the core of borderline pathology. This accounts for the phenomenological picture and characteristic relationship difficulties, and creates a long-term vulnerability to stress and life events.

Mentalizing is viewed as an essential human capacity underpinning interpersonal relations, which develops in the first few years of life in the context of safe and secure child–caregiver relationships. The infant finds its mind as represented in the mind of the other and develops a sense of self as a social agent which is the basis of understanding the minds of others. Through secure caregiver congruent marked mirroring the infant learns to differentiate and represent affect states and internalizes the soothing process as a basis for affect regulation and impulse control. The caregiver's mentalizing, regulatory, and joint attention activity is crucial to the development of effortful control required for both mentalizing and impulse control—in interaction with genetically determined temperamental factors.

This normal developmental process is severely disrupted in environmental conditions of neglect, emotional abuse, or physical or sexual maltreatment during childhood. The insecure infant is deprived of a crucial developmental learning opportunity. In non-congruent mirroring, internal states remain confusing, unsymbolized, and difficult to regulate. In this way early inadequate mirroring and disorganized attachment undermine the capacity to mentalize, leaving the individual extremely vulnerable to stressful psychosocial experiences—particularly in an attachment context.

When unable to mentalize, individuals revert to more primitive modes of thinking (psychic equivalence, teleological thinking, and pretend mode) which are recognizable in working with borderline patients.

In *psychic equivalence* the internal is equated with external—often a source of distress as fantasy projections and memories experienced as real and present (e.g. in flashbacks) and eclipsing the possibility of recognizing and exploring multiple perspectives. The capacity to decouple internal and external reality to pretend and imagine is an important developmental step towards true mentalizing when thoughts inner and outer are experienced as linked but separate, and thoughts and feelings are experienced as representations. However in *pretend mode* these become completely detached contributing to 'pseudomentalizing', emptiness, and dissociative states. In *teleological thinking* the sense of self as an agent is limited to physical actions in the world (as in first year of life). In this state patients demand concrete modification as the only true expression of the other's intention (notably care or concern), and accidents can only be experienced as intentional.

With disturbed or maltreating parents, the reality of hostile or frightening caregiver affect or representations of the child promotes hypervigilance and is a further disincentive to true mentalizing activity—it is not safe to explore the mind of the other. In addition to the lack of congruent representations to contribute to the infant's sense of agentive self, the exposure to non-self representations (often frightening or hostile) contributes to the infant internalizing an 'alien self' representation which disturbs their sense of coherence. This contributes to the sense of fragmentation BPD patients carry. The alien self can also be a source of terror and unbearable pain. The self can feel attacked from within and overwhelmed by a sense of badness impossible to mitigate by reassurance and experienced in psychic equivalence as actual badness. Attempts to get rid of this disturbing 'alien self' in teleological mode are seen as explaining suicide and self-harm—which may be a way to attack the alien self. In disturbed interpersonal interactions the alien self may be projected onto an abusing other. In this way 'self-destructive' behaviours are conceptualized in terms of an acutely disturbed self desperately trying to preserve a sense of coherence and existence.

BPD patients are also understood as having hyperactive attachment systems as a result of childhood trauma and biological disposition. This further inhibits the capacity to mentalize since activation of the attachment system is thought to temporarily inhibit or decouple mentalizing—accounting for the extreme interpersonal sensitivity of borderline patients and vulnerability to attachment stress.

Drawing on Schore (2003), Bateman and Fonagy (2004) have reviewed the available evidence for the neurobiological underpinnings of mentalization, and the impact of trauma on this. They emphasize the role of the prefrontal cortex in executive functions crucial to social cooperation and regulating interpersonal relationships. The medial prefrontal cortex and anterior cingulated gyrus are particularly activated in theory of mind and mentalizing tasks (Baron-Cohen *et al.* 2000) They highlight the vulnerability of prefrontal functioning to level of arousal—drawing on research that suggests that above a certain level of arousal there is a switch from prefrontal executive mode flexible reflective responding to more primitive posterior cortical/subcortical arousal with amygdala mediated memory encoding, hypervigilance, and fight/flight mode action centred responding (Arnsten 1998). They suggest those with insecure or disorganized attachment are highly sensitized to interpersonal interactions, being easily triggered to high arousal with a corresponding shift in predominant brain functioning. This contributes to the precariousness of mentalizing in borderline patients less able to modulate their level of arousal.

Assessment

It is important to bear in mind the context of assessment, since referral may be complicated by housing issues or concerns about parenting or acute risk. Exploring the patients' concerns from the start will facilitate developing rapport, and it is important to attend to this since patients may have a history of negative experiences with services, and arrive anxious or angry—anticipating rejection, criticism, or dismissal.

Assessment should make use of all available collateral information. An informant history (with permission) is particularly helpful in establishing whether there are enduring behavioural and emotional difficulties persistent from childhood or adolescence and across social, occupational, and interpersonal domains suggestive of a personality disorder, in contrast to episodic or chronic other psychiatric disorder.

A full psychiatric history and mental state examination is essential. This should include full personal history, family history, specific personality enquiry, detailed drug and alcohol history, and past psychiatric history.

Patients commonly present in crisis with mood swings, self-harm, or impulsive behaviour, typically triggered by an interpersonal event precipitating fears of abandonment. It is helpful to detail the event, associated thoughts and feelings, and actual and anticipated consequences, and to ask directly about associated drug or alcohol use, anger, and violence. Enquiring explicitly about the patient's understanding of their difficulties, impact on others, and what they think would help, will give a sense of their capacity to mentalize and be useful in thinking about referral for psychological treatment.

Diagnosis can be strengthened by using a standardized semi-structured interview such as the Personality Assessment Schedule (Tyrer *et al.* 1979), the Standardised Assessment of Personality (Mann *et al.* 1999, 2003), or the Structured Clinical Interview for DSM-IV Axis II Personality disorders (SCID-II) (First *et al.* 1997).

Risk assessment should be recorded and will be facilitated by an accurate risk history detailing frequency, severity, consequences of self-harm or dangerous behaviour, and precipitating factors (interpersonal or drugs and alcohol) which will frequently show patterns of self-harm and a degree of chronic risk. This enables the identification of times of more acute risk when the behaviour may deviate to guide management when the patient presents in crisis. A tool such as the Suicide and Self-harm Inventory (Bateman and Fonagy 2004) can help structure this. It is usually helpful to engage patients in filling out their risk assessment forms and important to explicitly consider risk to others—such as children—where relevant.

A *crisis plan* should be set up collaboratively and documented detailing the main problematic behaviours and factors increasing risk (drugs, alcohol, interpersonal events). It should detail whom the patient can contact in crisis, with an agreed staff response (including timescale), and covering out-of-hours situations and contingencies such as when the identified person is unavailable. The response may include a telephone conversation, brief emergency appointment, or hospital admission to manage the crisis acutely. This should be within the framework of an overall treatment plan that can be reviewed when the crisis has resolved. The crisis plan should be signed, dated, and made available to any clinical teams that the patient is likely to come into contact with.

Parenting and child protection issues

This is an important area to bear in mind when assessing women. Women with BPD may have complex histories, including teenage pregnancies, pregnancy from abuse or rape, infants adopted at birth, or children in care with varying degrees of contact and responsibility. Where children have been removed, or there is threat of this, it may be an over-riding preoccupation and source of distress and stir up intense feelings in relation to the woman's own parenting experiences. There may be statutory parenting concerns or formal assessment which may coincide with the request for assessment and treatment recommendations. Assessment should clarify other agencies currently involved, any concerns about risk, and current parenting support from friends, family, or statutory agencies.

Exploring a woman's thoughts about her child gives a sense of her capacity to mentalize about her child's needs, feelings, and intentions as separate from her own. There is interesting recent research investigating interactions between borderline mothers and their infants (Crandell *et al.* 2003; Hobson *et al.* 2005; Lyons-Ruth *et al.* 2007). Maternal insecurity and poor mentalizing limit the BPD mother's capacity to meet her child's emotional needs and impact on infant attachment and later psychological and cognitive development (Fonagy and Bateman 2007). In practical terms, BPD difficulties may affect her capacity to provide a stable home and ensure that basic needs for safety, health, and education are met. There may be more acute concerns about the impact of mood swings and disturbed and dangerous behaviour on the child. Moreover, the stresses of motherhood may precipitate a deterioration in maternal mental health with an escalation of disturbed behaviour and negative consequences for the child.

The Royal College of Psychiatrists council report 'Patients as Parents' (2002) details the impact of psychiatric illness on children, emphasizes the high risk of emotional abuse, and suggests guidelines for consultation with child care professionals. The report also details specific practice guidelines in relation to special circumstances including parental self-harm and parental hospitalization.

References

Adler G and Buie D (1979). Aloneness and borderline psychopathology: the possible relevance of some child developmental issues. *International Journal of Psycho-Analysis*, **60**, 83–96.

American Psychiatric Association (2000). *Diagnostic and Statistical Manual of Mental Disorders, fourth edition*. APA, Arlington, VA.

Arnsten AFT (1998). The biology of being frazzled. *Science*, **280**, 1711–2.

Baron-Cohen S *et al.* (eds) (2000). *Understanding Other Minds: Perspectives from Developmental Cognitive Neuroscience*. Oxford University Press, Oxford.

Bateman A and Fonagy P (2004). *Psychotherapy for Borderline Personality Disorder. Mentalization-based treatment.* Oxford University Press, Oxford.

Bartholemew K *et al.* (2001). Attachment. In WJ Livesley (ed) *Handbook of Personality Disorders: Theory, Research and Treatment*, pp. 196–230. Guildford Press, New York.

Beck AT and Freeman A (1990). *Cognitive Therapy of Personality Disorders.* Guilford Press, New York.

Black DW *et al.* (2006). Borderline personality disorder and traits in veterans: psychiatric comorbidity, healthcare utilization, and quality of life along a continuum of severity. *CNS Spectrums*, **11**, 680–9.

Blackburn R *et al.* (1990). Prevalence of personality disorders in a special hospital population. *Journal of Forensic Psychiatry*, **1**, 43–52.

Bradley R *et al.* (2005). The borderline personality diagnosis in adolescents. Gender differences and subtypes. *Journal of Child Psychology and Psychiatry*, **46**, 1006–19.

Bremner J *et al.* (1999). Neural correlates of memories of childhood sexual abuse in women with and without posttraumatic stress disorder. *American Journal of Psychiatry*, **156**, 1787–95.

Cardiasis W *et al.* (1997). Transitional objects and borderline personality disorder. *American Journal of Psychiatry*, **154**, 250–5.

Caspi A *et al.* (2002). Role of genotype in the cycle of violence in maltreated children. *Science*, **297**(5582), 851–4.

Caspi A *et al.* (2003). Influence of life stress on depression: moderation by a polymorphism in the 5-HTT gene. *Science*, **301**(5631), 386–9.

Cheng AT *et al.* (1997). Personality disorder and suicide. *A case control study. British Journal of Psychiatry*, **170**, 441–6.

Coccaro EF (1998). Biology of personality disorders. In: KR Silk (ed) *Neurotransmitter Function in Personality Disorders*, pp. 1–25. American Psychiatric Press, Washington, DC.

Coid J *et al.* (2006). Prevalence and correlates of personality disorder in Great Britain. *British Journal of Psychiatry*, **188**, 423–31.

Crandell LE *et al.* (2003). "Still-face" interactions between mother with borderline personality disorder and their 2-month-old infants. *British Journal of Psychiatry*, **183**, 239–47.

Crawford TN *et al.* (2001a). Dramatic-erratic personality disorder symptoms: I. Continuity from early adolescence into adulthood. *Journal of Personality Disorders*, **15**, 319–35.

Crawford TN *et al.* (2001b). Dramatic-erratic personality disorder symptoms: II. Developmental pathways from early adolescence to adulthood. *Journal of Personality Disorders*, **15**, 336–50.

Donegan NH *et al.* (2003). Amygdala hyperreactivity in borderline personality disorder: implications for emotional dysregulation. *Biological Psychiatry*, **54**, 1284–93.

First *et al.* (1997). *Structured Clinical Interview for DSM-IV Axis II Personality Disorders (SCID II) Clinical Version (SCID CV) (Users guide and interview).* Washington, DC., American Psychiatric Press, Inc.

Fonagy P (2006). The mentalization-focussed approach to social development. In: JG Allen and P Fonagy (eds) *Handbook of Mentalization-Based Treatment*, pp. 53–100. John Wiley & Sons, Chichester.

Fonagy P and Bateman A (2007). Mentalizing and borderline personality disorder. *Journal of Mental Health*, **16**, 83–101.

Fossati A *et al.* (2001). Temperament, character and attachment patterns in borderline personality disorder. *Journal of Personality Disorders*, **15**, 390–402.

Frank H and Paris J (1981). Recollections of family experience in borderline patients. *Archives of General Psychiatry*, **38**, 1031–4.

Fruzetti AE *et al.* (2005). Family interaction and the development of borderline personality disorder: a transactional model. *Developmental Psychopathology*, **17**, 1007–30.

Gabbard GO *et al.* (2006). A neurobiological perspective on mentalizing and internal object relations in traumatized patients with borderline personality disorder. In: JG Allen and P Fonagy (eds) *Handbook of Mentalization-Based Treatment*, pp. 123–40. John Wiley & Sons, Chichester.

Goldman SJ *et al.* (1993). Psychopathology in the families of children and adolescents with borderline personality disorder. *American Journal of Psychiatry*, **150**, 1832–5.

Gunderson JG (1996). The borderline patient's intolerance of aloneness: insecure attachments and therapist availability. *American Journal of Psychiatry*, **153**, 752–8.

Hariri AR *et al.* (2002). Serotonin transporter gene variation and the response of the human amygdala. *Science*, **297**, 400–3.

Herpetz SC *et al.* (2001). Evidence of abnormal amygdala functioning in borderline personality disorder: a functional MRI study. *Biological Psychiatry*, **50**, 292–8.

Hobson RP *et al.* (2005). Personal relatedness and attachment in infants of mothers with borderline personality disorder. *Development and Psychopathology*, **17**, 329–47.

Hoch P and Polatin P (1949). Pseudoneurotic forms of schizophrenia. *Psychiatry Quarterly*, **23**, 248–76.

Johnson JG *et al.* (1999). childhood maltreatment increases risk for personality disorders during early adulthood. *Archives of General Psychiatry*, **56**, 600–5.

Johnson JG *et al.* (2000). Associations between four types of childhood neglect and personality disorder symptoms during adolescence and early adulthood: findings of a community-based longitudinal study. *Journal of Personality Disorders*, **14**, 171–87.

Kernberg OF (1975). *Borderline Conditions and Pathological Narcissism.* Jason Aronson, New York.

Knight RP (1953). Borderline states. *Bulletin of the Menninger Clinic*, **17**, 1–12.

Lesch KP *et al.* (1996). Association of anxiety related traits with a polymorphism in the serotonin transporter gene regulatory region. *Science*, **274**, 1527–31.

Links PS *et al.* (1998). Prospective follow-up study of borderline personality disorder; prognosis, prediction of outcome, and axis II comorbidity. *Canadian Journal of Psychiatry*, **43**, 265–70.

Links PS *et al.* (1999). Impulsivity: core aspect of borderline personality disorder. *Journal of Personality Disorders*, **13**, 1–9.

Links PS *et al.* (2007). Affective instability and suicidal ideation and behaviour in patients with borderline personality disorder. *Journal of Personality Disorders*, **21**, 72–86.

Livesley W J *et al.* (1998) Phenotypic and genetic structure of traits delineating personality disorder. *Archives of General Psychiatry*, **55**, 941–8.

Lyons-Ruth K *et al.* (2005). Expanding the concept of unresolved mental states: hostile/helpless states of mind on the Adult Attachment Interview are associated with disrupted mother-infant communication and infant disorganization. *Developmental Psychopathology*, **17**, 1–23.

Lyons-Ruth K *et al.* (2007). A controlled study of Hostile-Helpless states of mind among borderline and dysthymic women. *Attachment and Human Development*, **9**, 1–16.

Lyoo IK *et al.* (1998). A brain MRI study in subjects with borderline personality disorder. *Journal of Affective Disorders*, **50**, 235–43.

Mahler MS (1971). A study of separation-individuation process and its possible application in borderline phenomenon in the psychoanalytic situation. *Psychoanalytic Study of the Child*, **26**, 403–24.

Mann A *et al.* (1999). An assessment of the Standardized Assessment of Personality as a screening tool for the International Personality Disorders Examination: a comparison of informant and patient accounts. *Psychological Medicine*, **29**, 985–89.

Mann P *et al.* (2003). Standardized Assessment of Personality — Abbreviated Scale (SAPAS): Preliminary validation of a brief screen for personality disorder. *British Journal of Psychiatry*, **183**, 228–32.

Masterson JF and Rinsley D (1975). The borderline syndrome: the role of the mother in the genesis and psychic structure of the borderline personality. *International Journal of Psychoanalysis*, **56**, 163–77.

Moran P *et al.* (2000). The prevalence of personality disorder among UK primary care attenders. *Acta Psychiatrica Scandinavica*, **102**, 52–7.

New AS *et al.* (2001). Suicide, impulsive aggression, and HTR1B genotype. *Biological Psychiatry*, **50**, 62–5.

Nickell AD *et al.* (2002). Attachment, parental bonding and borderline personality disorder features in young adults. *Journal of Personality Disorders*, **16**, 148–59.

Oldham JM (2006). Borderline personality disorder and suicidality. *American Journal of Psychiatry*, **163**, 20–6.

Paris J and Zweig-Frank H (2001). A 27-year follow-up of patients with borderline personality disorder. *Comprehensive Psychiatry*, **42**, 482–7.

Paris J *et al.* (1994). Psychological risk factors for borderline personality disorder in female patients. *Comprehensive Psychiatry*, **35**, 301–5.

Perry JC *et al.* (1986). A preliminary report on defences and conflicts associated with borderline personality disorder. *Journal of the American Psychoanalytic Association*, **34**, 863–93.

Rinne T *et al.* (2002). Hyperresponsiveness of hypothalamic-pituitary-adrenal axis to combined dexamethasone/corticotropin-releasing hormone challenge in female borderline personality disorder subjects with a history of sustained childhood abuse. *Biological Psychiatry*, **52**, 1102–12.

Schore AN (2001). Effects of a secure attachment relationship on right brain development, affect regulation, and infant mental health. *Infant Mental Health Journal*, **22**, 7–66.

Schore AN (2003). *Affect Regulation in the Repair of the Self*. WW Norton, New York.

Shachmow J *et al.* (1997). Biparental psychopathology and borderline personality disorder. *Psychiatry*, **60**, 171–81.

Shin LM *et al.* (1999). Regional cerebral blood flow during script driven imagery in childhood sexual abuse-related PTSD: A PET investigation. *American Journal of Psychiatry*, **156**, 575–84.

Skodol AE *et al.* (2002a). The borderline diagnosis I: psychopathology, comorbidity and personality structure. *Biological Psychiatry*, **51**, 936–50.

Skodol AE *et al.* (2002b). The borderline diagnosis II: biology, genetics and clinical course. *Biological Psychiatry*, **51**, 951–63.

Soloff PH *et al.* (2000a). Characteristics of suicide attempts of patients with major depressive episode and borderline personality disorder: a comparative study. *American Journal of Psychiatry*, **157**, 601–8.

Soloff P *et al.* (2000b). A fenfluramine-activated FDG-PET study of borderline personality disorder. *Biological Psychiatry*, **47**, 540–7.

Soloff P *et al.* (2003). Impulsivity and prefrontal metabolism in borderline personality disorder. *Psychiatry Research*, **123**, 153–63.

Stern A (1938). Psychoanalytic investigation and therapy in borderline group of neuroses. *Psychoanalytic Quarterly*, **7**, 467–89.

Torgersen S *et al.* (2000). A twin study of personality disorders. *Comprehensive Psychiatry*, Nov 2000, **41**(6), 416–25.

Tyrer P *et al.* (1979). Reliability of a schedule for rating personality disorders. *British Journal of Psychiatry*, **135**, 168–74.

Walsh F (1977). The family of the borderline patient. In: RR Grinker and B Werble (eds) *The Borderline Patient*, pp. 158–77. Jason Aronson, New York.

Widiger TA and Weissman MM (1991). Epidemiology of borderline personality disorder. *Hospital Community Psychiatry*, **42**(10), 1015–21.

World Health Organization (1992). *International Statistical Classification of Diseases and Related Health Problems (ICD-10)*. WHO, Geneva.

Zanarini MC (2000). Childhood experiences associated with the development of personality disorder. *Psychiatric Clinics of North America*, **23**, 89–101.

Zanarini MC and Frankenburg FR (1997). Pathways to the development of borderline personality disorder. *Journal of Personality Disorders*, **11**, 93–104.

Zanarini M *et al.* (1990). Discriminating borderline personality disorder from other axis II disorders. *American Journal of Psychiatry*, **147**, 161–7.

Zanarini MC *et al.* (1998). Axis 1 comorbidity of borderline personality disorder. *American Journal of Psychiatry*, **155**, 1733–39.

Zanarini MC *et al.* (2000). Biparental failure in the childhood experiences of borderline patients. *Journal of Personality Disorders*, **14**, 264–73.

Zanarini MC *et al.* (2003). The longitudinal course of borderline psychopathology; 6-year prospective follow-up of the phenomenology of borderline personality disorder. *American Journal of Psychiatry*, **160**, 274–83.

Zimmerman M and Mattia JI (1999). Axis I diagnostic co-morbidity and borderline personality disorder. *Comprehensive Psychiatry*, **40**, 245–52.

Zlotnick C *et al.* (2002). The role of gender in the clinical presentation of patients with borderline personality disorder. *Journal of Personality Disorders*, **16**, 277–82.

CHAPTER 14

Borderline personality disorder in women: treatment approaches

Sarah Majid

Most clinicians working with borderline personality disorder (BPD) take a pragmatic multimodal approach to treatment. Historically, patients were managed within general adult psychiatric services, and often considered problematic, untreatable, and only reluctantly accepted as suffering from a mental illness. There were, nonetheless, important treatment developments in therapeutic community settings. Over the past decade there has been increasing recognition and understanding of personality disorder as a disorder (Department of Health 2003) with inspiring new developments in psychological treatments and an expansion of specialist services The National Institute for Clinical Health and Excellence (NICE) guidelines for the treatment and management of BPD in the United Kingdom will further influence the range of National Health Service services and treatment approaches available. It emphasizes the role of psychological treatments, complex interventions, and crisis management, and recommends developing a care pathway for people with BPD (2009). It also reviews cost-effectiveness of psychological treatments (Brazier *et al.* 2006).

Medication

There is no specific medication for BPD, though it can help some patients through targeting specific symptoms and support psychotherapy work when integrated within an overall treatment programme. It is useful to consider whether the patient's symptoms are primarily in relation to *affect control* (mood lability, rejection sensitivity, intense anger, mood crashes, chronic emptiness, dysphoria, social anxiety), *impulsivity and sensation seeking* (aggression, self-harm, bingeing, risk-taking), or *cognitive perceptual disturbance*. Any comorbid

axis 1 disorders should be adequately treated. Please see NICE guidelines (2009) and American Psychiatric Association practice guideline (Gunderson 2001) for further details and review of evidence.

In prescribing, clinicians should consider transference and countertransference issues and the possibility of splitting (Gabbard 2005). Patients and clinicians can get caught up in idealizing medication as a solution to difficulties at a moment of intense need, despair, or suicide threat. Patients may experience prescribing concretely as the therapist giving or withholding care, though it may have value as a transitional object. Unfortunately BPD patients typically end up taking a number of drugs intermittently—each of questionable value and increasing the risk of overdose. Prescribing should occur within a stable therapeutic relationship, with clearly agreed target symptoms and trial period, and regular review of efficacy. Drugs which are not clearly helping should be stopped. Comorbid drug and alcohol use will also impact on efficacy and safety. Prescribing in women is further complicated by pregnancy, breastfeeding, and weight gain. As always, patients should be properly advised of the benefits and risks to make an informed treatment choice. Prescribing should be discussed with the whole team working with the patient to minimize splitting between clinicians and between psychotherapy and pharmacotherapy.

Antipsychotics

Antipsychotics can be helpful in women with paranoid ideas, transient psychotic episodes, or stress-induced hallucinations, illusions, derealization, and depersonalization. This can support psychotherapy for patients who are easily triggered to paranoid states in groups or intensely socially anxious (with anxiolytic doses).

The use of olanzapine to reduce paranoia, anxiety, interpersonal sensitivity, anger, and hostility in women with BPD is supported by a 6-month double-blind pla-cebo controlled trial (Zanarinii and Frankenberg 2001). Zanarini *et al.* (2004) suggested a combination of olan-zapine and fluoxetine as superior to fluoxetine alone in an eight-week trial of 45 women. A recent small trial suggests benefit from aripiprazole (Nickel *et al.* 2006),

Antidepressants

Antidepressants are commonly prescribed in BPD, fre-quently for comorbid depression. A specific role for selective serotonin reuptake inhibitors (SSRIs) in BPD in reducing anger, impulsive-aggressive behaviour, and affective lability is supported by a number of double blind randomized controlled trials (RCTs) such as the Rinne *et al.* (2002) study of 38 women, and consistent with the aetiological hypothesis of serotonergic dys-function. Some patients require increased doses up to 80 mg/day of fluoxetine. It is thought SSRIs may stimu-late neurogenesis in the hippocampus and reduce hyperactivity of the hypothalamic–pituitary–adrenal (HPA) axis by reducing hypersecretion of cortico-trophin releasing factor. A study of 30 borderline women given 150 mg/day fluvoxamine found a signifi-cant reduction of adrenocorticotropic hormone (ACTH) and cortisol response to combined dexameth-asone and corticotrophin-releasing hormone in women with childhood abuse (Rinne *et al.* 2003).There is also evidence for venlafaxine, though this is more dangerous in overdose. Some women may benefit from the addi-tional anxiolytic effect of mirtazapine.

Mood stabilizers

Carbamazepine and sodium valproate are sometimes used to reduce impulsive outbursts. Though there is some supporting evidence (Frankenberg and Zanarini 2002), it is weak and both carry risk of teratogenicity. Some small recent RCTs of topiramate and lamotrigine showed reduction in anger in women with BPD (Nickel 2004; Tritt 2005; Loew 2006). The NICE guideline high-lights this as an area for further research.

Hypnotics

Women with BPD frequently suffer insomnia and should be given basic sleep hygiene advice. Any hypnotic medication should be prescribed for short periods only, to restore sleep routine and limiting potential for abuse. A sedative antihistamine can be a useful alternative.

Guidelines for psychopharmacological management of borderline personality disorder

From Bateman and Fonagy (2004):

- Consider primary symptom complex (affect dysregulation, impulsivity, cognitive-perceptual disturbance)
- Consider meaning of prescribing in context of trans-ference and countertransference and the possibility of splitting
- Discuss treatment decision and implementation within whole team caring for patient
- Make clear recommendation but allow woman to take an informed decision without persuasion
- Agree trial period duration and do not prescribe another drug within this even if patient stops taking it (unless side effects intolerable)
- Prescribe within safety limits and consider the risk in overdose (e.g. weekly prescriptions)
- See patient at agreed intervals to review effect, titrate dose, and encourage compliance
- Stop drug if no benefit observed by staff or patient.

Psychoanalytic psychotherapy

Psychoanalytic thinking informs most current concep-tualizations and psychotherapeutic work with women with BPD. The capacity to use psychoanalytic psycho-therapy is complicated by reduced ego strength and reflective capacity, affective instability, and difficulty working with 'as if' interpretations. Though patients tend to be help-seeking and form intense relationships with their therapist, there are high drop-out rates (60%) and difficulty forming a therapeutic alliance (77%) (Frank 1992). The attachment context of ongoing treat-ment stirs up intense feelings and is typically compli-cated by acting out such as self-harm, substance misuse, and violence, and high demands of therapists with pres-sure to 'special treatment' and boundary violations.

Intensive psychoanalytic psychotherapy can be beneficial and contribute to lasting change in some patients, but needs to be long term and is extremely challenging for both therapist and patient, and should be done by experienced therapists or with expert super-vision. Interpretations can be particularly problematic.

In presenting an alternative view, the therapist can be experienced as abandoning or critical, amplifying anxiety and threat of fragmentation, and increasing the pressure to splitting and projection in an attempt to preserve psychic equilibrium in the face of overwhelming affects and fantasies—with the danger of a rapidly escalating disturbed paranoid state and behavioural outburst. Managing this requires attention to counter-transference–transference factors and flexibility of technique while working within the analytic frame. Analysts have also emphasized the importance of non-verbal factors in working with patients with such early developmental difficulties (Stewart 1992).

Valuable thinking about psychotherapy with BPD emerged from the Menninger project, a 25-year prospective study of psychoanalysis and supportive psychotherapy for patients with personality disorder (Wallerstein 1986). It suggested patients with low ego strength did better in supportive therapy and that the most disturbed patients (with borderline, paranoid features, drug and alcohol addiction) required a modified analytic approach using supportive-expressive therapy with attention to negative transference, focus on here and now interactions, a network of informal support, and periods of hospitalization (Kernberg 1972). Attention to the therapeutic alliance and transference emerge consistently as important in achieving good treatment outcomes in working with BPD (see Gabbard 2005). These insights are reflected in newer psychotherapies developed specifically for BPD, all of which offer a structured, supportive, here and now therapeutic approach, with attention to the therapeutic alliance and flexibility that can incorporate periods of hospital admission.

A number of studies support the usefulness of psychoanalytically-based treatment for BPD in individual, group, day hospital, and therapeutic community settings.

A trial of twice-weekly psychodynamic-interpersonal psychotherapy showed significant improvements in 48 patients with BPD, with reduction in episodes of self-harm and violence, time off work, number and length of hospital admissions, frequency of drug use, and self-report symptom index. This was sustained at five-year follow-up which also demonstrated substantial health-care cost savings (Meares *et al.* 1999). Guthrie (2001) demonstrated the effectiveness of 12-month psychodynamic-interpersonal therapy in an RCT for patients who self-harm.

Mentalization-based treatment

Mentalization-based treatment (MBT) was developed by Bateman and Fonagy (2004). In their model, unstable

or reduced capacity to mentalize is a core feature of BPD, explaining the observed clinical characteristics. Fostering the development of this capacity is believed to underlie all effective treatments of BPD, and is the primary focus in MBT. This approach can be applied in individual, group, and family therapy, and its effectiveness has been demonstrated in a partial day-hospital setting.

The relatively safe attachment relationship with a therapist and the therapeutic milieu is crucial in providing a secure base relationship context in which the individual can start to find their own mind through representations in the mind of the other. Feeling understood itself generates a sense of security which fosters further mental exploration. Therapists typically construct in their minds an image of the patient's mind, naming feelings and cognitions and spelling out implicit beliefs. For the patient this is a crucially different experience from that of a parent who is unresponsive or imposes their own disturbed or reactive experience. Therapists work collaboratively to foster mentalization in patients and sustain this in the face of inevitable challenges. Importantly, affective arousal can trigger a loss of mentalizing capacity and this is often marked in therapeutic contexts. Both mentalization and the failure to mentalize are understood as normal occurrences—and exploration of therapist failures to mentalize (alongside patient struggles) and the restoration of this—is a valuable aspect of therapy. Though personal history and experiences remain important in formulation, in MBT the key to improvement is promoting the capacity to mentalize rather than resolving problematic experiences or understanding unconscious conflict.

MBT applied in an individual or group setting involves a spectrum of interventions from supportive and empathic—through clarification and elaboration to basic mentalizing, interpretative mentalizing, and mentalizing the transference.

Mentalizing techniques for BPD

From Bateman and Fonagy (2006):

- Therapist stance: not knowing, active questioning, identifying, and accepting different perspectives; monitoring, acknowledging, and using own mistakes

- Identifying and exploring the consequences of patient's positive mentalization. (Includes praise for successful mentalizing)

- Clarification and affect elaboration. Includes open-ended questions, restating facts, and rewinding events moment by moment to trace actions back to feelings which are explored empathically

- 'Stop, Rewind, Explore': the therapist interrupts when mentalization fails to focus patient's attention on moment of rupture and reinstate it. (Often when an account has become muddling or appears to entail massive assumptions)

- Mentalizing the transference: relevant if feelings or motives in relation to the therapist are thought to underlie the patient's current mental state. It is an opportunity to validate the patient's experience, own therapist enactments, and explore alternative perspectives, e.g. encouraging the patient to consider what might be in the therapist's mind which might be different from their assumption. Any interpretations should be arrived at collaboratively and the patient's reaction explored.

Evaluation

A randomized controlled trial of 38 patients with BPD demonstrated the effectiveness of MBT applied in a psychoanalytically-orientated partial day-hospital programme for 18 months (Bateman and Fonagy 1999). The partial hospitalization included once weekly individual psychotherapy, thrice weekly group psychotherapy, once weekly expressive therapy, a weekly community meeting, and regular meetings with care coordinator and psychiatric medication review. The control group included regular psychiatric review with medication and admission as appropriate and outpatient and community follow-up. In the treatment group, the study showed significant reduction in suicide and self-harm attempts, number and duration of hospital admissions, use of psychotropic medication, self-report depression, anxiety, general symptom distress, and improvements in interpersonal function and social adjustment. In comparison, the control group showed limited change or deterioration in these variables. These improvements began after six months and continued to the end of treatment.

A follow-up study (Bateman and Fonagy 2001) showed these gains were maintained over 18 months after completing treatment and showed statistically significant continued improvement—suggesting that treatment enabled patients to better negotiate stresses and strains of everyday life without resorting to old coping strategies. For example, suicide attempt in the previous six months fell from 95% on admission to 5.3% at 18-month follow-up in the treatment group. Assessment of service utilization costs showed no difference between groups pre- and during treatment, but a trend for costs to decrease during the 18-month

follow-up in the treatment group. This shows that the intensive day-hospital treatment is not only significantly more efficacious—but no more costly than psychiatric care with predicted long-term savings longer term (Bateman and Fonagy 2003).

A more recent trial is investigating MBT applied in an outpatient twice weekly setting with patients receiving one individual and one group session per week for an 18-month treatment period. This is compared with patients randomly allocated to a control treatment of one individual and one group session per week supportive psychotherapy. The results are not yet available.

There have been interesting recent developments and applications of MBT in family work (SMART; Fearon *et al.* 2006) and mother–infant work (Minding The Baby; Sadler *et al.* 2006).

Transference-focused psychotherapy

Transference-focused psychotherapy (TFP) is a structured, manualized, time-limited outpatient psychodynamic psychotherapy based on Kernberg's psychoanalytic object relations-based conceptualization of borderline personality (Clarkin *et al.* 1999).

- Manualized

- Initial contract

- Two outpatient sessions per week

- One-year duration minimum

- Focus on immediate patient therapist interaction

- Active exploration of feelings, motivations and beliefs arising in this context, fosters reflection on mental state of self and other

- Non-judgemental clarification, confrontation, and interpretation

- Medication as required.

The treatment aims to contain suicidal and split-off behaviours, and to resolve identity diffusion through integrating projected aspects of self-fostering the development of a coherent sense of self and others. In psychoanalytic language this constitutes a move from paranoid-schizoid to depressive position functioning. This is done through promoting reflection on the mental states of self and other through active exploration of feelings, motivations, and beliefs as they arise in the therapeutic relationship, and within the safety of the therapeutic frame. These typically reflect activated, characteristic pathological object relations dyads in reference to the therapist (such as Abuser–Victim or Gratifying provider-dependent child). Clarification of the cognitive content of intense associated affective states provides containment, reduces acting out, and helps develop a capacity for reflection and affect modulation. It involves therapist awareness and containment of countertransference. Importantly, the therapist confronts contradictions in the patient's perceptions and affects in relation to themselves, and starts to interpret role reversals as they manifest in the here and now of the session. The therapist will interpret splitting and defensive motivations for this (e.g. defence against depressive anxieties or paranoid fear), alongside interpretation of underlying object relations dyads. The woman becomes increasingly aware of contradictions and oscillations between idealized and persecuting images of the therapist—and begins to accept the full range of her internal experience. This facilitates the gradual integration of idealized and persecutory experiences with a toning down of the intensity of affect and consolidation of self and object representations. The therapist generalizes experiences in therapy to relations outside, consolidating self and object representations and facilitating the woman's capacity to reflect, experience, and relate to self and others in a more healthy way.

Evaluation

An initial study of 23 borderline women treated for 12 months showed low drop out (19%) and significant reduction in suicide attempts and severity of self-harm. Women had fewer inpatient admissions, emergency room attendance, and inpatient days, and showed reduction in global symptoms with improved social functioning in friendships and work (Clarkin *et al.* 2001). More recently, a randomized controlled study of 90 patients with BPD comparing TFP with DBT and dynamic supportive therapy for one year showed significant improvements in depression, anxiety, global functioning, and social adjustment in all three groups. It showed significant improvement in suicidality with TFP and DBT only, and significant improvement in anger and impulsivity with TFP and supportive treatment. TFP was also significantly predictive of change in irritability and ratings of verbal and direct assault (Clarkin *et al.* 2004, 2007).

Dialectical behavioural therapy

Dialectical behavioural therapy (DBT) is an adaptation of CBT developed by Linehan (1991) working with parasuicidal women with BPD. It is manualized with supportive, behavioural, and cognitive components

and an emphasis on developing a positive therapeutic alliance (Linehan 1993). Typically, treatment is outpatient twice weekly for one year with one individual session (with homework) and one group session for educational skills training.

In Linehan's model, biological emotional vulnerability interacts with an invalidating family environment leading to core difficulties with emotional regulation and uncertainty about the validity of inner experience. DBT advocates a supportive and empathic therapeutic relationship, validating the woman's experience of themselves and building a positive therapeutic alliance.

DBT targets problem behaviours in BPD which are formulated using a behavioural functional analysis; an initial trigger leads to emotional dysregulation in the subject, who resorts to behaviours such as self-harm, drug, and alcohol use, binging and purging, isolation, suicidal ideas, or reckless behaviour to reduce or avoid painful emotions. This provides temporary relief—however, the continued use of this strategy reinforces emotional and behavioural problems. This vicious cycle is addressed collaboratively using a problem-solving approach to help the patient recognize the sequence and learn specific skills to interrupt the cycle at particular points.

DBT teaches new ways to manage emotional distress through improved capacity for self-recognition (as angry, sad, alone), greater tolerance of distress, and alternative strategies to regulate feelings without recourse to problem behaviours; stopping the problem behaviour stops the reinforcement. Vulnerability to cues triggering emotional dysregulation is addressed through behavioural exposure and stimulus control. Problem solving may suggest specific skills training such as strategies to improve interpersonal effectiveness.

Mindfulness training (developed out of Zen Buddhist mediation) has been developed as a core skill in DBT. Exercises include attention to the immediacy of experience, such as observing or describing thoughts or feelings as they arise, helping develop a capacity for self awareness and reflection and a tolerance of the experience of emotion. Importantly, arising mental contents are related to non-judgementally in contrast with an automatic 'bad—need to get rid of' attitude. Mindfulness is approached as a skill that will improve with practice—and it can be very positively reinforcing for women who feel at the mercy of uncontrollable mental experience to discover that their focus, concentration, and self-awareness can improve with regular practice over time.

The dialectical approach considers problem behaviours and the application of new skills within the wider system, recognizing the complexity of change. Factors within the patient and in their relationships that may impede change are understood in terms of inevitable dialectical tensions between contradictory positions. There is an explicit focus in DBT on the recognition of these, and the need to find a synthesis.

Evaluation

Linehan (1991) showed DBT to be effective in a randomized controlled trial of 44 women with BPD who had made at least two suicide attempts in the past five years, one within eight weeks. The control group (TAU) showed significantly increased rates of suicide attempts, inpatient days, and drop out. However, there were no differences in measures of depression, hopelessness, or reasons for living, and at one-year follow-up the treatment control differences were not sustained. Subsequent studies have confirmed efficacy in reducing parasuicide in outpatient and inpatient settings, but clinically significant change was not sustained at follow-up.

Cognitive therapy

In cognitive therapy BPD patients are formulated in terms of characteristic basic assumptions, dichotomous thinking, and a weak sense of identity leading to characteristic affects and behaviour that reinforce core beliefs in self-perpetuating cycles resistant to modification by individual experiences. Beck emphasizes the interaction between childhood environment and biological predispositions (temperament) resulting in the development of maladaptive cognitive, affective, motivational, action, and self-regulatory schemas, driving behavioural strategies that are dysfunctional in certain situations (Beck *et al.* 2004).

In women with BPD, typical basic assumptions include 'the world is dangerous and malevolent' with core beliefs such as 'I am powerless and vulnerable', 'I cannot cope alone', resulting in avoidance tackling problems and overdeveloped help-seeking and dependence behaviours, reinforcing vulnerability. These core beliefs, such as 'I am inherently unacceptable' and 'no one will ever love me', lead to chronic anxiety in relationships and self-punishment. These are intensified by dichotomous thinking, and rapid switches between extreme views compounding an unstable sense of identity. Goal confusion leads to ineffectiveness and poor motivation, further reinforcing helplessness, unacceptability, and dependence. For Beck, the borderline dilemma is feeling helpless in a hostile world without a source of security, vacillating between dependence and avoidance of others—unable to trust, rely, or feel safe in either position. Safran and Segal (1990) emphasize the interpersonal context, showing how schemas drive behaviours that provoke responses from others that confirm underlying assumptions.

Beck (2004) delineates standard cognitive and behavioural strategies to address dysfunctional schemas and behaviours including identifying goals, identifying and confronting schemas and core beliefs, and explicitly linking them to maladaptive behaviours. Dichotomous thinking is addressed through cognitive restructuring of beliefs associated with childhood and past traumas to help the patient develop more appropriate and adaptive behaviours to situations they currently face. Self-destructive behaviours and issues such as impulse and emotional control are specifically targeted.

Cognitive therapy has been adapted for working with BPD with longer treatments (often over a year) and availability for crisis contact between sessions. There is considerable attention to building a collaborative therapeutic alliance which is inevitably complicated by the patient's interpersonal difficulties. The therapeutic relationship may be used as a 'relationship laboratory' where powerful emotional reactions to the therapist are explored and 'transference' is understood cognitively in terms of underlying generalized beliefs and expectations. Misconceptions and misunderstandings are openly explored and therapists are encouraged to attend to countertransference feelings of anger, frustration, or attribution of malevolent intent. There is also explicit attention to issues stirred up by endings and breaks (Davidson 2000).

Young (1999) developed the concept of Early Maladaptive Schemas (EMS) that develop in response to unmet emotional needs in early dysfunctional family relationships, and are continually elaborated. Events activate these schemas, leading to distortions in thinking, powerful affect and problematic behaviour, and threatening a sense of identity. This results in schema coping behaviour as the patient's best attempt to stabilize. He also emphasizes schema maintenance, schema avoidance, and schema compensation.

Schema-focused therapy (SFT) has been developed as an intensive longer-term cognitive treatment for BPD (Young 2003). The model identifies four schema modes specific to BPD: detached protector, punitive parent, abandoned/abused child, and angry/impulsive child. It addresses these through a range of behavioural, cognitive, and experiential techniques that focus on the therapeutic relationship, daily life outside therapy (including homework assignments), and past (traumatic) experiences.

The aim is to facilitate the development of alternative schemas so that a patient's experience and behaviour is no longer dominated by dysfunctional schema.

Evaluation

Studies have demonstrated the benefits of manual assisted cognitive therapy and problem-solving therapy developed as brief crisis interventions after deliberate self-harm, and adapted for personality disorder (Evans *et al.* 1999; Huband *et al.* 2007). Other studies suggest benefits of cognitive therapy for BPD, with some evidence for improvement maintained at 18-month follow-up (Tyrer *et al.* 2003; Brown *et al.* 2004; Weinberg 2006).

Most recently, the BOSCOT trial (Davidson *et al.* 2006) randomized 106 BPD patients with BPD to 30 sessions of CBT plus TAU or TAU control group. The CBT focused on maladaptive core beliefs and over-/underdeveloped behavioural strategies (e.g. self-punishment/self-nurturance). Both treatment and control groups showed improvement at one year sustained after a further year follow-up in outcomes including inpatient hospitalization, suicidal behaviour, and use of accident and emergency treatment facilities. Patients with CBT had significantly less suicidal acts over the two years, dysfunctional beliefs, state anxiety, and symptom distress. No significant difference between groups was demonstrated in cost effectiveness or improvement in quality of life.

An interesting RCT of 88 BPD patients compared SFT with TFT, each delivered twice weekly for three years. This showed significant treatment effects with both treatments, with improved quality of life, reduction in BPDSI scores, and reduction in psychopathology and personality pathology with all effects apparent after one year. Survival analysis showed a significant effect in favour of SFT with greater improvement on abandonment fears, relationships, identity disturbance, impulsivity, parasuicidal behaviour, and dissociative and paranoid ideation (Giesen-Bloo *et al.* 2006)

Cognitive analytic therapy

Cognitive analytic therapy (CAT) was developed by Ryle as an integration of psychoanalytic and cognitive therapy. Like CBT it is time limited, problem orientated, structured and collaborative and uses behavioural methods and specific cognitive tools. Ryle revised and developed his original model specifically for patients with BPD (1997).

The therapist and patient work collaboratively to formulate the patient and set goals for therapy. The first four sessions identify *target problems* (TPs) (e.g. worthlessness, cutting, relationships) and *target problem procedures* (TPPs) which perpetuate them. TPPs include *traps* (vicious circles where negative beliefs generate behaviours with consequences that reinforce the beliefs), *dilemmas* (actions based on falsely dichotomous choices), and *snags* (ways in which the patient undermines their own fulfilment of aims). These are understood as dysfunctional ways of coping with feelings that perpetuate core pain, and are thought to originate in early relationship experiences which form a blueprint for subsequent relationships. These are conceptualized as *reciprocal roles* based on early relationships (neglecting–neglected) or on compensatory fantasy (perfectly caring–perfectly cared for) and recurrently manifest in the patient's relationships—including the therapeutic one. Each pole of the reciprocal role has an associated mood and self state. Patients move between these in response to internal and external triggers.

The therapist's understanding of the patient is shared through the reformulation letter explicitly linking target problems, target problem procedures, childhood experiences, and core pain. This narrative reconstruction of the patient's story from childhood to current difficulties can be very moving for patients who may feel truly heard, thought about, and understood for the first time. The therapy uses a wide range of techniques including diary writing, imagery, no-send letters, cognitive behavioural experiments, and reciprocal role interpretations to promote insight and behavioural change.

BPD is understood primarily in terms of rapidly switching dissociated self states that explain the characteristic intense unstable relationships, affect instability, and identity disturbance. For example, an idealizing–idealized pattern with behaviours seeking perfect care (and to avoid abandonment), precarious, and prone to switch to an abused-abusing state. Self-harm may be in a self-abusing or self-punishing role, or an attempt to escape an emotionally void blank state, or reclaiming an active role when faced with powerlessness. Anger may be the rage of an abused child or identification with an aggressive abuser role. Chronic feelings of emptiness are understood in terms of early unresolved deprivation, continuing failure to get emotional needs met, and ongoing insecurity.

This understanding of the patient is presented diagrammatically in the self states sequential diagram (SSSD) which plots the patient's self states, the transitions between them, and the behavioural procedures generated by each. This can be used by the therapist to reflect on events and mood shifts both outside the session and within. Typically a state shift may be triggered in the session so that the therapist is acutely and suddenly experienced as depriving or abusive at that moment threatening the therapeutic alliance. The SSSD becomes a valuable tool at this point for therapist and patient together to work out where they are on the map and reflect on the process and precipitant. As the patient becomes practised at recognizing her own states, state shifts, and identifying precipitants, the SSSD is something she can increasingly use outside sessions to help make sense of her subjective experience in relationships more widely. It is hoped that the continued self-monitoring will develop the patient's own capacity for reflection, reduce acting out associated with state/mood switches, and facilitate a more integrated sense of self.

Ryle understands BPD patients' difficulties as arising from deficits at three levels of development originating in childhood experiences of neglect, unpredictability, and commonly sexual or physical abuse. In combination with temperament and life events, these result in a restricted and distorted reciprocal role repertoire; dissociation between split-off aspects of self and limited capacity for self-reflection.

Ryle believes CAT provides a corrective emotional experience alongside intellectual understanding in promoting insight and behavioural change. He emphasizes the therapeutic relationship and explicit attention to transference and countertransference and issues stirred up by termination. The therapy for BPD is 24 sessions, with follow-up at one, two, three, and six months. The reformulation letter, the SSSD, and the goodbye letter are tools the patient takes away to help hold on to the work achieved in therapy. Ryle believes CAT helps patients develop a more integrated sense of themselves and their past, enabling a greater sense of control and responsibility for their lives supported by an internalized sense of the therapist.

A descriptive study of 27 patients offered 24 sessions plus four follow-up sessions over a year showed significant improvement in symptom and interpersonal outcome at six months post treatment (Ryle and Golynkina 2000), indicating the value of further randomized-controlled research to demonstrate efficacy.

Interpersonal therapy

This time-limited supportive therapy was developed for patients with depression and. focuses systematically on interpersonal sensitivity, role transitions, interpersonal disputes or losses, linking each to changes in mood. It has been recently adapted for patients with BPD with a small trial suggesting improvement in symptoms of depression and mental distress (Markowitz 2006). A trial comparing fluoxetine plus IPT for 39 patients (62% women) with BPD and comorbid MDD showed efficacy compared to fluoxetine alone in reducing depressive symptoms and self-rated psychological and social functioning quality of life measures (Bellino 2006).

Group therapy

Groups are very helpful in working with women with BPD. The group becomes a microcosm in which object relations and primitive phantasies and defences such as splitting and projection are externalized. Within the containment and facilitation of an ongoing group, patients can learn from each other and develop their reflective skills—often being very acute in their observations. It may be easier to accept confrontation and interpretation from fellow members than the therapist, and they can titrate their level of contact. Therapist interpretations may be more tolerable as part of a group theme, and with a dilution of dependency needs. Patients are encouraged to be responsible for thinking about themselves and each other and the 'group' as whole. In an outpatient psychotherapy setting, BPD patients are often seen in a mixed group with patients with neurotic or other personality disorder features where their immediacy of affect and directness of expression, and willingness to express dependency needs or feelings of rejection can be extremely valuable to others. See Garland (in press) for a thoughtful and coherent account of psychoanalytic work with borderline patients in a slow open long-term outpatient group. A randomized controlled trial by Munroe-Blum and Marziali (1995) showed significant improvement after 25 weekly sessions of interpersonal group therapy followed by five biweekly sessions. Gains were sustained at 12- and 24-month follow-up, and equivalent to the individual dynamic therapy 40 sessions control group. Group therapy is an important component in most specialist treatment programmes for personality disorder in therapeutic community, day hospital, and intensive outpatient settings. Patients usually have ongoing additional individual therapeutic contact which can help work through issues stirred up in the group context.

Family therapy

Family work may be important for couples or younger women or adolescents still living with their families. Relationships may be highly conflictual and it is important any professional contact with the wider family is with the explicit consent of the patient. The clinician needs to be sensitive in exploring family dynamics, giving space to the views of all family members—which may vary hugely. Characteristic interpersonal interactions may homeostatically maintain a pathological system in which the women or girl with BPD is 'ill' or 'bad'. Parental disturbance may be split off and projected into an adolescent who becomes projectively identified and expresses symptoms. Parents may have been neglectful or abusive and failed to provide structure or guidance required for healthy development. Or there may be over involvement with the daughter crucial in meeting parental needs, and lacking support to develop as an individual. Gunderson (2001) has also suggested a role for psychoeducational work with families of BPD patients to help them appreciate the complexities of the patient's struggle in relationships and in treatment.

Short-term mentalization and relational therapy (SMART) is a recently developed integrative family therapy that addresses problems in family relationships in terms of difficulties in mentalizing, exacerbated by stress and emotional arousal and setting up repetitive negative cycles of non-mentalizing interactions. The therapist fosters mentalizing in the family through modelling, active questioning, structured games, and homework. See Fearon et al. (2006).

Therapeutic communities

The therapeutic community was first described by Main as an institution in which the setting itself restores morale and promotes psychological treatment. The most well-known example is the Henderson Hospital whose structure and working practices demonstrate characteristic features of permissiveness, reality confrontation, democracy, and communalism. Permissiveness encourages the enactment of disturbed feelings and relationships which can then be examined by staff and patients alike. Staff/patient differences are minimized with patients having the majority vote in decision making—particularly regarding admission, disciplining, and discharge. There is daily large group therapy alongside a range of occupational activities. Dolan et al. (1992) showed a reduction in global severity index scores in 95 patients with severe personality disorder (est. 87% BPD). Though this was considered a costly residential setting, Dolan et al. (1997) demonstrated the cost-effectiveness of one year of residential treatment through reducing inpatient admissions, self

harm, psychological distress, and improving self-esteem in the year after treatment.

Main himself developed the Cassel Hospital, a residential psychodynamic psychotherapy setting offering a combination of intensive individual and once weekly group psychotherapy alongside community meetings, work groups, and structured activities, with psychotropic medication as required. A recent prospective study at the Cassel Hospital compared one-stage inpatient treatment with a two-stage step down programme consisting of 6 months of residential followed by 24–28 months of psychosocial outpatient/community treatment (Chiesa and Fonagy 2000). This involved continuing twice weekly group psychotherapy, once weekly psychosocial outreach nursing, regular psychiatric review, and networking with other healthcare agencies. Subjects allocated to the two-stage model showed significantly better improvement on most measures including self-harm, attempted suicide, psychiatric readmission rates, and more cost effective (Chiesa 2002), compared with both inpatient-only treatment and psychiatric outpatient treatment as usual. They also did significantly better at follow-up at one, three, and six years on global measures of mental health and social adjustment (Chiesa et al. 2006).

Recently there has been a move away from residential therapeutic community treatments to intensive psychodynamic day hospital services for the treatment of BPD.

A number of trials have demonstrated the efficacy of this approach with significant reductions in symptoms and health service utilization that are sustained at follow-up (Bateman and Fonagy 1999, 2001; Karterud et al. 2003). These typically provide a structured therapeutic milieu with a combination of individual and group psychodynamic treatments, other expressive groups (e.g. art therapy), and activity groups (e.g. gardening). There are clear rules about drug, alcohol use, and violence, and patients are involved in community responsibilities and decisions. There is an emphasis on ongoing supervision and team reflection on dynamics within the staff–patient group as a whole to contain working with patients. Based within psychiatric services, patients will have CPA review, psychotropic medication, and liaison with wider services working with the patient as required.

Inpatient treatment

Hospital admissions of BPD patients tend to be complicated by intense interpersonal dynamics with strong countertransference responses and splitting within staff teams. There is frequently a degree of acting out by staff as well as patients in the context of powerful projective processes. Patients may be given special care by some and hated and deprived by others. They may become attacking or refuse to engage in an overall treatment plan—resulting in hopelessness and futility amongst staff and pressure to discharge. For such reasons it is advisable for women with BPD to work through crises with increased outpatient or community support whenever possible. This may include daily contact with a home treatment or crisis resolution team and can help foster the patient's autonomy while staying sensitive to their level of distress and monitoring risk.

However, for some patients working in ongoing outpatient or partial hospital treatment, brief crisis admission may be necessary to manage acute risk if they become acutely suicidal, self-destructive, or transiently psychotic. The staff and hospital milieu can provide important concrete containment and an auxiliary ego function. Reflective practice groups are important in containing the emotional impact on staff of working with disturbed patients to preserve a thoughtful, therapeutic milieu. Although controlling strategies such as restraint, medication, and one-to-one monitoring may be required at times, the aim is to help the patient take responsibility for self-control. Staff can help patients identify precipitants of crisis, delay impulsive action, explore alternatives, and anticipate consequences of actions. Suicide attempters are often experienced as manipulative, but they are at increased risk of actual suicide. It is useful to engage patients actively in considering risk and criteria for safe discharge. During an admission, open communication between ward staff, and ongoing liaison with the wider team working with patients in the community is essential.

General principles in working with women with BPD

See Gabbard (2005):

- Individualized approach to patient care package. Consider role of carers
- Attention to the therapeutic alliance
- Awareness of psychodynamic factors such as transference, countertransference, splitting, and projection
- Clear, reliable, and consistent treatment boundaries—session times, team reviews etc.
- Flexibility of therapist intervention—supportive, expressive, interpretive—and availability

- Clear rules about violence, drug or alcohol use not permitted in treatment setting with identified consequences
- Monitor countertransference feelings to minimize countertransference acting out
- Accept intensity of patient's feelings and need to project. Avoid 'disidentification with aggressor'
- Promote mentalization. Elaborate on mental state that triggers enactment. Explore consequences of self-destructive behaviours. Explore alternatives to psychic equivalence
- Help patients own aspects of themselves that have been disavowed or projected onto others to help restore a sense of continuity. (Requires strong therapeutic alliance and empathic validation of patient's subjective experience prior to any interpretation.)
- Whole team and patient participation in treatment decisions
- Manage splitting between psychotherapy and pharmacotherapy
- Supervision, specialist training, and support of staff
- Crisis intervention plan—planning for out-of-hours needs and offering support while fostering autonomy
- Regular liaison with the range of services involved with the patient, joint review, distribution of CPA documentation, crisis intervention plan, and risk assessment
- Attention to endings and transitions.

References

Bateman AW and Fonagy P (1999). The effectiveness of partial hospitalization in the treatment of borderline personality disorder – a randomised controlled trial. *American Journal of Psychiatry*, **156**, 1563–69.

Bateman AW and Fonagy P (2001). The effectiveness of in the treatment of borderline personality disorder with psychoanalytically orientated partial hospitalization: an 18-month follow-up. *American Journal of Psychiatry*, **158**, 36–42.

Bateman AW and Fonagy P (2003). Health service utilisation costs for borderline personality disorder patients treated with psychoanalytically orientated partial hospitalization versus general psychiatric care. *American Journal of Psychiatry*, **160**, 169–71.

Bateman AW and Fonagy P (2006). Mentalizing and borderline personality disorder. In: JG Allen and P Fonagy (eds) *Handbook of Mentalization-Based Treatment*, John Wiley & Sons, Chichester.

Beck AT *et al.* (2004). *Cognitive Therapy of Personality Disorders*, 2nd edition. Guildford Press, New York.

Bellino S *et al.* (2006). Combined treatment of major depression in patients with borderline personality disorder: a comparison with pharmacotherapy. *Canadian Journal of Psychiatry – Revue Canadienne de Psychiatrie*, **51**, 453–60.

Brazier J *et al.* (2006). Psychological therapies including dialectical behaviour therapy for borderline personality disorder: a systematic review and preliminary economic evaluation, *Health Technology Assessment*, **10**, iii. Ix–iii, 117.

Brown GR *et al.* (2004). An open trial of cognitive therapy for borderline personality disorder. *Journal of Personality Disorder*, **18**, 257–71.

Chiesa M and Fonagy P (2000). The Cassel personality disorder study: methodology and treatment effects. *British Journal of Psychiatry*, **176**, 485–91.

Chiesa M *et al.* (2002). Health Service use costs by personality disorder following specialist and non-specialist treatment: a comparative study. *Journal of Personality Disorders*, **16**, 160–73.

Chiesa M *et al.* (2006). Six-year follow up of three treatment programs for personality disorder. *Journal of Personality Disorders*, **20**, 493–509.

Clarkin JF *et al.* (1999). *Transference-Focused Psychotherapy for Borderline Personality Disorder Patients*, Guildford Press, New York, NY.

Clarkin JF *et al.* (2001). The development of a psychodynamic treatment for patients with borderline personality disorder: a preliminary study of behavioural change. *Journal of personality Disorders*, **15**, 487–95.

Clarkin JF *et al.* (2004). The Personality Disorders Institute/Borderline Personality Disorder Research Foundation randomized control trial for borderline personality disorder: rationale, methods, and patient characteristics. *Journal of Personality Disorders*, **18**, 52–72.

Clarkin JF *et al.* (2007). Evaluating three treatments for borderline personality disorder: A multiwave study. *American Journal of Psychiatry*, **164**, 922–8.

Davidson KM (2000). *Cognitive Therapy for Personality Disorders: A Guide for Clinicians*, 2nd edition. Routledge, London; Arnold (Hodder), Hove.

Davidson K *et al.* (2006). The effectiveness of cognitive behaviour therapy for borderline personality disorder; results from the borderline personality disorder study of cognitive therapy (BOSCOT) trial. *Journal of Personality Disorders*, **20**(5), 450–65.

Department of Health (2003). *Personality Disorder; No Longer a Diagnosis of Exclusion*. DOH, London.

Evans K *et al.* (1999). Manual-assisted cognitive behaviour therapy (MACT): a randomised controlled trial of a brief intervention with bibliotherapy in the treatment of recurrent deliberate self-harm. *Psychological Medicine*, **29**, 19–25.

Fearon P *et al.* (2006). Short-term mentalization and relational therapy (SMART): an integative family therapy for children and adolescents. In: JG Allen and P Fonagy (eds) *Handbook of Mentalization-Based Treatment*, John Wiley & Sons, Chichester.

Frank AF (1992). The therapeutic alliances of borderline patients. In: JF Clarkin *et al.* (eds) *Borderline Personality Disorder; Clinical and Empirical Perspectives*, Guildford Press, New York.

Frankenberg FR and Zanarini MC (2002). Divalproex sodium treatment of women with borderline personality disorder and bipolar II disorder: a double-blind placebo-controlled pilot study. *Journal of Clinical Psychiatry*, **63**, 442–6.

Gabbard GO (2005). Cluster B personality disorders. Borderline. In: *Psychodynamic Psychiatry in Clinical Practice, The DSM-IV Edition. Revised*, pp. 427–81. American Psychiatric Press, Washington, DC.

Garland, CP. (2010) Psychoanalytic group therapy with severely disturbed patients; benefits and challenges. Ch. 5 In: Garland (ed) *The Groups Book: Psychoanalytic Group Therapy: Principles and Practices*, Karnac, London.

Giesen-Bloo J *et al.* (2006). Outpatient psychotherapy for borderline personality disorder. *Archives of General Psychiatry*, **63**, 649–58.

Gunderson JG (2001). *Borderline Personality Disorder; A Clinical Guide*. American Psychiatric Publishing, Washington DC.

Guthrie E *et al.* (2001). Randomised controlled trial of brief psychological intervention after deliberate self-poisoning. *British Medical Journal*, **323**, 135–7.

Huband N *et al.* (2007). Social problem-solving plus psychoeducation for adults with personality disorder: pragmatic randomised controlled trial. *British Journal of Psychiatry*, **190**, 307–13.

Karterud S *et al.* (2003). Day treatment of patients with personality disorders: experiences from a Norwegian treatment research network. *Journal of Personality Disorders*, **17**(3), 243–62.

Kernberg OF (1972). Final report of the Meninger Foundation's Psychotherapy Research Project. *Bulletin of the Menninger Clinic*, **36**, 181–95.

Linehan MM *et al.* (1991). Cognitive behavioural treatment of chronically parasuicidal patients *Archives of General Psychiatry*, **48**, 1060–4.

Linehan MM (1993). *Cognitive Behaviour Therapy of Borderline Personality Disorder*. Guildford Press, New York.

Loew TH *et al.* (2006). Toprimate treatment for women with borderline personality disorder: A double-blind, placebo-controlled study. *Journal of Clinical Psychopharmacology*, **26**, 61–6.

Markowitz JC *et al.* (2006). Interpersonal psychotherapy for borderline personality disorder: possible mechanisms of change. *Journal of Clinical Psychology*, **62**(4), 431–44.

Meares R *et al.* (1999). Psychotherapy with borderline patients I: A comparison between treated and untreated cohorts. *Australian and New Zealand Journal of Psychiatry*, **33**, 467–72.

Monroe-Blum H and Marziali E (1995). A controlled trial of short-term group treatment for borderline personality disorder. *Journal of Personality Disorders*, **9**, 190–8.

Nickel MK *et al.* (2004). Topiramate treatment of aggression in female borderline personality disorder patients: a double-blind, placebo-controlled study. *Journal of Clinical Psychiatry*, **65**, 1515–19.

Nickel MK *et al.* (2006). Aripiprazole in the treatment of patients with borderline personality disorder: a double-blind, placebo-controlled study. *American Journal of Psychiatry*, **163**, 833–38.

Rinne T *et al.* (2002). SSRI treatment of borderline personality disorder: a randomized placebo-controlled clinical trial for female patients with borderline personality disorder. *American Journal of Psychiatry*, **159**, 2048–54.

Rinne T *et al.* (2003). Fluvoxamine reduces responsiveness of HPA axis in adult female BPD patients with a history of sustained childhood abuse. *Neuropharmacology*, **28**, 126–32.

Ryle A (1997). *Cognitive Analytic Therapy and Borderline Personality Disorder: The Model and the Method*, Chichester.

Ryle A and Golynkina K (2000). Effectiveness of time-limited cognitive analytic therapy of borderline personality disorder: factors associated with outcome. *British Journal of Medical Psychology*, **73**(2), 197–210.

Sadler LS *et al.* (2006). Minding the Baby: A Mentalization-Based Parenting Program. In: JG Allen and P Fonagy (eds) *Handbook of Mentalization-Based Treatment*. John Wiley & Sons, Chichester.

Safran JD and Segal ZV (1990). *Interpersonal Process in Cognitive Therapy*. Basic Books, New York.

Stewart H (1992). *Psychic Experience and Problems of Technique*. Tavistock, London.

Tritt K *et al.* (2005). Lamotrigine treatment of aggression in female borderline-patients: a randomised, double-blind, placebo-controlled study, *Journal of Psychopharmacology*, **19**, 287–91.

Tyrer P *et al.* (2003). Randomized controlled trial of brief cognitive behaviour therapy versus treatment as usual in recurrent deliberate self harm: The POPMACT study. *Psychological Medicine*, **33**(6), 969–76.

Wallerstein RS (1986). *Forty-two Lives in Treatment: A Study of Psychoanalysis and Psychotherapy*. Guildford Press, New York.

Weinberg I *et al.* (2006). Manual assisted cognitive treatment for deliberate self-harm in borderline personality disorder patients. *Journal of Personality Disorders*, **20**, 482–92.

Young JE (1999). *Cognitive Therapy for Personality Disorders: Professional Resource Exchange*, 3rd edition. Professional Resource Exchange, Sarasota, FL.

Young JE *et al.* (2003). *Schema Therapy: A Practitioner's Guide*. Guildford Press, New York.

Zanarini MC and Frankenburg FR (2001). Olanzapine treatment of borderline patients; a double-blind, placebo-controlled study. *Journal of Clinical Psychiatry*, **62**(11), 849–54.

Zanarini MC *et al.* (2004). A preliminary randomized trial of fluoxetine, olanzapine, and the olanzapine-fluoxetine combination in women with borderline personality disorder. *Journal of Clinical Psychiatry*, **65**, 903–7.

CHAPTER 15

Women in forensic institutions

Lisa Wootton and Anthony Maden

Introduction

Women are always in a minority in forensic populations, whether in prisons or secure hospitals. As a consequence neither the institutions nor policymakers seem to know how to respond to them. The earliest response was to ignore them; women were an afterthought whose needs were overshadowed by the male offender population that dominated the landscape. At other times there was an overemphasis on psychopathology, reaching a peak when the United Kingdom (UK) government in the 1970s proposed rebuilding its main women's prison, Holloway, as a secure hospital. There was a tendency to see all the deviant behaviour of women as evidence of psychopathology, leading to Sim's charge that doctors located them 'at the centre of the professional gaze' (Sim 1990) when they came to examine and to medicalize prisoners.

Over the last decade policy has become more rational. The main advance has been to recognize that the mental health of offenders is continuous with the mental health of all women. Most women spend only brief periods in custody and it is unrealistic to imagine that either their health or broader social needs can be addressed in isolation from their lives outside the walls of the institution.

The new approach is neatly summarized in the title of the UK government's main policy document in this area: *Women's Mental Health: Into the Mainstream* (Department of Health 2002). As part of the general policy of social inclusion and reducing inequality, women are to be brought in from the margins. Awareness of gender differences should go along with acceptance of the principle of equality of access to healthcare. In practice these goals are to be achieved through an emphasis on individual needs assessment with services designed to meet the needs that emerge from the assessment.

Too often in the past the service has come first. Women have been squashed and squeezed into forensic services designed primarily for men. We have known for many years that 'women require different treatment and facilities to men if they are to have the opportunity to break the patterns of behaviour which have lead to their contact with the criminal justice system.' (Department of Health 2006a, p. 5). Now there is an opportunity to do something about the problem and we are beginning to see the first examples of services designed to meet women's needs. The rest of this chapter will consider what we know about women in forensic settings and how best we can develop responsive services.

The relationship between crime, gender, and mental disorder

Gender and crime

Women are generally less antisocial than men (Moffit *et al.* 2001). They are convicted of fewer crimes and the difference is particularly marked for violent or sexual crimes (Ministry of Justice 2007a). Women are more likely to be the victims rather than the perpetrators of violent crime, and 38% of violent crime is committed against women (Home Office 2007, p. 83).

In 2006, men were convicted or cautioned for 407 100 indictable offences compared to 99 900 for women, a ratio of 4:1. Theft and handling offences are the most common, see Table 15.1.

There are qualitative differences between the offending of men and women. Women are more likely to be involved in domestic violence, less likely to commit violence against strangers or acquaintances (Home Office 2007, p. 83).

Prospective longitudinal studies show that women's antisocial behaviour usually emerges in adolescence but fluctuates more than men's antisocial behaviour, mainly according to circumstances. Typical antisocial behaviour in young women is greatly influenced by social

Table 15.1 Female offenders found guilty or cautioned for indictable offences and percentage of each type of offence committed by women.

Offence type	Number of women (rounded to the nearest 100)	Percentage of total number of each type of offence committed by women
Violence against the person	17 900	18%
Sexual offences	200	3%
Robbery	100	11%
Burglary	200	7%
Theft and handling	50 200	29%
Fraud and forgery	8 800	33%
Criminal damage	2 900	13%
Drug offences	8 800	11%
Other offences	8000	13%
Motoring offences	300	5%
Total	99 900	20%

Source: Ministry of Justice (2007a, p. 92).

factors and male peers are a particularly important—and usually negative—influence (Moffit *et al.* 2001). The Cambridge study of delinquent development (Farrington 1994) showed that one of the main factors helping young men to stop offending was the stabilizing influence of a partner, and this recent work shows the influence sometimes operates in the opposite direction.

As in men, a history of conduct problems in adolescence is associated in women with several negative outcomes in adult life. Apart from adult antisocial behaviour they include relationship problems; depression; a tendency to self-harm and suicide; and poor physical health (Moffit *et al.* 2001). So whilst antisocial behaviour may be less common in young women there is nothing to suggest that it is any more benign. In fact there is evidence to suggest that the adult outcome may be worse as antisocial young women are such a small minority and may experience additional rejection because of their failure to conform to gender stereotypes.

Gender, mental disorder, and crime

In offenders with major mental disorder the balance between men and women is much less skewed. The additional offending risk conferred by having a major mental disorder is greater for women than for men and this narrows the gap in offending between the sexes (Hodgins *et al.* 1996). Even so, women account for only a minority of those in secure institutions for mentally disordered offenders. They have generally accounted for less than 20% of the population in high secure hospitals, and a greater proportion in this setting were judged to be misplaced in that they did not need to be in such high security (Lart *et al.* 1999).

Women in prison

The prison population

The prison population in England and Wales is at a record high (Ministry of Justice 2008), having increased by 41% between 1996 and 2006 (Ministry of Justice 2007b). During the same period the female prison population increased by 94% (Ministry of Justice 2007b, p.92), admittedly from a very low baseline. The reasons are complex and relate partly to women receiving lengthy sentences for their involvement in drug smuggling.

These changes mean that while women remain less likely than men to be sent to prison they make up an increasing proportion of those in prison (currently 5.4%) (Ministry of Justice 2007c). The number of women in prison has almost doubled since 1996 but remains small at 4430. The percentage of women within the prison population is similar in other English-speaking countries (Bartlett 2007a).

The most common convictions for sentenced women in prison are acquisitive, followed by drug and then violent offences. For men, violent and acquisitive offences are equally common and outnumber drug offences. Sentenced women in prison are almost twice as likely as sentenced men to have been convicted of a drug offence and are less likely to have been convicted of a violent offence (although this gap has been narrowing). Table 15.2 shows the offences for which women in prison had been convicted, in 2007, and the comparison figures for men.

Women in prison are a disadvantaged group and often have complex and interdependent problems. There is a high prevalence of adverse childhood experiences (O'Brien *et al.* 2003; Department of Health 2006a), poor educational attainment (O'Brien *et al.* 2003), and work histories (Social Exclusion Unit 2002), and high rates of mental disorder and substance misuse (Maden *et al.* 1994; O'Brien *et al.* 2003). The experience of being in prison can compound these problems;

Table 15.2 The offences that have been committed by women and men in prison on immediate custodial sentences (i.e. excluding fine defaulters), 2007

Offence type	Women	Men
Violence against the person	22%	28%
Sexual offences	1%	12%
Robbery	9%	13%
Burglary	6%	8%
Theft and handling	11%	5%
Fraud and forgery	8%	2%
Drug offences	29%	15%
Motoring offences	1%	2%
Other offences	12%	9%
Offence not recorded	< 1%	< 1%

Source: Ministry of Justice (2007b).

women are separated from their children and social networks and they are within a hierarchal and potentially authoritarian institution where they are often victimized (O'Brien *et al.* 2003).

Mothers in prison

Forty-three per cent of women are living with their children immediately prior to imprisonment, about half of these as a lone parent, and relationships with partners frequently break down while women are in custody (O'Brien *et al.* 2003). Each year up to 17 000 children are separated from their mothers by imprisonment, and only 5% of them remain in their own family home after their mother's imprisonment (Department of Health 2006a). A study at Holloway prison found that in women with mental disorder transferred to hospital, almost half of the women who had borne children were still their primary carers (Rutherford *et al.* 2004).

The Prison Service provides a limited number of places in mother and baby units which take babies up to the age of 18 months. However, the admission criteria tend to select out mothers with mental disorder. Within the units, mental disorder remains under-diagnosed and treated, potentially putting mothers and their children at risk (Birmingham *et al.* 2006a).

The behaviour of women in prison

Women in prison receive more adjudications than men for all types of punishable offences, including violence (Ministry of Justice 2007b, p. 110). In part this may be the result of less serious breaches of the rules: comparison

with male prisoners is difficult due to the differing nature of the regimes; women, for example, are afforded more physical freedom than men with a similar security classification (Maden 1996). Women who have had three or more punishments are more likely to have attempted suicide than those with only one or two, suggesting a possible link between women causing breaches of discipline and mental illness (Department of Health 2006a).

Self-harm and suicide in prison are of considerable public and institutional concern. Twenty-six per cent of sentenced female prisoners report having committed an act of self-harm or having made a suicide attempt in the last year (O'Brien *et al.* 2003). The rate of completed suicide in custody was higher for women than men between 1999 and 2004 but is now similar, at about 1 per 1000 population per year (Ministry of Justice 2007b, p. 114).

Mental disorder amongst women in prison

Mental disorder is common in prisons (Fazel and Danesh 2002) and female prisoners are particularly at risk (Maden *et al.* 1994; O'Brien *et al.* 2003) (see Table 15.3).

Women in prison suffer higher rates of mental disorder than women in the community and their male counterparts in prison. They are a particularly vulnerable group who suffer additional stresses within prison.

The prevalence figures tell only part of the story and interpretation is complicated. The debate has sometimes been conducted in simplistic terms, according to which all mentally disordered women should be removed from prison to hospital. This extreme position

Table 15.3 Rates of disorder among women prisoners

Mental health problem	Sentenced prisoners	Remand prisoners
Psychosis	1.6%	4.5%
Personality disorder	18%	15.5%
Alcohol abuse/ dependence	9%	8.5%
Drug abuse/ dependence	26%	33.5%
Neurotic disorder	16%	43.7%
Mental handicap	2.3%	2.4%
Other disorders	1.2%	5.6%
No diagnosis	43%	22.9%

Source: Maden (1996) and Maden *et al.* (1995).

in the debate over medicalization of female offending is unsustainable in principle (drug addiction is not usually a reason for hospitalization so why should it become so in prison?) and for practical reasons (there are not enough beds).

The real challenge is to assess and meet the full range of healthcare need in prisoners, whether it be for transfer to hospital or some form of help in prison, but the task is not straightforward. It is relatively easy to count heads in prevalence surveys but there is no standardized measure of the need for treatment. As a result surveys rarely address this dimension of the problem, and when they do they use idiosyncratic estimates or self-report of previous treatment.

In addition to presenting with high rates of mental disorder and comorbidity (Bartlett 2007a), women are more likely than men to have had psychiatric treatment in the past and to be receiving treatment in prison (Maden 1996). This presumably reflects, in part, the increased needs of this population but may also reveal a willingness by professionals to respond to evidence of psychological distress in women and for the women themselves to have a more positive attitude towards treatment. In their survey of women prisoners, Maden *et al.* (1996) measured attitudes to treatment and found significantly more women wanted treatment. For every inmate given a diagnosis, they also made a recommendation for treatment: ranging from no treatment to transfer to hospital. No treatment was more likely to be recommended for men (odds ratio (OR) 0.4, 95% confidence interval (CI) 0.3–0.5), there was not a significant difference between the sexes in the number recommended for transfer to hospital (OR 1.6, 95% CI 0.8–3.0) but women were more likely to be recommended for outpatient treatment (OR 2.4, 95% CI 1.8–3.4).

Treatment in prison

Treatment within the prison system can take a number of forms, for example, addressing mental disorder, substance misuse, or offending behaviour. These areas of need are not independent of one another, although the services provided may be almost entirely independent despite being located within the same institution. Mental disorder is treated by healthcare, substance misuse by the CARAT service (Counselling, Assessment, Referral, Advice and Throughcare), and offending behaviour by the cognitive behavioural 'treatments' which are part of the Offending Behaviour Programmes Unit.

On 1 April 2003, the NHS formally took over the provision of healthcare within the prison service in England and Wales and government policy is based on the idea of providing equivalence of care between the community and prison (Department of Health 1999a). However, in many ways prison is not equivalent to the community: prisoners are a highly selected population with a number of characteristics complicating their treatment; they are living in a custodial environment and there is no equivalent in the community to a prison healthcare wing (Wilson 2004; Birmingham *et al.* 2006b).

Despite the high rates of mental disorder, few women are transferred out of prison to a hospital bed: less than 2% of new receptions in a study at HMP Holloway (Rutherford *et al.* 2004). The women who are accepted may face long waits before transfer, and those with personality disorder and those requiring higher levels of security wait even longer. Factors associated with difficulty obtaining an inpatient bed include: having a personality disorder; reporting a history of sexual and or physical abuse; being chronically self-harming; and having a history of substance misuse (Gorsuch 1999).

The CARAT service was established as the universal drug treatment service in every prison in England and Wales in 1999. They assess prisoners, give advice about drug misuse, and refer to appropriate drug services: clinical services, CARAT services, rehabilitation programmes, and therapeutic communities. These services are provided chiefly by external drug agencies, prison officers, and healthcare staff working in partnership. CARAT figures show that women are more likely to refer themselves, spend more on drug use, and are more likely to have had treatment before (May 2005).

Over the last few decades there has been an increase in the evidence base for cognitive-based interventions for offending behaviour (McGuire 1995, 2002). These programmes are generally delivered by forensic psychologists and prison staff. However, the majority of the evidence relates to men and while the programmes are often considered suitable for female prisoners, a recent evaluation of female prisoners showed no significant reduction in one- or two-year reconviction rates for those who had had treatment compared to a matched sample who had not (Home Office 2006). Male prisoners with personality disorder also have available to them a prison run on the lines of a therapeutic community; no such service exists for women.

The Dangerous Severe Personality Disorder Service, however, does have a facility for women: the Primrose Project with 10 beds. This new service intends to draw on the best practice from both the Prison Service and the National Health Service (NHS) to develop a hybrid model of health intervention for women who have care needs that extend beyond that which current mental health services can address, and for whom transfer to the NHS is not deemed appropriate (Department of Health 2006b).

The challenge is to bring all these services together in order to help women who have multiple and complex difficulties, which are not neatly subdivided to fit in with service provision; moreover many women are in prison only for a short period. A history of trauma is a good example of a complicating factor, one which is common, can impact on all these areas, and is not necessarily specifically addressed by any of these services. Perhaps inevitably it is the women with the most complex difficulties for whom the provision is often the poorest. Furthermore, continuity of service between the prison and community rarely exists.

The Corston Report recommends that custodial sentences should be reserved for women who commit serious and violent offences and pose a threat to the public, and that existing women's prisons should be replaced with suitable, geographically dispersed, small, multifunctional custodial centres (Corston 2007). Were this to be implemented, it would mean a complete transformation of current provision.

Women in secure psychiatric services

Characteristics of women in secure psychiatric services

The number of women in prison may be small, but the number of women in secure psychiatric services is even smaller and they are outnumbered by men at all levels of security. However, proportionally women are more likely to receive a psychiatric disposal for criminal behaviour than men (Maden 1996; Lart et al. 1999). As with the case of women in prison, the evidence base primarily describes the population and does not extend to effective treatments (Lart et al. 1999; Bartlett 2000, 2007b).

Compared to their male counterparts in secure forensic services, the women appear more 'psychiatric' and less 'criminal' (Bartlett 1993): they are more likely to be admitted as transfers from other hospitals, following non-criminalized behavioural disorder (for example, assaults which have not lead to prosecutions or self-harm), they have fewer previous criminal convictions, and more previous psychiatric admissions (Coid et al.

2000). They are also more likely to be admitted under the legal category of 'Psychopathic Disorder' and to have a history of arson (Coid et al. 2000). Like women in prison there is a high prevalence rate of adverse childhood experiences, including physical and sexual abuse, poor educational attainment, and work histories (Bland et al. 1999). Compared with women in prison, there are fewer mothers, and those that are mothers are unlikely to have an expectation of caring for their children on discharge (Bland et al. 1999). Self harm is also common (Lart et al. 1999): in a case note study at Broadmoor (Bland et al. 1999) only 16% of the women did not have a history of self-harm. Comorbid substance abuse/dependence is also common (Lart et al. 1999).

The higher prevalence of the category of 'Psychopathic Disorder' among the female detained population has raised the question of whether it constitutes a medicalization of antisocial behaviour which would be criminalized in men (Bartlett et al. 2001). Some have debated whether the psychiatric response to women is excessive, or that to men inadequate. In fact, if we return to our starting principles, the question is unlikely to lead to a useful answer. The crucial issue is whether individual patients get the needs assessment and the tailored treatment they require. Even a cursory glance at the women's wards of high security hospitals in the 1980s showed that many of their patients were far from having their needs met but fortunately the world has changed since then.

Service provision

Whilst women are generally considered less of a threat to the outside world there is general agreement that they present more of a challenge within secure hospitals. The small number of women in high and medium security account for a disproportionate number of assaults on staff and other patients, deliberate self-harm, and episodes of seclusion. Women are said to have less need for perimeter security and more need for internal or relational security.

As a consequence, women were central to the discussions in the 1990s about the future of high security hospitals. Many patients in high security were judged not to need all aspects of high security. They could be looked after safely in medium security if adaptations were made to meet their particular needs, for example, tolerance of a longer stay than the usual two-year ceiling.

A high proportion of these misplaced patients were women and their main specific needs were for high staffing ratios and skilled nursing care in medium security. Their treatment needs were not being adequately met at the appropriate level of physical security (Milne *et al.* 1995; Lart *et al.* 1999) and as a result many women suffered from the unnecessary constraints of being detained in high security.

All was not well in medium security either. Women, as a minority in high secure and medium secure services, lacked privacy and were vulnerable to victimization by male patients (some of whom had histories of sexual and physical violence towards women) (Bartlett *et al.* 2001).

After years of debate the late 1990s saw drastic action in these areas. Two of the three high security hospitals no longer admit women. The remaining high secure beds are now concentrated in a single hospital, Rampton, which takes advantage of the concentration of patients in one place to provide a more specialized services. It is no longer considered acceptable to try and fit women into a service primarily designed for men (Department of Health 1999b, 2002, 2003).

As the number of beds in high security has fallen, a new service development aims to provide a more appropriate service. Women's Enhanced Medium Secure Services (WEMSS) provide a more accessible, locally-based service where the emphasis is on skilled nursing care and psychological therapies rather than perimeter security. There are currently three pilot WEMSS services, the largest of which is the Orchard in West London with 45 beds, it opened in 2007 (The Orchard – Enhanced Medium Secure Mental Health Unit at St Bernard's Hospital, Ealing). These services have been designed to cater specifically to the needs of women and aim to provide a therapeutic environment that is able to safely contain and manage distress and disturbance, while providing appropriate therapeutic interventions (Green 2007).

Being for women only, WEMSS units are in line with a general trend in the NHS to separate inpatient facilities for men and women. Debate about this issue continues. The common ground is that separate services are needed but there is fierce argument about their extent. On the one hand it is argued that women who have been victimized throughout their lives need protection when at their most vulnerable. On the other it is accepted that such protection is necessary when mental health problems are at their most acute, but the task of recovery and rehabilitation entails coming to terms with the world through controlled exposure.

There is, of course, no simple answer and the debate is an example of the general tension in mental health between protection from stress and allowing recovery by attempting more ambitious tasks, always with the possibility of failure. There is little research in the area. One exception is a study that shows (unsurprisingly) that while there may be other benefits, single-sex units do not eliminate the problem of victimization (Mezey *et al.* 2005).

Treatment

Perhaps unsurprisingly, medication is the most common form of explicit treatment over and above a secure hospital environment. In their study at Broadmoor, Bland *et al.* (1999) found while 72% of women had a diagnosis of mental illness, almost all women were receiving antipsychotics (97%), and most were also receiving antidepressants (91%). A third (32%) were receiving or had received formal psychotherapy. The literature review by Lart *et al.* (1999) concluded that there was unmet need for responses to personality disorder, substance dependence, and trauma therapy relating to histories of abuse. They made a number of recommendations including a shift towards relational security which would enable more individualized levels of security to develop in response to women's needs. These recommendations have been incorporated into WEMSS, which provide 'high levels of therapy in a non-oppressive environment, coupled with effective observation of patients' (The Orchard – Enhanced Medium Secure Mental Health Unit at St Bernard's Hospital, Ealing, p. 1).

Behaviour after discharge: reoffending

Research regarding the outcomes after discharge from secure forensic units has tended to focus on reconvictions. Women are less likely to re-offend than men (Buchanan 1998; Coid *et al.* 2007), however, some or all of the gender differences in offending may be explained by the fact that women are more likely to harm themselves, less likely to have a history of alcohol and drug problems, and less likely to have a previous criminal history (Milne *et al.* 1995).

Conclusion

Women and men are different: this includes differences in the nature and prevalence of mental disorder and antisocial behaviour, but also differences in their lives, expectations, and responsibilities. This is captured by recent policy documents relating to gender and mental health and prison services (Department of Health 1999b, 2002, 2003, 2006a; Corston 2007). They conclude that gender needs to be integral to our services, not an afterthought; our services need to be holistic, and we need to listen to the women themselves in order to facilitate this. However putting this into practice is more difficult. The evidence base for effective treatment in this population is lacking (Lart *et al.* 1999; Bartlett 2000, 2007b), and we need to think about how we give disempowered women a meaningful voice within hierarchical and coercive systems.

References

Bartlett A (1993). Rhetoric and reality: what do we know about English special hospitals? *International Journal of Law and Psychiatry*, **16**, 27–51.

Bartlett A (2000). *Expert Paper: Social Division and Difference: Women*. NHS National Programme on Forensic Mental Health Research and Development. http://www.liv.ac.uk/fmhweb/publications.htm

Bartlett A (2007). *Second Expert Paper: Social Division and Difference: Women*. NHS National Programme on Forensic Mental Health Research and Development. http://www.liv.ac.uk/fmhweb/publications.htm

Bartlett A (2007a). Women in prison: concepts, clinical issues and care delivery. *Psychiatry*, **6**, 444–8.

Bartlett A *et al.* (2001). Do women need special secure services? *Advances in Psychiatric Treatment*, **7**, 302–9.

Birmingham L *et al.* (2006a). The mental health of women in prison mother and baby units. *Journal of Forensic Psychiatry and Psychology*, **17**(3), 393–404.

Birmingham L *et al.* (2006b). Prison medicine: ethics and equivalence. *British Journal of Psychiatry*, **188**(1), 4–6.

Bland J *et al.* (1999). Special women, special needs: a descriptive study of female Special Hospital patients. *Journal of Forensic Psychiatry*, **10**(1), 34–45.

Buchanan A, (1998). Criminal conviction after discharge from Special (High Secure) Hospitals: Incidence in the first 10 years. *British Journal of Psychiatry*, **172**, 472–6.

Coid J *et al.* (2000). Women admitted to secure forensic psychiatry services: I Comparison of women and men. *Journal of Forensic Psychiatry*, **11**(2), 275–95.

Coid J *et al.* (2007). Patients discharged from medium secure forensic psychiatry services: reconvictions and risk factors. *British Journal of Psychiatry*, **190**, 223–9.

Corston J (2007). *The Corston Report: a report by Baroness Jean Corston of a review of women with particular vulnerabilities in the criminal justice system*. Home Office, London.

Department of Health (1999a). *The Future Organisation of Prison Healthcare*. Department of Health, London.

Department of Health (1999b). *Secure futures for women: making a difference*. Department of Health, London.

Department of Health (2002). *Women's Mental Health: Into the Mainstream. Strategic Development of Mental Health Care for Women*. Department of Health, London.

Department of Health (2003). *Mainstreaming Gender and Women's Mental Health: Implementation Guidance*. Department of Health, London.

Department of Health (2006a). *Women at Risk: the mental health of women in contact with the criminal justice system*. Department of Health, London.

Department of Health (2006b). *Dangerous and Severe/Complex Personality Disorder High Secure Services: Planning and delivery guide for women's DSPD services (Primrose Programme)*. Department of Health, London.

Farrington DP (1994). *Cambridge Study in Delinquent Development (Great Britain), 1961–1981*. Inter-University Consortium for Political and Social Research, Ann Arbor, MI.

Fazel S and Danesh J (2002). Serious mental disorder in 23 000 prisoners: a systematic review of 62 surveys. *Lancet*, **359**, 545–50.

Gorsuch N (1999). Disturbed female offenders: helping the 'untreatable'. *Journal of Forensic Psychiatry*, **10**(1), 98–118.

Green R (2007). New Therapeutically Enhanced Medium Secure Services for Women In England. *International Association of Forensic Mental Health Services Newsletter*.

Hodgins S *et al.* (1996). Mental disorder and crime. Evidence from a Danish birth cohort. *Archives of General Psychiatry*, **53**(6), 489–96.

Home Office (2006). *Cognitive Skills Programmes: Impact on reducing reconviction among a sample of female prisoners*. Home Office, London.

Home Office (2007). *Crime in England and Wales 2006/7*. Home Office Statistical Bulletin, London.

Lart R *et al.* (1999). *CRD Report 14 — Women and secure psychiatric services: A literature review 1999*. Centre for Reviews and Dissemination.

Maden T (1996). *Women, Prisons and Psychiatry: Mental Disorder Behind Bars*, Butterworth-Heinemann, Oxford.

Maden T *et al.* (1994). Psychiatric disorder in women serving a prison sentence. *British Journal of Psychiatry*, **164**, 44–54.

Maden A *et al.* (1995). *Mental Disorder in Remand Prisoners*. Department of Forensic Psychiatry, Institute of Psychiatry. London.

Maden A *et al.* (2006). Gender differences in reoffending after discharge from medium-secure units: National cohort study in England and Wales. *British Journal of Psychiatry*, **189**(2), 168–72.

May C (2005). *The CARAT drug service in prisons: findings from the research database*. Home Office, London.

McGuire J (1995) *What Works. Reducing reoffending: guidelines from research and Practice*. Wiley, Chichester.

McGuire J (2002). *Offender Rehabilitation and Treatment: Effective Programmes and Policies to Reduce Reoffending*. Wiley, Chichester.

Mezey G *et al.* (2005). Safety of women in mixed-sex and single-sex medium secure units: Staff and patient perceptions. *British Journal of Psychiatry*, **187**(6), 579–82.

Milne S *et al.* (1995). Sex differences in patients admitted to a regional security unit. *Medicine Science and the Law*, **35**, 57–60.

Ministry of Justice (2007a). *Criminal Statistics 2006: England and Wales*. Ministry of Justice, London.

Ministry of Justice (2007b). *Offender Management Caseload Statistics 2006.* Ministry of Justice Statistical Bulletin: London.

Ministry of Justice (2007c). *Population in Custody December 2007.* Ministry of Justice: London.

Ministry of Justice (2008). *Prison population and accommodation briefing for 22nd February 2008.* National Offender Management Service.

Moffit TE *et al.* (2001). *Sex differences in antisocial behaviour,* Cambridge University Press, Cambridge.

O'Brien M *et al.* (2003). Psychiatric morbidity among women prisoners in England and Wales. *International Review of Psychiatry,* **15**, 153–7.

Rutherford H *et al.* (2004). The transfer of women offenders with mental disorder from prison to hospital. *Journal of Forensic Psychiatry & Psychology,* **15**(1), 108–23.

Sim J (1990). *Medical Power in Prisons: The Prison Medical Service in England, 1774–1989 (Crime, Justice and Social Policy).* Open University Press, Milton Keynes.

Social Exclusion Unit (2002). *Reducing Re-offending by Ex-prisoners.* Social Exclusion Unit, London.

The Orchard – Enhanced Medium Secure Mental Health Unit at St Bernard's Hospital, Ealing. http://www.nhs-procure21. gov.uk/content/downloads/071015%20-%20The%20 Orchard%20-%20West%20London%20Mental%20 Health%20-%20JC.pdf

Wilson S (2004). The principle of equivalence and the future of mental health care in prisons. *British Journal of Psychiatry,* **184**(1), 5–7.

CHAPTER 16

The social care needs of women with mental illness

Adil Akram and Andrew Kent

Why is it important to consider the social care needs of women separately from those of men?

> Gender is a complex variable because men and women differ not only biologically, but also in their life experiences.
>
> Leibenluft (1996)

Social care needs make an important contribution to the quality of life of men and women with mental health problems (Lehman *et al.* 1982; 1983; UK700 Group 1999). Such needs include housing, food, money, social interaction, relationships, childcare, education, and care of self and the home. Many of these needs are amenable to influence and intervention from health and social care services, and the interventions targeting improved quality of life for people living with severe mental illness should take account of these needs (UK700 Group 1999).

There is an argument that health and social services are designed to be 'gender blind' or 'gender neutral' and therefore women's needs are already effectively considered, without having to make a distinction by gender. This leads to the assumption that men and women's social care needs are the same. As Curtis (2005), risking a truism, points out women are not the same as men, and supposedly 'gender blind' services are essentially male orientated and focused, with women in the default position of the 'other'. Women with severe mental illness are 'othered' to an even greater extent (Montgomery 2005); their needs not acknowledged or incorporated into the mainstream, despite being a socially active group.

Authors such as Kohen (2001), argue for 'gender sensitive understanding in psychiatric services'. We agree and argue that social needs should also be understood from a woman's perspective as women's health may be more strongly associated with social environment than men's (Cooper *et al.* 1999). The different life experiences of women inform and influence their health experiences. Ramsay and her colleagues (2001) suggest that this influences the differing ways mental health problems can present in men and women and has implications for their management.

An improved understanding of the specific social care needs of women could lead to the development of practical solutions that can be implemented by case managers and have the potential to have a real impact on quality of life. This is in keeping with the current 'recovery'-based philosophy that increasingly pervades mental healthcare delivery, aiming to restore the individual to as full a life as possible, by normalizing rehabilitative social roles. Recent United Kingdom (UK) government policy documents (see Box 16.1) have highlighted mental health and social care inequalities and built on a raft of related policies over the past two decades (Ramsay *et al.* 2001).

What are the social care needs that are specific to women?

Areas of specific social care need for women include mental illness in pregnancy, antenatal and postnatal care, motherhood, custody of children, sexual, physical, and emotional abuse, stigma, and specific mental illnesses (Kohen 2001). These needs are almost wholly exclusive to women and often neglected in favour of more generic needs transcending gender such as housing, food, money, and employment. Being *gender blind* does not necessarily lead to being *gender fair* as this tends to lead to a male-focused perspective or set of social needs priorities. The categorization of needs under 'clinical' or 'social' labels is itself not particularly

Box 16.1   Recent UK policy documents promoting the assessment of the social care needs of women

2000	*Secure Futures for Women: Making a Difference* (Department of Health)
2000	*Safety, Privacy and Dignity in Mental Health Units* (NHS Executive)
2000	*Future Female – A 21st Century Gender Perspective* (The Women's National Commission/The Future Foundation)
2000	*Treating Women Well – Women and the NHS* (The Women's National Commission)
2004	*National Service Framework for Children Young People and Maternity Services* (Department of Health)
2003	*Mental Health and Social Exclusion Report* (Department of Health)
2003	*Women's' Mental Health: Into the Mainstream, Strategic Development of Mental Healthcare for Women* (Department of Health)
2006	*Making the Grade? Executive Summary* (End Violence against Women Campaign)
2007	*Antenatal and Postnatal Mental Health* (NICE)
2007	*Confidential Enquiry into Maternal and Child Health* (CEMACH)
2008	*Care of Pregnant Women with Complex Social Factors* (NICE).

helpful as it becomes relatively arbitrary which aspects of a woman's experience are given recognition under which heading. For example, is the sexual health of a woman with mental illness a social or clinical issue? We argue that it is *both*, and to ignore the complex interplay of social and clinical need results in a selectively greater disadvantage to women.

Women's experience of health services and pregnancy

Women are the major users of National Health Service (NHS) health services in general and report ill health more frequently than men (The Women's National Commission Health Group 2000). Women are likely to present differently to healthcare services compared to men (Goldberg and Huxley 1992). Specific mental illnesses occur in women in relation to childbirth. As stated by the Royal College of Psychiatrists (2000): 'Perinatal mental health problems are common, many are serious and they can have long-lasting effects on

maternal health and child development.' These disorders are highlighted in ICD-10 (World Health Organization 1992) as disorders of 'Pregnancy, Childbirth and the Puerperium' and comprise of maternity or 'baby' blues, postnatal depression, and puerperal psychosis. About 10 or 15 women in 100 will experience postnatal depression and about 1 in 500 will experience puerperal psychosis (Blumenthal 1995; Oates 2003). Of note, the later two conditions are often mistaken for maternity blues, which itself may affect up to 85 out of 100 women and initially may look similar in clinical presentation.

Social factors are thought to play a major aetiological role in the development of postnatal depression, whereas biological factors are more strongly associated with puerperal psychosis (Royal College of Psychiatrists 2000). Specific psychosocial factors increasing risk for postnatal depression include young maternal age, relationship difficulties with partner or family, lack of social network, and substance misuse (O'Hara *et al.* 1996).

Within the first month of delivering a baby, there is a 35 times increased risk of hospital admission for a psychotic illness (Kendell *et al.* 1987). Suicide is a leading cause of maternal death in the UK (CEMACH 2007). Despite these striking findings, there is a lack of mother and baby unit beds nationally (Nicholls and Cox 1999; Royal College of Psychiatrists 2000). Recent National Institute of Health and Clinical Excellence (NICE) guidelines (2007) for perinatal care promote access to specialist inpatient units in addition to pre-pregnancy planning, early monitoring, and support of women with a history of mental illness.

Complex social factors have been strongly implicated in pregnancies with poor outcomes, including the death of the child or the mother. The UK national confidential enquiries into maternal and child health (CEMACH 2007) have identified women living in deprived areas as having a fivefold greater mortality than women in affluent areas. Babies born into these circumstances were found to be twice as likely to die compared to babies born to women living in the least deprived areas of the UK (NICE 2008). Other social factors linked to maternal death are also included in Box 16.2.

Women's experience of mental illness

Women are also over-represented in specific domains of mental illness, as shown in Table 16.1.

Table 16.1 highlights data from the National Co-morbidity Survey Replication showing an increased

Box 16.2 Complex social factors implicated in maternal death (NICE 2008)

♦ Domestic abuse

♦ Being single

♦ Being unemployed

♦ Having an unemployed partner

♦ Recent migration into UK

♦ Speaking no English

♦ Contact with child protection or social services.

Table 16.2 Lifetime prevalence estimates of DSM-IV eating disorders

Sex	Anorexia nervosa	Bulimia nervosa	Binge eating disorder
Female	0.9%	1.5%	3.5%
Male	0.3%	0.5%	2.0%

Table 16.1 Odds ratios for lifetime risk of DSM-IV psychiatric disorder based on gender

Sex	Any anxiety disorder	Any mood disorder	Any disorder
Female	1.6	1.5	1.1
Male	1.0	1.0	1.0

lifetime risk for women of any psychiatric disorder over men (Kessler *et al.* 2005), with significantly elevated rates for anxiety disorders and mood disorders.

Importantly, women are significantly more likely to be diagnosed with three or more disorders (odds ratio 1.24, p<0.05) compared to men (Kessler *et al.* 1994a). This suggests that there is a heavy burden of psychiatric comorbidity carried by women over their lifetimes. It is likely that social factors contribute proportionately more towards precipitating, perpetuating, and maintaining ill health in this group. Healthcare services need to address these unmet social care needs, as well as the comorbidity and adverse effects on social functioning that arise, particularly in light of the effects on quality of life (UK700 Group 1999) and the likely transgenerational effects conferred.

The landmark studies of Brown and Harris (1978) and Harris *et al.* (1987) also highlight the importance of adequate social supports to protect women from depression. Social stressors loading a woman's risk for depressive illness identified by these studies included: lack of a confiding relationship; no employment outside of the home; three or more children under the age of 15 at home; and an unhappy marriage.

Social factors have also been linked to the difference in onset of psychotic illness such as schizophrenia in women. Seeman (1995) suggests that as social support

declines in later life as children leave home, this contributes to the late second peak of incidence of schizophrenia exclusively seen in women (also at the time of menopausal oestrogen decline) (Lewine and Seeman 1995). Women with a dual diagnosis of schizophrenia and illicit substance misuse also had more social contact problems compared to men (Brunette and Drake 1997).

Eating disorders occur in markedly larger numbers in women, by a ratio of 10:1. Table 16.2 highlights the higher prevalence of all eating disorders in women (Hudson *et al.* 2007). This is likely to be mediated by social influences and expectations around women to look slim at all costs.

Other gender disparities also become apparent within mental health services. Older women are much more likely to have recurrent major depressive episodes (Kessler *et al.* 1994b), yet evidence suggests that older women with severe enduring mental illness may receive less intensive input compared to other groups (Perkins and Rowland 1991). In addition, there is underfunding and lack of provision of services for women such as eating disorders and perinatal psychiatric services, despite NICE guidelines highlighting their importance.

Women with mental illness and sexual health

Little research has been conducted in the UK on the sexual health needs of women with severe mental health problems. However, research from overseas indicates that women with severe mental health problems are more likely than others to experience adverse outcomes across a range of health domains and that when these occur they are likely to be transgenerational—affecting not only the woman but also her children, with substantial personal and societal costs.

Women with severe mental health problems have more lifetime sexual partners, higher rates of unprotected sex, coerced sex, sexually transmitted infections (STIs), a poorer knowledge of sexual health, and attend fewer appointments for cervical screening, mammography and HIV testing. Studies show they have more unwanted pregnancies, terminations, and children taken into care, and that they are at greater risk of violence in pregnancy and have higher rates of obstetric complications, but are less likely to receive appropriate antenatal care (McEvoy *et al.* 1983; Coverdale and Arruffo 1989; Cournos *et al.* 1994; Miller and Finnerty 1996; Sacker *et al.* 1996; Coverdale *et al.* 1997; Miller and Finnerty 1998; Lindamer *et al.* 2003).

The views of women with severe mental health problems on reproductive and sexual health issues have been identified as poorly studied, with cultural differences ignored (Krumm and Becker 2006). There is hardly any data on the attitudes and views of mental healthcare professionals in respect of these needs, although one review has argued that sexual health services should be offered in conjunction with mental health services, as separate clinics act as a barrier preventing vulnerable women seeking appropriate help and advice (Miller 1997). One small qualitative study conducted in the UK suggests that women with severe mental health problems would welcome more attention to their physical health needs in general by mental health professionals, and that they feel that their reproductive and sexual health needs in particular are often ignored and invalidated (Birch *et al.* 2005).

Importance and relevance to the NHS

Half of all pregnancies in the UK are unplanned and the number of terminations is increasing (Department of Health 2003a). Studies from Norway and the United States (US) have suggested that the fertility of women with severe mental illness has increased with deinstitutionalization (Odegard 1980; Nicholson *et al.* 1996). Reproductive rates amongst women with serious mental illness such as schizophrenia were similar to healthy controls in US studies (Miller and Finnerty 1996; Sacker *et al.* 1996), but subjects had less awareness of birth control methods (Miller and Finnerty 1996). Improving access to preconception planning and reproductive healthcare to vulnerable groups, including women with severe mental health problems, has repeatedly been identified as an NHS priority. Most recently, the National Service Framework for Children, Young People and Maternity Services (Department of Health 2004) highlighted the ongoing need for better access to pre-conception advice and maternity services for vulnerable women, and the needs of women

with severe mental health problems were specifically identified.

The National Service Framework for Mental Health (Department of Health 1999), the Strategy for Sexual Health (Department of Health 2003a), and Mental Health and Social Exclusion Report (Department of Health 2003b) all emphasize the need to improve healthcare services for people with severe mental health problems. The Department of Health has specifically identified the need to develop services to meet women's needs in 'Women's Mental Health: Into The Mainstream' (2003c) and promotes understanding illness 'from a woman's perspective'. The joint statement 'A common purpose: Recovery in future mental health services' (Royal College of Psychiatrists 2007) highlights the importance of developing and integrating a recovery based approach into mental healthcare services. This emphasizes involving patient expertise from direct experience of living with illness in developing research and services to meet needs.

One US study found that despite their greater need, women with severe mental health problems may actually receive fewer gynaecological services than other women (Lindamer *et al.* 2003). This lack of adequate sexual healthcare access or provision may have additional, personally devastating consequences for women, on top of the distress associated with living with a mental health problem. This has widespread implications for the individual and society, creating an economic and social burden in terms of subsequent increased NHS costs of relapse, termination of pregnancy, treatment for STIs, and substantial social service provision to look after unwanted children who themselves may become vulnerable to consequent serious social and mental health problems.

Women and violence

Violence against women is a significant social problem having widespread effects across society. Violence against women is defined by the United Nations (1993) as:

> Violence against women refers to any act of gender-based violence that results in, or is likely to result in, physical, sexual or psychological harm or suffering to women, including threats of such acts, coercion or arbitrary deprivation of liberty, whether occurring in public or private life. Violence against women shall be understood to encompass, but not be limited to, the following:
>
> (a) Physical, sexual and psychological violence occurring in the family, including battering, sexual abuse of female children in the household, dowry-related violence, marital rape, female genital mutilation and other

traditional practices harmful to women, non-spousal violence and violence related to exploitation;

(b) Physical, sexual and psychological violence occurring within the general community, including rape, sexual abuse, sexual harassment and intimidation at work, in educational institutions and elsewhere, trafficking in women and forced prostitution;

(c) Physical, sexual and psychological violence perpetrated or condoned by the State, wherever it occurs.

Almost half of all adult women in England and Wales have experienced violence of one form (Walby 2004). One in four women have experienced domestic violence (Walby and Allen 2004), and this makes up one-third of all violent crime against women. Women suffering with severe mental illness appear even more likely to be victims of serious violence, including rape, sexual assault, and domestic violence compared to the general population (Coverdale *et al.* 1997; Miller 1997).

Nothwithstanding the personally devastating consequences of violence, violence against women represents a major economic cost to the nation, with the direct and indirect costs of domestic violence alone in the UK estimated to be £23 billion (Walby 2004). Violence against women is a common factor contributing to the development of mental health problems in women and costs the NHS an estimated £1.4 billion a year (End Violence Against Women Campaign 2006). Rape has the highest health-related costs of any violent crime at approx £75 000 per case (Dubourg *et al.* 2005), whilst the rate of convictions in the UK has dropped from 1 in 13 (33%) in 1977 to 1 in 20 (5.3%) in 2004 (End Violence Against Women Campaign 2006).

The campaign to end violence against women acknowledges that it is impossible to address this issue from a gender neutral perspective (End Violence Against Women Campaign 2006). This is because men are recognized as still occupying a relative position of power over women in contemporary society, and this is reinforced by the prevailing social and economic climate (Gold 1998).

Women and families

The traditional model of the family unit has changed dramatically over the past 40 years. There has been a sharp increase in the number of cohabiting couples, single parents, and divorced or remarried parents in the UK. This trend is reflected across the developed world. The UK General Household Survey (2002) found that the percentage of lone mother families rose from 7% in 1971 to 24% in 2002. In contrast, the percentage of families in the UK consisting of married or cohabiting couples with children dropped from 92% in 1971 to 73% in 2002 (see Fig. 16.1).

The percentage of families headed by mothers who never married has increased from 1% in 1971 to 12% in 2002. The percentage of families headed by mothers

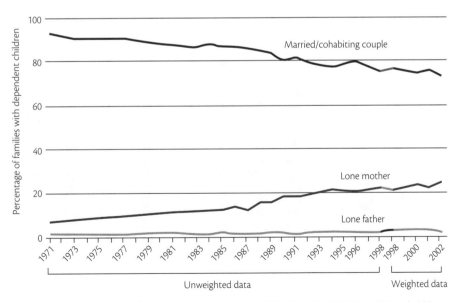

Fig. 16.1 Families with dependent children by family type: Great Britain, 1971–2002. From the 2002 General Household Survey, published in 2004.

who were previously married, and are now divorced, widowed, or separated, has risen from 6% to 12% during the same period.

The proportion of women aged 18 to 49 that were married has declined continuously since 1979, from almost three-quarters (74%) to less than a half (49%) in 2002. During this same period, the proportion of single women has more than doubled from 18% in 1979 to 38% in 2002.

Being a parent is a major social role of crucial importance not only to the family, but also to society. As suggested by Ramsay and her colleagues (2001), 'parenting can act as a buffer to adversity' for children from negative social influences. Parenting can also instil a sense of resilience, status, and well-being in women with mental or physical problems that may reduce their social function or status in other areas. Unfortunately, the positive aspects of being a parent are often overlooked by service providers for the very women who may benefit most. For example, Pound and Abel (1996) found that mothers who have had poor parenting experiences may be least likely to receive social support to help them when they become parents. Women suffering with severe mental illness have fertility rates equivalent to the background population and many are mothers (Miller 1998). Services can view this as more of a problem than an advantage, and ignore the potentially

therapeutic and motivating role that motherhood can confer.

Women and housing

Figures from the UK General Household Survey (2002) show that since 1971 there have also been significant changes in the composition of UK households. These have included an increase in the proportion of one-person households, and of households headed by a lone parent.

Between 1971 and 1998, the overall proportion of one-person households almost doubled from 17% to 31%, and the proportion of households consisting of one person aged 16 to 59 tripled from 5% to 15%.

The proportion of non-married women who were cohabiting at the time of the 2002 survey has increased from 11% in 1979 to 29% in 2002 (see Fig. 16.2). Among single women, the proportion cohabiting has almost quadrupled (from 8% in 1979 to 31% in 2002).

Already 14% of households are occupied by women living on their own and by 2011 there will be almost 8 million households with one person, one-third of all households (The Women's National Commission/The Future Foundation 2000).

A significant minority of women are homeless. Marshall and Reed (1992) state that these women suffer

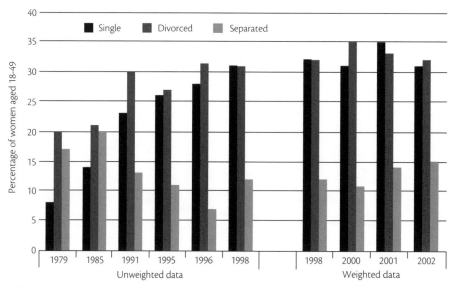

* Widows have not been included because their numbers are so small

Fig. 16.2 Percentage of single, divorced, and separated women aged 18–49 cohabiting by legal marital status: Great Britain, 1979–2002. From the 2002 General Household Survey, published in 2004.

higher levels of mental illness despite lower levels of substance misuse. Subgroups of women who may be pregnant, have children, or have a mental illness are entitled to housing provided by local councils. However, the availability and quality of this housing stock varies and access to services and supporting benefits is also a major problem for these particularly vulnerable groups.

Women and an ageing population

Life expectancy for women has doubled over the 20th century. As seen in Fig. 16.3, there will be a 30% increase in the proportion of women over 55 by 2021.

Women will be faced, in the future, with increasing risks related to poverty, care provision, and age discrimination. The proportion of women living with mental illness into older age will also increase and this group will be particularly vulnerable in terms of social care needs. Older women are more likely than men to be dependant on help from others for activities of daily living. They are less likely to be able to go out alone and live independently (Debate of the Age 1998).

This is already a large burden in terms of cost and it is set to rise. Barring any major advances in medical science equalizing male life expectancy, women will continue to make up the majority of the older adult population, yet their private pensions are less than 10% of men's when they retire.

Women from black and minority ethnic groups

Social care needs appear to make an even greater contribution to mental health in black and minority ethnic groups. The UK700 study found social, clinical, and unmet needs accounted for a larger variance in quality of life amongst African-Caribbean participants compared to participants from other ethnic groups. This suggests that interventions based on addressing these needs '. . . may have a greater effect on improving quality of life in the disproportionate number of African-Caribbean patients who are treated for severe mental illness in the UK' (UK700 Group 1999).

Women of black African and Caribbean origin have a higher risk of maternal death than women from other groups. The difference is striking, with maternal mortality rates of 62.4 and 41.1 per 100 000 pregnancies respectively, compared to 11.1 per 100 000 for white women (NICE 2008).

Complex social factors also influence perinatal mortality. The stillbirth and neonatal mortality rate is approximately twice that in babies born to women of black African or Caribbean origin compared to white women (NICE 2008). Contributors may include difficulty accessing antenatal care and lack of appropriate service provision.

Poverty has been demonstrated to have a major impact on mental health. This is linked to women from

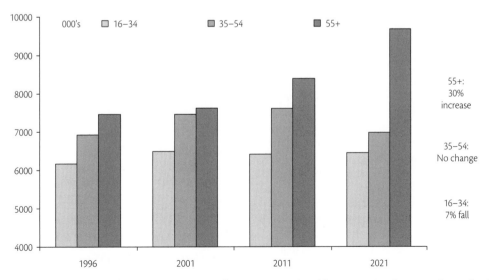

Fig. 16.3 On the whole, the impact of future trends are positive for women. Reproduced from *Future Female – A 21st Century Gender Perspective* (The Women's National Commission/The Future Foundation 2000).

minority populations who are often in the lowest paid jobs. Pakistani and Bangladeshi women are more likely to work part-time then other groups (Commission for Racial Equality 1997). These groups experience four times the rate of poverty than white women (Berthoud 1998) and 30% of Asian women are dissatisfied with NHS services (The Women's National Commission Health Group 2000). People from black and minority ethnic groups reported less patient satisfaction overall with the NHS services they received (Healthcare Commission 2008).

Women in prison

The number of women in UK prisons is rising. Many of these women suffer with mental health problems and are vulnerable as a result. The 'Women in Prison' website (2008) outlines the magnitude of the problem:

◆ 70% of women prisoners have mental health problems

◆ 37% have attempted suicide

◆ 20% have been in the care system as children compared to 2% of the general population

◆ At least 50% report being victims of childhood abuse or domestic violence

◆ Nearly a third of women prisoners who have owned/rented accommodation before prison lose their homes as a result of imprisonment

◆ 65% reoffend on release

◆ A prison bed costs between £25 000 and £45 000 a year

◆ The most common offences for which women are sent to prison are theft and handling stolen goods

◆ The women's prison population went up by 173% in the decade to 2004.

'Fourteen per cent of all female prisoners have experienced a psychotic illness in the previous 12 months' (Singleton *et al.* 1998). Prison is often the end result of a culmination of the social and psychological insults experienced by some vulnerable groups of women over their lifetime such as poverty, abusive relationships, isolation and violence.

National guidelines advise that the quality of mental health services available for people in prison should be equivalent to those available to the public. 'Prisoners are entitled to the same level of healthcare as that provided in society at large. Those who are sick, addicted, mentally ill or disabled should be treated . . . to the same standards demanded within the National Health

Service.' (HM Inspectorate of Prisons 1996). At present, the current model of mental healthcare delivery occurs via in reach teams of specialists. Unfortunately, there does not appear to be equivalence in terms of mental healthcare between the community mental health team (CMHT) and 'in-reach' models. This is despite the NHS taking over the healthcare of prisoners from the Prison Health Service in 2006. The report 'Short-changed: spending on prison mental healthcare' (Sainsbury Centre for Mental Health 2008), outlines the reasons for the disparity, including the greater prevalence of mental illness in the prison population, geographical variations in practice, logistical difficulties and an organizational culture that differs. This report also highlights the 'postcode lottery' of NHS funding allocated, with prisoners in London receiving twice as much resources per head compared to the East Midlands, despite no basis in terms of differing needs or costs.

> Taking the most hurt people out of society and punishing them in order to teach them how to live within society is, at best, futile. Whatever else a prisoner knows, she knows everything there is to know about punishment because that is exactly what she has grown up with. Whether it is childhood sexual abuse, indifference, neglect; punishment is most familiar to her.
>
> Chris Tchaikovsky, former prisoner and founder of 'Women in Prison'

Social roles and mental well-being

Health inequalities and socioeconomic deprivation are closely related. Cooper and colleagues (1999) suggest that women's health is even more strongly associated with the social environment than men's. A social life comprising of fulfilling social roles around family, friends, work, and community may help to promote psychological health and alleviate the effects of stress in women. By contrast, people with few quality social roles have the poorest psychosocial health (Ramsay *et al.* 2001). Women are the main carers of children and elderly relatives (The Women's National Commission Health Group 2000). This caring role often occurs in isolation from wider social supports and goes unacknowledged behind closed doors, but often has an impact on the mental health of the women involved.

Women and changing social needs in the future

Fig 16.4 summarizes the differing social factors impacting on women today and for the foreseeable future.

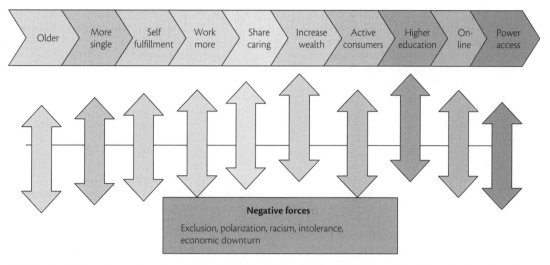

Fig. 16.4 Projected change in age of female population. England and Wales, 1996-based. Reproduced from *Future Female – A 21st Century Gender Perspective* (The Women's National Commission/The Future Foundation 2000).

As stated by the report from The Women's National Commission/The Future Foundation (2000), the overall trends appear to be positive, although the negative forces acting on them are highlighted and could lead to setbacks. An understanding of these forces and the complex interplay of the socioeconomic factors will allow us to develop insightful and effective strategies to deliver meaningful change to women living with a mental illness.

Conclusion

Women with severe mental health problems often have complex social care needs. These needs make a significant adverse contribution to their quality of life. They also contribute to the morbidity and mortality of a wide range of problems that selectively affect women. When social care needs exist, they should be addressed wherever possible within an overarching care plan. It is not enough that services are gender blind, services must be gender fair.

References

Berthoud R (1998). *Incomes of Ethnic Minorities. ISER Report 98–1*. Institute for Social and Economic Research, Joseph Rowntree Foundation, Colchester.

Birch S *et al.* (2005). The physical healthcare experiences of women with mental health problems: Status versus stigma. *Journal of Mental Health*, **14**(1), 61–72.

Blumenthal SJ (1995). Improving women's mental and physical health: Federal initiatives and programs. *American Psychiatric Press Review of Psychiatry*, **14**, 181–204.

Brunette MF and Drake RE (1997). Gender differences in patients with schizophrenia and substance abuse. *Comprehensive Psychiatry*, **38**, 109–16.

Brown GW and Harris TO (1978). *Social Origins of Depression: A Study of Psychiatric Disorder in Women*. Tavistock, London.

Commission for Racial Equality (1997) Employment and Unemployment. CRE factsheets. CRE, London.

CEMACH (2007). *The Confidential Enquiry into Maternal and Child Health (CEMACH). Saving Mothers' Lives: reviewing maternal deaths to make motherhood safer – 2003–2005. The Seventh Report on Confidential Enquiries into Maternal Deaths in the United Kingdom*. CEMACH, London.

Cooper H *et al.* (1999). *The Influence of Social Support and Social Capital on Health*. Health Education Authority, London.

Cournos F *et al.* (1994). Sexual activity and risk of HIV infection among patients with schizophreniA. *American Journal of Psychiatry* **151**(2), 228–32.

Coverdale JH and Arruffo JA (1989). Family planning needs of female chronic psychiatric outpatients. *American Journal of Psychiatry*, **146**, 1489–91.

Coverdale JH *et al.* (1997). Family planning needs and STD risk behaviours of female psychiatric outpatients. *British Journal of Psychiatry*, **171**, 69–72.

Curtis V (2005). Women are not the same as men: specific clinical issues for female patients with bipolar disorder. *Bipolar Disorder*, **7**(Suppl. 1), 16–24.

Debate of the Age (1998). *Ageing and the future for health and social care*. Age Concern England, London.

Department of Health (1999). *National Service Mental Health Framework for Mental Health*. Department of Health, London.

Department of Health (2000a). *Secure Futures for Women: Making a Difference. Report of the High Security Psychiatric Commission Board.* Department of Health, London.

Department of Health (2000b). *In-Patients Formally Detained in Hospitals under the Mental Health Act 1983 and Other Legislation.* Department of Health, London.

Department of Health (2003a). *Strategy for Sexual Health.* Department of Health, London.

Department of Health (2003b). *Mental Health and Social Exclusion Report.* Department of Health, London.

Department of Health (2003c). *Women's Mental Health: Into The Mainstream, Strategic Development of Mental Healthcare for Women.* Department of Health, London.

Department of Health (2004). *National Service Framework for Children Young People and Maternity Services.* Department of Health, London.

Dubourg R *et al.* (2005). *The economic and social costs of crime against individuals and households 2003/4, Home Office online report 30/05.* Home Office, London. http://www.homeoffice.gov.uk/rds/pdfs05/rdsolr3005.pdf

End Violence Against Women Campaign (2006). *Making the Grade? Executive Summary.* Amnesty International, UK

General Household Survey (2002) http://www.statistics.gov.uk/ssd/surveys/general_household_survey.asp.

Gold JHCM. (1998). Gender differences in psychiatric illness and treatments: a critical review. *Journal of Nervous and Mental Disease*, **186**(12), 769–75.

Goldberg D and Huxley P (1992). *Common Mental Disorders.* Routledge, London.

Harris T *et al.* (1987). Loss of parent in childhood and adult psychiatric disorder: the role of social class position and premarital pregnancy. *Psychological Medicine*, **17**(1), 163–83.

Healthcare Commission (2008). *Report on self reported experience of patients from black and minority ethnic groups.* Healthcare Commission, London.

HM Inspectorate of Prisons (1996). *Patient or prisoner?* Home Office, London.

Hudson JI *et al.* (2007). The prevalence and correlates of eating disorders in the National Comorbidity Survey Replication. *Biological Psychiatry*, **61**(3), 348–58.

Kendell RE *et al.* (1987). Epidemiology of puerperal psychoses. *British Journal of Psychiatry*, **150**, 662–73.

Kessler RC *et al.* (1994a). Lifetime and 12-month prevalence of DSM-III-R psychiatric disorders in the United States: Results from the National Comorbidity Survey. *Archives of General Psychiatry*, **51**, 8–19.

Kessler RC *et al.* (1994b). Sex and depression in the national comorbidity survey. II: Cohort effects. *Journal of Affective Disorders*, **30**(1), 15–26.

Kessler RC *et al.* (2005). Lifetime prevalence and age-of-onset distributions of DSM-IV Disorders in the National Comorbidity Survey Replication. *Archives of General Psychiatry*, **62**, 593–602.

Kohen D (2001). Psychiatric services for women. *Advances in Psychiatric Treatment*, **7**, 328–34.

Krumm S and Becker T. (2006). Subjective views of motherhood in women with mental illness – a sociological perspective. *Journal of Mental Health*, **15**(4), 449–60.

Lehman AF (1983). The wellbeing of chronic mental patients: assessing their quality of life. *Archives of General Psychiatry*, **40**, 369–73.

Lehman AF *et al.* (1982). Chronic mental patients: the quality of life issue. *American Journal of Psychiatry*, **10**, 1271–6.

Leibenluft E (1996). Sex is complex. *American Journal of Psychiatry*, **153**(8), 969–72.

Lewine RJ and Seeman MV (1995). *Gender, Brain and Schizophrenia. Gender and Psychopathology.* American Psychiatric Press, Washington, DC.

Lindamer LA *et al.* (2003). A comparison of gynaecological variables and service use among older women with and without schizophrenia. *Psychiatric Services*, **54**(6), 902–4.

Marshall EJ and Reed JL (1992). Psychiatric morbidity in homeless women. *British Journal of Psychiatry*, **160**, 761–8.

McEvoy JP *et al.* (1983). Chronic schizophrenic women's attitudes towards sex, pregnancy, birth control and childbearing. *Hospital and Community Psychiatry*, **34**, 536–9.

Miller LJ and Finnerty M (1998). Family planning knowledge, attitudes and practices in women with schizophrenic spectrum disorders. *Journal of Psychosomatic Obstetrics and Gynaecology* **19**(4), 210–17.

Miller LJ and Finnerty M (1996). Sexuality, pregnancy, and childrearing among women with schizophrenia-spectrum disorders. *Psychiatric Services*, **47**(5), 502–6.

Miller LJ (1997). Sexuality, reproduction, and family planning in women with schizophrenia. *Schizophrenia Bulletin* **23**(4), 623–35.

Montgomery P (2005). Mothers with a serious mental illness: a critical review of the literature. *Archives of Psychiatric Nursing*, **19**(5), 226–35.

NHS Executive (2000). *Safety, Privacy and Dignity in Mental Health Units.* Department of Health, London.

NICE (2007). *Antenatal and Postnatal Mental Health.* NICE, London.

NICE (2008). *Care of pregnant women with complex social factors.* NICE, London.

Nicholson J *et al.* (1996). 'Sylvia Frumkin' has a baby: A case study for policymakers. *Psychiatric Services*, **47**, 497–501.

Nicholls KR and Cox JL (1999). The provision of care for women with postnatal mental disorder in the United Kingdom: an overview. *Hong Kong Medical Journal*, **5**, 43–7.

O'Hara MW and Swain AM (1996). Rates and risk of postpartum depression – a meta-analysis. *International Review of Psychiatry*, **8**, 87–98.

Oates M (2003). Perinatal psychiatric disorders: a leading cause of maternal morbidity and mortality. *British Medical Bulletin*, **67**, 219–29.

Odegard O (1980). Fertility of psychiatric first admissions in Norway 1936–75. *Acta Psychiatrica Scandinavia*, **62**, 212–20.

Perkins RE and Rowland LA (1991). Sex differences in service usage in long-term psychiatric care. Are women adequately served? *British Journal of Psychiatry*, **158**(suppl. 10), 75–9.

Pound A and Abel K (1996). Motherhood and Mental Illness. In: K Abel *et al.* (eds) *Planning Community Mental Health Services for Women. A Multiprofessional Handbook*. pp. 20–35. Routledge, London.

Ramsay R *et al.* (2001). Needs of women patients withmental illness. *Advances in Psychiatric Treatment*, **7**, 85–92.

Royal College of Psychiatrists (2000). *Council Report CR88: Perinatal Maternal Mental Health Services*. Royal College of Psychiatrists, London.

Royal College of Psychiatrists, CSIP, SCIE (2007). *A common purpose: Recovery in future mental health services (Joint position paper 08)*. Royal College of Psychiatrists, London.

Sacker A *et al.* (1996). Obstetric complications in children born to parents with schizophrenia: A meta analysis of case control studies. *Psychological Medicine*, **26**, 279–87.

Sainsbury Centre for Mental Health (2008). *Short-changed: Spending on Prison Mental Healthcare*. Sainsbury Centre for Mental Health, London.

Seeman MV (1995). *Gender Differences in Treatment Response in Schizophrenia. Gender and Psychopathology*. American Psychiatric Press, Washington, DC.

Singleton N *et al.* (1998). *Psychiatric morbidity among prisoners in England and Wales*. Office for National Statistics, London.

The Women's National Commission Health Group (2000). *Treating Women Well – Women and the NHS*. The Women's National Commission, Cabinet Office, HM Government, London.

The Women's National Commission/The Future Foundation (2000). *Future Female – A 21st Century Gender Perspective*. The Future Foundation, London.

UK700 Group (1999). Predictors of quality of life in people in people with severe mental illness. *British Journal of Psychiatry*, **175**, 426–32.

United Nations (1993). Resolution 48/104. *General Assembly Declaration on the Elimination of Violence Against Women*. Article 1 & Article 2. UN, Geneva.

Walby S (2004). *The Cost of Domestic Violence*. Department of Trade and Industry, London.

Walby S and Allen J (2004). *Domestic Violence, Sexual assault and Stalking: Findings from the British Crime Survey*. Home Office, London.

'Women in Prison' website (June 2008) http://www. womeninprison.org.uk

World Health Organization (1992). *Tenth Revision of The International Classification of Diseases (ICD-10): Classification of Mental and Behavioural Disorders: Clinical Descriptions and Diagnostic Guidelines*. WHO, Geneva.

Perinatal Psychiatric Disorders

Jona Lewin

CHAPTER 17

Perinatal psychiatric disorders

Jona Lewin

Introduction

The earliest description of puerperal mental illness can be found in medical texts in the 17th century (Brockington 1996), but it was the seminal paper by Kendell *et al.* (1987), which drew attention to the significance of puerperal mental illness as the authors showed that hospital admissions in the puerperium are 22 times greater than in the two years preceding childbirth. This increase of psychopathology for women in the perinatal phase was confirmed in a recent population-based register study of psychiatric admission during the first year after giving birth in Denmark (Munk-Olsen *et al.* 2006). The authors found that the prevalence of severe mental disorders during the first three months after childbirth was 1.03/1000 births for mothers and 0.37/1000 birth for fathers. For primiparas, the first weeks and months after delivery had an increased risk of first admission with any mental disorder, and from 10–19 days postpartum had the highest risk, in comparison with women who had given birth 11–12 months prior. This increased risk remained regardless of the age of mother. For women having second children, the increased risk of the postpartum mental disorders was present but lower than that for primiparous women; no association between time since birth and mental disorders was found after the birth of the third child. For mothers, increased risk of admission with unipolar disorders persisted during the first five months postpartum, but only up to 30 days for schizophrenia like disorders and up to 60 days for bipolar affective disorders.

Traditionally, disorders specific to childbirth have been divided into three categories: postnatal blues, postnatal depression, and puerperal psychosis. Postnatal blues has also been regarded as a normal variation of emotional change occurring after childbirth (Miller and Ruckstalis 1999).

There has been much debate about whether or not postnatal depression and puerperal psychosis are distinct from depression or psychosis occurring at other times. ICD-10 only allows categorization if criteria for other psychiatric disorders are not met, and DSM-IV, despite providing coding to denote a relationship to pregnancy or childbirth, also tends to play down any distinctive difference. It can be argued that this has led to under-recognition of these disorders, provides a barrier to effective research and communication, and ignores recent evidence in favour of distinctive features in aetiology, presentation, and treatment. Recommendations for remedying this problem have emerged from a workshop on the classification of postnatal mood disorders (Paykel 1999).

However, there appears to be a consensus amongst most psychiatrists that postpartum disorders are not distinct nosological entities with neither postpartum depression nor postnatal psychosis having specific aetiology (Riecher-Rössler and Rohde 2003; Brockington 2004).

According to Riecher-Rössler and Rohde (2003), giving birth to a child with all its biological and psychosocial consequences seems to act as a major stressor, which—within the general vulnerability–stress model—can trigger the outbreak of all classical disorders in predisposed women.

In their study, Munk-Olsen *et al.* (2006) noted an increase of a wide range of psychiatric conditions in the postnatal period. A few years ago, Paykel (2002) appealed for a specifier, which could apply to any disorder and applies to the onset within the first three postpartum months.

In this chapter I will describe the most common psychiatric conditions in the perinatal phase, which include perinatal depression, puerperal psychosis, bipolar affective disorder, post-traumatic stress disorder, anxiety and panic disorder, and eating disorder. It has been noted that despite varying symptomatology, women with schizophrenia rarely experience relapses of their symptoms after childbirth (Meltzer and Kumar 1985).

Towards the end of this chapter I will discuss in brief the relationship between mental illness and infanticide.

Perinatal depression

Fifty to eighty-five per cent of women experience the 'maternal blues', which is characterized by mild depressive symptoms, anxiety, irritability, mood swings, tearfulness, increased sensitivity, and fatigue The 'blues' typically peak on the fourth and fifth postpartum day, and usually resolve spontaneously by postnatal day ten (Pitt 1973; Gold 2002).

Perinatal depression encompasses depressive episodes, which occur either during pregnancy or during the first 12 months after delivery. In a population-based sample of 1555 women in Sweden, anxiety and depression were more prevalent during mid-trimester (~30%) than postpartum (16%). History of psychiatric disorder, being single, and obesity were risk factors for new-onset postpartum psychiatric disorder (Andersson *et al.* 2006).

A systematic review published in 2004 (Bennett *et al.* 2004) showed the prevalence at first, second, and third trimesters to be 7.5%, 12.8%, and 12%, respectively. A more recent systematic review and meta-analysis of perinatal depression found the prevalence of depression in the first trimester at 11.0%, which dropped to 8.5% in the second and third trimester. After delivery the prevalence of depression rose to its highest level in the third month at 12.9%. In the fourth through seventh months postpartum the prevalence of depression declined slightly staying in the range of 9.9–10.6%, after which it declined to 6.5% (Gavin *et al.* 2005).

Apart from the effects on psychological health, antenatal depressive symptoms have been associated with increased risk of obstetric interventions such as epidural analgesia, operative deliveries, and admissions to neonatal units (Chung *et al.* 2001).

Postnatal depression has been associated with lower quality interaction between mothers and their infant (Stein *et al.* 1991), with subsequent greater child insecurity in attachment relationships (Marmorstein *et al.* 2004) and higher levels of psychiatric disturbances amongst their children (Murray and Stein 1989).

Puerperal psychosis

Puerperal psychosis arises after one in 500–1000 births. Although the absolute risk for any woman is low, relative to other times in a woman's life, this period carries the highest risk. The illness has its onset in the early postnatal period, usually within the first month, but most commonly within the first one to two days (Kendell *et al.* 1987).

With appropriate treatment most women will make a complete recovery but remain at very high risk of future puerperal episodes. Some studies have shown that women with a previous history of puerperal psychosis or bipolar disorder have a 20–30% risk of puerperal recurrence, but the risk rises to over 50% when family history is also a contributing factor. The strong association with bipolar disorder implies a genetic disposition, and recent evidence has emerged of a specific familial risk for puerperal episodes in bipolar disorder (Jones and Craddock 2005). Other authors have estimated that nearly two-thirds of women suffering from postpartum psychosis will experience a relapse after subsequent deliveries (Newport *et al.* 2002).

Although earlier studies suggested Caesarean section, birth of female infant, and pre-term deliveries to be associated with postpartum psychosis, recent studies have confirmed only primiparity, older maternal age, and being a single mother as risk factors (Nager *et al.* 2005; Yun *et al.* 2005). The significance of primiparity was confirmed in a recent publication of a study of 129 women with bipolar affective puerperal psychosis. They found that primiparity was an independent risk factor for postpartum psychosis. Whether women who have postpartum psychosis in their first pregnancy might have less inclination for a second pregnancy has not been addressed (Blackmore *et al.* 2006).

The onset of postpartum psychosis is usually rapid. The peak of the illness often falls within the first two weeks after delivery. Women usually develop paranoid, grandiose, or bizarre delusions, mood swings, confused thinking, and grossly disorganized behaviour that represents a dramatic change from previous functioning (Brockington 1996).

While the majority of cases are affective in nature, several studies describe atypical presenting features such as mixed affective states and confusion Non-affective or schizophrenic presentations are much less common. Typically, the presentation is one of rapid fluctuations of mood, perplexity, confusion, and markedly altered behaviour (Wisner *et al.* 1994). Two of 1000 women with postpartum psychosis may commit suicide, and these women often use irreversible and aggressive means (Lewis 2004).

The wide range of psychiatric symptomatology of puerperal psychosis has given rise to heated debate about the categorization of this condition. Dean and Kendell (1981) showed that most of the women admitted for postpartum psychoses within 90 days of delivery fulfilled research diagnostic criteria for an affective disorder. Similarly Brockington *et al.* (1981) found an excess of manic symptoms and less schizophrenia symptoms in study subjects than in controls.

In their seminal study, Kendell *et al.* (1987) found that the majority of puerperal women requiring hospital admission met research diagnostic criteria for manic or depressive disorders and the authors submit that puerperal psychoses are manic depressive illnesses and unrelated to schizophrenia.

Brockington *et al.* (1981) and Klompenhouwer and van Hulst (1991) have stated that confusion and lability of mood are characteristic for psychotic women in the puerperium. Klompenhouwer and Hulst (1991) argue that, according to research criteria, the large majority of patients with puerperal psychotic disorders cannot be classified within the Kraepelinian dichotomy of schizophrenia and affective disorders, but has to be classified as schizoaffective or unspecified functional psychosis. Pfuhlmann *et al.* (2000) stated that these atypical clinical features do not even fit the category 'schizoaffective psychoses'. He proposed to classify this condition as cycloid psychoses—within a classification developed by Leonhard.

Lewin (2006) pointed to the similarities between puerperal psychosis and acute and transient psychotic episodes as defined in ICD-10. Both are separate from schizophrenia, schizoaffective disorder, or affective disorder, based on the clinical manifestation, and lack a consensus of definition and seem to challenge the Kraepelinian dichotomy (Kohl 2004; Marneros 2006a). Acute and transient psychosis affects mainly females (Marneros 2006) and Lewin (2006) hypothesized a possible link between puerperal psychosis and acute and transient psychoses.

Rohde and Marneros (2000) re-evaluated the diagnoses of 61 women with first onset of psychosis after delivery and found that according to ICD-10 criteria 29.5% should be classified as having acute and transient psychosis. The other diagnoses were schizoaffective disorder, affective disorder, schizophrenia, and organic psychoses. In a later correspondence Marneros (2006b) stated that the frequency of acute and transient psychoses in this sample was much higher than expected compared to the general population prevalence and suggested that this might be a reason for the frequent observation that puerperal psychoses are mainly acute, short episodes with 'colourful' psychopathology and good prognosis.

Bipolar affective disorder

It has been well established that in women with previously diagnosed bipolar disorder, the risk of a relapse is increased during the puerperium (Sharma and Mazmanian 2003). Pre-existing bipolar disorder is one of the greatest risk factors for puerperal psychosis. Recent studies have estimated that over 60% of women with bipolar affective disorder will experience relapse in the first six postnatal months if not taking mood-stabilizing agents (Viguera *et al.* 2000). In addition, a study examining first-episode bipolar affective disorder reported a sevenfold risk occurring in the 2nd to 28th day after delivery (Terp and Mortensen 1998). These findings suggest that biological factors and most likely the hormonal changes following childbirth are largely responsible for the onset of episodes of affective disorder following childbirth.

Bipolar affective disorder is a recurrent condition, with more than 90% of individuals who have experienced one episode of mania experiencing many episodes, with cases equally common in men and women (Dell and O'Brian 2003). Bipolar disorder has an early age at onset in both men and women, with approximately 60% experiencing initial onset in adolescence or early adulthood with an average age at onset of 21 years. Women have an increased risk of rapid cycling and mixed episodes (Amsterdam *et al.* 2002).

Treatment of pregnant women with bipolar disorder poses difficult clinical dilemmas as most commonly used antimanic medications, i.e. lithium and antiepileptic medications, carry fetal teratogenic risks (Viguera *et al.* 2000).

Post-traumatic stress disorder

The incidence of post-traumatic stress disorder (PTSD) may vary from 3% in the general population to 7.7% in economically deprived groups within the first year after delivery (Ayers and Pickering 2001; Loveland *et al.* 2004; Soderquist *et al.* 2006). In a longitudinal follow-up study in a general population (Ayers and Pickering 2001), the incidence of PTSD at six weeks postpartum was 2.8%, while chronic PTSD at six months postpartum was 1.5%.

History of psychological problems, trait anxiety, obstetric procedures, feelings of loss of control, and lack of partner support are known risk factors of post-traumatic stress symptoms related to childbirth (Olde *et al.* 2006). Postpartum PTSD occurs more commonly after instrumental vaginal delivery or emergency Caesarean section than after normal vaginal delivery, while the risk is lower after elective Caesarean section (Ryding *et al.* 1998a, 1998b).

Spontaneous miscarriage and perinatal death can also result in PTSD (Engelhard *et al.* 2001) and up to 29% of women develop PTSD after a stillbirth (Turton *et al.* 2001). Women, who become pregnant within one year after having a stillbirth, have a higher risk of developing PTSD (Turton *et al.* 2001).

Comorbid diagnoses are common amongst those with the diagnosis of PTSD; women with PTSD have a fivefold and threefold increase in risk, respectively, of having a major depressive episode and generalized anxiety disorder (Loveland *et al.* 2004). PTSD is also associated with suicidal risk, and about one-third of women report thoughts of self-harm (Smith *et al.* 2006).

Anxiety and panic disorders

The postpartum period is a time of vulnerability for the development of anxiety disorder, as women are often overwhelmed by changing roles, multiple demands on their time, financial burdens, and lack of sleep. In contrast to the prevalence of anxiety disorders at 5% in the general population, a cohort study revealed that anxiety occurred in 30% of women during the second trimester of pregnancy and in 16% in the postpartum period. A history of psychiatric disorder and being single were common risk factors for new-onset postpartum anxiety disorders, while the absence of previous psychiatric illness is a favourable factor for postpartum recovery from antepartum anxiety (Andersson *et al.* 2006).

Two categories of anxiety in the perinatal period have been described; subsyndromal situational anxiety and clinically significant comorbid anxiety, which was experienced by almost 50% of women with depression during pregnancy and postpartum (Ross *et al.* 2003). In a community survey of 68 postpartum women, 4.4% met DSM-IV criteria for generalized anxiety disorder, 28% had subsyndromal difficulties with generalized anxiety, and about one-third had symptoms of depression (Wenzel *et al.* 2003).

Depression and anxiety commonly coexist and depending on the domain of anxiety, 10–50% of women reporting anxiety symptoms were found to have comorbid depressive symptoms (Wenzel *et al.* 2005). Hart and McMahon (2006) showed that anxiety symptoms have negative effects on pregnancy outcome, such as less optimal maternal–fetal quality of attachment and more negative attitudes towards motherhood.

Panic disorder is one of the most prevalent psychiatric disorders according to the Epidemiological Catchment's Area Population Survey (Regier *et al.* 1990). Lifetime prevalence for panic disorder is estimated at 2.25% and women are 2.5–3 times more likely than men to meet criteria for panic disorder. Panic disorder is not only common but is also considered to be a chronic and debilitating illness associated with significant comorbidity (Ballenger *et al.* 1998; Yonkers 1998).

It has been estimated that 3–12% of women experience symptoms related to panic disorder at some time during pregnancy and the postpartum period (Wenzel *et al.* 2001; Smith MV *et al.* 2004). According to available data, 11–29% of women with panic disorder report the onset during pregnancy (Nonacs and Cohen 2003).

It appears that pregnancy has a variable effect on the risk of relapse in panic disorder. Some researchers suggest that panic disorder may tend to go into remission during pregnancy and it is hypothesized that this may be caused by hormonal changes in pregnancy (Villenponteaux *et al.* 1992; Sutter-Dallay *et al.* 2004).

Villenponteaux *et al.* (1992) carried out a retrospective survey study and reported that most women experienced a decrease in panic symptoms during pregnancy, although it was noted that there was variability between and within individuals. Cohen *et al.* (1994a) collected preliminary data based on a retrospective study of 49 women with pregravid panic disorder and reported that the course of panic disorder during pregnancy was variable with a subset of sever cases showing clear relapse. Northcott and Stein (1994) reported that most pregnant women (63%) in their cohort of patients with panic disorder described an exacerbation of symptoms in the postpartum period. Sholomskas *et al.* (1993) also demonstrated higher rated of panic disorder onset in the postpartum period.

Although there is conflicting data regarding the relationship between pregnancy and relapse in panic disorder, there appears to be a consensus in the literature that the postpartum period represents a time of a high risk of relapse for patients with panic disorder (Cohen *et al.* 1994b, 1996).

Eating disorder

Anorexia nervosa has a prevalence of up to seven per 1000 in the United Kingdom population and is common in adolescent girls and young women. Bulimia nervosa has a prevalence of 0.5–1% and tends to affect a slightly older age group. Women with atypical eating disorder have abnormal eating behaviour, but do not meet the criteria for anorexia nervosa or bulimia nervosa. There are no data of the prevalence of this disorder, but it is thought that it is more common than bulimia nervosa (NICE 2004).

Pregnancy with the accompanying weight gain and change in body shape can adversely affect women with eating disorders or conversely eating disorders may improve during pregnancies because of the women's' worries about its adverse effects on the unborn baby (Rocco et al. 2005).

This question was addressed in a recent prospective cohort study of 12 254 women with a history of eating disorder, an active disorder, obesity, or no eating disorder, which reported that women with an eating disorder generally improved throughout pregnancy. However, these women reported continuing concern and anxiety about their weight, dieted more often, used more laxatives, exercised more, and practised more self-induced vomiting than the other groups of pregnant women (Micali et al. 2007). Several studies have found that women with eating disorders are at increased risk of relapse of the disorder postnatally, especially those with a history of anorexia nervosa or a high frequency of binge eating at conception (Morgan JF et al. 1999; Blais et al. 2000).

There is evidence that women with eating disorders are at increased risk of postnatal depression. A retrospective case–control study of 94 women with eating disorders found that a third of them developed postnatal depressed (Morgan et al. 2006). This issue was addressed by another large retrospective questionnaire study of women with one or more pregnancies. Mazzeo et al. (2006) found that those women with eating disorders were more likely to report depression during pregnancy and postpartum than at other times. Women with an eating disorder are more likely to have an underlying affective disorder (up to 40%), and this together with the added stresses of pregnancy (body image change, weight gain, loss of control) is thought to make these women more vulnerable to postnatal depression (Ward 2008).

Women with eating disorders have an increased risk of physical complications of their pregnancies. It has been shown that women with a history of eating disorder have a significantly increased risk of hyperemesis during pregnancy, preterm delivery, and small-for-gestational-age infants (Sollid et al. 2004; Kouba et al. 2005). A controlled study comparing 122 women with active bulimia during pregnancy with 82 control subjects with inactive disease found that the risks for postnatal depression, miscarriage, and preterm delivery were significantly increased twofold to threefold (2.8, 2.6, and 3.3 significantly higher respectively) (Morgan et al. 2006).

Infanticide

Infanticide by the mother is rare and has been associated with severe mental illness. Reports in the psychiatric literature on infanticide are based on fairly small numbers.

Marleau et al. (1995) sketched the sociodemographic and psychological profiles of 17 mothers who had either killed a child (n=14) or had attempted to do so (n=3). There were no neonaticides in their group and of the 18 victims, six were infanticides, and 12 were filicides. Affective disorders were noted in almost all the mothers (major depressive disorder in six, dysthymia in 16, schizoaffective disorder in two). Only two mothers did not have an axis 1 disorder, according to DSM-IV. Personality configurations according to DSM-IV criteria for axis II were largely borderline (n=5) or dependent (n=4).

McKee and Shea (1998) reviewed 20 women, who had been charged with murdering their children and who were referred to a forensic psychiatric hospital. They reported a prevalence of psychosis as 40% and of major depression as 25%. In a small study of six filicides, Stanton et al. (2000) noted that all mothers exhibited severe mood disorders. The children's ages ranged from a few weeks to seven years.

Although infanticide is an extreme form of infant and child abuse, all episodes of mental illness during and after childbirth have adverse effects on fetus and child developments.

Conclusions

Perinatal psychiatric disorders comprise a range of psychotic and neurotic conditions, some arise for the first time during this period and others are relapses of previous disorders. All of these disorders have adverse effects on the women's quality of life and ability to function during pregnancy and after having given birth. With timely support and treatment by qualified multidisciplinary mental health teams, and support from an informal system, relapses and exacerbations of psychiatric conditions can be prevented or ameliorated. This will not only minimize the psychological suffering of new mothers, but will also reduce the risk of the development of attachment difficulties between mother and infant and reduce the risk of any adverse effects on the development of the infant.

References

Amsterdam JD *et al.* (2002). Bipolar disorder in women. *Psychiatry Annals*, **32**, 397–404.

Andersson L *et al.* (2006). Depression and anxiety during pregnancy and six months postpartum: a follow-up study. *Acta Obstetrica et Gynecologica Scandinavica*, **85**, 937–44.

Ayers S and Pickering AD (2001). Do women get posttraumatic stress disorder as a result of childbirth? A prospective study of incidence. *Birth*, **28**, 111–18.

Ballenger JC *et al.* (1998). Consensus statement on panic disorder from the international consensus group on depression and anxiety. *Journal of Clinical Psychiatry*, **59**(suppl 8), 47–54.

Bennett HA *et al.* (2004). Prevalence of depression during pregnancy: Systematic review. *Obstetrics and Gynecology*, **103**, 698–709.

Blackmore ER *et al.* (2006). Obstetric variables associated with bipolar affective puerperal psychosis. *British Journal of Psychiatry*, **188**, 32–6.

Blais MA *et al.* (2000). Pregnancy: Outcome and impact on symptomatology in a cohort of eating-disordered women. *International Journal of Eating Disorders*, **27**, 140–9.

Brockington IF *et al.* (1981). Puerperal psychosis. *Phenomena and Diagnosis*, **38**, 829–33.

Brockington IF (1996). *Motherhood and Mental Illness*. Oxford University Press, New York.

Brockington I (2004). Postpartum psychiatric disorders. *Lancet*, **363**, 303–10.

Chung TK *et al.* (2001). Antepartum depressive symptomatology is associated with adverse obstetric and neonatal outcomes. *Psychosomatic Medicine*, **63**, 830–4.

Cohen LS *et al.* (1994a). Impact of pregnancy on panic disorder: A case series. *Journal of Clinical Psychiatry*, **55**, 284–288.

Cohen LS *et al.* (1994b). Postpartum course in women with pre-existing panic disorder. *Journal of Clinical Psychiatry*, **55**, 289–92.

Cohen LS *et al.* (1996). Course of panic disorder during pregnancy and the puerperium: A preliminary study. *Biological Psychiatry*, **39**, 950–4.

Dean C and Kendell RE (1981). The symptomatology of puerperal illnesses. *British Journal of Psychiatry*, **139**, 128–33.

Dell DL and O'Brien BW (2003). Suicide in pregnancy. *Obstetrics and Gynecology*, **102**, 1306–9.

Engelhard IM *et al.* (2001). Posttraumatic stress disorder after pregnancy loss. *General Hospital Psychiatry*, **23**, 62–6.

Gavin NI *et al.* (2005). Perinatal depression. A systematic review of prevalence and incidence. *Obstetrics and Gynecology*, **106**, 1071–83.

Gold LH (2002). Postpartum disorders in primary care: diagnosis and treatment. *Primary Care*, **29**, 27–41.

Hart R and McMahon CA (2006). Mood state and psychological adjustment to pregnancy. *Archives of Women's Mental Health*, **9**, 329–37.

Jones I and Craddock N (2005). Bipolar disorder and childbirth: the importance of recognising risk. *British Journal of Psychiatry*, **186**, 143–6.

Kendell RE *et al.* (1987). Epidemiology of puerperal psychoses. *British Journal of Psychiatry*, **150**, 662–73.

Klompenhouwer JL and van Hulst AM (1991). Classification of postpartum psychosis: a study of 250 mother and baby admissions in the Netherlands. *Acta Psychiatrica Scandinavica*, **84**, 255–61.

Kohl C (2004). Postpartum psychosis: closer to schizophrenia or the affective spectrum? *Current Opinion in Psychiatry*, **17**, 87–90.

Kouba S *et al.* (2005). Pregnancy and neonatal outcomes in women with eating disorders. *Obstetrics and Gynecology*, **105**, 255–60.

Lewin J (2006). Acute and transient psychotic disorders and puerperal psychosis. *British Journal of Psychiatry*, **189**, 468.

Lewis G (2004). *Why Mothers Die 200–2002*. RCOG Press, London.

Loveland *et al.* (2004). Posttraumatic stress disorder in pregnancy: Prevalence, risk factors, and treatment. *Obstetrics and Gynecology*, **103**, 710–17.

Marleau JD *et al.* (1995). Infanticide committed by the mother. *Canadian Journal of Psychiatry – Revue Canadienne de Psychiatrie*, **40**, 142–9.

Marneros A (2006a). Beyond the Kraepelinian dichotomy: acute and transient psychotic disorders and the necessity for clinical differentiation. *British Journal of Psychiatry*, **189**, 1–2.

Marneros (2006b). Acute and transient psychotic disorders and puerperal psychosis. Author's reply. *British Journal of Psychiatry*, **189**, 468.

Marmorstein NR *et al.* (2004). Psychiatric disorders among offspring of depressed mothers: associations with paternal psychopathology. *American Journal of Psychiatry*, **161**, 1588–94.

McKee GR and Shea SJ (1998). Maternal filicide: A cross-national comparison. *Journal of Clinical Psychology*, **54**, 679–87.

Mazzeo SE *et al.* (2006). Associations among postpartum depression, eating disorders, and perfectionism in a population-based sample of adult women. *International Journal of Eating Disorders*, **39**, 202–11.

Meltzer ES and Kumar P (1985). Puerperal mental illness, clinical features and classification: a study of 142 mother-and-baby admission. *British Journal of Psychiatry*, **147**, 647–54.

Micali N *et al.* (2007). Eating disorders symptoms in pregnancy: A longitudinal study of women with recent and past eating disorders and obesity. *Journal of Psychosomatic Research*, **63**, 297–303.

Miller LJ, Ruckstalis M (1999). Hypotheses about postpartum reactivity. In: LJ Miller (ed) *Postpartum Mood Disorder*, pp. 262–5. American Psychiatric Press, Washington, DC.

Morgan JF *et al.* (1999). Impact of pregnancy on bulimia nervosa. *British Journal of Psychiatry*, **174**, 135–40.

Morgan JF *et al.* (2006). Risk of postnatal depression, miscarriage, and preterm birth in bulimia nervosa: Retrospective controlled study. *Psychosomatic Medicine*, **68**, 487–92.

Northcott C and Stein M (1994). Panic disorder in pregnancy. *Journal of Clinical Psychiatry*, **55**, 539–42.

Munk-Olsen T *et al.* (2006). New parents and mental disorders: A population-based register study. *Journal of the American Medical Association*, **296**, 2582–9.

Murray L and Stein A (1989). The effects of postnatal depression on the infant. *Bailliere's Clinical Obstetrics and Gynaecology*, **3**, 921–33.

Nager A *et al.* (2005). Are sociodemographic factors and year of delivery associated with hospital admission for postpartum psychosis? A study of 500 000 first-time mothers. *Acta Psychiatrica Scandinavica*, **112**, 47–53.

NICE (National Institute for Health and Clinical Excellence) (2004). *Eating disorders. Core interventions in the treatment and management of anorexia nervosa.* NICE, London.

Newport DJ *et al.* (2002). The treatment of postpartum depression: minimizing infant exposures. *Journal of Clinical Psychiatry*, **63**, 31–44.

Nonacs R and Cohen LS (2003). Assessment and treatment of depression and anxiety during pregnancy: an update. *Psychiatric Clinics of North America*, **26**, 1–8.

Olde E *et al.* (2006). Posttraumatic stress following childbirth: A review. *Clinical Psychology Review*, **26**, 1–16.

Paykel ES (1999). Classification of postpartum disorders in ICD 10 and DSMIV: recommendations prepared by Satra Broock Workshop on Classification of Postnatal Mood Disorders. *Newsletter 9*, The Marce Society.

Paykell ES (2002). Mood disorders: review of current diagnostic systems. *Psychopathology*, **35**, 94–9.

Pfuhlmann B *et al.* (2000). Differential diagnosis, course and outcome of postpartum psychoses: a catamnestic investigation (in German). *Nervenarzt*, **71**, 386–92.

Pitt B (1973). "Maternity blues". *British Journal of Psychiatry*, **122**, 431–3.

Regier DA *et al.* (1990). The epidemiology of anxiety disorders: The Epidemiologic Catchment Area (ECA) experience. *Journal of Psychiatric Research*, **24**, 3–14.

Riecher-Rössler A and Hofecker FM (2003). Postpartum depression: Do we still need this diagnostic term? *Acta Psychiatrica Scandinavica*, **108**, 51–6.

Rocco PL *et al.* (2005). Effects of pregnancy on eating attitudes and disorders: A prospective study. *Journal of Psychosomatic Research*, **59**, 175–9.

Rohde A, Marneros A (2000). Bipolar disorders during pregnancy. In: A Marneros and J Angst (eds) *Bipolar Disorders 100 Years After Manic Depressive Insanity*. Kluwer Academic Publishers, Dordrecht.

Ross LE *et al.* (2003). Measurement issues in postpartum depression part 1: Anxiety as a feature of postpartum depression. *Archives of Women's Mental Health*, **6**, 51–7.

Ryding EL *et al.* (1998a). Predisposing psychological factors for posttraumatic stress reactions after emergency caesarean section. *Acta Obstetrica et Gynecologica Scandinavica*, **77**, 351–2.

Ryding EL *et al.* (1998b). Psychological impact of emergency Cesarean section in comparison with elective Cesarean section, instrumental and normal vaginal delivery. *Journal of Psychosomatic Obstetrics and Gynecology*, **19**, 135–44.

Sharma V and Mazmanian D (2003). Sleep loss and postpartum psychosis. *Bipolar Disorders*, **5**, 98–105.

Sholomskas D *et al.* (1993). Postpartum onset of panic disorder: A coincidental event? *Journal of Clinical Psychiatry*, **54**, 476–80.

Smith MV *et al.* (2004). Screening for and detection of depression, panic disorder, and PTSD in public-sector obstetric clinics. *Psychiatric Services*, **55**, 407–14.

Smith MV *et al.* (2006). Symptoms of posttraumatic stress disorder in a community sample of low-income pregnant women. *American Journal of Psychiatry*, **163**, 881–4.

Soderquist J *et al.* (2006). The longitudinal course of posttraumatic stress after childbirth. *Journal of Psychosomatic Obstetrics and Gynecology*, **27**, 113–19.

Sollid CP *et al.* (2004). Eating disorder that was diagnosed before pregnancy and pregnancy outcome. *American Journal of Obstetric and Gynecology*, **190**, 206–10.

Stanton J *et al.* (2000). A qualitative study of filicide by mentally ill mothers. *Child Abuse and Neglect*, **24**, 1451–60.

Stein A *et al.* (1991). The relationship between post-natal depression and mother-child interaction. *British Journal of Psychiatry*, **158**, 46–52.

Sutter-Dallay AL *et al.* (2004). Women with anxiety disorders during pregnancy are at increased risk of intense postnatal depressive symptoms: A prospective survey of the MATQUID cohort. *European Psychiatry*, **19**, 459–63.

Terp I and Mortensen P (1998). Post-partum psychoses: clinical diagnoses and relative risk of admission after parturition. *British Journal of Psychiatry*, **172**, 521–6.

Turton P *et al.* (2001). Incidence, correlates and predictors of posttraumatic stress disorder in the pregnancy after stillbirth. *British Journal of Psychiatry*, **178**, 556–60.

Viguera AC *et al.* (2000). Risk of recurrence of bipolar disorder in pregnant and nonpregnant women after discontinuing lithium maintenance. *American Journal of Psychiatry*, **157**, 179–84.

Villeponteaux VA *et al.* (1992). The effects of pregnancy on pre-existing panic disorder. *Journal of Clinical Psychiatry*, **53**, 201–3.

Ward VB (2008). Eating disorders in pregnancy. *British Medical Journal*, **336**, 93–6.

Wenzel A *et al.* (2001). The occurrence of panic and obsessive symptoms in women with postpartum dysphoria: A prospective study. *Archives of Women's Mental Health*, **4**, 5–12.

Wenzel A *et al.* (2003). Prevalence of generalized anxiety at eight weeks postpartum. *Archives of Women's Mental Health*, **6**, 43–9.

Wenzel A *et al.* (2005). Anxiety symptoms and disorders at eight weeks postpartum. *Journal of Anxiety Disorders*, **19**, 295–311.

Wisner KL *et al.* (1994). Symptomatology of affective and psychotic illnesses relating to childbirth. *Journal of Affective Disorders*, **30**, 77–87.

Yonkers KA *et al.* (1998). Is the course of panic disorder the same in women and in men? *American Journal of Psychiatry*, **155**, 596–602.

Yun Y *et al.* (2005). Obstetric complications and transition to psychosis in an 'ultra' high risk sample. *Australian and New Zealand Journal of Psychiatry*, **39**, 460–6.

CHAPTER 18

Postnatal depression

Nora Turjanski

Introduction

Pregnancy has been described as a developmental phase when a woman acquires a representation of self as a mother, a sense of ability to perform mothering behaviours whilst she develops an emotional tie to the child (Hart and McMahon 2006). A disruption of this process by a disturbance of emotional well-being or of mental health affects the mother, infant, and family. Since the 1950s, obstetric care in the Western world has become gradually aware of this and more attentive to the welfare of women during pregnancy and delivery (Kemker and Gamboa 2006). Identifying and managing perinatal depression started gathering pace in the 1990s (Lumley 2005).

The puerperium, following childbirth is a period of adjustment. Difficulties might arise from the birth experience, exhaustion, and pain. The first few weeks of the baby's life are associated with severe sleep deprivation, a high level of emotional demand, and anxieties about breastfeeding and the baby's health. During the puerperium a woman needs to contend with body and hormonal changes, recovery of figure, loss of libido, and a possible change in the family and the couple relationships (Brockington 1998).

Changes in mood around the time of child birth are described across many cultures and settings (Oates *et al.* 2004) and overall, pregnancy is no longer considered a protective factor.

Untreated psychiatric illness might have harmful effects on the unborn baby. This probably results from women's decreased self-care and decreased compliance with obstetric antenatal care. Associations between maternal psychopathology and certain obstetric outcomes, such as infant autonomic functioning, preterm birth, birth weight, and lower APGAR scores have been reported (Zuckerman *et al.* 1989; Perkin *et al.* 1993,

Chung *et al.* 2001; Dierckx *et al.* 2009). Depression and stress during pregnancy might delay intrauterine growth (Kelly *et al.* 2002). However, research results have been inconsistent. Evans and colleagues (2007) showed no association between depression and low birth weight, once confounding factors were excluded.

Perinatal mood disorders might induce negative cognitions about motherhood, result in disengaged parenting, and affect the quality of the attachment to the fetus and the mother–child relationship (Lyons-Ruth *et al.* 1986; Murray 1992; Anderson *et al.* 1994; Hart and McMahon 2006; Moehler *et al.* 2006). The psychological development of the child requires an appropriate parent–child interaction. The quality of care given during the first years of life influences children's mental health outcomes and their cognitive development (Oates 1995; Murray *et al.* 1996; Sinclair *et al.* 1998; Hay *et al.* 2001; Heron *et al.* 2004; Josefsson and Sydsjo 2007).

Not just because of its consequences, but in relationship to its cause, many researchers consider that perinatal psychopathology should be differentiated from similar symptoms when developed separately from childbirth. It remains unclear whether depression at this stage of life is influenced by specific biological factors related to childbirth or results from general psychosocial circumstances. It is thought that mild to moderate anxiety and depression might be influenced by psychosocial conditions, while the most severe disorders might relate to biological factors (Oates 2005).

Biological and neurotransmitter hypotheses to explain perinatal depression have involved several hormones, neurotransmitters, and their precursors, as it is the case with other forms of depression. Specific research on perinatal depression has focused on oestrogen, progesterone, cortisol, and thyroid hormones changes, as well as serotonin and its precursor tryptophan (Baïlara *et al.* 2006; Kemker and Gamboa 2006). Possibly, hormonal changes associated with childbirth induce depression if women have an intrinsic vulnerability (Bloch *et al.* 2000). Exposure to high gonadal steroids, followed by abrupt withdrawal precipitated depressive symptoms in women with a history of postnatal depression but not in controls (Bloch *et al.* 2000). Other biological hypotheses include a dysregulation of the hypothalamic–pituitary–adrenal axis already present during pregnancy. It is known that stress can accelerate labour. Stress affects pregnancy through stimulation of cortisol and placental corticotrophin-releasing hormone (CRH) (Kemker and Gamboa 2006). A recent study showed a direct association between blood levels of CRH in the second trimester and development of postnatal depression (Yim *et al.* 2009). Other studies have looked at the role of serotonin. Associations between depressive symptoms and polymorphic variations in the expression of the serotonin transporter gene, a possible regulator of serotonergic function, have been reported (Sanjuan *et al.* 2008). At present, it remains unclear what is the relative value of these factors in the aetiology of perinatal depression.

Prediction and detection of mood disorders

In England, the maternity care plan includes a booking appointment at 12 weeks followed by approximately ten antenatal visits and two to four weeks of midwife care postnatally, before transfer to the health visitor.

This plan provides ample opportunities for prediction and detection of psychiatric disorders. Despite this, depression in the perinatal period is under recognized and untreated. Several studies showed that only between 20–25% of women with psychopathology were identified in obstetric clinics (Kelly RH *et al.* 2001, Smith *et al.* 2004). The presence of domestic violence increased detection rates of depression (Smith *et al.* 2004). During the puerperium, tiredness, exhaustion, and emotional struggles may mask the presentation of depression. Additional barriers to detection include lack of training in mental health, anxiety about how to deal with these patients, as well as likely resource implications (Buist 2003). Health professionals might minimize symptoms of depression or, on the contrary, misuse the term postnatal depression to label a different psychiatric disorder. Distress or transient emotional difficulties may be misinterpreted as depression and hastily referred to psychiatrists. Hence, there is a need to improve the detection of perinatal depression in primary care settings and obstetric clinics.

Prediction is the identification of current or past risk factors which increase the probability of developing a specific disorder. Detection is the identification of a disorder.

Prediction

There is no reliable predictive instrument to use in routine clinical practice. Prediction of perinatal mood disorders is based on the presence of certain risks for both the ante- and postnatal period.

The development of depression during pregnancy is associated with a previous history of depression or postnatal depression. Patients who discontinue appropriate maintenance antidepressants may relapse in both the antenatal and postnatal period. However, it is not unusual to observe a general low threshold for antidepressant prescription. Other risk factors include family history of mood disorders, marital dysfunction, and younger age of the mother (Kemker and Gamboa 2006). Psychosocial circumstances especially socioeconomic deprivation may increase the risk of antenatal depression (Abel 2007).

Risk factors for postnatal mood disorders have been better studied. The strongest risk factor is the presence of depressed mood or anxiety during pregnancy (Kim *et al.* 2008; Milgrom *et al.* 2008).

It is important to consider the presence of a personal or family history of depression and its characteristics. Postnatal depression may have some biological specificity, especially when it develops immediately following childbirth. A previous history of depression is associated with a 30% chance of postpartum relapse, but this risk increases to 50% if the previous episode was postpartum (Kemker and Gamboa 2006). Additionally, it has been shown that women who present with a new onset of depression postpartum have a higher risk of further relapses following childbirth. A history of depression unrelated to pregnancy is associated mainly with further relapses unconnected to childbirth (Cooper and Murray 1995). When onset of depression is restricted only to the first month postpartum, 42% of women with a positive family history of postnatal depression experienced depression following their first delivery (Forty *et al.* 2006). On the other hand, longitudinal follow-up of women with an unrestricted onset of postnatal depression showed a globally higher risk for a recurrent depressive disorder (Josefsson and Sydsjo 2007). The chance of relapse might relate to the severity and duration of the previous episode and the presence of additional risk factors during the new pregnancy. (Elliott *et al.* 2000; NICE 2007).

Other risks include level of social support, life events, low socioeconomic status, and unwanted pregnancy (O'Hara and Swain 1996; Beck 2001; Robertson *et al.* 2004; NICE 2007). Emotional and practical social support appear to be protective while social isolation is detrimental (Robertson *et al.* 2004). Additionally, vulnerable personality and difficulties with partner might be significant. There is no link with a Caesarean section (Carter *et al.* 2006; Milgrom *et al.* 2008).

The difficulty is that these risks factors are non specific and widely distributed in the general population (Oates 1995). A longitudinal study initiated mid-pregnancy followed two cohorts of women with high and low risk of developing depression based on some of the criteria discussed (Verkerk *et al.* 2003). Approximately 25% of those considered to be at high risk developed depression in the ante- or the postnatal period while only 6% of the low-risk group were affected at any point of the study (Verkerk *et al.* 2003). This latter figure is not dissimilar to the global 12-month prevalence for major depressive disorder in the general population without differentiation by gender (Kessler *et al.* 2003). Around 50% of the patients who developed depression were already affected by week 32 of pregnancy and 80% of them within the first three months postpartum (Verkerk *et al.* 2003).

Detection

A reliable method of identifying depression by non-mental health professionals would be highly useful. Several scales have been assessed, few which are specific to postnatal depression (NICE 2007). The Edinburgh Postnatal Depression Scale (EPDS) has been developed to detect mothers suffering from postnatal depression in primary healthcare settings (Cox *et al.* 1987). It was designed as a screening instrument but has become a detection tool. Mainly used in the postnatal period, one study has validated its use antenatally (Murray and Cox 1990).The EPDS is a self-questionnaire that rates how the woman has been feeling for the past week. It contains ten short statements rating levels of enjoyment, blame, sadness, anxiety, and thoughts of self-harm. Most women complete the scale in less than five minutes. It is strongly influenced by anxiety. The validation study showed that mothers who scored above a cut-off point of 12.5 were likely to be suffering from a depressive illness. Although the EPDS uses cut-off points, mood disorders are considered to be along a continuum without categorical distinctions (Murray and Carothers

1990; NICE 2007). The EPDS is best suited to identify severe depression but not to measure its severity and the score should not override clinical judgement. The sensitivity of this instrument varies according to the settings, being higher when used in research. The assessment of minor depression is associated with decreased sensitivity and specificity. Another problem is that it is easy to distort the answers when women are concerned about the consequences of having a psychiatric diagnosis (NICE 2007). The EPDS is widely used and has been translated into many languages. Interestingly, an internet administered EPDS with a 12 cut-off score, showed good internal consistency when compared with a pen and paper version (Spek *et al.* 2008).

Alternatively, case finding may be achieved with specific sets of questions. Whooley (1997) suggested that two focused questions from the Patient Health Questionnaire could be used to detect depression in primary and secondary settings. These questions are: 'During the last month, have you often been bothered by feeling down, depressed, or hopeless?' and 'During the last month have you often been bothered by having little interest or pleasure in doing things?'. These two questions have high sensitivity but low specificity. Specificity improved by adding a third question developed by Arroll and colleagues: 'Is this something with which you would like help? (Arroll *et al.* 2005; NICE 2007). More recently a postpartum study using three questions from the EPDS (based on detection of worries, blame, and anxiety) showed a 95% sensitivity to screen for depression in primary care (Kabir *et al.* 2008).

In conclusion, at present there is insufficient evidence to recommend any screening tools. Existing guidelines suggest that these questions may be used at a woman's first contact with primary care, at her booking visit, and postnatally (NICE 2007).

Mood disorders during pregnancy

Perinatal disorders do not constitute a special group in ICD-10 and usual clinical guidelines are applied to their diagnosis.

In the past, pregnancy was considered to be a protective factor for mental health disorders. Recently, research has focused on psychiatric disturbances during this period but results have been conflicting. Population studies suggest that, overall, the rate of mood disorders is lower in pregnant than in non-pregnant women. As previously stated, this is not the case for women with existing risk factors (Van Bussel *et al.* 2006; Vesga-Lopez *et al.* 2008). Some studies suggested that depression is increased at specific periods of the pregnancy, either during the first, second, or the third trimester (Bennet *et al.* 2004; Heron *et al.* 2004; Gavin 2005). The Avon longitudinal study of parents and children showed a higher rate of depression in the last trimester of pregnancy (13.5% at 32 weeks) than in the postpartum phase (9% at eight weeks postnatal) (Evans *et al.* 2001). More women became depressed during pregnancy than in the transition from the pregnancy to the puerperium (Evans *et al.* 2001).

The exact prevalence of anxiety during pregnancy is unclear (Ross and McLean 2006; Abel 2007), though it is commonly seen in clinical practice, especially during the first and last trimester. Women may have difficulties adjusting to the pregnancy, in particular if this has been unplanned. As delivery approaches, some women's fears about childbirth and how to cope with a new born baby increase. Physical discomfort during both the first and third trimester may be a contributory factor (Kemker and Gamboa 2006; Abel 2007). Of notice are ruminative thoughts in patients with either well-established or previously unrecognized obsessive–compulsive disorder, which appears to worsen during pregnancy. This is a particularly important diagnosis as ruminations might contain intrusive ideas of harming the baby, which are distressing and rarely enacted (Abel 2007). Appropriate recognition of these symptoms allows educating the patient, as well as implementing treatment if indicated, hence reducing distress. If not properly identified and treated, mothers may avoid contact with the infant and the condition result in inappropriate intervention by social services.

Mood disorders in the postnatal period

Puerperal depression is a form of major depressive disorder which is universally recognized. However, the duration of the puerperium is ill defined. This disorder onset is within the first four weeks postpartum according to the DSM-IV or six weeks according to the ICD-10. Clinically, onset extends to up to one year following childbirth.

Studies reported a variable prevalence. A meta-analysis showed a prevalence of 13% (O'Hara and Swain 1996) with most cases starting in the first three months postpartum (Cooper and Murray 1998; Kemker and Gamboa 2006).

There are three main presentations of postpartum depressive symptoms: baby blues, depression, and psychosis.

Epidemiological data indicates that 50% of women experience baby blues, 13–15% have postnatal depression (12 months postpartum), and 0.5/1000–2/1000 have puerperal psychosis. Referral to a psychiatrist in the first year postpartum is much higher than at any other point in women's life (Oates 1995).

Baby blues present as a transient emotional lability of mood, but without the persistence and severity of depression. Women experience tearfulness, irritability, sleeplessness, decreased concentration, and transient elated mood. Care of the baby is not impaired and there are no depressive cognitions (Musters *et al.* 2008). These symptoms last for approximately one week and might be related to rapid changes in progesterone levels (Pitt 1973; Kendell *et al.* 1981; Harris and Lovett 1994). Women need monitoring to ensure this is not the onset of postpartum depression.

Postpartum depression often presents with low mood and marked anxiety and ruminations about the well-being of the baby. Several of the usual diagnostic features of depression such as decreased energy, and altered sleep and libido are common after childbirth, therefore is important to establish whether depressive cognitions, hopelessness, tiredness, and reduced self-esteem are present (Musters *et al.* 2008). Women may present with a general sense of being an inadequate mother. There may be intrusive thoughts about abandoning or harming the baby or self, which have to be specifically explored. As described, the highest incidence is during the first month postpartum but it remains increased for three months.

Postnatal depression can progress to psychosis, the most severe form of mood disorder. Postpartum psychosis is a manifestation of either unipolar or, more frequently, bipolar disorder with either a new onset or a relapse in the postpartum period (See Chapter 19). Traditionally described as presenting a latent, symptom-free period of a few days, recent research suggest that in women with pre-existing bipolar affective disorder, symptoms develop rapidly during the first week of puerperium. Subtle alterations in mood may be already present during the last phase of pregnancy (Heron *et al.* 2008). Disorders with a manic component develop earlier than those with depression (Heron *et al.* 2008). Postpartum psychosis tends to present with marked affective components, and disorganization of thought and behaviour (Kemker and Gamboa 2006).

A psychotic mother might place her children at high risk. This may be due to the delusional disorder or result from accidental injury and neglect caused by uncontrolled behaviour.

Particular at-risk groups

Pregnant immigrant women

In immigrant women, the reported rates of depression approach 40% during the pregnancy and puerperium (Zelkowitz *et al.* 2008). These women might present with a combination of risk factors including previous psychological trauma, a new alien culture, marital difficulties, language barrier, and difficult socioeconomic circumstances. Additional markers of increased vulnerability to develop puerperal depression are: multitude of somatic complaints, high perinatal anxiety, and premigration stress (Zelkowitz *et al.* 2004, 2008). Often, traumatic experiences have been closely guarded and post-traumatic stress disorder remains untreated. Social isolation and lack of support from the extended family tends to compound the problem and predispose to depressive symptoms.

Teenage pregnancy

The United Kingdom (UK) has the highest rate of teenage pregnancy in the European Union. There are complex socioeconomic reasons for this situation. Pregnancy might be associated with an unstable background, sexual abuse, and impulsive behaviour, and with alcohol or drug abuse (Bayatpour *et al.* 1992). Depending on the age, these women tend to have a higher risk of physical complications during pregnancy. The adverse psychosocial circumstances are associated with increased levels of depression (Barnet *et al.* 1995; Abel 2007).

Assisted conception

These women might present with higher levels of anxiety during pregnancy and have early parenting difficulties, while postnatal self-confidence might be lower (Hammaberg *et al.* 2008).

Previous stillbirth

A previous stillbirth is a significant risk factor for depression, post-traumatic stress disorder, and anxiety during a subsequent pregnancy and puerperium (Hughes *et al.* 1999; Turton *et al.* 2001).

These symptoms also affect fathers during their partner's pregnancy though to a lesser degree (Turton 2006).

Bereavement

Perinatal loss because of stillbirth, miscarriage, or severe disability in the infant has been associated with development of affective and post-traumatic stress disorders in both the women and her partner. It is relevant to consider the presence of previous mental health disorders and strength of coping mechanisms. Couples require appropriate professional intervention, counselling, and education.

Other groups which might have an increased psychosocial risk of developing perinatal depression are inner-city black Caribbean women (Edge 2007), pregnant women with the human immunodeficiency virus infection, pregnant women exposed to domestic violence, and those using alcohol and illicit drugs.

Management of perinatal affective disorders

Pharmacological treatment during pregnancy and the puerperium is discussed in Chapter 19 of this book.

Prevention

There is no current evidence that psychological and psychosocial interventions can prevent postnatal depression, even in high-risk groups (Dennis and Creedy 2004). Additional professional support, such as intensive home visits by health professionals, provided postnatally to a selected group of high-risk women may have protective effects (Dennis and Creedy 2004, 2005).

There is no evidence that treatment with gonadal steroids can prevent development of postnatal depression (Dennis *et al.* 2008). Prophylactic use of antidepressants in a targeted group of women with a confirmed history of postpartum depression may be useful, though the evidence base for this approach is scarce (Wisner *et al.* 1994, Musters *et al.* 2008).

Management of antenatal depression

Due to lack of research, there is no evidence to endorse psychological or psychosocial treatment of antenatal depression (Dennis *et al.* 2007), though clinical practice suggests it is beneficial. Trials assessing usefulness of treatments such as massage therapy and acupuncture have been too small (Dennis and Allen 2008).

Management of postnatal depression

In terms of psychological input, mild to moderate depression can be addressed by self-help strategies, supportive counselling, and brief structured psychotherapy such as cognitive behavioural or interpersonal therapy. The overlap between symptoms of depression and the general level of exhaustion in the first week postpartum are a confounder when interventions are assessed. Despite this, there is some evidence that psychological and psychosocial interventions are effective in the treatment of postnatal depression (Dennis and Hodnett 2007). A recent study showed some beneficial effects when health visitors were trained to detect depression and treat patients with a cognitive behavioural or a person-centred approach, compared with standard care. Further research should clarify whether the improvement observed in the treated group related to the psychological intervention or to an increased level of empathy from the trained group of professionals (Morrell *et al.* 2009). Both control and intervention group improved their scores by six months, presumably as women's tiredness and general coping mechanisms increased. Furthermore, another study which provided over-the-telephone peer support showed that empathic understanding can improve EPDS scores at 12 weeks (Dennis *et al.* 2009). However, this study used a low cut-off score of 9 which might have diluted the diagnosis of depression.

Severe depression might incorporate pharmacological treatment alongside psychological treatment (NICE 2007). Access to psychological input might be difficult or delayed but it is imperative to treat these women promptly with appropriate medication if required (Munster *et al.* 2008).

Interpersonal therapy might be particularly useful to address depression in inner-city pregnant adolescents, where social circumstances, establishment of boundaries, validation of pregnancy, and addressing choices about keeping the baby have a particular importance (Shanok and Miller 2007; Miller *et al.* 2008).

Other non-pharmacological treatments include light therapy which has shown some promise in a pilot study (Corral *et al.* 2007).

There is little evidence that gonadal steroids can be used in the treatment of postnatal depression, there is some evidence for synthetic progestin, but no evidence for naturally occurring progesterone. Oestrogens appear to have only modest value to treat this condition (Dennis *et al.* 2008).

The large majority of mild to moderate mental health disorders, and specifically depression, present in primary care and maternity services. Usually general practitioners (GPs) treat mood disorders as in any other time of the patient's life. Perinatal mental health services have a role in supporting primary care, especially when issues of pharmacological treatment surface.

In patients with severe disorders, perinatal psychiatrists or general adult psychiatrists with an interest in perinatal mental health should take the lead as complexities and risks to both mother and baby increase. High-risk patients should be referred even when well. Ideally, patients with previously established severe mental health pathology should be encouraged to plan their pregnancies. Thus, appropriate interventions and monitoring can be established jointly with the psychiatric team.

Treatment of moderate or severe depression and of possible relapse of severe psychopathology should remain multidisciplinary with fluid communication amongst all parties. These may include the women's partner, other relatives or friends, the community mental health team, GP, obstetric team (midwifes, neonatologist, health visitors, etc.) and social services if required. It is essential to have a birth plan agreed in advance. This plan should give consideration to the pregnancy, delivery, puerperium, and breastfeeding phases. It should contain a comprehensive risk assessment to women, baby, and other children if indicated. It should detail availability of professional support for routine consultations and in an eventual crisis. The birth plan should explore available support from partner and others, consideration of possible stress load from house chores, other children, and quality of the social environment. It should address sleep deprivation and possible strategies to ameliorate this. The plan has to encompass management strategies such as counselling and medication and it should be endorsed by all parties. Preservation of contact between mother and baby is paramount if at all possible. The birth plan may need to consider admission to hospital.

Service provision

Primary, secondary, and specialist perinatal care should be available according to the severity of the disorder and with prompt access to psychological input. This may result from in-house obstetric counsellors, psychological input attached to primary care, the community mental health team, or be a component of inpatient treatment. Specific interventions may include care from the children and family psychiatric services and work regarding attachment and bonding.

Patients may require inpatient care. Increasingly women tend to be admitted to mother and baby units. These units care for women with moderate to severe mental illnesses and their infants up to 12 months old. The main purpose of the admission is treatment of the acute illness whilst avoiding disruption of the developing mother–child relationship. Another component of the admission is the assessment of the patient's mothering abilities. Admission to a mother and baby unit is generally associated with high levels of satisfaction (Neil *et al.* 2006). Units with clear links to community services are seen as more successful than those standing in isolation (Kohen 2001). (See Chapter 21.)

Alternatively, women could be admitted to a crisis house or to a psychiatric unit if pregnant or when admission with the baby is not the preferred option. Single-gender wards are favoured (Kohen 1999), though in practice this may not be always available. Consideration of women's particular physical needs, care for their dignity in the immediate postpartum, preservation of the relationship with the baby, and liaison with the obstetric team are essential.

The Confidential Enquiries into Maternal Deaths have been important drivers that influenced perinatal mental health care in the UK. The enquiry conducted between 1997 and 1999 identified suicide as one of the leading causes of maternal death in UK (Lewis and Drife 2001). Similar findings resulted from the 2000–2002 enquiry (Oates 2005). The majority of suicides died violently. Half of the women had a previous psychiatric history. Possible diagnosis at time of death included psychosis, depression, anxiety, and drug and alcohol dependency. Four suicides were combined with infanticides. The most common profile denoted a period of high risk between late pregnancy and three months following delivery. It identified those most at risk as a white, older woman in her second or subsequent pregnancy, married, and living in comfortable circumstances. There was a high likelihood of a previous history of mental illness and ongoing contact with psychiatric services (Oates 2005). Importantly, 32% of deaths were due to physical illness mistakenly attributed to psychiatric disorders. Nevertheless, maternal suicide is rare, particularly in pregnancy, and overall suicide rates are lower than in the general female population (Appleby 1991; Oates 2005). Similar findings have been replicated in Australia (Austin *et al.* 2007).

The latest enquiry, conducted between 2003 and 2005 saw maternal deaths due to suicide relegated to be the second leading course of indirect maternal death. It remains to be seen whether this is an artefact or results from a sustained and progressive change in clinical practice (Lewis 2007).

These confidential enquiries have informed recommendations for practice and national guidelines which have been implemented across the country. The National Institute for Health and Clinical Science (NICE) released a series of guidelines linking care in the perinatal period and mental health. The last one was published in January 2007 (NICE 2007).

Service provision for perinatal care in the UK is unevenly distributed (NICE 2007). Furthermore, a review of maternity services by the Healthcare Commission in 2008 highlighted some failings which may influence women's emotional well-being and mental health. These are: poor communication and support to women postnatally; a suboptimal continuity of care during the perinatal period; and inequalities in access to perinatal mental health services. NICE recommend instigating a stepped care approach focusing on mother, baby, and nuclear family needs. Access to appropriate services and continuity of care are essential. The implementation of patient care pathways which should include all tiers of care and link inpatient and outpatient facilities may help to improve treatment (NICE 2007).

References

Abel KM (2007). Perinatal and gynaecological disorders. In: GG Lloyd and E Guthrie (eds) *Handbook of Liaison Psychiatry*, pp. 632–72. Cambridge University Press, Cambridge.

American Psychiatric Association (1994). *Diagnostic and Statistical Manual of Mental Disorders (DSM-IV)*, American Psychiatric Association, Washington, DC.

Anderson VN *et al.* (1994). Mood and transition to motherhood. *Journal of Reproductive and Infant Psychology*, **12**, 69–77.

Appleby L (1991). Suicide during pregnancy and in the first post-natal year. *British Medical Journal*, **302**, 137–40.

Arroll B *et al.* (2005). Effect of the addition of a 'help' question to two screening questions on specificity for diagnosis of depression in general practice: diagnostic validity study. *British Medical Journal*, **331**, 884.

Austin MP *et al.* (2007). Maternal mortality and psychiatric morbidity in the perinatal period: challenges and opportunities for prevention in the Australian setting. *Medical Journal of Australia*, **186**(7), 364–7.

Baïlara KM *et al.* (2006). Decreased brain tryptophan availability as a partial determinant of post-partum blues. *Psychoneuroendocrinology*, **31**, 407–13.

Barnet B *et al.* (1995). Association between postpartum substance use and depressive symptoms, stress, and social support in adolescent mothers. *Pediatrics*, **96**, 659–66.

Bayatpour M *et al.* (1992). Physical and sexual abuse as predictors of substance use and suicide among pregnant teenagers. *Journal of Adolescent Health*, **13**(2), 128–32.

Beck CT (2001). Predictors of postpartum depression: an update. *Nursing Research*, **50**(5), 275–85.

Bennett HA *et al.* (2004). Prevalence of depression during pregnancy: systematic review. *Obstetrics and Gynecology*, **103**(4), 698–709.

Bloch M *et al.* (2000). Effects of gonadal steroids in women with a history of postpartum depression. *American Journal of Psychiatry*, **157**, 924–30.

Brockington I (1998). Puerperal disorders. *Advances in Psychiatric Treatment*, **4**, 312–19.

Buist A (2003). Promoting positive parenthood: emotional health in pregnancy. *Australian Journal of Midwifery*, **16**(1), 10–14.

Carter FA *et al.* (2006). Cesarean section and postpartum depression: a review of the evidence examining the link. *Psychosomatic Medicine*, 68, 321–30.

Chung TKH *et al.* (2001). Antepartum depressive symptomatology is associated with adverse obstetric and neonatal outcomes. *Psychosomatic Medicine*, **63**, 830–4.

Commission for Healthcare Audit and Inspection (2008). *Towards better births: A review of maternity services in England.* www.healthcarecommission.org.uk.

Cooper PJ and Murray L (1995). Course and recurrence of postnatal depression. Evidence for the specificity of the diagnostic concept. *British Journal of Psychiatry*, **166**, 191–5.

Cooper PJ and Murray L (1998). Fortnightly review: Postnatal depression. *British Medical Journal*, **316**, 1884–6.

Corral M *et al.* (2007). Morning light therapy for postpartum depression. *Archives of Women's Mental Health*, **10**(5), 221–4.

Cox JL *et al.* (1987). Development of the 10-item Edinburgh Postnatal Depression Scale (EPDS). *British Journal of Psychiatry*, **150**, 782–876.

Dennis CL (2005). Psychosocial and psychological interventions for prevention of postnatal depression: systematic review. *British Medical Journal*, **331**, 15.

Dennis CL and Allen K (2008). Interventions (other than pharmacological, psychosocial or psychological) for treating antenatal depression. *Cochrane Database Systematic Review*, 4, CD006795.

Dennis CL and Creedy D (2004). Psychosocial and psychological interventions for preventing postpartum depression. *Cochrane Database Systematic Review*, 4, CD001134.

Dennis CL and Hodnett E (2007). Psychosocial and psychological interventions for treating postpartum depression. *Cochrane Database Systematic Review*, 4, CD006116.

Dennis CL *et al.* (2007). Psychosocial and psychological interventions for treating antenatal depression. *Cochrane Database Systematic Review*, 18(3), CD006309.

Dennis CL *et al.* (2008). Oestrogens and progestins for preventing and treating postpartum depression. *Cochrane Database Systematic Review*, **8**(4), CD001690.

Dennis CL *et al.* (2009). Effect of peer support on prevention of postnatal depression among high risk women: multisite randomised controlled trial. *British Medical Journal*, **338**(a3064), 280–4.

Dierckx B *et al.* (2009). Maternal psychopathology influences infant heart rate variability: Generation R Study. *Psychosomatic Medicine*, **71**(3), 313–21.

Edge D (2007). Ethnicity, psychosocial risk, and perinatal depression–a comparative study among inner-city women in the United Kingdom. *Journal of Psychosomatic Research*, **63**(3), 291–5.

Elliott SA *et al.* (2000). Promoting mental health after childbirth: a controlled trial of primary prevention of postnatal depression. *British Journal of Clinical Psychology*, **39**, 223–41.

Evans J *et al.* (2001). Cohort study of depressed mood during pregnancy and after childbirth. *British Medical Journal*, **323** (7307), 257–60.

Evans J *et al.* (2007). Depressive symptoms during pregnancy and low birth weight at term: longitudinal study. *British Journal of Psychiatry*, **191**, 84–5.

Forty L *et al.* (2006). Familiality of postpartum depression in unipolar disorder: results of a family study. *American Journal of Psychiatry*, **163**(9), 1549– 53.

Gavin NI *et al.* (2005). Perinatal depression: a systematic review of prevalence and incidence. *Obstetrics and Gynecology*, **106**(5, 1), 1071–83.

Hammarberg K *et al.* (2008). Psychological and social aspects of pregnancy, childbirth and early parenting after assisted conception: a systematic review. *Human Reproduction Update*, **14**(5), 395– 414.

Harris B *et al.* (1994). Maternity blues and major endocrine changes: Cardiff puerperal mood and hormone study II. *British Medical Journal*, **308**, 949–53.

Hart R and McMahon CA (2006). Mood state and psychological adjustment to pregnancy. *Archives of Women's Mental Health*, **9**(6), 329–37.

Hay DF *et al.* (2001). Intellectual problems shown by 11-year-old children whose mothers had postnatal depression. *Journal of Child Psychology and Psychiatry*, **42**(7), 871–89.

Heron J *et al.* (2004). The course of anxiety and depression through pregnancy and the postpartum in a community sample. *Journal of Affective Disorders*, **80**(1), 65–73.

Heron J *et al.* (2008). Early postpartum symptoms in puerperal psychosis. *BJOG; An International Journal of Obstetrics and Gynaecology*, **115**(3), 348–53.

Hughes P *et al.* (1999). Stillbirth as a risk factor for anxiety and depression in the next pregnancy: does time since loss make a difference? *British Medical Journal*, **318**, 1721–4.

Josefsson A and Sydsjo G (2007). A follow-up study of postpartum depressed women: recurrent maternal depressive symptoms and child behaviour after four years. *Archives of Women's Mental Health*, **10**, 141–5.

Kabir K *et al.* (2008). Identifying postpartum depression: are 3 questions as good as 10? *Pediatrics*, **122**(3), e696–e702.

Kelly RH *et al.* (2002). Psychiatric and substance use disorders as risk factors for low birth weight and preterm delivery. *Obstetrics and Gynaecology*, **100**(2), 297–304.

Kelly RM *et al.* (2001). The detection and treatment of psychiatric disorders and substance use among pregnant women cared for in obstetrics. *American Journal of Psychiatry*, **158**, 213–19.

Kemker S and Gamboa M (2006). Pregnancy. In: M Blumenfield and JJ Strain (eds) *Psychosomatic medicine*, pp. 603–30. Lippincott, Williams and Wilkins, Philadelphia, PA.

Kendell RE *et al.* (1981). Mood changes in the first 3 weeks after childbirth. *Journal of Affective Disorders*, **3**, 317–26.

Kessler RC *et al.* (2003). National Comorbidity Survey Replication. The epidemiology of major depressive disorder: results from the National Comorbidity Survey Replication (NCS-R). *Journal of the American Medical Association*, **289**(23), 3095–105.

Kim YK *et al.* (2008). Prediction of postpartum depression by sociodemographic, obstetric and psychological factors: a prospective study. *Psychiatry and Clinical Neurosciences*, **62**(3), 331–40.

Kohen D (1999). Specialised in-patient psychiatric service for women. *Psychiatric Bulletin*, **23**, 31–3.

Kohen D (2001). Psychiatric services for women. *Advances in Psychiatric Treatment*, **7**, 328–34.

Lewis G (ed) (2007). *The Confidential Enquiry into Maternal and Child Health (CEMACH). Saving Mothers' Lives: reviewing maternal deaths to make motherhood safer – 2003–2005. The Seventh Report on Confidential Enquiries into Maternal Deaths in the United Kingdom.* CEMACH, London.

Lewis G and Drife J (2001). *Why Mothers Die 1997–1999. The Fifth Report of the Confidential Enquiries into Maternal Deaths in the United Kingdom.* RCOG Press, London.

Lumley J (2005). Attempts to prevent postnatal depression. *British Medical Journal*, **331**, 5.

Lyons-Ruth K *et al.* (1986). The depressed mothers and her one year old infant: environment, interaction, attachment and infant development. In: EZ Tronick and T Field (eds) *Maternal Depression and Infant Disturbance. New Directions for Child Development*, pp. 61–82. Jossey-Bass, San Fransisco, CA.

Milgrom J *et al.* (2008). Antenatal risk factors for postnatal depression: a large prospective study. *Journal of Affective Disorders*, **108**(1–2), 147–57.

Miller L *et al.* (2008). Interpersonal psychotherapy with pregnant adolescents: two pilot studies. *Journal of Child Psychology and Psychiatry*, **49**(7), 733–42.

Moehler E *et al.* (2006). Maternal depressive symptoms in the postnatal period are associated with long-term impairment of mother-child bonding. *Archives of Women's Mental Health*, **9**, 273–8.

Morrell CJ *et al.* (2009). Clinical effectiveness of health visitor training in psychologically informed approaches for depression in postnatal women: pragmatic cluster randomised trial in primary care. *British Medical Journal*, **338**, 276–80.

Murray D and Cox JL (1990). Screening for depression during pregnancy with the Edinburgh Depression Scale (EPDS). *Journal of Reproductive and Infant Psychology*, **8**, 99–107.

Murray L (1992). The impact of postnatal depression on infant development. *The Journal of Child Psychology and Psychiatry*, **33**, 543–61.

Murray L and Carothers AD (1990). The validation of the Edinburgh Post-natal Depression Scale on a community sample. *The British Journal of Psychiatry*, **157**, 288–90.

Murray L *et al.* (1996). The cognitive development of 5 year old children of postnatally depressed mothers. *Journal of Child Psychology and Psychiatry*, **37**, 927–35.

Musters C *et al.* (2008). Management of postnatal depression. *British Medical Journal*, **337**, a736, 399–403.

NICE (National Institute for Health and Clinical Excellence) (2007). *Antenatal and Postnatal Mental Health.* The British Psychological Society and The Royal College of Psychiatrists.

Neil S *et al.* (2006). A satisfaction survey of women admitted to a Psychiatric Mother and Baby Unit in the northwest of England. *Archives of Women's Mental Health*, **9**, 109–12.

Oates M (1995). Risk and childbirth in psychiatry. *Advances in Psychiatric Treatment*, **1**, 146–53.

Oates M (2005). Deaths from suicide and other psychiatric causes. In: Lewis G and Drife J (eds) *Confidential Enquiry: Why mothers die? 2000–2002. The Sixth Report on Confidential Enquiries into Maternal Deaths in the United Kingdom.* CEMACH, London.

Oates RM *et al.* (2004). Postnatal depression across countries and cultures: a qualitative study. *British Journal of Psychiatry*, **184**, s10–s16.

O'Hara MW and Swain AM *et al.* (1996). Rates and risk of postpartum depression – a meta-analysis. *International Review of Psychiatry*, **8**, 37–54.

Perkin MR *et al.* (1993). The effect of anxiety and depression during pregnancy on obstetric complications. *British Journal of Obstetrics and Gynaecology*, **100**, 629–34.

Pitt B (1973). Maternity blues. *British Journal of Psychiatry*, **122**, 431–3.

Robertson E *et al.* (2004). Antenatal risk factors for postpartum depression: a synthesis of recent literature. *General Hospital Psychiatry*, **26**(4), 289–95.

Ross LE and McLean LM (2006). Anxiety disorders during pregnancy and the postpartum period: A systematic review. *Journal of Clinical Psychiatry*, **67**(8), 1285–98.

Sanjuan J *et al.* (*2008*). Mood changes after delivery: role of the serotonin transporter gene. *British Journal of Psychiatry*, **193**(5), 383–8.

Sinclair D and Murray L (1998). Effects of postnatal depression on children's adjustment to school, teachers report. *British Journal of Psychiatry*, **172**, 58–63.

Shanok AF and Miller L (2007). Depression and treatment with inner city pregnant and parenting teens. *Archives of Women's Mental Health*, **10**, 199–210.

Smith MV *et al.* (2004). Screening for and detection of depression, panic disorder, and PTSD in public-sector obstetric clinics. *Psychiatric Services*, **55**(4), 407–14.

Spek VRM *et al.* (2008). Internet administration of the Edinburgh Depression Scale. *Journal of Affective Disorders*, **106**(3), 301–5.

Turton P *et al.* (2006). Psychological impact of stillbirth on fathers in the subsequent pregnancy and puerperium. *British Journal of Psychiatry*, **188**(2), 165–72.

Turton P *et al.* (2001). Incidence, correlates and predictors of post-traumatic stress disorder in the pregnancy after stillbirth. *British Journal of Psychiatry*, **178**, 556–60.

Van Bussel JC *et al.* (2006). Women's mental health before, during, and after pregnancy: a population-based controlled cohort study. *Birth*, **33**(4), 297–302.

Verkerk GJM *et al.* (2003). Prediction of depression in the postpartum period: a longitudinal follow-up study in high-risk and low-risk women. *Journal of Affective Disorders*, **77**, 158–66.

Vesga-López O *et al.* (2008). Psychiatric disorders in pregnant and postpartum women in the United States. *Archives of General Psychiatry*, **65**(7), 805–15.

Wisner KL and Wheeler SB (1994). Prevention of recurrent post-partum major depression. *Hospital and Community Psychiatry*, **45**(12), 1191–6.

Whooley MA *et al.* (1997). Case-finding instruments for depression. Two questions are as good as many. *Journal of General Internal Medicine*, **12**, 439–45.

World Health Organization (1992). *International Statistical Classification of Diseases, 10th Revision (ICD-10)*, WHO, Geneva.

Yim S *et al.* (2009). Risk of postpartum depressive symptoms with elevated corticotropin-releasing hormone in human pregnancy. *Archives of General Psychiatry*, **66**(2), 162–9.

Zelkowitz P *et al.* (2004). Factors associated with depression in pregnant immigrant women. *Transcultural Psychiatry*, **41**(4), 445–64.

Zelkowitz P *et al.* (2008). Stability and change in depressive symptoms from pregnancy to two months postpartum in childbearing immigrant women. *Archives of Women's Mental Health*, **11**(1), 1–11.

Zuckerman B *et al.* (1989). Depressive symptoms during pregnancy: Relationship to poor health behaviors. *American Journal of Obstetrics and Gynecology*, **160**, 1107–11.

CHAPTER 19

Puerperal psychosis

Ian Jones, Jessica Heron, and
Emma Robertson Blackmore

Introduction

> A young woman in child-bed not well purged after birth
> and delivery, fell into a great delirium suddenly without
> any disease afore going. She was angry most with her best
> friends, husband and mother, but she spoke many things
> religiously . . . .
>
> Felix Plater, 1602 (in Brockington 1996)

The link between childbirth and mental illness has
been recognized for hundreds, if not thousands, of
years. The concept of puerperal or postpartum psychosis (PP) has a long history, but has fallen into disrepute
in the age of modern classifications that do not recognize this disorder as a nosological entity. Even in the
21st century, however, the triggering of severe episodes
of illness by childbirth remains a significant public
health problem, tragically illustrated by a number of
cases in which women suffering from puerperal
psychosis have killed themselves or harmed their baby
(Jones and Craddock 2005). Suicide is a leading cause
of maternal death in the UK and it is clear that a high
proportion of maternal suicides occur in women with
an acute onset of psychosis in the early postpartum
period (CEMACH 2007).

Although as a concept, PP is controversial, the occurrence of severe episodes of psychiatric illness with onset
in the immediate postpartum is clearly of great clinical
importance. The stakes are high and the early recognition and prompt treatment of women who become ill
is vital.

In this chapter we will pose, and attempt to answer,
a number of questions in relation to PP. We will first
consider what constitutes an episode of this disorder
and its typical clinical presentation. We will then move
on to discuss its epidemiology, nosology, aetiology, and,
finally, focus our attention on management, and in particular how to identify and manage women at risk.

Clinical features

A wide range of psychiatric conditions occur in relationship to childbirth but mood disorders have perhaps
received the most attention. PP is often seen as the
extreme of a postpartum mood disorder spectrum with
the baby blues and postnatal depression completing
the trio.

The 'blues', 'highs', and postnatal depression

More than 50% of women experience transient mood
symptoms following childbirth, often labelled the baby
or maternity 'blues'. In addition to depressed mood,
high mood symptoms are also common at this time.
A significant number of women, perhaps 10–20%,
experience a brief subclinical hypomanic-like episode
in the first postpartum week sometimes termed the
'highs' (Heron et al. 2005). These conditions typically
last only a few days, do not require intervention, and
should not be labelled as a disorder.

Episodes of clinical depression occur commonly both
in pregnancy and following delivery and may cause significant disruption to the woman and her family.
Studies in a variety of settings and employing differing
definitions of postnatal depression have been conducted
and show that 10–15% of mothers experience clinically
significant depressive symptoms at some time during
the first six months following childbirth, although a
lower figure receive treatment (O'Hara and Swain 1996;
Musters et al. 2008).

Puerperal psychosis

While there may not be a problem with recognizing the
'core' of this phenomenon and in its use in everyday
practice, there are difficulties in defining its boundaries,
with a range of definitions employed both clinically and
in research.

The term puerperal or postpartum psychosis usually refers to a severe mental illness with a dramatic onset shortly after childbirth—the majority in the first few postpartum days (Heron *et al.* 2007). A wide range of diagnoses can present with psychotic features in the puerperium, and include acute confusional states due to a variety of causes (e.g. post-eclamptic or infective), alcohol withdrawal, chronic psychosis (e.g. schizophrenia), psychotic depression, mania, schizophreniform, and schizoaffective episodes. The term puerperal psychosis is reserved for episodes with an acute onset in the puerperium although previous episodes of illness may have occurred. Continuing symptoms of a chronic psychosis such as schizophrenia and 'organic' disorders such as acute confusional states and alcohol withdrawal are typically excluded. This leaves a group of acute onset affective psychoses including manic, depressive, and schizoaffective forms.

The time of onset following delivery must also be considered and it is important to recognize that an episode may not come to medical attention for a considerable time following the first occurrence of symptoms. Time frames have varied widely in research studies, from a very tight definition with onset within two weeks of delivery, to studies that have included all women found to be psychotic within the first postpartum year. It is usual, however, to limit the concept of PP to those episodes with an acute episode shortly following delivery, within weeks rather than months, and in a recent study the vast majority of episodes of PP (well over 90%) had their onset within the first two postpartum weeks (Heron *et al.* 2007).

Typical symptoms of puerperal psychosis

The symptoms of PP include a wide variety of psychotic phenomena such as delusions and hallucinations, the content of which is often related to the new child. Affective (mood) symptoms, both elation and depression, are prominent as is a disturbance of consciousness marked by an apparent confusion, bewilderment, or perplexity. The clinical picture often changes rapidly with wide fluctuations in the intensity of symptoms and severe swings of mood.

As we discussed earlier, studies of symptoms are complicated by marked variations in inclusion criteria and definitions of the puerperal period, but consistently demonstrate that the majority of puerperal psychotic episodes are affective, with mania particularly common in the two weeks following childbirth (Brockington 1996). For example, Brockington and colleagues (1981) examined the symptoms experienced in 58 puerperal episodes compared to 52 episodes of non-puerperal psychotic illness occurring in women of childbearing age. They found that systematization of delusions, persecutory ideas, auditory hallucinations, odd affect, and social withdrawal were less common in the puerperal patients whereas manic symptoms—elation, rambling speech, flight of ideas, lability of mood, distractibility, euphoria, and excessive activity—were all more frequent and severe.

Epidemiology

The question of how often PP occurs in the general population is not easy to answer due to the various definitions of the condition that have been applied. The studies of Kendall and colleagues in the 1970s and 1980s identified new onset psychotic episodes in one in 250 deliveries in Camberwell and found an admission rate of one in 500 deliveries in Edinburgh (Kendell *et al.* 1976; Kendell *et al.* 1987). The latter figure is perhaps the origin of the often quoted incidence rate but in fact reflected a wide range of diagnoses in the women admitted. Limiting to clearly psychotic diagnoses gives a rate of approximately one in 1000 deliveries but it is also likely that some episodes of mania that would appropriately be labelled as PP may not have resulted in admission—particularly if facilities for conjoint admission with the baby were not available. There is consistency in the literature with regard to admission rates, however, with the large Danish register studies of more than a million deliveries also finding rates of approximately one in 1000 (Terp and Mortensen 1998; Munk-Olsen *et al.* 2006).

Relationship to bipolar disorder

Although a wide variety of clinical features are seen in episodes of PP, there is strong evidence for a close relationship with bipolar disorder. As we have seen, symptoms of mania are common in puerperal psychotic episodes and further evidence for the link comes from studies examining the natural history of puerperal psychotic episodes—the condition has an excellent prognosis but women remain at high risk of developing further puerperal and non-puerperal affective episodes (Robling *et al.* 2000; Robertson *et al.* 2005). Women diagnosed with bipolar disorder are at particular risk in the puerperium with episodes following 25–50% of deliveries (Jones and Craddock 2001) but perhaps the strongest evidence of a specific relationship with bipolar disorder comes from registry studies in the general population.

A range of studies have demonstrated that the puerperium is a time of increased risk for severe manic or psychotic mood disorder. In the studies of Kendall in Camberwell and Edinburgh, women were at a 22-fold increased risk of suffering an episode of affective psychosis in the four weeks following delivery and the risk was even higher (relative risk (RR)= 35) when only first deliveries were considered (Kendell *et al.* 1976, 1987). The study of Terp and Mortensen, however, linking Danish birth and psychiatric admission registers for over one million births found seemingly different results (Terp and Mortensen 1998). It reported only a small increase in the risk of admission with an episode of functional psychosis in the three months following delivery (RR= 1.09, 95% confidence interval (CI) = 1.03– 1.16) although this figure was much higher for first admissions (RR= 3.21, 95% CI= 2.96–3.49). When individual disorders were considered, however, the findings were far closer to those of the earlier studies. The risk of psychosis following childbirth was not distributed evenly across the functional psychoses—the chances of being admitted with an episode of schizophrenia were actually lower than at other times, while women with bipolar disorder were at a particularly high risk. Indeed the highest relative risk (6.82) was obtained for first episode bipolar manic depressive psychosis 2–28 days following delivery and, although not reported in the original paper, an even higher figure (approaching 20) was obtained if only the first two weeks of the puerperium were considered. Moreover, the analysis of diagnostic subgroups in the Danish study ignored a large number of women who had a diagnosis of ICD-8 'puerperal psychosis' as no equivalent non-puerperal diagnosis was available. Given that it is likely that the majority of women receiving the PP diagnosis would have a bipolar spectrum disorder, the relative risk for bipolar disorder is likely to be an underestimate of the increased risk. The true magnitude of risk to bipolar women is underlined by further analysis of the Danish data published recently that reports the relative risk for an admission with bipolar disorder in the month following first pregnancies to be 23—over four times higher than the relative risk for admission with schizophrenia (Munk-Olsen *et al.* 2006).

Classification of severe postpartum episodes

The nosology of severe psychiatric disorders in relation to childbirth is controversial and confused, which has led to problems in both research and clinical practice. Although some have argued that PP is a condition in its own right, there is little evidence to support this conclusion and it is more appropriate to view childbirth as a *trigger* of psychotic episodes.

Questions remain, however, regarding both the specificity of childbirth as a stressor and about the strength of its effect. The issue is whether childbirth is a powerful and specific trigger of certain forms of psychiatric episodes or a non-specific stressor like any other life event, acting to trigger a wide variety of psychotic illness. The non-specific nature of puerperal episodes has become the predominant view over recent decades; at least in part this is reflected in, and moulded by, the way these episodes are treated by the ICD and DSM classification systems.

PP was included in ICD-8, but its use was qualified by the instruction to only use this diagnosis when the use of another category was not possible. The category disappeared in ICD-9 and -10, with only a ragbag 'mental and behavioural disorders associated with the puerperium, not elsewhere classified' available for episodes with onset within six weeks of delivery and only if they do not meet the criteria for disorders classified elsewhere.

In the DSM classification there is a similar story. DSM-II included a category of PP but again carried the instruction to use only if 'all other possible diagnoses have been excluded'. By DSM-IV, although the category had disappeared, a 'postpartum onset specifier' was included in the mood disorders chapter for onsets within four weeks of delivery. In the DSM, therefore, episodes of PP are treated as mood disorders with a postpartum trigger.

Despite the classification systems not recognizing PP as a separate nosological entity, the term postpartum or puerperal psychosis has remained in clinical use and there is an argument that this nosological confusion has hindered research into this important disorder. A particular issue may have been that the clinical presentation of these episodes, with prominent mood and psychotic symptoms, does not sit comfortably with the Kraeplinian dichotomy that has dominated psychiatric thinking for the last century. However, recent evidence necessitates a reappraisal of the dichotomy (Craddock and Owen 2005) and this change in approach may have implications for the status of PP in the years to come.

The status of puerperal psychosis

As we have seen, the status of PP and its clinical boundaries remain subject to debate but given the literature discussed earlier a number of issues are clear. There is no reason to believe that PP is a condition in own right but neither is there a non-specific relationship between childbirth and a whole range of psychiatric disorders.

Rather, the weight of evidence supports a close link to bipolar illness, and it is clear that women with a bipolar diathesis represent a group at a particularly high risk of episodes in the puerperium.

Aetiology

It is appropriate, therefore, in clinical practice and research, to consider most episodes of PP as representing women with a bipolar disorder diathesis acted on by a specific puerperal trigger. Understanding the nature of this trigger will be of great benefit. It will allow for the development of treatments for PP and perhaps even enable the prevention of illness in those women at high risk. It may also enable us to understand more about the aetiology of mood disorders in general. What then, is currently known about the nature of the trigger?

Changes in medication

Perhaps the simplest and intuitively appealing explanation is that the excess of episodes of bipolar illness seen after delivery could be accounted for by the fact that bipolar women often come off medication, such as lithium, prior to conception or in early pregnancy because of concerns over toxicity to the fetus. Viguera and colleagues (2000) examined this hypothesis and employed survival analysis to examine the course of 42 women with previous bipolar episodes who stopped lithium due to pregnancy compared to 59 age-matched non-pregnant lithium discontinuers. Rates of recurrence were very similar for both groups up to 40 weeks but following delivery a large and highly significant difference in recurrence rates was observed (70% vs 24% recurrence). The increased risk of recurrence following childbirth for bipolar women is not, it appears, merely a result of women stopping mood stabilizing medication.

Psychosocial factors

Another possible explanation is that childbirth is acting as a general, non-specific psychosocial stressor like any other life event. While it is clear that becoming a mother is a complex and often difficult psychosocial transition and clearly plays a major role in many episodes of postnatal depression, psychosocial factors have not been shown to play a major role in vulnerability to psychosis in the puerperium. Four studies have examined high-risk women and are consistent in finding no association between stressful life events and the occurrence of a PP episode (McNeil 1988; Brockington *et al.* 1990; Dowlatshahi and Paykel 1990; Marks *et al.* 1991).

Genes

Recent evidence has demonstrated that genetic factors increase vulnerability to the puerperal triggering of bipolar episodes. The evidence from family studies suggests that vulnerability to affective disorders is increased in the relatives of women with puerperal psychosis (Jones *et al.* 2001). Moreover, studies have suggested that episodes of PP are a marker for a more familial form of bipolar disorder (Jones and Craddock 2002) and that a specific vulnerability to the puerperal triggering of bipolar illness is familial (Jones and Craddock 2001). Further support for the involvement of genetic factors comes from the report of familial clustering of puerperal psychotic episodes associated with consanguinity which raises the possibility of a recessive gene contributing to susceptibility (Craddock *et al.* 1994). The relationship between genetic factors influencing puerperal triggering and those for the bipolar diathesis remain unclear. It is possible that one or more susceptibility genes for bipolar illness also lead to a vulnerability to puerperal triggering. Alternatively, the genetic factors influencing puerperal vulnerability may be completely distinct from those that determine the bipolar diathesis and act as course modifiers. It is likely that only when the genetic factors are found will the relationship be resolved.

Molecular genetic studies of PP are ongoing with interesting findings at the serotonin transporter gene (Coyle *et al.* 2000) and linkage evidence pointing to the long arm of chromosome 16 (Jones *et al.* 2007). It is hoped that ongoing genome-wide association studies may reveal the individual genetic factors implicated by the studies mentioned; however, it is clear that sample sizes need to be far bigger than those at present to achieve the power needed to identify genes of small to modest effect (Ferreira *et al.* 2008).

Parity

Another clue to the aetiology of this condition is the well-established effect of parity—episodes being more common following first babies (Robertson Blackmore *et al.* 2005). The reason for the excessive risk in primiparous women is not clear. An important bias is that women with a severe postpartum episode may be less likely to go on to have further children but this is unlikely to be the main explanation (Kendell *et al.*1987; McNeil 1988). Another possible explanation is that first pregnancies and the transition to new motherhood are a greater psychological stress than subsequent deliveries but, as discussed earlier, psychosocial factors do not seem to play an important role. The possibility remains that the effect of primiparity is, at least in part, due to biological differences. Hormonal, immunological, and other biological differences between first and subsequent pregnancies are therefore interesting targets for further investigation into the aetiology of PP (Robertson Blackmore *et al.* 2005).

Obstetric factors

A further area that has received attention is the possibility that certain obstetric factors are associated with episodes of PP, with both obstetric complication and Caesarean section rates found to be higher in some studies. Robertson and colleagues compared affected and unaffected deliveries in over 50 women with PP and found that experiencing a complication during delivery more than doubled the risk of PP (Robertson Blackmore *et al.* 2005). Other factors which have been examined such as sex of the child, gestation of pregnancy have not been consistently supported as risk factors (McNeil and Blennow 1988; Videbech and Gouliaev 1995; Kirpinar *et al.* 1999).

Hormones

The lack of evidence implicating psychosocial factors and consideration of the abrupt onset of illness during a time of major physiological change suggests that biological, possibly hormonal, factors are of fundamental importance. The role of several hormones (e.g. progesterone, prolactin, follicular stimulating hormone [FSH], and luteinizing hormone [LH]) have been considered but oestrogen has perhaps received the greatest attention. A number of studies have examined a range of hormonal measures in women with postpartum affective episodes and controls (Hendrick *et al.* 1998; Bloch *et al.* 2003) but no consistent well-replicated hormonal differences have been demonstrated. It is likely, therefore, that women with puerperal psychotic episodes do not show gross abnormalities in endocrine physiology but rather a vulnerability to puerperal triggering represents an abnormal response to the normal hormonal fluctuations of pregnancy and childbirth.

The evidence pointing to reproductive hormones in the aetiology of puerperal triggering is predominantly circumstantial. One study, however, provides more direct evidence for the involvement of oestrogen and progesterone in the puerperal triggering of affective symptoms. Bloch and colleagues (2000) employed a paradigm in which they simulated the supraphysiologic gonadal steroid levels of pregnancy and withdrawal to a hypogonadal state in eight women with, and eight women without, a history of postpartum depression. They found that five of the eight women with a history of postpartum depression and none of the women in the comparison group developed significant mood symptoms during the withdrawal period.

Sleep

A plausible hypothesis that has received a little attention in the literature is that the sleep deprivation of delivery and the immediate postpartum period is responsible for puerperal triggering of illness (Sharma and Mazmanian 2003; Sharma *et al.* 2004). It is know that rhythm disturbances such as sleep loss can trigger the onset of mania in bipolar patients and, unsurprisingly, sleep loss is common for new mothers.

Management

As we have seen, the concept of PP encompasses a wide range of clinical presentations on the affective disorders spectrum from typical manic episodes through mixed presentations to psychotic depressions. The management of women will, therefore, depend on a number of factors, including the symptoms experienced by the women, her level of disturbance, and her previous response to medication. There are, however, some general points which can be made.

Management of the acute episode of puerperal psychosis

Although ideally women who need inpatient care for a mental disorder within 12 months of childbirth should be admitted to a specialist mother and baby unit (NICE 2007), the provision of services is patchy in the United Kingdom and non-existent in many countries throughout the world. For the majority of women with PP requiring admission there is no option other than a general adult ward without their baby. Developments such as home treatment may provide an alternative, but the severity, inherent risks, and rapidly changing picture seen typically in an episode of PP do not, in our opinion, make it an ideal candidate for treatment at home.

The whole range of psychotropic medication may need to be employed including antipsychotics, mood stabilizers, and benzodiazepines. For clear depressive presentations antidepressants may be required, although the underlying bipolarity of many episodes must be considered and similar caveats as for the treatment of bipolar depression more generally are appropriate. With regard to breastfeeding, the severity of the illness and the chaotic presentation means that breastfeeding often becomes impossible. If breastfeeding is contemplated, factors in the baby such as prematurity and systemic illness should be considered in addition to the particular properties of the medication itself. Electroconvulsive therapy can be effective in the treatment of PP (Reed *et al.* 1999) and there is certainly an argument that the quicker the mother's symptoms can be brought under control the less the disruption of the mother and baby bond.

Management of women at risk

Women with bipolar disorder are known to be at particularly high risk for PP. Other important risk factors include: having experienced a previous episode of PP; having a first-degree relative who has experienced an episode of PP; and having a first-degree relative with bipolar disorder (Jones and Craddock 2005). Women at high risk according to these criteria may be well, not in contact with mental health services, and may fail to recognize the seriousness of the situation. It is clear, therefore, that all antenatal woman should be asked about these risk factors and protocols put in place to ensure that women at potential risk receive a formal risk assessment and management plan (Jones and Craddock 2005; NICE 2007). How screening and risk management is delivered will differ according to local circumstances but is clear that all women with a history of bipolar or severe postpartum episodes must be identified by antenatal services.

The risks of illness following childbirth should be discussed with all women with bipolar disorder of childbearing years, and the need for contraception and the importance of seeking help if contemplating pregnancy (or if unexpectedly becoming pregnant) emphasized. At least 50% of pregnancies are unplanned and therefore consideration should be given to potential pregnancy in making decisions about medication in all women of childbearing potential. This has led to the recommendation that sodium valproate should not be used in this group of women if it can be avoided due to its particular teratogenic and developmental effects (NICE 2007).

Decisions about continuing or stopping medications prior to, or during, pregnancy are difficult and should be the result of a detailed and individualized cost–benefit analysis. Although there are significant concerns about the reproductive safety of many of the medications used to manage individuals with bipolar disorder,

there appears to be particular problems with regard to sodium valproate and all other options need to be considered rather than exposing the fetus to this medication. Stopping medication is not without its own risks, however, and in a recent study women with bipolar disorder who stopped medication in pregnancy were more than twice as likely to experience a recurrence than those who remained on medication (Viguera *et al.* 2007). No universal recommendations can be made and it must be emphasized that the decision ultimately must rest with the woman and her family. Stopping medication should always be a carefully considered decision and never a reflex response and the decision to start medication for women who become symptomatic in pregnancy or when breastfeeding must be the result of weighing up both the potential risks from taking medication, and the risks posed by the illness itself.

For women at risk, perhaps the most important aspect of management is to maintain close contact and keep under review during the perinatal period. It may also be important to address other avoidable factors that may increase risk—decreasing general levels of stress for example and paying attention to sleep in late pregnancy and the early postpartum weeks. Lastly, for women with a history of bipolar disorder who have discontinued medication during or prior to pregnancy the introduction of prophylactic medication in the immediate postpartum period should be considered. Some evidence exists for the use of lithium in this context (e.g. Stewart *et al.* 1991) but the few studies conducted have been open and retrospective and there are practical problems with obtaining therapeutic levels quickly to cover the period of risk. These issues have led some perinatal psychiatrists to use typical or atypical neuroleptics as prophylaxis, and despite some anecdotal reports of success with this strategy, nothing has yet been reported in the literature.

Prognosis and risk of recurrence

The short-term prognosis for PP is generally good. However, women need to be counselled about the risks of a further puerperal or non-puerperal episode and about plans to minimize this risk. Recurrence rates following subsequent pregnancies are 40–57% and in excess of 60% of women go on to have further non-puerperal episodes (Kirpinar *et al.* 1999; Terp *et al.* 1999; Robling *et al.* 2000; Robertson *et al.* 2005). Despite the high risk of recurrence, women and their families can do much to reduce this and to minimize the effects of an episode should it occur. Many women who have experienced PP go on to extend their families and this is clearly a reasonable decision for them to make. It is not appropriate, as perhaps happened too frequently in the past, for women in these circumstances to be told not to have further children.

References

Bloch M *et al.* (2000). Effects of gonadal steroids in women with a history of postpartum depression. *American Journal of Psychiatry*, **157**(6), 924–30.

Bloch M *et al.* (2003). Endocrine factors in the etiology of postpartum depression. *Comprehensive Psychiatry*, **44**(3), 234–46.

Brockington IF *et al.* (1981). Puerperal psychosis: phenomena and diagnosis. *Archives of General Psychiatry*, **38**, 829–33.

Brockington IF *et al.* (1990). Stress and puerperal psychosis. *British Journal of Psychiatry*, **157**, 331–4.

Brockington IF (1996). Puerperal psychosis. In: *Motherhood and Mental Health*, pp. 200–84. Oxford University Press, Oxford.

CEMACH (The Confidential Enquiry into Maternal and Child Health) (2007). [online] Available at http://www.cemach.org.uk. [Accessed August 29 (2008)].

Coyle N *et al.* (2000). Variation at the serotonin transporter gene influences susceptibility to bipolar affective puerperal psychosis. *Lancet*, **356**, 1490–1.

Craddock N *et al.* (1994). Bipolar affective psychosis associated with consanguinity. *British Journal of Psychiatry*, **164**, 359–64.

Craddock N and Owen MJ (2005). The beginning of the end for the Kraepelinian dichotomy. *British Journal of Psychiatry*, **186**, 364–6.

Dowlatshahi D and Paykel ES (1990). Life events and social stress in puerperal psychosis: absence of effect. *Psychological Medicine*, **20**, 655–62.

Ferreira MA *et al.* (2008). Collaborative genome-wide association analysis supports a role for ANK3 and CACNA1C in bipolar disorder. *Nature Genetics*, **40**, 1056–8.

Hendrick V *et al.* (1998). Hormonal changes in the postpartum and implications for postpartum depression. *Psychosomatics*, **39**(2), 93–101.

Heron J *et al.* (2005). Postnatal euphoria – are "the highs" an indication of bipolarity? *Bipolar Disorders*, **7**(2), 103–10.

Heron J *et al.* (2007). No 'latent period' in the onset of bipolar affective puerperal psychosis. *Archives of Womens Mental Health*, **10**(2), 79–81.

Jones I and Craddock N (2002). Do puerperal psychotic episodes identify a more familial subtype of bipolar disorder? Results of a family history study. *Psychiatric Genetics*, **12**, 177–180.

Jones I *et al.* (2001). Molecular genetic approaches to puerperal psychosis. *Progress in Brain Research*, **133**, 321–32.

Jones I *et al.* (2001). Familiality of the puerperal trigger in bipolar disorder: results of a family study. *American Journal of Psychiatry*, **158**, 913–17.

Jones I *et al.* (2005). Bipolar disorder and childbirth: the importance of recognising risk. *British Journal of Psychiatry*, **186**, 453–4.

Jones I *et al.* (2007). Bipolar affective puerperal psychosis – genome-wide significant evidence for linkage to chromosome 16. *American Journal of Psychiatry*, **164**(7), 1099–104.

Kendell RE *et al.* (1976). The influence of childbirth on psychiatric morbidity. *Psychological Medicine*, **6**(2), 297–302.

Kendell RE *et al.* (1987). Epidemiology of puerperal psychoses. *British Journal of Psychiatry*, **150**, 662–73.

Kirpinar I *et al.* (1999). First-case postpartum psychosis in Eastern Turkey: a clinical case and follow-up study. *Acta Psychiatrica Scandinavica*, **100**, 199–204.

Marks MN *et al.* (1991). Life stress and postpartum psychosis: a preliminary report. *British Journal of Psychiatry*, **158**, 45–9.

McNeil TF (1988). A prospective study of postpartum psychoses in a high risk group. 4. Relationship to life situation and experience of pregnancy. *Acta Psychiatrica Scandinavica*, **77**, 645–53.

McNeil TF and Blennow (1988). A prospective study of postpartum psychoses in a high risk group. 6. Relationship to birth complications and neonatal abnormality. *Acta Psychiatrica Scandinavica*, **78**, 478–84.

Munk-Olsen T *et al.* (2006). New parents and mental disorders: a population-based register study. *Journal of the American medical Association*, **296**(21), 2582–9.

Musters C *et al.* (2008). Management of postnatal depression. *British Medical Journal*, **337**, a736.

NICE (National Institute for Clinical Excellence) (2007). Antenatal and postnatal mental health: clinical management and service guidelines. [online]. Available at. www.nice.org.uk/Guidance/CG45 (Accessed 29 August (2008)).

Oates M (2003a). Perinatal psychiatric disorders: a leading cause of maternal morbidity and mortality. *British Medical Bulletin*, **67**, 219–29.

Oates M (2003b). Suicide: the leading cause of maternal death. *British Journal of Psychiatry*, **183**, 279–81.

O'Hara MW and Swain AM (1996). Rates and risk of postpartum depression-a meta-analysis. *International Review of Psychiatry*, **8**(1), 37–54.

Reed P *et al.* (1999). A comparison of clinical response to electroconvulsive therapy in puerperal and non-puerperal psychosis. *Journal of Affective Disorders*, **54**(3), 255–60.

Robertson E *et al.* (2005). Risk of puerperal and non-puerperal recurrence of illness following bipolar affective puerperal (post-partum) psychosis. *British Journal of Psychiatry*, **186**, 258–9.

Robertson Blackmore E *et al.* (2006). Obstetric factors associated with bipolar affective puerperal psychosis. *British Journal of Psychiatry*, **188**, 32–6.

Robling SA *et al.* (2000). Long-term outcome of severe puerperal psychiatric illness: a 23 year follow-up study. *Psychological Medicine*, **30**(6), 1263–71.

Sharma V *et al.* (2003). Sleep loss and postpartum psychosis. *Bipolar Disorders*, **5**(2), 98–105.

Sharma V *et al.* (2004). The relationship between duration of labour, time of delivery, and puerperal psychosis. *Journal of Affective Disorders*, **83**(2–3), 215–20.

Stewart DE *et al.* (1991). Prophylactic lithium in puerperal psychosis. The experience of three centres. *British Journal of Psychiatry*, **58**, 393–7.

Terp IM, Mortensen PB (1998). Post-partum psychoses. Clinical diagnoses and relative risk of admission after parturition. *British Journal of Psychiatry*, **172**, 521–6.

Terp IM *et al.* (1999). A follow-up study of postpartum psychoses: prognosis and risk factors for readmission. *Acta Psychiatrica Scandinavica*, **100**, 40–6.

Videbech P, Gouliaev G (1995). First admission with puerperal psychosis: 7–14 years of follow-up. *Acta Psychiatrica Scandinavica*, **91**, 167–73.

Viguera AC *et al.* (2000). Risk of recurrence of bipolar disorder in pregnant and nonpregnant women after discontinuing lithium maintenance. *American Journal of Psychiatry*, **157**, 179–84.

Viguera AC *et al.* (2007). Risk of recurrence in women with bipolar disorder during pregnancy: prospective study of mood stabilizer discontinuation. *American Journal of Psychiatry*, **164**(12), 1817–24.

CHAPTER 20

Obstetric liaison services

Gillian Wainscott and Giles Berrisford

Introduction

It has been recognized since ancient times that pregnancy is not always associated with psychological well-being and there are many accounts in historical literature of mothers having serious problems with their mental health, both during pregnancy and in the post-partum period. It was only in the last decades of the last century that proper emphasis was given to the fact that mental health is as important as physical health during pregnancy and in the postpartum period with respect to both morbidity and mortality.

Successive Confidential Enquiries into Maternal Deaths (1994–1996, 1997–1999, 2000–2002) identified that psychiatric mortality is the most common cause of maternal death: more common than direct causes of maternal death such as sepsis, haemorrhage, thrombosis, or eclampsia. As a result of each of these enquiries, recommendations have been made that management protocols should be in place in every Trust for pregnant women with a history of mental health problems to ensure that care plans are devised to reduce risk during this vulnerable time.

It is possible that these recommendations are starting to impact upon the care women are receiving. The most recent Confidential Enquiry (2003–2005) revealed a significant decrease in the number of suicides in the first year postpartum, with reduction from 58 suicides during the years 2000–2002, to 37 during the years 2003–2005 (Lewis 2007, p.157). This improvement is most encouraging although it is difficult to measure which changes in perinatal mental healthcare have produced this improvement.

Unfortunately, the remaining deaths from indirect causes of psychiatric illness are characterized by similar hallmarks as those seen in previous Confidential Enquiries. Specifically, failings were seen with poor identification of previous psychiatric history (79 of the 98 women who died as an indirect cause of their mental illness had a past psychiatric history, yet this was identified in just 55 of the cases). Where it was identified, a management plan was devised and implemented in only 24 cases (Lewis 2007, p. 159). This seems to highlight the fact that there is some improvement still to be made with the accurate identification and appropriate management of these women.

Recent National Institute for Health and Clinical Excellence (NICE) guidelines for antenatal and postnatal mental health recognized that perinatal mental health service provisions are 'patchy' and non-standardized (NICE 2007, p. 243). The importance of developing a written care plan during the first trimester for pregnant women with a current or past history of severe mental illness was endorsed and it was recommended that this should be done in collaboration with specialist perinatal mental health services (Guideline's Clinical Practice Recommendations) (NICE 2007, p. 119). The three key areas of identification, planning, and communication were reinforced. In order to achieve the last two aims, the creation of clinical networks is outlined. The objective of these networks is to provide a specialist multidisciplinary perinatal psychiatric service with direct input in the form of consultation and advice to maternity services, the objective of which is to ensure that care plans can be effectively coordinated and that a clear pathway of care for service uses can be implemented.

The exact method for achieving these objectives is not stipulated. What is recognized is that specialist perinatal mental health services will have an important part to play in achieving the objectives, particularly in areas of high morbidity. A crucial component is undoubtedly effective liaison between the general medical and the mental health services. An effective method of developing this is through the antenatal mental health liaison clinic.

The function of an antenatal mental health liaison clinic

The antenatal mental health liaison clinic will ensure that close links are established at the interface between maternal and psychiatric services. This is in part achieved simply by the close proximity of the services, which occurs when the liaison clinic is run alongside the routine antenatal clinic. The existence of the clinic raises awareness of the importance of psychiatric morbidity. Stigma is reduced as mothers pass easily through the various stages of antenatal care with a psychiatric consultation being no less intimidating than having blood taken or a scan performed.

Recognition of vulnerable mothers is dependent in the main on proper training being given to community midwives. Screening questions in various parts of the documentation, including the hand-held notes, are specifically designed to identify those women who are at risk, but the correct interpretation of the answers to these questions is dependent on the nominated midwife having an informed understanding of meaning of the answers. Good communication from general practitioners (GPs) is a mandatory requirement as it is not unknown for women with more serious mental health problems to hide this from obstetric and midwifery staff for fear this might compromise the progress of their pregnancy and maybe encourage referral to the Local Authority due to child protection concerns.

Clear protocols need to be in place as to what should happen once vulnerable mothers have been identified. In the case of doubt as to whether a referral is appropriate, mental health service professionals are on hand to discuss these cases and to give appropriate advice. The closer links between maternal and psychiatric services ensure that better communication is more likely. This enables better management planning, in the form of plans which are devised by all stakeholders, and therefore can be adhered to by all healthcare professionals. It is of note that in half of the deaths resulting from psychiatric disorder, major deficiencies in communication were noted (Lewis 2007, p.162).

In summary, therefore, much work has been done to identify the contributing factors to why women die in the perinatal period. In terms of mental health, key lessons have been learned about raising the awareness of all healthcare professionals involved in the care of pregnant women as to the dangers posed by serious mental illness. This appears to be having an impact upon the numbers of deaths we are seeing as a result of mental illness during this time. More can be done. The current areas of focus revolve around the need for improved communication and the development of effective management plans. One method of achieving this is through the development of antenatal mental health clinics. This helps to encourage the detection of mental illness and through increased communication results in the implementation of holistic and cogent management plans.

The establishment of an antenatal mental health liaison clinic

Following the publication of the second Confidential Enquiry into Maternal Deaths, and the occurrence in 2002 of two maternal deaths in Birmingham, and in advance of further strategic documents such as NICE guidelines, successful collaboration between midwifery and obstetric staff and a perinatal psychiatry team led to the formation of a group whose remit was to implement recommendations from the Confidential Enquiry through the setting up of a care pathway whereby vulnerable mothers could be identified and care plans put in place to ensure their mental needs were catered for during pregnancy and the immediate postpartum period.

Two essentials were immediately identified, namely the need for improved communication between agencies including primary care, midwifes and obstetricians, and community mental health teams and also training.

It was recognized that mothers at risk of having particular difficulties with mental health problems during pregnancy and immediately postpartum could be categorized easily into:

1 Those with a history of serious mental illness:

  a Those who were currently well but were at high risk of relapse, e.g. women with a history of bipolar disorder

  b Those women who were currently unwell. These women usually still needed treatment throughout their pregnancy and invariably were under the care of a community mental health team. In these cases, communication with the community mental health team was vital for two reasons.

    i In order to ensure that the mental health workers were aware that their patient was pregnant—often the woman was reluctant to disclose this to her care coordinator in that team for fear of being judged or being told that it was not advisable that they should continue with the pregnancy ii To give advice regarding optimum medication prescribed during pregnancy. Attitudes, even amongst clinicians, to medication during pregnancy are very variable and often based on feelings rather than evidence. This may result in the immediate discontinuation of medication or reducing dose of medication to subtherapeutic levels, or changing medication back to the more 'old-fashioned' remedies in the mistaken belief that medication that has been around for longer is *ipso facto* safer during pregnancy. Such 'knee-jerk' reactions often lead to relapse of illness during the later stages of pregnancy or postpartum

2 Those women who present with a first episode of illness during pregnancy

3 Mothers who abuse substances, including so-called recreational drugs, other illicit substances, and alcohol.

Training issues

Traditionally, GPs refer pregnant women to antenatal departments as soon as pregnancy is diagnosed. Any referral letter emphasizes physical health problems and may not make reference to mental health problems, especially if episodes of illness have occurred many years previously, e.g. in the case of women suffering from bipolar affective disorder. During the booking process midwives ask a number of questions screening for a variety of health problems. These questions may include one on mental health issues. The wording of the question used initially was vague and a positive answer might indicate a minor adjustment reaction to an adverse life event and more serious mental health problems have been missed. In training, midwives undertaking the booking have been encouraged to be more specific in their questioning and to ask whether the woman had received treatment from a specialist mental health team, including inpatient care, and whether they continued to take medication. These recommendations have been endorsed in the 2007 NICE guidelines on antenatal and postnatal mental health, where in addition to asking about past or present severe mental illness, e.g. schizophrenia and bipolar disorder; psychosis in the postnatal period, and severe depression, it has been suggested that enquiry should be made as to family history, especially in the patient's mother, looking for a history of puerperal psychosis or bipolar affective disorder.

It has been heartening to see where training needs in this respect have been identified and espoused by the Strategic Health Authority with the compilation of training CDs, showing midwives how best to enquire sensitively for a past history of mental health problems and to learn to pick up cues regarding current mental state.

Referral pathways

Community midwives were encouraged to discuss women in need that they had identified with a specialist midwife who had been specifically appointed to coordinate the care of disadvantaged women. This midwife had received more intensive mental health training and was better able to signpost care for the woman in need to the appropriate resource. She acted as a filtering system ensuring that women vulnerable to mental health problems or mental illness were seen by the perinatal psychiatry team. These women were seen in the mental health clinic held within the antenatal department without the need for formal referral, thus lessening any stigma attached to the presence of mental health problems and subscribing to the general philosophy that mental health was as important as physical health during pregnancy. Previous experience had shown that if such women were referred on to another department, e.g. in a psychiatric unit, attendance was poor as the women felt stigmatized and labelled as being mad and the very women who needed most to be seen did not attend.

Women had the right to refuse to be seen within the mental health clinic. In such cases the history was discussed between the specialist midwife and the perinatal psychiatry team and, depending on the potential seriousness of the problem, more strenuous attempts were made by the midwives to encourage attendance at the mental health liaison clinic. In all cases GPs and, if appropriate, community mental health teams were informed of the referral to the liaison clinic and the outcome of consultation.

Women with drug and alcohol problems posed a particular challenge. Frequently they led chaotic lifestyles and presented to midwifery services late in pregnancy. Many had had previous involvement with social services specifically for child care issues, and often because of this, and the fear that social service involvement during the current pregnancy would lead to removal of the baby at birth, attendance at antenatal clinics was often erratic and led to attempts by the women to change the booked place of delivery. These women were referred to the substance misuse team who attended the antenatal department at the same time as the perinatal psychiatry team, but less frequently, but worked in close conjunction with them. They had the benefit of outreach workers who were able to visit the women in their own homes and facilitate their attendance at the antenatal clinic, including the mental health clinic, particularly when comorbidity was present. The workers from the substance misuse team were especially expert in giving advice to mothers regarding the prescription of medications, such as methadone, and were able to collaborate with neonatalogists regarding the management of withdrawal symptoms in the newborn.

The occurrence of a first episode of illness was not an uncommon event and often the community midwife was best placed to identify this in an expectant mother and ensure referral to the mental health liaison clinic. Pregnant women show a reluctance to admit to mental health problems to their primary care workers for a variety of reasons, and prominent amongst these is the fear that the local authority will become involved, perhaps with the ultimate sanction of removal of the baby. In the event of a pregnant woman developing a mental illness, treatment, both pharmacological and psychological, may well be necessary. There is still a reluctance to prescribe medications in pregnancy, and whilst it is acknowledged that this should be undertaken with caution and by a clinician who is well-versed in this therapeutic area, the adverse effects of untreated illness during pregnancy, as regards both the outcome of pregnancy and the effects on the unborn child, are often not recognized or given the importance they warrant. Most frequently this refers to depressive disorders and anxiety states but other conditions include post-traumatic stress disorder where the woman has previously experienced a harrowing or life-threatening birth process, women with a history of eating disorder when some of the symptoms of this disorder may be reawakened as the body shape changes, and obsessive–compulsive disorder.

Psychological therapy, either individual or group therapy, has been shown to be of considerable benefit in a variety of mental health problems during pregnancy and this can be facilitated through the perinatal psychiatry service. There is often an apprehension that waiting times for psychological therapies are excessively long. NICE guidelines have made the firm recommendation that women during pregnancy (and the postpartum period) should be seen for treatment normally within one month of the initial assessment and no longer than three months afterwards. Every effort should be made by clinicians to ensure that resources are in place to ensure these recommendations can be implemented.

The more seriously unwell woman may be referred on to the local community mental health team and more intensive care provided through an attached home treatment service. In the rarer event of a pregnant woman requiring inpatient treatment, the only recourse is to liaise with general psychiatrists and arrange admission to an acute general psychiatric ward as there are currently very few units in the country dedicated for the inpatient care of pregnant women with serious mental illness. It is known that if a woman is exposed to stress from whatever cause then this has a very negative impact on the progress of the pregnancy and puts the unborn child at risk, yet the only available facility to admit pregnant women is into an environment of an acute ward that is highly disturbed and threatening. In these instances it is important that the perinatal psychiatry team remains involved to give advice regarding medication during pregnancy, and to be part of the care plan after delivery, which may include admission of the mother with the baby to a psychiatric mother and baby unit.

Implementation of the antenatal mental health liaison clinic

Birmingham is the second city in England with a population in excess of one million. The City Hospital where the first antenatal mental health clinic in Birmingham was established is within the inner-city area with a high index of deprivation and a diverse multi-ethnic population including large numbers of women seeking asylum. Over 4000 women are delivered at the City Hospital each year. It was initially intended that the liaison clinic would take place every month but it soon became apparent that the demand exceeded this provision and clinics are now held on a weekly basis with a senior psychiatrist specializing in perinatal psychiatry, usually a consultant, in attendance together with a community psychiatric nurse from the perinatal psychiatry service.

In the first year of operation, 114 mothers were referred to the clinic and this referral rate has remained fairly constant over subsequent years with 122 mothers being referred in 2007. The ethnic diversity of the population served is reflected in the numbers of mothers whose ethnic origin is the Asian subcontinent, these numbers exceed the numbers of mothers who are regarded as white Caucasian. This leads to the need for interpreters and an understanding of the particular cultural issues pertaining to these women. It has always been a high priority to try to identify women with mental health needs from the ethnic minorities given the reticence within some cultures to acknowledge mental health problems.

The numbers of women who are seeking asylum remain high, and has been consistently around 10% of the total numbers of mothers referred each year. These mothers, in addition to language- and cultural-specific needs often bring with them memories of violent and traumatic experiences and not infrequently the child has been conceived as a result of a rape.

Whilst NICE guidelines have emphasized that social factors, such a poor relationship with a partner, should not be used for the routine prediction of the development of a mental disorder, basic demographic details of the women seen have been collected in order to understand the characteristics of the population seen. This information has been remarkably constant over the years and in all respects has been consistent with the social profile of the catchment area of the hospital.

Less than a half of the women were married and just under one-third, single. The remainder of the women said they were cohabiting with a partner who may or may not be the father of the expected child.

One-third of the women seen described themselves as housewives—these were usually married women from the Asian subcontinent. Only 20% of women said they were either in full-time or part-time employment prior to the pregnancy.

The reporting of domestic violence increased over the years and in 2007, 47% of women attending the clinic disclosed that they had been subject to some form of domestic violence during their lives. The greater rate of disclosure might have been due to an actual increase in the rate of violence. Alternatively, over the years this has become a less taboo subject and hence there might be a greater willingness for the group to disclose their experiences. With training, clinic staff may have developed greater expertise in asking about this sensitive area and locally there has been investment in 'safe houses' and refuges where women can be accommodated and feel safe following the disclosure of violence.

Mental health profile of women attending the mental health clinic

Consistently over the years around 80% of women seen had a previous history of mental illness. Of these:

- 64% had a mood disorder, including 10% with a previous episode of postnatal depression. The mood disorders ranged from bipolar affective disorder through varying degrees of depressive disorder and mixed/anxiety depressive disorder
- 4% had suffered a psychotic illness
- 9% had been admitted a psychiatric hospital previously

- 20% did not have a documented diagnosis but did report previous episodes of mental illness treated in either primary or secondary care
- 3% suffered other conditions such as eating disorder, obsessive–compulsive disorder, post-traumatic stress disorder where symptoms consequent to previous traumatic births were reawakened, were also identified.

Of these women with a history of psychiatric problems, nearly one-half were currently well and may not have sought psychiatric support of their own volition. The antenatal clinic was an ideal setting to offer psychoeducation and to include assessment of risk of relapse, especially in patients with a past history of bipolar disorder, and also to provide support to enable management plans to be formulated in the event of them becoming unwell.

A number of women presented with a new episode of illness. The majority of these were mood disorders but one episode of psychosis first presentation and one case of post-traumatic stress disorder was seen. New illnesses were frequently identified by the midwives during the booking process and routine antenatal consultations and reflected the effectiveness of the training given. The midwives themselves were reassured that having raised the possibility of mental health problems there was a resource immediately available where women could be seen promptly.

Outcome measures

After initial assessment various treatment options were discussed and this included medication and psychological therapies. This included individual work with a community psychiatric nurse or group therapy in the form of attendance at a specific antenatal mental health support group which combined elements of anxiety management, and coping with depression and other mental health problems through cognitive therapy. In mothers whose risk of serious illness after delivery was high, consideration was given to placing their names on the waiting list for admission to the inpatient unit of the mother and baby unit as a contingency plan. The care plans, with appropriate contact telephone numbers, were carefully documented in the hand-held pregnancy notes kept by the mother, the obstetric notes, and communicated by letter to the GP and to the local community mental health team if relevant.

If there were no obvious risk issues women were discharged from the clinic. This occurred generally in 10% of cases. Mostly women were seen at intervals during their pregnancy in the mental health liaison clinic (75% of cases) for their mental state and effectiveness of the care plan to be monitored. In around 10% of cases a community psychiatric nurse visited the mother at home to offer additional support, and in a further 10% of cases, help from a community mental health team was enlisted if the patient was not already known to them.

Conclusions

An antenatal mental health clinic provides an ideal setting for the identification of women either with, or at risk of, developing mental illness. A collaborative, informal, multi-agency working environment promotes closer working and helps reduce the stigma of mental health services for pregnant women.

Training of midwives is of benefit in giving confidence to them in their interactions with patients with mental health problems, and easy accessibility to mental health services gives reassurance that any problems picked up will be dealt with promptly and effectively.

For those mothers who are unwell, the clinic offers an alternative point of access to psychiatric services which is less intimidating. Medication and other therapeutic options can be discussed with a team confident in the management of a pregnant woman with a mental illness.

The success of the clinic is evidenced through the knowledge that no unexpected crisis situations developed and the absence of any fatality due to psychiatric cause. It has also enabled access to continuing psychiatric care where this has been indicated.

References

Lewis G (ed) (2007). *The Confidential Enquiry into Maternal and Child Health (CEMACH). Saving Mothers' Lives: reviewing maternal deaths to make motherhood safer – 2003–2005. The Seventh Report on Confidential Enquiries into Maternal Deaths in the United Kingdom*. CEMACH, London.

NICE (2007). *Antenatal and Postnatal Mental Health*. NICE, London.

CHAPTER 21

Psychiatric mother and baby units

Trevor Friedman

Introduction

This chapter will describe the background to the development of psychiatric mother and baby units in the setting of perinatal and general adult psychiatric services. It will also deal with the evidence for their effectiveness in treating and improving the experience of mentally ill mothers.

Development of mother and baby units

Psychiatric mother and baby units were developed in Great Britain in the 1950s. This was a time of great change in psychiatric care with the development of the National Health Service in 1948 leading to a major reorganization in the way that psychiatric care was provided. Psychiatric care had previously depended mostly upon the presence of large psychiatric hospitals run by physician superintendents, often with little in the way of doctors with specialist psychiatric training other than in areas of London and other parts of the country. This time also saw a move by organizations such as the National Association for the Welfare of Children in Hospital to ensure that mothers were able to be with their sick children on paediatric wards.

It would seem in the setting of the change of ethos, both politically and medically (Main 1948), towards more patient-centred care and keeping mothers with their children, that mother and baby units opened in London, Shenley, and Banstead (Margison and Brockington 1982). The theoretical basis for the benefit of such services was also influenced by Bowlby's work (1973) on the adverse affects of separation on the mother–infant relationship. There was a general move in the 1950s towards the keeping together of mothers and infants in all medical settings because of this and the general belief and understanding in the importance of bonding between mother and infant.

The further development of mother and baby units over subsequent years often depended upon the interests of particular specialists in developing such services. The majority of mother and baby units are located in the British Isles with some in the Antipodes (Buist *et al.* 2004) and a few else worldwide. The presence of this marked variation in the provision of mother and baby units raises the question as to the evidence for their necessity and benefit. One would suppose that if the impact upon health outcomes and satisfaction for the mother and baby were extensive one would expect such services to be provided worldwide in those countries with developed healthcare services. There may be factors to do with the health service organization and delivery of care that have prevented their development worldwide.

The demands for the provision of mother and baby units and the ability to keep mother and baby together during times of serious mental illness have generally been supported by the medical professional and service user groups. The number of mother and baby units has waxed and waned over the years and until recent times has depended generally upon the enthusiasm of individual specialists in perinatal psychiatry and their teams to develop such services. The rationale for provision of services and different styles of service will be discussed later in this chapter but in recent years the need to show the evidence base for such decisions and for the provision of what can be a costly service has increased the threat to some services.

Provision of services

There have been a number of studies of the availability of mother and baby services over the years. A study by Prettyman and Friedman in 1991 of England and Wales indicated about 20% of health districts had dedicated facilities for mothers and their babies, whilst approximately a half admitted mothers with babies to acute general psychiatric wards. A number of areas were reviewing their facilities and there appeared to be a general move towards providing more joint admission but there were still large areas of the country without the ability to jointly admit mothers with their babies.

There is sometimes a debate as to the definition of a mother and baby unit. There are clearly some units which have a separate identity with specialist staff, including special equipment and arrangements for nursery and child feeding. Sometimes single side rooms are designated as mother and baby units without the comprehensive package of care described.

A later survey by Oluwatayo and Friedman (2005) carried out a similar survey of 78 Mental Health Trusts in England. This was a larger survey of perinatal psychiatry services that indicated that just over a third of Trusts had specific mother and baby beds, with approximately two-thirds of these being dedicated units. Most psychiatric services considered their resources inadequate and in that survey less than half of the Mental Health Trusts provided any specialist perinatal services and only a few provided a comprehensive service. The survey found a reduction in the number of dedicated inpatient units for perinatal women in England since 1999 and it was felt that this might be related towards the shift to community provision as an alternative to admission. These issues were further reviewed as part of the National Institute of Health and Clinical Excellence (NICE) guidelines on clinical management in antenatal and postnatal mental health published in 2007 (NICE 2007). The NICE guidelines as part of their review carried out a survey of services for pregnant women and those in the perinatal period. A brief questionnaire was sent to all Primary Care Trust chief executives in England and chief executives of National Health Trusts in Wales. They received a response from just under half of all health authorities. There was a further study of specialist mental health services which received a good response rate and this stated that 31% of respondents were direct providers of either specialist mother and baby unit or had designated beds specifically for women in the antenatal or postnatal period. A further 40% made use of mother and baby beds outside of their Trust. At the same time 52% reported using general psychiatric beds without a facility for admitting infants. This data suggested a number of Trusts were making use of several different services and were admitting mothers to different types of care.

These surveys indicate that whilst there appears to be general consensus that such facilities should be able there has not been the development of a comprehensive service across the United Kingdom (UK) ensuring that all mentally ill mothers could be admitted with their children.

National guidelines

There have been a number of reports and recommendations concerning perinatal mental health services. The Royal College of Psychiatrists Council report (2000) made a series of recommendations including the necessity of a local perinatal mental health strategy to provide effective treatment on a comprehensive basis. Included in these recommendations was that mother and baby units be established to allow admission of mothers with their babies. It was understood that because of economies of scale that it may be necessary for these to serve the needs of a number of health authorities.

In that report it was felt unlikely that anything above the largest health authority would have sufficient numbers of women requiring admission following childbirth to justify the setting up of a specialist mother and baby unit. There was a need for a critical mass of births and it was suggested that a number of health authorities could jointly purchase a unit to serve a population large enough to ensure the admissions necessary to maintain the skills of the staff and to provide the resources necessary for the patients' care.

The rates of puerperal psychosis have generally been stated as one in 500 births (Brockington 1998) but more recent experience suggests that the figure may be lower than this; a health area of a million people might have a birth rate of 12 000–15 000 births suggesting 20–30 cases of puerperal psychosis per year. There are other diagnoses leading to admission but it is this group where it might be felt to be essential to have provision for joint admission. This issue of the relative rarity of admissions following childbirth necessitating large catchment areas is a significant issue in the organization and efficiency of such services.

The NICE guidelines on clinical management and service guidance for antenatal and postnatal mental health published in 2007 reviews the range of services and treatment for pregnant women. It identified the functions of the inpatient services as including: managing mental health problems during pregnancy; the assessment of mental illness in the postnatal period, including risk assessment and the assessment of ability of the mother to care for the infant; provision of expert care of women requiring admission; the expert provision of safe care for the infants and women admitted; and support for the women in caring for and developing a relationship with her baby. The care of these women is complicated by the need to work with and liaise with other services including maternity and obstetric services, GPs, and maternity-based and community mental health services. The comprehensive maternity services in the UK, which are unique in having dedicated health visitors and midwife home visits after birth, have also probably contributed to the development of perinatal psychiatry services. Other countries, notably the United States, have many different and disparate services providing (or not providing!) care during this period, which makes the organization of psychiatry services complex compared with the UK where almost all women pass through the National Health Service maternity services.

The NICE guidelines discuss that a key factor in the decision to admit a woman with an infant is consideration of the welfare of the infant; whether the infant is better to stay with his or her mother, or whether the infant should be cared for by another family member whilst the mother is receiving inpatient treatment. In areas with specialist units the infant is normally admitted with their mother. There are often logistic issues in relation to geographical proximity which may be important in relating to visiting times and contact with family and social networks. This is clearly a factor in relation to support after discharge and linking in with local services.

The NICE guidelines state that there should be careful planning about the development of mother and baby units, involving key stakeholders taking into account population needs and the influence of related services. The NICE guidelines reiterate that there are few formal evaluations of the provision of mother and baby units and the cost effectiveness of this style of care provision. Indeed, there are no economic analyses of these specialist inpatient units or specialist perinatal teams.

In Scotland the Scottish Intercollegiate Guidelines Network (SIGN 2002) produced a national clinical guideline on the management of postnatal depression and puerperal psychosis. This involved a comprehensive review of the management of psychiatric conditions during pregnancy and puerperium in relation to mother

and baby units. This review of the literature describes several studies where mother and baby admissions occur (Buist et al. 1990; Kumar et al. 1995) and whilst they describe advantages in avoiding separation of mother and infant and establishing positive attachment and providing support, they are generally descriptive papers rather than clinical trials. The recommendation of this group was that the option to admit mother and baby together to a specialist unit should be available to all mothers. It also stated that mothers and babies should not be routinely admitted to general psychiatric wards. The evidence for this was not based upon trial data but upon expert opinion and so this was at the lowest grade of evidence to support this recommendation.

The framework for mental health services in Scotland (Scottish Executive 2004) in relation to perinatal mental illness, including hospital admission, contains a detailed framework for mental health services and the assessment that should occur and this endorses the right of mothers to have their babies with them during admission if this is what they wish.

Studies of outcomes from mother and baby units

An early paper by Kumar et al. 1995 is a study of the characteristics of 160 admissions to a mother and baby unit. In this study 56% of the admissions occurred within two weeks of delivery and the average duration of admission was two months. Twenty patients had schizophrenia, 56 had affective psychoses, and 24 had non-psychotic disorders. The demographic and obstetric characteristics of these groups were similar but the affective psychosis group were more likely to have acute illnesses and an earlier onset of admission occurring within two weeks of delivery. Women with non-psychotic disorders were also more likely to become unwell within two weeks of delivery but tended to be admitted later. In this study only 7% of the affective psychotic and non-psychotic women were discharged separated from their infants and they found that the women with schizophrenia required greater input of nursing resources than mothers with other illnesses and that 50% were discharged without their infants.

In the UK there was a large collection of mother and baby admission data through the Marcé clinical database (Salmon 2004). This lead to an examination of maternal, clinical, and parenting outcome related to diagnosis and associations with poor outcomes (Salmon et al. 2003). Information was collected on over 1000 mother and baby admissions including 224 mothers with schizophrenia, 155 with bipolar disorder, 409 with non-psychotic depression. There was generally a good clinical outcome in 78% of cases but there were particular predictors of poor outcome. In particular, the factors that predicted poor outcome were a diagnosis of schizophrenia, behavioural disturbance during admission, low social class, and psychiatric illness in the woman's partner or a poor relationship with a partner. In those with poor outcome on all these four variables, 66% suffered schizophrenia. Women with schizophrenia showed more behavioural disturbance, were more likely to experience hallucinations and delusions, and were more likely to be of low social class. They were also less likely to have a partner although more likely to have a partner with psychiatric illness.

There is a limited literature in relation to studies examining outcome and benefits of mother and baby units. A Cochrane review of mother and baby units and schizophrenia (Joy and Saylan 2007) discusses the issue of admitting mothers with schizophrenia and their babies together might be felt to be particularly important because of the difficulties for women with schizophrenia in forming attachment to their children. The children of mothers with schizophrenia may also be at more risk of losing their mother as primary carer as it is often considered that they are unable to cope (Howard 2003). Mother and baby units may also help in engaging people with serious mental illness into the services (Klompenhouwer and van Hulst 1991; Appleby and Dickens 1993; Kumar and Hipwell 1994; Barnett and Morgan 1996).

The paper reviews the concerns about admitting mothers to psychiatric units due to risk of institutionalization, exposure to multiple carers, and potential physical harm from deluded mothers. Various anecdotal evidence and findings suggest the actual incidents of harm to babies in mother and baby units as very rare (Margison and Brockington 1982; Buist 1990; Salmon 2004). This paper states that there is not a good explanation as to why there are few mother and baby units in other Western countries (Kumar 1995; Cawley 1999) outside of the UK. The paper suggests that it may be in part related to differences in family structure and ences and differences in healthcare and occasionally different cultures, as well as the lack of firm evidence to support the cost effectiveness of such units.

The Cochrane review attempted to include all relevant randomized controlled trials of admission versus non-admission to mother and baby units of mothers with schizophrenia. The review was unsuccessful in finding controlled trials addressing this issue. Forty-four papers

were identified but there was only one control study which had to be excluded, from Baker *et al.* (1961) which compared 20 mothers treated in a mother and baby unit with 20 mothers treated on acute admission ward but without admission of a baby. In this study, which was not randomized, over half the mothers in the standard care group (13 out of 20) were able to take their children home whereas all the mothers on the mother and baby unit were reported as being able to take full care of their baby on their return home. The mother and baby unit group were reported as being more seriously ill on admission but were discharged with fewer symptoms. This comparative descriptive study suggested that the admission to mother and baby units was helpful; although this study took place over 40 years ago and diagnostic and clinical practices have changed since then. The conclusion of the review was that they did not find reliable objective evidence for the efficacy of mother and baby units in schizophrenia and these findings were similar to other reviews.

In studies that included women's views to admission, they expressed a wish to use a mother and baby unit rather than a standard ward (Margison and Brockington 1982; Kumar 1995; Neil 2006), but these papers also state that at the moment it is very unclear if they have any beneficial affect in terms of mother recovery, risks to the infant, or the development of mother and child bond compared with other models of care. The conclusion for policy makers and managers from these studies was that units for mentally ill mothers and their babies are expensive and their effects and benefits over other packages of care are uncertain. These studies show that units are preferred by patients, which is important, but concern is raised whether this is a sufficient reason for unevaluated investment, and the reviews state that if newer units are being constructed whilst older packages of care are being phased out, then this should afford an opportunity for evaluation.

There is an interesting study looking at psychiatric morbidity and mental health treatment needs in prison mother and baby units (Birmingham *et al.* 2006). There are four prison mother and baby units in England and Wales, although these clearly are not specifically for the treatment of psychiatric disorders, but are used for women who have babies whilst in custody. Fifty-five participants were recruited (93% of group). It was noted that 60% of the women had mental disorders with a third having a diagnosis of personality disorders but interestingly no one had a psychotic disorder. Thus the group in mother and baby units in prisons tend to have more stable backgrounds than their prison counterparts and women serving sentences for drug offences are favoured. A selection process appears to select out women with psychiatric morbidity and other difficulties that may make them unsuitable for placement in prison mother and baby units.

The case has also been made for using mother and baby units to assess parenting capacity in mothers with mental health problems—often in collaboration with social services departments. There are a number of studies (Seniveratne 2003) looking at parenting assessment in a psychiatric mother and baby unit. A case note study of 62 referrals for an inpatient parenting assessment during a six-year period found that fewer than half the mothers were discharged together with their babies at the end of the assessment period and that at follow-up less than a third were still caring for their children. Mothers with depression were more likely to remain primary carers. The general finding was that it illustrated the need for more integrated coordination between professionals in mental health and children's services to ensure early planning for mothers and infants at risk as this appears to benefit the outcome of keeping mother and baby together.

Service organization

There continues to be widespread debate as to the organization of perinatal mental health services. It would seem from a review of the literature that the position of admitting psychiatrically sick mothers with their babies appears to have become part of the culture and psychiatric practice within the UK and one or two other countries noticeably Australia and New Zealand (Brockington 2004). At the same time there are very large areas of the world where this practice is almost unknown. It is obviously important to understand the reasons for this in trying to consider the benefits and drawbacks of such a service that have lead to such a wide differences in the organization of treatment.

It would seem to some extent that differences in services may reflect cost and funding of such services. Mother and baby units in the UK were initially started as part of local initiatives by individual clinicians and not dependant upon funding through insurance schemes which would have found such admissions more expensive than those requiring admission of the mother alone.

The use of mother and baby units also arose at the time when there was far less community care and people with significant psychiatric illness were routinely admitted to hospital. The general rates of admission to psychiatric units have fallen significantly due to changes in clinical practice and the development of more comprehensive services in the community. In particular, the use of assertive outreach teams and crisis resolution teams which are able to offer home treatment on a more regular basis has reduced the number of admissions to psychiatric units. These services will presumably also impact upon the necessity of admitting sick mothers with their babies where home treatment has been shown to be a practical alternative to admission (Oates 1996).

This is an important issue because there has always been a tension related to the rates of psychiatric morbidity amongst new mothers and the number of beds required to service a population. Mother and baby units have generally been developed in large conurbations and even then have often needed to offer admissions over larger geographical areas to maintain viability. There is a tension between the desire to have specialist units with skilled staff able to care for both mothers and babies whilst at the same time wanting to keep mothers and their babies close to home and to integrate with local services. If the rates of sick mothers requiring admission fall further this threatens the viability of larger mother and baby units and more flexible and imaginative responses will be required.

Mother and baby units depend to an extent on the cultural and social background of the populations that are being served. The decision to admit mothers to psychiatric wards with their babies will depend to an extent on the support of families and local communities. There may be cultures where extended families are more willing or able to take on sick mothers or to care for their babies whilst they are admitted to hospital. The increasing use of crisis teams and their associated early discharge services may allow periods of admission to reduce and for mothers only to be admitted during acutely disturbed periods. There is also an issue within the management of mother and baby units as to whether babies should be present when their mothers are acutely psychiatrically unwell or enormously behaviourally disturbed. At these times it is often impractical or unwise for mothers to have close contact with their babies and it may be better for them to be cared for by their families.

There is no doubt from surveys and feedback from patients that generally there is a desire amongst patient groups and staff to try and admit mothers with their babies. There is a strong desire for such services to continue and it is for decision makers to weigh up the balance between the wants and desires of patients, staff, and their supporters, and the increased financial cost associated with specialist mother and baby units. This is a dilemma in the United States where there has been insufficient evidence to support the development of mother and baby units (Wisner 1996).

There is clearly a need for better research data as to the benefits and costs of running such units compared with other models of care. It is difficult to decide upon the benefits of mother and baby units because they should exist within the wider remit of a specialized perinatal psychiatry service. In this way they form part of a delivery of care that can integrate with other parts of psychiatric and general medical services. The difficulty is that certain ways of organizing services may be beneficial in one part of the country but not in another. There is a move towards providing managed clinical networks for perinatal mental health services and this should enable a more rational method of organizing such specialist services.

References

Appleby L and Dickens C (1993). Mothering skills of women with mental illness. *British Medical Journal*, **306**, 348–9.

Baker AA et al. (1961). Admitting schizophrenic mothers with their babies. Lancet, **ii**, 237–39.

Barnett B and Morgan M (1996). Postpartum psychiatric disorders: who should be admitted to hospital? *Australian and New Zealand Journal of Psychiatry*, **30**(6), 709–14.

Birmingham L et al. (2006). The mental health of women in prison mother and baby units. *Journal of Forensic Psychiatry and Psychology*, **17**(3), 393–404.

Bowlby J (1973). *Attachment and Loss (Vol. 2), Separation: Anxiety and Anger.* Hogarth Press and the Institute of Psycho-Analysis, London.

Brockington I (1998). Puerperal disorders. *Advances in Psychiatric Treatments*, **4**, 312–19.

Brockington I (2004). Postpartum psychiatric disorders. *Lancet*, **363**, 303–10.

Buist A et al. (1990). Review of a mother-baby unit in a psychiatric hospital. *Australian and New Zealand Journal of Psychiatry*, **24**, 103–8.

Buist A et al. (2004). Mother-baby psychiatric units in Australia – the Victorian experience. *Archives of Women's Health*, **7**, 81–7.

Cawley S et al. (1999). Who needs a mother and baby unit? *Nursing Standard*, **13**, 33–6.

Howard L et al. (2003). Predictors of social services supervision of babies of mothers with mental illness after admission to a psychiatric mother and baby unit. *Social Psychiatry and Psychiatric Epidemiology*, **38**, 450–5.

Joy CB and Saylan M (2007). Mother and baby units for schizophrenia. *Cochrane Database of Systematic Reviews*, **1**, CD006333.

Klompenhouwer JL and Van Hulst AM (1991). The classification of postpartum psychosis: a study of 250 mother and baby admissions in the Netherlands. *Acta Psychiatrica Scandinavia*, **84**, 225–261.

Kumar R et al. (1995). Clinical survey of a psychiatric mother and baby unit: characteristics of 100 consecutive admissions. *Journal of Affective Disorders*, **33**, 11–22.

Kumar R and Hipwell AE (1994). Implications for the infant of maternal puerperal psychiatric disorders. In: Rutter M et al. (eds) *Child and Adolescent Psychiatry*, third edition. Blackwell, Oxford.

Main T (1948). Mothers and children in psychiatric hospital. *Lancet*, **11**, 845.

Margison F and Brockington IF (1982). Psychiatric mother and baby units. In: IF Brockington and R Kumar (eds) *Motherhood and Mental Illness*, pp. 223–228. Academic Press, London.

Neil S et al. (2006). A satisfaction survey of women admitted to a psychiatric mother and baby unit in the northwest of England. *Archives of Women's Mental Health*, **9**, 109–12.

Oates M (1996). Psychiatric services for women following childbirth. *International Review of Psychiatry*, **8**, 87–98.

Oluwatayo F and Friedman T (2005). A survey of perinatal psychiatric services in England and Wales. *Psychiatric Bulletin*, **29**, 177–179.

NICE (2007). *Antenatal and Postnatal Mental Health.* National Institute for Health and Clinical Excellence, London.

Prettyman RJ and Friedman T (1991). Care of women with puerperal and psychiatric disorders in England and Wales. *British Medical Journal*, **302**, 1245–6.

Royal College of Psychiatrists (1992). Report of the General Psychiatry Section Working Party on Postnatal Illness. *Psychiatric Bulletin*, **16**, 519–22.

Royal College of Psychiatrists (2000). *Perinatal Maternal Mental Health Services.* Royal College of Psychiatrists, London.

Salmon M et al. (2003). Clinical and parenting skills outcomes following joint mother-baby psychiatric admission. *Australia and New Zealand Journal of Psychiatry*, **37**, 556–62.

Salmon MP et al. (2004). A national audit of joint mother and baby admissions to UK psychiatric hospitals: an overview of findings. *Archives of Women's Mental Health*, **7**, 65–70.

Seneviratne G et al. (2003). Parenting assessment in a psychiatric mother and baby unit. *British Journal of Social Work*, **4**, 535–55.

SIGN (2002). *Postnatal Depression and Puerperal Psychosis.* Scottish Intercollegiate Guidelines Network, Edinburgh.

Scottish Executive (2004). *Framework for mental health services in Scotland: perinatal mental illness/postnatal depression hospital admission and support services. NHS HDL, (2004).* 6. Scottish Executive Health Department, Edinburgh.

Wisner KL et al. (1996). Clinical dilemmas due to the lack of inpatient mother-baby units. *International Journal of Psychiatry in Medicine*, **26**, 479–93.

Women and Substance Abuse

CHAPTER 22

Women and alcohol

John Roche, Eilish Gilvarry, and Ed Day

Introduction

The second half of the 20th century saw an enormous change in the role of women in society, and with this came a shift in their relationship with alcohol. The number of women in paid employment has steadily risen in the developed world since the 1960s, and this has increased access to alcohol. More opportunities to drink have coincided with an increase in social acceptability of alcohol consumption and drunkenness in women. In the United Kingdom (UK) cheap alcohol and targeted advertising have combined with a rise in the number of women in their 20s and 30s with few family responsibilities and high disposable income to fuel an increase in consumption (Plant and Plant 2006). For example, female undergraduate students may feel pressured to drink as much as men to be socially accepted (Young *et al.* 2005).

These issues are significant, as there appear to be gender differences in alcohol-related morbidity, with women tending to drink less than men though they are more prone to alcohol-related problems. In addition there are specific problems that only occur in women, for example, issues around pregnancy. In this chapter the epidemiology of the problem is summarized and areas of specific consideration with regard to women and alcohol are explored.

Terminology

Patterns of alcohol consumption and related harm can be classified in different ways. In the UK a unit of alcohol contains 8 g of pure ethanol, and the latest government guidance recommends that 'adult women should not regularly drink more than 2–3 units of alcohol a day' (HM Government 2007). Alcohol consumption at this level is referred to as 'sensible drinking', whereas drinking above these levels is 'hazardous'. 'Harmful drinking' is 'drinking at levels that lead to significant harm to physical and mental health'. The Office for National Statistics (ONS) define a 'binge' as drinking more than twice the recommended maximum amount in one session, i.e. more than six units for a woman. Another common definition of a binge is 'drinking to get drunk'.

The World Health Organization (WHO), in the International Classification of Diseases 10th Revision (ICD-10) (WHO 1997) defines 'acute intoxication' as:

a condition that follows the administration of a psychoactive substance resulting in disturbances in level of consciousness, cognition, perception, affect or behaviour, or other psycho-physiological functions and responses. The disturbances are directly related to the acute pharmacological effects of the substance and resolve with time, with complete recovery, except where tissue damage or other complications have arisen.

Dependence syndrome is defined (WHO 1997) as:

a cluster of behavioural, cognitive, and physiological phenomena that develop after repeated substance use and that typically include a strong desire to take the drug, difficulties in controlling its use despite harmful consequences, a higher priority given to drug use than to other activities and obligations, increased tolerance, and sometimes a physical withdrawal state.

Epidemiology

Historically men have always consumed more alcohol than women. In recent years, however, the gap has been closing amongst 16–24-year-olds, particularly heavy episodic drinking (GENACIS 2005). This suggests that general levels of drinking amongst women are increasing, with the relaxation of traditional social controls on women's drinking cited as a key reason, accompanied by a shift in traditional gender roles.

Obtaining reliable data on alcohol use is difficult—surveys consistently record less alcohol consumption than would be expected based on alcohol sales. This is partly due to a tendency for people to underestimate the amount of alcohol they consume. The best data we have suggest that in 2005 women drank on average 6.5 units per week, with 37% drinking up to three units and 20% drinking over three units of alcohol at least once per week. The proportion of women drinking more than 14 units per week was 10% in 1988, 17% in 2002, and 13% in 2005 (ONS 2005).

The Alcohol Needs Assessment Research Project (ANARP) found that 38% of men and 16% of women (age 16–64) in England had an alcohol use disorder, and within this, 32% of men and 15% of women were hazardous or harmful alcohol users. Twenty-one per cent of men and 9% of women were binge drinkers, and the overall prevalence of alcohol dependence was 3.6%, with 6% of men and 2% of women met the criteria for alcohol dependence. The prevalence of hazardous drinking varied across regions, ranging from 18–29%, and alcohol dependence varied from 1.6–5.2%. The incidence of alcohol use disorders declined with increasing age. Black and ethnic minorities had a similar prevalence of alcohol dependence, but a considerably lower prevalence of harmful/hazardous drinking (Drummond *et al.* 2005). Responses to the ONS Opinions Study in 2008 highlighted that UK women consume less alcohol than their male counterparts, are more likely to drink wine and spirits, are more likely to drink in their home or someone else's home, and are slightly more likely than men to drink alone.

The European School Survey Project on Alcohol and other Drugs (ESPAD) study of 15- and 16-year-old students across Europe showed that in 2007 females drank more on the latest drinking day than males in Iceland and approximately equal amounts in Finland, Norway, and Sweden. Boys drank slightly more than girls in the UK, Denmark, the Netherlands, and the Slovak Republic. Elsewhere the gender gap was more in keeping with the general trend of males of all ages drinking significantly more than their female counterparts (Hibell *et al.* 2009). Considering the increased bioavailability of equivalent doses of alcohol in women, this marks an alarming trend of increased alcohol use in young females.

The pattern of development of alcohol problems differs between men and women. Randall *et al.* (1999) found that women first get drunk at a later age (26.6 versus 22.7 years), develop drinking problems at a later age (27.5 versus 25.0 years), and exhibit loss of control over drinking at a later age (29.8 versus 27.2 years). However, despite starting to drink later in life, the development of ensuing problems was more rapid.

The authors called this 'telescoping', and suggested it could be due to biological differences in the response to alcohol, increased prevalence of psychiatric comorbidity, or sociocultural differences such as women being more likely to be identified as having an alcohol problem than men.

Physiological differences

Alcohol appears to affect women differently to men. Gender may affect the absorption, distribution, metabolism, and excretion of any drug, and these differences are likely to be mediated by levels of adipose tissue, protein binding, and action of the cytochrome P450 system, all of which differ between men and women. Hormonal changes and the menstrual cycle have been implicated in affecting the pharmacodynamics and pharmacokinetics of alcohol. There is a dose-dependent relationship of alcohol causing an elevation of liver enzymes, and women are more sensitive to this. Drinking alcohol with food may reduce this effect in women, but not in men (Stranges *et al.* 2004).

For an equal alcohol intake, women develop higher blood alcohol levels than men despite a faster rate of elimination. Women have a higher fat concentration and lower water concentration than men, both of which lead to higher blood alcohol levels. There is also delayed gastric emptying of alcohol. The gender difference is more pronounced following oral rather than intravenous administration, thus demonstrating there is a difference in the degree of 'first-pass' metabolism (Baraona *et al.* 2001). Women have less alcohol dehydrogenase in the stomach resulting in less oxidation and therefore more alcohol being ultimately absorbed (Frezza *et al.* 1990). Women with alcohol dependence have even less stomach alcohol dehydrogenase activity which reduces first-pass metabolism further still (Baraona *et al.* 2001), although this gender difference disappears at about the age of 50 (Seitz *et al.* 1993). It has also been proposed that women's organs and tissues are more vulnerable to the effects of alcohol and that this is mediated by higher oestrogen concentration (Day *et al.* 1998).

Women differ from men in that they have lower gastric alcohol dehydrogenase activity, a decreased volume of ethanol distribution, and an enhanced rate of ethanol oxidation in the liver. These differences would be expected to produce more hepatotoxic products such as acetaldehyde and oxygen radicals which would contribute to an increased vulnerability to medical consequences of alcoholism (Baraona 2001).

Physical health

Alcohol has a significant impact on physical health. For men and women long-term heavy alcohol consumption is associated with increased risk of liver disease, nutritional deficiencies, obesity, pancreatitis, cerebrovascular accidents, neurological diseases including epilepsy and dementia, peripheral neuropathy, cardiomyopathy, pulmonary infections, acute respiratory distress syndrome, endocrine abnormalities, and disorders relating to the musculoskeletal system, skin, and the haemopoietic system. Acute intoxication may lead to confusion, coma, and death, as well as a lack of inhibitions which increase the risk of physical and sexual violence. Withdrawal may lead to seizures or delirium tremens (Barclay et al. 2008). Alcohol use in the elderly can lead to osteoporosis. One study found that women aged 67–90 who drank more than 10 units per day had greater bone loss than women with minimal alcohol intake (Hannan et al. 2000).

There have been alarming recent increases in the rates of death from alcoholic liver disease in the UK. In 1997–2001 the rates of mortality for alcohol cirrhosis in women of all ages were 7.7/100 000 per year in England and Wales, and 16.1/100 000 per year in Scotland. This represented an increase of 35% in England and Wales and 63% in Scotland compared with the period 10 years before, and was in stark contrast to the falling rates across the rest of Europe (Leon and McCambridge 2006).

Alcohol is increasingly linked to many forms of cancer. One large study showed that the death rate from cancer was 30% higher in middle-aged and elderly women reporting one or more drinks per day compared with non-drinkers (Thun et al. 1997). Alcohol is one of a number of lifestyle and environmental risk factors identified for breast cancer. Ginsburg et al. (1996) showed that moderate alcohol consumption increased the circulating levels of oestrogen in postmenopausal women by 300%. A pooled analysis of six prospective cohort studies, including over 300 000 women evaluated for up to 11 years, concluded that alcohol consumption is associated with a linear increase in the incidence of breast cancer for intakes less than eight units per day (Smith-Warner et al. 1998). However, other work has suggested that there is an inverse relationship between moderate alcohol consumption and breast cancer survival (Barnett et al. 2008).

Psychiatric comorbidity

Alcohol problems and psychiatric illness commonly coexist and the relationship between them is complex.

In the UK the COSMIC study (Comorbidity of Substance Misuse and Mental Illness Collaborative Study) was published in 2003. It reported that a majority of alcohol patients (85.5%) had a psychiatric disorder: 19.4% had a psychotic disorder, 80.6% had an affective or anxiety disorder, and 53.2% had a personality disorder (Weaver et al. 2003).

In the United States (US) the most consistently reported co-occurring disorders in heavy drinkers are other substance use disorders, and mood, anxiety, and schizophrenic disorders (Kessler et al. 1997). In the National Comorbidity Survey, lifetime risk for major depression in women compared with men was 1.7. Alcohol-dependent women were 4.4 times more likely to have an affective disorder compared to women in the general population, and 3.1 times more likely to have an anxiety disorder. Higher rates were also reported of social phobia, simple phobia, and post-traumatic stress disorder (PTSD) compared to alcoholic men. Forty per cent of alcoholic women report a previous suicide attempt compared to 8.8% of matched non-alcoholic women (Gomberg 1989). The risk for alcohol dependence was 4.8 times higher for depressed women and 3.1 times higher for depressed men compared with the general population, and the odds ratio for alcohol dependence was 3.1 and 2.2 among women and men with comorbid anxiety disorders (Kessler et al. 1997).

Another study found that women with a history of depression are 2.6 times more likely to be heavy drinkers than those without a history of depression. Even after adjusting for age, history of personality disorder, and father's history of drinking this figure remained high at 2.2 (Dixit et al. 2000). There is evidence that anxiety disorders have an aetiological role in alcohol use disorders, with social anxiety, phobias, and PTSD further elevating this risk (Merikangas et al. 1998). Whilst men with alcohol use disorders are four times more likely to complete suicide than other men, women with alcohol use disorders have a suicide risk 20 times greater (Harris 1997).

PTSD almost doubles the risk of a substance misuse disorder from 8–25% to 22–43%.(Jacobsen 2001), and between one-third and two-thirds of women with a substance misuse disorder meet criteria for PTSD often stemming from childhood physical or sexual abuse. This compares with 10–30% of men with a substance misuse disorder, and their PTSD typically stems from combat or crime trauma (Najavits 1997). In a twin study, childhood sexual abuse increased later alcohol dependence by a factor of 3.0 after controlling for confounding familial factors. Childhood intercourse increased relative risk to 6.5 (Kendler et al. 2000).

Eating disorders, notably bulimia nervosa, have a high correlation with alcohol use disorders with prevalence rates at about one-third. This is similar to comorbidity with PTSD and major depressive disorder, and these may well be confounding factors in the relationship (Dansky *et al.* 2000). Alcohol-dependent women also report higher levels of domestic violence. The severity of alcohol dependence symptoms is proportional to the number of violent assaults that a woman has experienced.

Screening and identification

Although women generally drink less than men, they experience more severe sequelae and their transition from initial abuse to dependence is more rapid (Randall 1999). Alcohol screening questionnaires have been shown to be superior to laboratory tests for detecting heavy drinking (Bernadt *et al.* 1982). However, partly due to excluding women in their development, alcohol screening questionnaires used in primary care have a tendency to be less sensitive in women. One study found that the CAGE questionnaire performed particularly poorly and suggested using lower cut-off points in women. Possible reasons for this reduced sensitivity could be stigma leading to under-reporting of alcohol use, the fact that women develop alcohol problems at lower consumption levels than men, and women are less likely to experience overt social consequences such as financial or legal problems secondary to their drinking (Bradley *et al.* 1998).

The Alcohol Use Disorders Identification Questionnaire (AUDIT) developed by the WHO is considered the best screening tool and has been used across various countries. Using ICD-10 alcohol use disorders as a gold standard it has a sensitivity greater than 0.9 and specificity greater than 0.8 (Saunders 1993), and its utility seems not to be affected by gender or ethnicity (Steinbauer 1998). In the UK, detection rates of alcohol use disorders are low. The General Practice Research Database showed that general practitioners identified one in 67 male and one in 82 female hazardous drinkers, and only one in 28 males and one in 20 females with alcohol dependence (Drummond *et al.* 2005).

Treatment and outcomes

Most research has shown a relatively low proportion of women to men in alcohol treatment services compared to the ratio of women to men with alcohol problems. For instance, the Australian National Household Study showed that in the general population there was a 2:1 ratio between high-risk drinking in men and women, whereas in alcohol treatment services this ratio ranged from 3:1 to 10:1 (Swift *et al.* 1996). More recent data from the ANARP study in the UK showed a Prevalence Service User Ratio (PSUR) of 12 in women and 21 in men. This meant that 8.5% of the 'in need' alcohol-dependent women were accessing services, compared with 4.8% of men. This engagement with services varied across regions with the highest uptake in the North West and the lowest in the North East (Drummond *et al.* 2005).

A review of research relating to women entering and staying in alcohol treatment in the US (Greenfield *et al.* 2007) found that women were less likely to enter treatment than men, but that once in treatment prognosis was comparable. There did appear to be some factors that hindered women's entry into treatment more than men, such as poor economic situation, lower education levels, and fewer social supports. The large Project MATCH study found that women tended to relapse less severely than men and be more willing to seek help following relapse. They had more abstinent days and drank less per drinking day than their male counterparts (Project MATCH Research Group 1997).

A review of psychosocial treatments for alcoholism found that there was little evidence that existing treatment is less beneficial for women then men, although employment outcomes may be worse for women. Enhanced therapies with childcare and individualized therapy are associated with better outcomes, but this may well be due to situational rather than gender effects. Likewise, treatment for PTSD is likely to be beneficial for men as women. A small number of trials have failed to produce strong evidence in favour of women-only treatment (Winhusen 2003).

In the pharmacologic treatment of alcohol misuse, the major areas of concern in women are those related with pregnancy. The use of benzodiazepines may lead to congenital malformations after exposure in the first trimester and floppy infant syndrome after exposure in the third trimester. Carbamazapine, naltrexone, and valproate are contraindicated in pregnancy. Disulfiram is best avoided, and there is no data for acamprosate (Bogenschutz and Geppert 2003).

There are a variety of reasons why women may be less able or less inclined to seek treatment—gender and cultural insensitivity in programme content, perceived threat of legal sanction including loss of child custody, lack of child care, and transportation, inadequate or no health insurance coverage, caretaker roles for dependent family members, and societal intolerance and stigmatization of alcohol- and drug-dependent women (Chasnoff 1991). One study reported that women were more likely to encounter opposition to entering treatment from their family and friends (Beckman and Amaro 1986). Women have been arrested and criminally charged for substance use during pregnancy, and instead of seeking help some women opt to deliver their children at home for fear of this (Paltrow 1998).

There is no clear strategy focusing explicitly on women and alcohol in the UK. In the latest guidelines *Safe. Sensible. Social.* (HM Government 2007) the only gender-specific inclusions are consistency of advice on pregnancy and the difference in guideline safe amounts.

Alcohol and pregnancy

Alcohol use during pregnancy negatively impacts in a number of ways: increased risk of infertility, miscarriage, prematurity, stillbirth, and structural congenital malformations. It can lead to preterm labour, affect fetal growth and development, and can lead to fetal alcohol spectrum disorders (FASD) (Taylor 2006). Alcohol-related damage is considered to be the leading cause of non-genetic intellectual disability in the Western World (Abel *et al.* 1987). Alcohol is teratogenic and these disorders present in diverse ways within a spectrum: fetal alcohol syndrome (FAS), partial fetal alcohol syndrome (PFAS), alcohol-related birth defects and alcohol-related neurodevelopmental disorders. However, there is uncertainty surrounding the range of conditions associated with alcohol and the reliability of diagnostic criteria. The manifestations are of structural problems, behavioural, and neurocognitive development problems. The full syndrome presents as: central nervous system anomalies often leading to cognitive and developmental disabilities, behavioural problems, difficulties with executive functioning, facial dysmorphology, and growth deficiency. The spectrum of disorders may present with variations of the classic triad of FAS.

The data on the incidence of this spectrum is unreliable. In the UK, the general incidence of FAS is considered to be approximately 0.2/1000 live births, in the US, 0.5–2/1000 live births. The damage caused by alcohol is dependent on the amount and pattern of alcohol consumed, the stage of pregnancy, with critical periods being the first and third trimester, genetic factors, other substance use, particularly tobacco, and factors such as poverty and nutrition. The occurrence of FAS is associated with frequency of binge drinking, though only approximately 5% of children born to mothers who drink heavily during pregnancy present with the full syndrome (Gray *et al.* 2006).

In the US, surveys have shown that between 9–15% of pregnant women drink once a month or more (Ebrahim 1999). A similar survey in the UK of antenatal attendees, reported that 45% consumed no alcohol, 44% consumed less than one unit per week, 10% consumed up to one unit per day, and 1% more than one unit per day (RCOG 2006). In the UK, of those that continued to drink, 71% consumed less than one unit of alcohol per week and only 3% had drunk more than seven units a week (ONS 2006). However, the evidence of the effects of alcohol resulting from low to moderate levels of alcohol intake during pregnancy is inconclusive (Gray *et al.* 2006). Moreover, the authors of this report noted that the evidence was not robust enough to exclude any risk at low levels, with other reports suggesting low levels associated with later behavioural problems and effects on children's mental health (BMA Board of Science 2007).

There is variation in guidance given to pregnant women on alcohol use and level of risk. In the US, the advice is clear: women who are pregnant or who may become pregnant should abstain from alcohol, with much work aimed at universal preventative measures, such as public health campaigns and labelling of alcohol drinks. NICE (2008) recommend alcohol should certainly be avoided in the first three months of pregnancy, and after this period if a woman does drink whilst pregnant then she should ideally consume no more than two units on two occasions per week and avoid binge drinking. RCOG (UK 2006) note the increasing evidence on the harmful effects of alcohol on the fetus; though observe that there is no evidence on the harm from 'low levels' of alcohol, defined as no more than one or two units of alcohol a week.

Preventative measures include information and advice to pregnant women, screening, brief interventions, and treatment for those with alcohol-related problems. Pregnancy is a key time when alcohol use disorders can be identified, with motivation for treatment likely to be enhanced at this time. Much of the treatment for those with abuse/dependence is similar to that of the non-pregnant woman, including possible detoxification and psychosocial interventions. However, a Cochrane review (Lui *et al.* 2008) found that no randomized controlled trails had yet investigated psychosocial interventions specifically addressing alcohol in pregnancy, this is clearly an area warranting further research.

Conclusions

Alcohol, the nation's favourite drug, is associated with numerous health and social problems, and these often affect women differently to men. It is clear that the prevalence of alcohol use disorders in women is climbing, particularly when compared to men. This is leading to severe consequences; for example, the significant increase in alcohol cirrhosis mortality among women in Scotland.

Women are coming to the attention of services more readily than in the past, possibly due to the increased acceptance and awareness of alcohol consumption and related problems amongst women in today's culture. There is limited evidence suggesting any particular form of treatment is more effective in females specifically. More research is needed in this area. The issue of alcohol use during pregnancy and the advice to be given to women at this time remains unclear, with the high prevalence of drinking during pregnancy being at odds with the cautious advice to abstain.

With the increasing prevalence and changing cultural norms, greater emphasis should be put on identification, treatment, and research issues specifically directed at women.

References

Abel AK and Sokel R (1987). Incidence of fetal alcohol syndrome and economic impact of FAS related anomalies. *Drug and Alcohol dependence*, **19**, 51–70.

Alcohol Concern (2008). Women and alcohol – a cause for concern? *Acquire*, **52**.

Baraona E *et al.* (2001). Gender differences in pharmacokinetics of alcohol. *Alcoholism: Clinical and Experimental Research*, **25**, 502–7.

Barclay GA *et al.* (2008). The adverse effects of alcohol misuse. *Advances in Psychiatric Treatment*, **14**, 139–51.

Barnett GC *et al.* (2008). Risk factors for the incidence of breast cancer: do they affect survival from the disease? *Journal of Clinical Oncology*, **26**, 3310–16.

Beckman L and Amaro H (1986). Personal and social difficulties faced by women and men entering alcoholism treatment. *Journal of Studies in Alcohol*, **47**, 135–45.

Bernadt MW *et al.* (1982). Comparison of questionnaire and laboratory tests in the detection of excessive drinking and alcoholism. *Lancet*, **1**, 325–8.

BMA Board of Science (2007). *Fetal Alcohol Spectrum Disorders: A Guide To Health Professionals*. BMA, London.

Bogenschutz MP and Geppert CMA (2003). Pharmacologic treatments for women with addictions. *Obstetrics and Gynaecology Clinics of North America*, **30**, 523–44.

Bradley KA *et al.* (1998). Alcohol screening questionnaires in women. *Journal of the American Medical Association*, **280**(2), 166–71.

Chasnoff IJ (1991). Drugs, alcohol, pregnancy, and the neonate: Pay now or pay later. *Journal of the American Medical Association*, **266**, 1567–8.

Dansky BS *et al.* (2000). Comorbidity of bulimia nervosa and alcohol use disorders: results from the National Women's Study. *International Journal of Eating Disorders*, **27**, 180–90.

Day AJ *et al.* (1998). Deglycosylation of flavonoid and isoflavonoid glycosides by human small intestine and liver beta-glucosidase activity. *FEBS Letters*, **436**, 71–5.

Dixit AR and Crum RM (2000). Prospective study of depression and the risk of heavy alcohol use in women. *American Journal of Psychiatry*, **157**, 751–8.

Drummond *et al.* (2005). *Alcohol Needs Assessment Research Project (ANARP): The 2004 National Needs Assessment for England*. Department of Health, London.

Ebrahim S *et al.* (1999). Comparison of binge drinking among pregnant and non-pregnant women, United States, 1991–1995. *American Journal of Obstetrics and Gynecology*, **180**, 1–7.

Frezza M *et al.* (1990). High blood alcohol levels in women. The role of decreased gastric alcohol dehydrogenase activity and first pass metabolism. *New England Journal of Medicine*, **322**, 95–9.

GENACIS Project Final Report (2005). *Gender, Culture and Alcohol Problems: A Multi-National Study*. Institute for Medical Informatics, Berlin.

Ginsburg E *et al.* (1996). Effects of alcohol ingestion on estrogens in post menopausal women. *Journal of the American Medical Association*, **276**, 1747–51.

Gomberg ES (1989). Suicide risk among women with alcohol problems. *American Journal of Public Health*, **79**, 1363–5.

Gray R and Henderson J (2006). *Review of the Fetal Effects of Prenatal Alcohol Exposure. Report to the Department of Health*. University of Oxford, Oxford.

Greenfield SF *et al.* (2007). Substance abuse treatment entry, retention, and outcome in women: a review of the literature. *Drug and Alcohol Dependence*, **86**, 1–21.

Hannan MT *et al.* (2000). Risk factors for longitudinal bone loss in elderly men and women: The Framingham osteoporosis study. *Journal of Bone and Mineral Research*, **15**, 710–20.

Harris C and Barraclough B (1997). Suicide as an outcome for mental disorders. *British Journal of Psychiatry*, **170**, 205–28.

Hibell B *et al.* (2009). *The 2007 ESPAD Report - Substance Use Among Students in 35 European Countries*. The Swedish Council for Information on Alcohol and Other Drugs (CAN), Stockholm.

HM Government (2007). *Safe. Sensible. Social, The Next Steps in the National Alcohol Strategy*. Department of Health, London.

Home Office (2009). *Crime in England and Wales 2007/08: Supplementary Tables: Nature of burglary, vehicle-related theft, personal and other household theft, vandalism, and violent crime*. Home Office, London.

Jacobsen LK *et al.* (2001). Substance use disorders in patients with posttraumatic stress disorder: a review of the literature. *American Journal of Psychiatry*, **158**, 1184–90.

Kendler KS *et al.* (2000). Childhood sexual abuse and adult psychiatric and substance use disorders in women. *Archives of General Psychiatry*, **57**, 953–9.

Kessler RC *et al.* (1997). Lifetime co-occurrence of DSM-III-R alcohol abuse and dependence with other psychiatric disorders in the National Comorbidity Survey. *Archives of General Psychiatry*, **54**, 313–21.

Leon DA and McCambridge J (2006). Liver cirrhosis mortality rates in Britain from 1950 to 2002: an analysis of routine data. *Lancet*, **367**, 52–6.

Lui S *et al.* (2008). Psychosocial interventions for women enrolled in alcohol treatment during pregnancy. *Cochrane Database of Systematic Reviews*, **3**, CD006753.

Merikangas KR *et al.* (1998). Comorbidity of substance misuse disorders with mood and anxiety disorders: results of the International Consortium in Psychiatric Epidemiology. *Addictive Behaviours*, **23**, 893–907.

Navajits LM *et al.* (1997). The link between substance abuse and posttraumatic stress disorder in women. *American Journal on Addictions*, **6**(4), 273–83.

NICE (2008). *Antenatal Care: Routine Care For The Health Pregnant Woman*. NICE, London.

ONS (2005). *General Household Survey*. The Stationery Office, London.

ONS (2006). *Statistics on Alcohol: England 2006*. The Stationery Office, London

Paltrow LM (1998). Punishing women for their behaviour during pregnancy: An approach that undermines the health of women and children. In: CL Wetherington and PM Roman (eds) *Drug Addiction Research and the Health of Women*, pp. 467–501. National Institute on Drug Abuse, Rockville, MD.

Plant MA and Plant ML (2006). *Binge Britain*. Oxford University Press, Oxford.

Project MATCH Research Group (1997). Matching alcoholism treatments to client heterogeneity: project MATCH posttreatment drinking outcomes. *Journal of Studies of Alcohol*, **58**, 7–29.

Randall CL *et al.* (1999). Telescoping of landmark events associated with drinking: a gender comparison. *Journal of Studies on Alcohol*, **60**, 252–60.

Royal College of Obstetricians and Gynaecologists (2006). *RCOG Statement No. 5 – Alcohol consumption and the outcomes of pregnancy*. Royal College of Obstetricians and Gynaecologists, London.

Saunders JB *et al.* (1993). Development of the Alcohol Use Disorders Identification Test (AUDIT): WHO collaborative project on early detection of persons with harmful alcohol consumption. *Addiction*, **88**, 791–804.

Seitz HK *et al.* (1993). Human gastric alcohol dehydrogenase activity: effects of age, sex and alcoholism. *Gut*, **34**, 1433–7.

Smith-Warner SA *et al.* (1998). Alcohol and breast cancer in women. A pooled analysis of cohort studies. *Journal of the American Medical Association*, **279**, 535–40.

Steinbauer JR *et al.* (1998). Ethnic and sex bias in primary care screening tests for alcohol use disorders. *Annals of Internal Medicine*, **129**, 353–62.

Stranges S *et al.* (2004). Differential effects of alcohol drinking pattern on liver enzymes in men and women. *Alcoholism, Clinical and Experimental Research*, **28**(6), 949–56.

Swift W *et al.* (1996). Characteristics of women with alcohol and other drug problems: findings of an Australian national survey. *Addiction*, **91**, 1141–50.

Taylor DJ (2006). *Alcohol consumption and the outcomes of pregnancy. Statement No 5*. Royal College of Obstetricians and Gynaecologists, London.

Thun MJ *et al.* (1997). Alcohol consumption and mortality among middle-aged and elderly U.S. adults. *New England Journal of Medicine*, **337**, 1705–14.

Weaver T *et al.* (2003). Comorbidity of substance misuse and mental illness in community mental health and substance misuse services. *British Journal of Psychiatry*, **183**, 304–13.

WHO (1992). *The International Classification of Diseases, (ICD-10): Classification of Mental and Behavioural Disorders: Clinical Descriptions and Diagnostic Guidelines. Tenth Revision*. WHO, Geneva.

Winhusen TM and Kropp F (2003). Psychosocial treatments for women with substance misuse disorders. *Obstetrics and Gynecology Clinics of North America*, **30**, 483–99.

Young AM *et al.* (2005). Drinking like a guy: frequent binge drinking among undergraduate women. *Substance Use & Misuse*, **40**, 241–67.

CHAPTER 23

Women and drugs

Ed Day and Erin Turner

Introduction

The abuse of psychoactive drugs by women can be an emotive issue, particularly when drug use is felt to conflict with 'traditional' female roles such as child rearing. Despite the fact that drug use is not a particularly new phenomenon, very little research attention has been paid to the unique characteristics of female drug users until recently. This chapter will briefly describe the epidemiology, aetiology, and treatment of illicit drug use, whilst focusing on aspects of the issue that are experienced differently by women.

Terminology

Addiction is not an all-or-none phenomenon, and can be thought of as existing along a spectrum of severity from misuse to harmful use/abuse to dependence. The point at which an individual moves from one category to another is often not clear, and it is not necessary to pass through all of the stages before reaching dependence. Classificatory systems such as ICD-10 or DSM-IV provide definitions for these terms (World Health Organization 1992; American Psychiatric Association 1994). 'Misuse' indicates that the substance is either not legal, or else is used in a way that does not comply with medical recommendations 'Harmful use' or 'abuse' is defined as a pattern of substance use that is causing damage to health but does not meet the criteria for dependence.

The term 'dependence' describes a chronic, recurring condition with physical, psychological, and social dimensions. It is characterized by a loss of control over one's substance use, and is usually associated with unsuccessful attempts to cut down or control use. Substances are taken in larger amounts or over a longer period than was intended, and considerable time is spent in obtaining, using, or recovering from the effects of the drugs. This leads to a reduction in other social, occupational, or recreational activities, but use continues despite the drug-related problems. Physical tolerance to the substance and a withdrawal syndrome on reduction or cessation of use are usually present. Most psychoactive substances, if used regularly, can produce some degree of dependence.

Epidemiology

It is reported that some 185 million people worldwide—3.1% of the global population or 4.3% of people aged 15 years and above—were consuming illicit drugs in the late 1990s (WHO/UNODC/UNAIDS Position Paper 2004). Around 4 million people use illicit drugs each year in the United Kingdom (UK), and the most commonly used drugs are cannabis, ecstasy and cocaine. In 2006, data from the United States (US) and the European Union suggested that 25–40% of all adults had tried cannabis at some point in their lives, 4–14% cocaine, 3% ecstasy, 3.5% amphetamines, and 0.8–1.5% heroin (European Monitoring Centre for Drugs and Drug Addiction 2007; Substance Abuse and Mental Health Services Administration 2007). Furthermore, 20% had made illicit use of prescribed medications, in particular pain killers, tranquilizers, stimulants, and sedatives. (Substance Abuse and Mental Health Services Administration 2007).

Although opiate addicts of the 19th century were very likely to be middle-class women who began their dependence through medical treatment, men have been considered much more likely to use, abuse, and become dependent on drugs in the last century (Zilberman and Blume 2005). Recent surveys of drug use in the general population in developed countries point to higher rates of use in men. In the US, the Epidemiological Catchment Area study surveyed the mental health status of a representative sample of adults and found that 25% of women reported any lifetime illicit drug use, compared to 36% of men. A similar ratio of women to men was found in the National Psychiatric Morbidity Survey 2000 in the UK (20% of women had ever previously used an illicit drug, compared with 33% of men [1: 1.7]) (Singleton *et al.* 2001). However, when younger people are surveyed, the gender differences are much smaller. For example, UK estimates of the numbers of people aged 11–15 years who report drug use in the past year indicate no significant gender difference (22% of boys and 20% of girls). These findings suggest that the rates of drug use among women relative to men may increase in the future (Zilberman and Blume 2005).

As we move along the spectrum of drug problems from use to abuse or dependence, so the ratio of women to men decreases. Hickman *et al.* (2004) used epidemiological methods to determine the prevalence of injecting drug use in three UK cities, and found ratios of men to women of between 2.5–4:1, depending on age cohort and location. Populations of individuals in treatment in the UK consistently show a 1:3 ratio of women to men (National Treatment Agency for Substance Misuse 2005). Possible reasons for these findings will be discussed later, although it is important to remember that female drug users are not a homogenous group, and other factors such as ethnicity, social class, and primary drug of use also have an impact on prevalence rates.

Aetiological factors

The aetiology of drug abuse and dependence is multifactorial, but there are some interesting differences between men and women in the likely interplay of genetic and environmental causative factors. Data from large-scale twin studies suggest that the pattern of genetic and environmental risk factors for psychoactive drug dependence is similar in males and females (Kendler *et al.* 2007). However, animal research points to differences between men and women in their biological responses to drugs. For example, in laboratory studies of animals given the opportunity to self-administer intravenous cocaine or heroin, females began self-administration sooner and administered larger amounts of the drugs (National Institute on Drug Abuse 1999). In humans, women have also been noted to show a greater subjective response to intranasal cocaine than men (Kosten *et al.* 1996), but cocaine-dependent women also have fewer abnormalities in blood flow to the brain than cocaine-dependent men. These findings may be mediated by changes in sex hormones, and oestrogen in particular (Kaufman *et al.* 2001).

The environmental factors associated with the initiation and development of drug use, abuse, and dependence also differ between men and women. Childhood trauma, and in particular childhood physical and sexual

abuse, is a significant predisposing risk factor for drug taking in women. A dose–response relationship has been reported in women between the severity of self-reported childhood sexual abuse and risk for developing drug abuse (Kendler *et al.* 2000). Furthermore, not only is prior assault a risk factor in the development of drug abuse, but drug use in turn is associated with further victimization (Kilpatrick *et al.* 1997). Drug using women often report multiple sources of violence, and although drug use is a way of numbing oneself to the trauma, it also erodes a sense of self-worth, importance, competence, and control (Rosenbaum *et al.* 2005). A recent UK review of the impact of abuse on engagement and retention rates for women in substance use treatment has highlighted 'the need for assessment of domestic abuse to inform practice responses and the need for staff training in order to identify and address domestic abuse in an informed way' (Galvani *et al.* 2007).

Female heroin misusers are more likely to live with another drug user, and have a drug-using sexual partner than male heroin abusers (Gossop *et al.* 1994). Initial heroin use in women has been found to be highly influenced by a male sexual partner (Hser *et al.* 1987). Other illicit drugs may have other sociocultural factors associated with their initiation in women. Stimulant drugs can be used as a weight-control measure, and social pressure for the perfect body may be more focused on women than men.

Course of the problem

Initiation into illicit drug use does not lead inevitably to regular and problematic use for everyone. Vulnerability to use is highest among young people, and individuals addicted to opioids and stimulants often become dependent on these drugs in their early twenties and remain intermittently dependent for decades. Biological, psychological, sociological, and economic factors determine when a person will start taking drugs. However, once dependence is established there are usually repeated cycles of cessation and relapse extending over decades (National Consensus Development Panel on Effective Medical Treatment of Opiate Addiction 1998). In one long-term outcome study that conducted a 24-year follow-up of 581 male opioid users, 29% were currently abstinent, but 28% had died, 23% had positive urine tests for opioids, and 18% were in prison (Hser *et al.* 1993). Women have been reported to have an earlier age of initial use of illicit drugs, younger age at first treatment, and more rapid development of dependence (Greenfield *et al.* 2003).

Drug-related problems

Women have a greater vulnerability than men to physical, mental, and social consequences of substance use. In the UK National Treatment Outcome Research Study (NTORS), women reported more frequent cocaine use than men, greater health problems, and increased likelihood of having a drug-using partner and responsibility for children (Stewart *et al.* 2003). Drug use, abuse, and dependence may cause a range of physical complications, often associated with intravenous use. Sharing injecting equipment may lead to the transmission of infections such as hepatitis B, hepatitis C, or HIV. The number of AIDS cases in women has increased threefold since the mid 1980s (Greenfield *et al.* 2003). Drugs such as opioids, stimulants, or cannabis can cause disruptions of the menstrual cycle, and cocaine-dependent women may experience galactorrhoea, amenorrhoea, and infertility, possibly due to the effect on prolactin levels. Women may also be more sensitive to the cardiovascular effects of stimulant drugs (Greenfield *et al.* 2003).

Mental health disorders are common in those with drug abuse or dependence. The odds of a mental health disorder were 4.5 times higher than the odds of those without a history of a drug disorder in the Epidemiologic Catchment Area (ECA) study (Regier *et al.* 1990). The rates of affective disorders and anxiety are higher in women than men in the general population (Chandler and McCaul 2003), and rates of psychiatric comorbidity (particularly affective, anxiety, and eating disorders) are also higher among women with drug misuse disorders than men. This is significant as a co-occurring psychiatric disorder has the potential to exaggerate the negative health and social consequences of drug abuse or dependence. Rates of suicide attempts are higher in drug-dependent women than in alcohol-dependent women or drug-dependent men (Zilberman *et al.* 2003).

Injecting drug use

Injecting drug use has symbolic importance to both drug users and the general public as a whole, as the move to intravenous use often represents more serious levels of use. Women are less likely than men to inject, but have a higher incidence of sharing needles and injecting equipment. Women who do inject may do so more often, and with higher doses than men (Oretti and Gregory 2005). Women sharing injecting paraphernalia may do so because they do not consider sharing with a sexual partner harmful. This may explain the

studies which report higher rates of HIV and hepatitis B and C infection among women.

There are mixed reports as to whether there is a difference between men and women in the length of time that drugs are used by other routes before the transition to injecting (Oretti and Gregory 2005). Research has often shown that people are initiated into injecting by someone else, and women appear to be more frequently injected first by a sexual partner (Crofts *et al.* 1996). When it comes to drugs, women often have an inequitable power relationship with men, and are more likely to obtain drugs from their sexual partner than are men. The practice of peer injecting illicit drugs places women recipients at risk of physical, economic, and emotional abuse from their male intimate partner injectors (Wright *et al.* 2007). Women also appear to have more difficulties with injecting than men, and have more resulting health problems, e.g. deep vein thrombosis, abscesses, and other local complications.

Drug misuse and pregnancy

The National Pregnancy and Health Survey gathered self-report data from 2613 women who had given birth in 1992 which found that over 5% admitted using illicit substances during pregnancy. It is difficult to interpret such data due to the twin problems of under-reporting due to shame and fear of stigmatization, and a frequent failure of health professionals to enquire about, or recognize, drug dependence. However, as approximately one-third of drug users are female, and that the majority of these are of childbearing age, the potential scope and significance of the problem is self-evident.

Concealed pregnancy is more common in women who abuse drugs, and late presentation to healthcare services is common. A complex interplay of factors may explain these findings, including the high incidence of menstrual abnormalities in this group, and the (erroneous) belief in the heroin subculture that a woman is unlikely to become pregnant while using heroin. Hence neglect of contraception is common, and amenorrhoea, morning sickness, and fatigue mistaken for signs of withdrawal or contaminated drugs.

Even if the woman is aware that she is pregnant, medical services are often avoided due to feelings of shame or fear. Interviews with pregnant women suggest that the main barriers to accessing antenatal care in this group are lack of transportation, lengthy waits for appointments, having too many other problems (e.g. housing or legal issues), the belief that prenatal care is unnecessary, fear of medical examination, lack of childcare for other children, and fear of judgemental staff (Mikhail *et al.* 1999). The trauma of having gone through previous child protection proceedings will inevitably lead to reluctance to contact healthcare agencies. Late presentation is a particular problem as early engagement in antenatal care is important to improve outcome and general well-being of mother and baby.

Pregnancy-related health risks for the mother and baby

Poor baseline physical health amongst problem drug users is accentuated during pregnancy, and obstetric management is complicated by anaemia, cardiac disease, depression and anxiety, blood-borne viruses and other sexually transmitted diseases, poorly controlled hypertension and diabetes, pneumonia, abscesses, poor dental hygiene, pneumonia, and tuberculosis (Kaltenbach *et al.* 1998). In addition, many have to cope with single parenthood, lack of social support, poverty, homelessness, lack of education, domestic violence, stress, and low self-esteem. These problems often render the woman less receptive to treatment and can interfere with their ability to get to appointments on time, prioritize their own health above their drug use and other housing or relationship difficulties, and can often jeopardize the therapeutic relationship. Engaging in prostitution and theft to fund their drug habit will often take precedence over seeking antenatal care.

There are a number of drug-related effects on the child, some caused directly by the drug, others linked to factors associated with a drug-taking lifestyle such as malnutrition, poverty, infection, and the intoxication–withdrawal cycle. The vast majority of heroin users are also cigarette smokers, which has been linked to decreased infant birth weight, intrauterine growth retardation, and prematurity. Injecting drug users expose their unborn child to the risk of a blood-borne viral infection. Mothers who are infected with HIV and hepatitis B and C can pass these infections to their baby *in utero* through vertical transmission, during childbirth, or through breastfeeding. HIV infection carries a significant mortality for infants, and hepatitis B and C can lead to chronic liver disease, cirrhosis, and death for an infected child.

As a general principle, substance misuse during the first trimester of pregnancy can affect fetal organogenesis, whereas use in the second and third trimesters can result in growth retardation and impairments in the newborn. Continued drug use close to term can cause premature birth, neonatal abstinence syndrome, and has been linked with sudden infant death syndrome

(SIDS). Specific effects of a range of illicit substances can be found elsewhere (Day *et al.* 2005).

Management issues of drug misuse in pregnancy

It is important to note that drug use in itself does not render a mother unloving or incapable of looking after her child. Qualitative research with pregnant drug-using women shows that they have a strong responsibility for their children, and nurturing is a key goal. There is an awareness that drugs are a drain on their attention on their children's needs or finances, and various strategies are attempted to maintain mothering standards (Rosenbaum *et al.* 2005). A balanced, holistic, and non-judgemental approach should be adopted by healthcare professionals in dealing with these vulnerable women, whilst maintaining an awareness of the needs of the child. The welfare of the unborn child must be considered from the outset, with social services involvement if it is deemed necessary. This presents a conflict of interests as contacting social services may put strain on the therapeutic relationship, so it must be done sensitively, making the mother aware of the referral.

Women of childbearing age already engaged in drug services should be offered contraceptive advice, including education on safe sexual practice. Needle exchange programmes, advice on safer injecting practice, and testing for and immunization against blood-borne viruses are extremely important harm reduction measures. The provision of healthy lifestyle and dietary advice, including support in reducing tobacco and alcohol consumption, are important goals.

A detailed assessment and comprehensive care plan when a pregnant woman presents at services is essential. The woman's physical, mental, and social health must be considered in the initial assessment and in formulating the management plan. Every effort should be made to ensure multidisciplinary working, with good communication between health professionals, namely the drug specialist, the general practitioner, midwife, health visitor, obstetrician, and social services. In view of the complexities of need and numbers of different professionals involved, it is wise to appoint a care coordinator, one of whose roles would be to organize case conferences. The mother and her partner should be involved in all decision-making. Of key importance is maintenance of contact with the woman throughout her pregnancy and in the antenatal period, therefore particular emphasis should be placed on building a trusting relationship with the woman and offering support where necessary. The recommended treatment for women using opioids during pregnancy is methadone stabilization and maintenance. There is a body of evidence showing that the outcome for the baby is improved with methadone compared to heroin alone (Finnegan 1991).

Treatment

Drug dependence is a complicated problem, and therefore, effective treatment services incorporate several components. Although some people resolve their problems without recourse to specialist treatment (Sobell *et al.* 2000), there is a strong evidence base that shows that the outcomes of treatment for drug use and crime are positive and clinically meaningful (Gossop 2006). Pharmacological, psychological, and social interventions are combined in a variety of different ways by treatment services, but there are two broad modalities of treatment: those with a focus on reducing harm and stabilization, and those focused on assisting the user to become abstinent from all addictive substances. In reality, this is a somewhat arbitrary split, as most patients require a different approach at different stages of their addiction 'career'.

Harm reduction and maintenance

Although long-term abstinence from all drugs is likely to produce the best outcome, this approach is not always acceptable to the individual. Setting more limited treatment targets can be effective at both an individual and population level, and the 'harm reduction' model has evolved in the last 30 years. Injecting any drug carries a significant risk of infection, and advice about improved injection technique and cleaning of equipment can be effective in reducing this risk, particularly when combined with the provision of clean needles and syringes via local needle exchange schemes.

Maintenance or 'substitute' prescribing implies the use of a legally prescribed drug of known purity and quality instead of an illegal drug. Methadone maintenance therapy (MMT) has been used for 40 years in the management of heroin dependence, and research has demonstrated clear benefits in reducing illicit opioid use, HIV infection, and criminal activity (Marsch 1998; National Institute for Health and Clinical Excellence 2007). The prescription of methadone, or latterly buprenorphine, can act as an inducement for the patient to attend a treatment programme where other problems that originally led to drug use may be addressed (e.g. housing, relationship, or employment difficulties).

Maintenance treatment may last indefinitely, but ultimately reduction of the dose of methadone and detoxification will be possible.

Psychological treatments have two broad aims: firstly to assist individuals in making changes in their drug using behaviour, and secondly to address coexisting mental health disorders (Wanigaratne *et al.* 2005). Effective techniques for altering drug-using behaviour include motivational enhancement therapy, cognitive behavioural techniques (including skills training and relapse prevention), the community reinforcement approach, contingency management, and behavioural-couples therapy (Wanigaratne *et al.* 2005).

Achieving abstinence

An alternative to 'maintaining' the patient on a medication is to assist them in stopping altogether. Outpatient 'drug-free' services are common in the US, partly due to the structure of the licensing system for opioid medication, and partly due to higher levels of stimulant use. They vary in the type and intensity of services offered, and are often more suitable for individuals who are employed or who have extensive social support. Low-intensity programmes may offer little more than education and encouragement, and group counselling is emphasized in many. Other outpatient models, such as intensive day treatment, can be comparable to residential programmes in services and effectiveness (Adler *et al.* 2003). In the UK, it is increasingly rare that community outpatient services just offer abstinence-based approaches, and most will support harm reduction, maintenance, or abstinence goals as appropriate.

Narcotics Anonymous (NA) is a direct descendent of Alcoholics Anonymous (AA), and may have a greater number of drug users involved in its programme worldwide than any other treatment initiative (Gossop 2006). NA regards addiction as a relapsing illness with complete abstinence as the only treatment goal. By working through each of the 12 steps the individual comes to acknowledge to themselves and other people the harm substance use has caused to themselves and others, and where possible to make amends (Wanigaratne *et al.* 2005). Residential/therapeutic community services owe their origins to the influence of AA, and they share a common focus on abstinence as the over-riding goal of treatment (Gossop 2006). They see recovery from addiction as requiring a profound restructuring of thinking, personality, and lifestyle, involving more than just giving up drug-taking behaviour.

Treatment of drug use disorders in women

The importance of gender-specific and gender-sensitive issues has only recently been highlighted in research in the drug treatment field. Women are represented in consistently lower numbers than men in all countries with developed treatment systems for substance misuse. Furthermore, there is a relatively low proportion of women in treatment compared with the prevalence of these disorders in women in the general population (Greenfield *et al.* 2003). One explanation might be that women tend to define their problems as physical or mental health problems and so seek care in the physical or mental health sectors (Greenfield *et al.* 2003).

There is also a range of possible barriers to entering treatment for women. Childcare issues are a major problem, and surveys of drug misuse treatment in the US have estimated that only 13% of services offer child-care services, and this figure is even lower in the UK. In 2007, only five residential treatment services in England or Wales accepted women accompanied by their children. Services in the US have also had a hesitancy to treat pregnant women, although this group are prioritized in the UK (National Treatment Agency for Substance Misuse 2006). Women with substance misuse problems have a real fear of their children being removed by social services and other professionals (Galvani *et al.* 2007). Treating clinicians have to strike a difficult balance between helping women and protecting 'at-risk' children, and at times popular media attention has served to demonize pregnant drug users—e.g. the 'crack baby' issue in the 1980s—see Rosenbaum and Murphy (2005, p. 1079). Resistance to treatment can also come from a sexual partner, and can be overt (i.e. violence) or more subtle (i.e. refusing to look after children, or assist in transportation) (Rosenbaum and Murphy (2005).

However despite these issues, an overview of women in treatment by the National Treatment Agency for Substance Misuse (2005) found that:

> While there are clear indications that women enter treatment at different points in their drug using careers, with different needs and different problems, there is no clear evidence to suggest that women are generally under-represented in treatment services in England. The indications from other markers would suggest that, if anything, women in the UK may be more likely to seek treatment than their male equivalents, and that they do so earlier in their problem drug-using careers.

Substance misuse treatment services designed specifically for women, such as provision of childcare services, prenatal care services, women-only treatment, mental health services, and supplemental services and workshops addressing women-focused topics, can be beneficial in improving treatment outcomes. Improved outcomes include changes in substance use, mental health symptoms, perinatal/birth outcomes, employment, self-reported health status, and HIV risk reduction (Brady and Ashley 2005). Unfortunately, although the substance abuse treatment system has increasingly recognized the need for such services, they are still available only to a limited number of clients. In the late 1990s only 6% of all US services served women only, 37% offered special programmes for women, and 19% special programmes for pregnant women (Brady and Ashley 2005).

Outcomes of drug misuse

Longer substance abuse treatment episodes and successful completion of treatment are usually related to positive outcomes (Simpson and Sells 1990). Research suggests that gender is not necessarily a predictor of retention, completion, or outcome once an individual begins treatment (Greenfield *et al.* 2003). However, there are predictors of treatment retention and some of these are specific to women. Among women enrolled in treatment, service type and some pretreatment characteristics such as referral source, psychological functioning, personal stability, and number of children may be important predictors of length of stay or treatment completion. Gender-specific programmes may enhance treatment retention among some subgroups of women (Greenfield *et al.* 2003).

References

Adler M *et al.* (2003). The treatment of drug addiction: a review. In: AW Graham *et al.* (eds) *Principles of Addiction Medicine*, third edition, pp. 419–28. American Society of Addiction Medicine, Chevy Chase, MD.

American Psychiatric Association (1994). *Diagnostic and Statistical Manual of Mental Disorder*. APA, Washington, DC.

Brady TM and Ashley OS (2005). *Women in substance abuse treatment: results from the alcohol and drug services study (ADSS)*. Substance Abuse and Mental Health Services Administration, Office of Applied Studies, Rockville, MD.

Chandler G and McCaul ME (2003). Co-occurring psychiatric disorders in women with addictions. *Obstetrics and Gynecology Clinics of North America*, **30**, 469–81.

Crofts N *et al.* (1996). The first hit: circumstances surrounding initiation into injecting. *Addiction*, **91**(8), 1187–96.

Day E and George S (2005). Management of drug misuse in pregnancy. *Advances in Psychiatric Treatment*, **11**(4), 253–61.

European Monitoring Centre for Drugs and Drug Addiction (2007). *Annual Report 2007: The State of the Drugs Problem in Europe*. EMCDDA, Lisbon.

Finnegan LP (1991). Treatment issues for opioid-dependent women during the perinatal period. *Journal of Psychoactive Drugs*, **23**(2), 191–201.

Galvani S and Humphreys C (2007). *The Impact of Violence and Abuse on Engagement and Retention Rates for Women in Substance Use Treatment*. National Treatment Agency for Substance Misuse, London.

Gossop M *et al.* (1994). Sex differences in patterns of drug taking behaviour. A study at a London community drug team. *British Journal of Psychiatry*, **164**(1), 101–4.

Gossop M (2006). *Treating Drug Misuse Problems: Evidence of Effectiveness*. National Treatment Agency for Substance Misuse, London.

Greenfield SF *et al.* (2003). Epidemiology of substance use disorders in women. *Obstetrics and Gynecology Clinics of North America*, **30**, 413–46.

Hickman M *et al.* (2004). Injecting drug use in Brighton, Liverpool, and London: best estimates of prevalence and coverage of public health indicators. *Journal of Epidemiological Community Health*, **58**(9), 766–71.

Hser Y *et al.* (1987). Sex differences in addict careers. 1. Initiation of use *American Journal of Drug Alcohol Abuse*, **13**(1&2), 33–57.

Hser Y *et al.* (1993). A 24-year follow-up of California narcotics addicts. *Archives in General Psychiatry*, **50**, 577–84.

Kaltenbach K *et al.* (1998). Opioid dependence during pregnancy. *Obstetrics and Gynaecology Clinics of North America*, **25**(1), 139–51.

Kaufman MJ *et al.* (2001). Cocaine-induced cerebral vasoconstriction differs as a function of sex and menstrual cycle phase. *Biological Psychiatry*, **49**(9), 774–81.

Kendler KS *et al.* (2000). Childhood sexual abuse and adult psychiatric and substance use disorders in women: an epidemiological and co-twin control analysis. *Archives of General Psychiatry*, **57**, 953–9.

Kendler KS *et al.* (2007). Specificity of genetic and environmental risk factors for symptoms of cannabis, cocaine, alcohol, caffeine, and nicotine dependence. *Archives of General Psychiatry*, **64**(11), 1313–20.

Kilpatrick DG *et al.* (1997). A 2-year longitudinal analysis of the relationships between violent assault and substance use in women. *Journal of Consulting and Clinical Psychology*, **65**(5), 834–47.

Kosten TR *et al.* (1996). Gender differences in response to intranasal cocaine administration to humans. *Biological Psychiatry*, **39**, 147–8.

Marsch LA (1998). The efficacy of methadone maintenance interventions in reducing illicit opiate use, HIV risk behaviour and criminality: a meta-analysis. *Addiction*, **93**(4), 515–32.

Mikhail BI *et al.* (1999) Perceived impediments to prenatal care among low-income women. *Western Journal of Nursing Research*, **21**(3), 335–5.

National Consensus Development Panel on Effective Medical (1998) Treatment of Opiate Addiction. Effective medical treatment of opiate addiction. *Journal of the American Medical Association*, **280**(22), 1936–43.

National Institute for Health and Clinical Excellence (2007). *Methadone and buprenorphine for the management of opioid dependence. NICE Technology Appraisal Guidance*. National Institute for Health and Clinical Excellence, London.

National Institute on Drug Abuse (1999). *Gender differences in drug abuse risks and treatment. NIDA Notes 15(4)*. NIDA, Bethesda, MD.

National Treatment Agency for Substance Misuse (2005). *Women in Drug Treatment Services. Report No. 6*. NTA, London.

National Treatment Agency for Substance Misuse. (2006) *Models of Care for the Treatment of Adult Drug Misusers. Update 2006*. National Treatment Agency for Substance Misuse, London.

Oretti R and Gregory P (2005). Women and injecting. In: R Pates *et al.* (eds) *Injecting Illicit Drugs*, pp. 59–68. Blackwell, Oxford.

Regier DA *et al.* (1990). Comorbidity of mental disorders with alcohol and other drug abuse. Results from the epidemiologic catchment area (ECA) study. *Journal of the American Medical Association*, **264**, 2511–18.

Rosenbaum M and Murphy S (2005). Women's research and policy issues. In: Lowinson JH *et al.* (eds) *Substance Abuse: A Comprehensive Textbook*, pp. 1075–92. Lippincott Williams & Wilkins, Philadelphia, PA.

Simpson D and Sells SB (1990). *Opioid Addiction and Treatment: A 12-Year Follow-Up*. Robert E. Krieger Publishing Co, Malabar, FL.

Singleton N *et al.* (2001). *Psychiatric Morbidity Among Adults Living in Private Households*. TSO, London.

Sobell LC *et al.* (2000). Natural recovery from alcohol and drug problems: methodological review of the research with suggestions for future directions. *Addiction*, **95**(5), 749–64.

Stewart D *et al.* (2003). Similarities in outcomes for men and women after drug misuse treatment: result of the National Treatment Outcome Research Study (NTORS). *Drug and Alcohol Review*, **22**(1), 35–41.

Substance Abuse and Mental Health Services Administration (2007). *Results from the 2006 National Survey on Drug Use and Health: National Findings*. Office of Applied Studies; Report No.: NSDUH Series H-32, No. SMA 07–4293. DHHS Publication, Rockville, MD.

Wanigaratne S *et al.* (2005). *The Effectiveness of Psychological Therapies on Drug Misusing Clients. Report No.: 11*. National Treatment Agency for Substance Misuse, London.

WHO/UNODC/UNAIDS Position Paper (2004). *Substitution maintenance therapy in the management of opioid dependence and HIV/AIDS prevention*. World Health Organization, Geneva.

World Health Organization (1992). *The ICD-10 Classification of Mental and Behavioural Disorders. Tenth revision.* WHO, Geneva.

Wright NMJ *et al.* (2007). Is peer injecting a form of intimate partner abuse? A qualitative study of the experiences of women drug users. *Health & Social Care in the Community,* **15**(5), 417–25.

Zilberman ML *et al.* (2003). Discriminating drug-dependent women from alcoholic women and drug-dependent men. *Addictive Behaviors,* **28**(7), 1343–9.

Zilberman ML, Blume SB (2005). Drugs and Women. In: JH Lowinson *et al.* (eds) *Substance Abuse: A Comprehensive Textbook,* pp.1064–75. Lippincott Williams & Wilkins, Philadelphia, PA.

CHAPTER 24

The sociocultural and personal dimension of eating disorders

Mervat Nasser

Eating disorders: the sociocultural argument

Food is considered a 'cultural system', and eating patterns are acknowledged as culturally shaped and socially controlled (Caplan 1997). Roland Barthes viewed food as symbolic of the entire social environment and regarded it a language or a form of communication between people (Barthes 1975). Hence, food practices have little to do with hunger or health needs than with the conditions of subjective identity and social relationships.

Food restraint, fear of fatness, and the pursuit of thinness are modern terms that are now used interchangeably to refer to the pathological dieting behaviour integral to anorexia nervosa. The anorexic syndrome was first reported in the latter part of the 19th century by William Gull (1874) in Britain and Charles Lasègue (1873) in France; both described a distinct state of self-starvation peculiar to young women and likely to be caused by a host of emotional factors. It was noted, however, that nearly half of the anorexic population exhibited symptoms of binge eating following periods of self-starvation. Russell (1979) referred to this group as having 'bulimia nervosa' and described it as a variant of anorexia nervosa characterized with periodic over-eating, self- induced vomiting, or purging to compensate for the effects of over-eating. Both anorexia and bulimia nervosa were later subsumed under 'eating disorders'—a term that was introduced to acknowledge the full spectrum of eating psychopathology. The concept has been incorporated in both the American Diagnostic Manual (DSM-IV, American Psychiatric Association 1993) and the International Classification of Mental and Behavioural Disorders (ICD-10, WHO 1992).

Eating disorders are considered unique among psychiatric disorders in the degree to which social and cultural factors influence their epidemiology and development. The nature of the eating disorder syndrome and the fact that it clearly merges with the prevalent and the culturally acceptable behaviour of dieting called for an interpretation that is grounded in the culture we live in. The phenomenon was therefore understandably linked to the cultivation of a certain type of body ideal and the promotion of thinness values through media, fashion, and diet industry. Subclinical cases or partial syndrome that merge with normal dieting behaviour were generally estimated to be five times more common than the full-blown syndromes (Dancyger and Garfinkel 1995).The finding was consistent with the 'spectrum hypothesis' of eating disorders and ran parallel to reported steady increase in the rate of their occurrence in the latter half of the 20th century (Lucas *et al.* 1991).

The sociocultural model of eating disorders was further supported by the susceptibility of certain subcultural groups to develop these disorders, such as dancers, models, and athletes, where the demand for thinness is endemic (Garner and Garfinkel 1980; King and Mezey 1987; Weight and Noakes 1987).

This epidemiological research has also shown a clear and consistent 'gender bias' where women were found to be ten times more at risk for such disorders than men. 'Fat' is considered integral to women's biology, and has the tendency to concentrate in certain areas of the woman's body, particularly those with sexual significance like the breasts and hips. Also a threshold of body fat is an essential requisite for menstruation.

In view of this skewed distribution, feminist theorists posited that these disorders represent an answer to the dilemma women face today, being torn between old and new expectations of their gender role. The thinness ideal came to be seen as metaphorical synthesis between the old notions of attractiveness and fashionability and the new modern values of autonomy, achievement, and self-control (Orbach 1986; Malson 1998). This conflict over gender role produces in women a sense of 'gender ambivalence', i.e. a term used to describe the societal ambivalence of the female role and the ambiguities felt by women, particularly during periods of historical and cultural transition (Silvertein and Perlick 1995; also see Chapter 28, this volume). Even among the small proportion of men who develop such disorders, a disproportionate number have doubts or uncertainties about their sexuality and gender identity problems (Williamson 1999).

Another finding that emerged in the 1990s, was the apparent increase in the prevalence of eating disorders in proportion to the level of 'urbanization' in any given society (Rathner and Messner 1993; Hoek *et al.* 1995), This was explained on the basis of social mobility and changes within family structure with tendency towards nuclearization. Also, as cities urbanized, eating patterns, food preferences, and meal times seem to change with the inevitable rise in the rates of obesity and a subsequent increase in weight consciousness and disordered patterns of eating (Nasser and Katzman 1999).

So, within this framework, cultural, subcultural, and intracultural risks in the pathogenesis of eating disorders are easily discernable. The apparent absence of these disorders in non-Western cultures and societies; added—at first—another support and made some regard the phenomenon of eating disorders as exclusively bound to the Western culture (Prince 1983) (see Box 24.1).

Eating disorders: the global perspective

The culture-boundedness/specificity of eating pathology stood first on the assumption that societal mandates regarding thinness were rooted in Western cultural values and conflicts. The theory of culture-boundedness was based on the scarcity of these disorders as judged by the few published reports in this respect. This was thought to reflect perceived differences in aesthetic standards between West and non-West. In contrast to the Western ideal of thinness, non-Western societies were seen to favour plumpness and associate with it positive attributes of wealth,

---

> **Box 24.1** Eating disorders: the sociocultural argument
>
> Epidemiological evidence: a steady increase over the past 50 years.
>
> - Nature of psychopathology: symbolic of notions of thinness cherished and promoted by culture.
> - Continuum of morbidity: spectrum of severity/merges with culturally acceptable behaviours.
> - Gender specific: women at risk/conflicting gender roles.
> - Subcultural variations: more prevalent in dancers, models, and athletes.
> - Intracultural variations: more prevalent in urban than rural areas.
> - Cross-cultural variations: assumed rare in non-Western cultures (different aesthetic values, differentials of wealth, preservation of traditional gender roles).

---

fertility, and femininity. The fact that the majority of these societies also belong to Third World economies, made them appear protected from developing a disorder commonly associated with wealth and affluence. Also, the role of women in non-Western societies continued to be seen within a restricted framework of the stereotyped and the traditional, and therefore considered immune from the challenges of modernity that women in the West face (Nasser 1997, 2000).

In spite of these considerations, there is now an increasing body of evidence that challenges the rarity of these disorders in non-Western cultures and societies. Research among different ethnicities living in the United Kingdom (UK) and United States (US) showed the presence of these disorders in such groups. Also a surge of publications in the 1990s, from different countries in the world suggests that eating disorders are increasingly becoming a global phenomenon. Most of these studies aimed to explore the impact of immigration, acculturation, and overall cultural change in the pathogenesis of these disorders.

Eating disorders in ethnic minority groups

The experience of women from other ethnicities and cultures with disordered eating behaviours has accumulated after the publication of several case reports in both the UK and the US (Jones *et al.* 1980; Andersen and Hay 1985; Thomas and Szmukler 1985; Hsu 1987;

Lacey and Dolan 1988). These authors observed the psychological problems of those girls who were reported to have high aspirations and clear achievement orientation. They were also described as being conflicted over their 'racial identity' with a powerful urge to fit into the host society, hoping for integration through conforming to the prevailing ideal of thinness/beauty. Hence, immigration and acculturation were regarded in a great number of these studies to be behind the immigrants' susceptibility to developing weight concerns. A correlation was found between the level of acculturation and morbid concern over weight (Smith and Krejci 1991; Davis and Katzman 1998). Dieting behaviour was found to be equal among black and white females in the US (Gray *et al.* 1987), and dysfunctional eating patterns were found to be more prevalent in the African-Caribbean population in Britain than their white counterparts (Reiss 1996).

In some of these cases, the desire to fit into a culturally desirable weight was not only a licence to approval/acceptance but also served the need of the immigrants to correct a negative stereotyped image of their race (Davis and Katzman 1999). The issue of 'racial identity' and its relationship to eating disorders was further studied among black South African women after the fall of the apartheid regime, where the reported increase of eating disorders following the political change was linked to a sense of shifting identity and altered self-conception among those South African females (Szabo *et al.* 1995; Le Grange *et al.* 1998).

From these reports and studies it is clear that women from minority groups—contrary to the initial assumption—could be at a higher risk of developing eating psychopathology than originally assumed. The following are the risk factors encountered in these groups:

- Confused/disturbed racial identity
- High level of acculturation and assimilation of the prevailing aesthetic standard
- Desire for acceptance/approval through conforming to the host society's values
- Desire for success, achievement, and the fulfilment of higher aspirations
- A strong need to correct a negative and traditionally stereotyped racial image.

Eating disorders across cultures, ethnicities, and societies

The majority of research into eating disorders across cultures was modelled on community surveys carried out in the West. Most of these studies were structured around a recurring binary hypothesis aiming to identify if eating psychopathology did exist in non-Western societies or not, as well as the relationship between exposure to Western cultural norms and values and increased vulnerability to such disorders. Some of the earliest studies were carried out in Egypt (Nasser 1986, 1994; Dolan *et al.* 1990), Greece (Fichter *et al.* 1983), and Turkey (Fichter *et al.* 1988), where high rate of disordered eating behaviour was found among those who appeared to be more influenced by the idealized Western cultural norms in this respect.

In Israel, where both Arab and Jewish school girls were examined, the Kibbutz women were found to have the highest risk for eating morbidity followed by the Arab Muslims (Apter *et al.* 1994). The effect of combined religious influence and exposure to Western culture values was later explored in a number of studies with evidence of equal or higher rates of disordered eating behaviour in Muslim women in the UAE and Iran (Abou-Saleh *et al.* 1998; Nabakht and Dezkhan 2000).

Studies of the eating disorders in Asian groups, was initially part and parcel of studies carried out on 'Asian' immigrants in the UK or in other countries in the West. The Asians constitute the largest immigrant population in the UK and comprise Indians, Pakistanis, and Bangladeshis. The most notable of these studies is the one conducted by Mumford and Whitehouse (1988) on Asian schoolgirls in Bradford which showed Asian girls to have higher risk to eating disorders than the Caucasian group, particularly girls from traditional/Islamic backgrounds. However, in another study conducted in Lahore, Pakistan, the girls who were most Westernized appeared to be more at risk of developing an eating disorder (Mumford *et al.* 1991).More cases of bulimic behaviour were also found among Asian schoolgirls than Caucasians in further studies conducted on mixed population of school girls in the UK (Ahmed *et al.* 1994; McCourt and Waller 1995).

Cultural variations on how 'Asian' is defined between the US and UK, suggest that studies of Asian populations in these countries actually differ in the types of samples they are examining. While in the UK, these investigations typically involve individuals who are ethnically south Asian (i.e. from India, Pakistan, and Sri Lanka, etc.), in the US the term 'Asian American' refers to East Asian and South Asian countries. When Asian women attending American schools in the United States were compared to those in Hong Kong, the former group showed evidence of increased vulnerability to abnormal eating behaviours (Davis and

Katzman 1998). Also, disordered eating patterns and body dissatisfaction were, on the whole, reported to be on the increase in Hong Kong (Katzman 1995; Lee and Lee 1996). It was argued however, that the over-reliance on the 'fear of fatness' as a diagnostic criterion in eating psychopathology could have led to an overall underestimation of the magnitude of these problems in societies like China, India, and Japan (Katzman and Lee 1997). They added that the weight/thinness-focused approach to the eating disorder phenomenon failed to take into account the cultural meaning of 'self-starvation' in a society like China, for instance, where the food denial is symbolic of loss of voice in a social world perceived to be oppressive (Lee 2001). The same was argued in a survey of eating disorders in Singapore (Pok and Tian 1994).

On the other hand, Japan reported an increased tendency towards anorexic behaviours since the Second World War, attributed to changes in traditional family structure in the post-war period (Ishikawa 1965). This was followed by several studies which confirmed this trend (Suematsu *et al.* 1985; Kamata *et al.* 1987; Mukai *et al.* 1994). The level of urbanization was found to affect this incidence with higher rates of these disorders in cities than in rural areas of Japan (Ohzeki *et al.* 1990).

A similar situation was found in Latin America with eating disorders emerging as a significant problem in urban areas in particular. Cases of anorexia nervosa were reported in Chile and Brazil (Pumarino and Vivanco1982; Nunes *et al.* 1991), and in Argentina an 'epidemic of eating disorders' in Buenos Aries was reported in the 1990s and was related to ambiguities and conflicting cross-currents regarding national and that of female identity in particular (Meehan and Katzman 2001)

However, one of the most interesting findings of transcultural research in the field of eating disorders was the emergence of eating psychopathology in Eastern Europe following the politico-economic change. Eating disorders that were largely unreported in Eastern Europe before the collapse of the communist regimes began to appear in eastern European literature. High rates of abnormal eating attitudes as measured by the Eating Attitude Test Questionnaire (EAT) were reported in Hungary, Poland, and the Czech Republic (Szabo and Tury 1991; Krch 1994; Rathner *et al.* 1995; Warczyk-Bisaga and Dolan 1996) and for detailed review of this published research refer to Nasser (1997), Nasser and Katzman (1999) and Gordon (2001) (Fig. 24.1).

It is important, however, to mention that several doubts were raised about the validity of using the

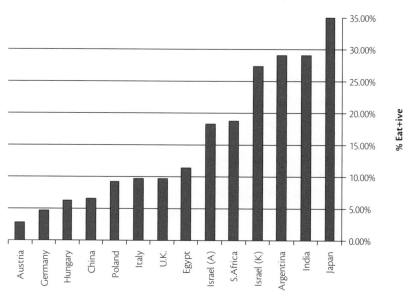

Fig. 24.1 Percentage of dieting/abnormal eating attitudes worldwide

Countries

EAT in different cultural settings, particularly its susceptibility to cultural misinterpretation (King and Bhugra 1989). Despite those concerns the use of EAT in these studies proved to be helpful in facilitating research and allowing possible comparisons to be made between cultures in this respect (Nasser 1995, Nasser 1999).

Eating disorders: marker of culture change

From what has been advanced so far, it is possible to argue that countries in the grip of cultural changes as well as immigrants and minority groups on the fringe of mainstream cultures, are at certain risk for developing disordered forms of eating.

Immigration and increased migration to the cities is a common feature of today's world; this is normally accompanied with increased social mobility as well as changes within family structures. Following urbanization there is a notable change in individual lifestyle, particularly with reference to work and dietary habits. The urbanized world is also increasingly becoming more 'uniform' by reason of several globalizing forces, including mass media, information technologies, and the adoption of market economy. Market forces, in turn leads to the standardization of an aesthetic ideal and the marketing of this ideal.

The transition in some countries from State-controlled economy to markets has arguably undermined the collective social structure and resulted in the disappearance of some of the social networks that provided women with protection in their education, employment, and childcare rights. This is seen to be behind the 'gender ambivalence' felt by women of former socialist regimes, in addition to increased consumerism and material aspirations.(Catina and Joja 2001; Nasser and Katzman 2003). It was suggested that the increase in commercialism and the changing gender roles, coupled with the depletion of State-offered benefits (such as education, employment, and healthcare), may result in the commodification of the human body and its modification to fit with the global standardizations of beauty, marketability, and adaptability (Rathner 2001).

Another dimension to the 'change in culture' is the emergence of 'online cultures', reflected in a change of how an individual relates to one's own nation as a geographic entity which carries with it a threat to the sense of national identity (Morley and Robins 1995; Nasser and Katzman 1999, 2003).

There is no doubt that there are inherent advantages in the potentially unlimited choices, but to negotiate these choices the individual needs to learn how to reformulate an identity amidst an influx of visual information and images. However, at times of change or when 'identity definition or redefinition' is called for, the individual was noted to have a tendency to shift the locus of power to the body and reformulate the new identity in bodily terms. This results in various forms of 'body control', including eating disorders which make them, in turn, symptomatic of the 'transition' in culture and not culture per se (Nasser and DiNicola 2001). This means that the underlying sociocultural dynamics of eating psychopathology lies in 'cultural change'. This can be broken down to the following forces:

- ◆ Increased levels of urbanization, migration, and immigration
- ◆ Lifestyle changes—change in work/dietary habits
- ◆ Deregulation of media and economy
- ◆ Global standardization of beauty and commodification of the human body
- ◆ Gender ambivalence and increased confusion over gender roles
- ◆ Revision of traditional family structures
- ◆ Revision of traditional national boundaries through universal media and cyber culture.

Implications for prevention and intervention

As one examines the movement of eating disorders from individual neurosis to cultural marker of distress, caused by transitional and conflicting cultural forces, it becomes increasingly important to identify ways of operationalizing treatment and prevention strategies. By organizing our research and clinical questions around ways of assisting women in self-determination, control, and connection rather than simply documenting media and weight insults, we may be able to progress beyond the limitations of our current strategies and provide alternatives for women struggling with eating disorders as a 'answer' to complex personal, social, and personal problems. Nasser and Katzman (1999) suggested that the prevention of eating problems will be enhanced by the provision of new social supports and the careful work of providing new ways of belonging at the work and school level. They also recommended a shift in emphasis towards competencies rather than pathology in prevention and treatment strategies.

However, the question remains as to how to generate dialogue and engage individuals who share the same predicament worldwide? Perhaps the answer lies in taking advantages of the existing information technology. Electronic connections may provide a new way of achieving female connectedness, one in which women may be able to help other women whom they would not have been able to access in the past. Linked by computer technology, women may be able to overcome their social and political isolation and gain new insights into formulae for success and survival (Nasser 1999).

Similar techniques are currently being used in the management of eating disorders, focusing on psychoeducation and self-help cognitive strategies. These interactive web-based multimedia programmes are likely to make specialist therapies available to many more people who traditionally would have been unable to access such help. Recognition of these new mechanisms is likely to stimulate research devoted to a transnational perspective for the prevention and management of eating disorders.

References

Abu-Saleh M *et al.* (1998). Anorexia nervosa in an Arab culture. *International Journal of Eating Disorders*, 23, 207–12.

Ahmed S *et al.* (1994). Eating attitudes among Asian school girls: the role of perceived parental control. *International Journal of Eating Disorders*, 15(1), 91–7.

American Psychiatric Association (1993). *Diagnostic and Statistical Manual of Mental Disorders*, Fourth edition. Washington, DC.

Andersen A and Hays A (1985). Racial and socioeconomic influences in anorexia nervosa and bulimia. *International Journal of Eating Disorders*, 4, 479–87.

Apter A *et al.* (1994). Cultural effects on eating attitudes in Israeli subpopulations and hospitalised anorectics. *Genetic, Social, and General Psychology Monographs*, 120(1), 83–99.

Barths R (1975). European Diet from Pre-industrial to Modern Times. In: E Foster and R Foster (eds) *Towards a Psychosociology of Contemporary Food Consumption*. Harper Row, New York.

Caplan P (1997). *Food, Health and Identity*. Routledge. London and New York.

Catina A and Joja O (2001). Emerging markets: submerging women. In: M Nasser *et al.* (eds). *Eating Disorders and Cultures in Transition*, pp. 111–27. Routledge, Taylor and Francis Group, London and New York.

Dancyger I and Garfinkel P (1995). The relationship of partial syndrome of eating disorders to anorexia nervosa and bulimia nervosa. *Psychological Medicine*, 25, 1018–25.

Davis C and Katzman MA (1998). Chinese men and women in USA and Hong Kong: Body and self esteem ratings as a prelude to dieting and exercise. *International Journal of Eating Disorders*, 23, 99–102.

Davis C and Katzman MA (1999). Perfection as acculturation. *International Journal of Eating Disorders*, 25, 65–70.

Dolan B *et al.* (1990). Eating behaviours and attitudes to weight and shape in British women from three ethnic groups. *British Journal of Psychiatry*, 157, 523–8.

Fichter M *et al.* (1983). The epidemiology of anorexia nervosa: a comparison of Greek adolescents living in Germany and Greek adolescents in Greece. In: PL Darby *et al.* (eds) *Anorexia Nervosa: Recent Developments in Research*, pp. 95–105. Liss, New York.

Fichter M *et al.* (1988). Anorexia nervosa in Greek and Turkish adolescents. *European Archives of Psychiatry and Neurological Sciences*, 237, 200–8.

Ford K *et al.* (1990). Cultural factors in the aetiology of eating disorders: evidence from body shape preference of Arab students. *Journal of Psychosomatic Research*, 34(5), 501–7.

Gray J *et al.* (1987). The prevalence of bulimia in a black college population. *International Journal of Eating Disorders*, 6, 733–40.

Garner DM and Garfinkel PE (1980). Sociocultural factors in the development of anorexia nervosa. *Psychological Medicine*, 10, 483–91.

Gordon R (2001). Eating disorders East and West: A culture-bound syndrome unbound. In: M Nasser *et al.* (eds) *Eating Disorders and Cultures in Transition*, pp. 40–66. Brunner-Routledge (Taylor & Francis Group), London and New York.

Gull W (1874). Anorexia nervosa. *Clinical Society's Transactions* **vii**, 22.

Hoek H *et al.* (1995). Impact of urbanisation on detection rates of eating disorders. *American Journal of Psychiatry*, 152(9), 1272–85.

Hsu LK (1987). Are eating disorders becoming more common in blacks? *International Journal of Eating Disorders*, 6, 113–24.

Ishikawa K (1965). Ueber die Eltern von anorexia-nervosa-Kranken. In: JE Meyer and H Feldmann (eds) *Anorexia Nervosa*. Verlag, Stutgart.

Jones DJ *et al.* (1980). *Epidemiology of anorexia nervosa in Monroe County*, New York. 1960–1976. *Psychosomatic Medicine*, 42, 551–8.

Kamata K *et al.* (1987). Binge eating among female students. *Japanese Journal of Psychiatry and Neurology*, 41, 151–2.

Katzman MA and Lee S (1997). Beyond body image: the integration of feminist and transcultural theories in understanding self starvation. *International Journal of Eating Disorders*, 22, 385–94.

Katzman AM (1995). Asia on my mind: are eating disorders a problem in Hong Kong? *Eating Disorders: the Journal of Treatment and Prevention*, 3, 378–80.

Krch F (1994). 'Needs and possibilities of prevention of eating disorders in the Czech Republic.' Presented at IV International Conference on Eating Disorders, New York.

King M and Bhugra D (1989). Eating disorders lessons from a cross –cultural study. *Psychological Medicine*, **19**, 955–8.

King M and Mezey G (1987). Eating behaviours of male racing jockeys. *Psychological Medicine*, **17**, 249–53.

Lacey JH *et al.* (1988). Bulimia in British blacks and Asians. A catchment area study. *British Journal of Psychiatry*, **152**, 73–9.

Lasègue C (1873). De l'anorexie hysterique. *Archives Generales de Medicine*. Reprinted in RM Kaufman and M Heiman eds. *Evolution of Psychosomatic Concepts: Anorexia Nervosa, a Paradigm* (1964), pp 141–55. International University Press, New York.

Le Grange D *et al.* (1998). Eating attitudes and behaviors in 1,435 South African Caucasian and non-Caucasian college students. *American Journal of Psychiatry*, **155**, 250–4.

Lee S (1995). Self-starvation in context: towards a culturally sensitive understanding of anorexia nervosa. *Social Science Medicine*, **41**, 25–36.

Lee S (2001). Fat phobia in anorexia nervosa: Whose obsession is it? In: M Nasser *et al.* (eds) *Eating Disorders and Cultures in Transition*, pp. 40–66. Brunner-Routledge (Taylor & Francis Group), London and New York.

Lee S and Lee A (1996). Disordered eating and its psychosocial correlates among Chinese adolescent females in Hong Kong. *International Journal of Eating Disorders*, **20**, 177–83.

Lucas A *et al.* (1991). 50-year trends in the incidence of anorexia nervosa in Rochester, Minnesota: a population based study. *American Journal of Psychiatry*, **148**, 917–22.

McCourt J and Waller G (1995). Developmental role of perceived parental control in eating psychopathology of Asian and Caucasian school girls. *International Journal of Eating Disorders*, **17**, 277–82.

Malson H (1998). *The Thin Woman: Feminism, Post-structuralism and the Social Psychology of Anorexia Nervosa*. Routledge, London.

Meehan O and Katzman MA (2001). Argentina: the social body at risk. In: M Nasser *et al.* (eds) *Eating Disorders and Cultures in Transition*, pp. 146–71. Brunner-Routledge (Taylor & Francis Group), London and New York.

Morley D and Robins K (1995). *Spaces of Identity, Global Media, Electronic Landscapes and Cultural Boundaries*. Routledge, London and New York.

Mukai T *et al.* (1994). Eating attitudes and weight preoccupation among female high school students in Japan. *Journal of Child Psychology and Psychiatry*, **33**, 677–88.

Mumford DB and Whitehouse AM (1988). Increased prevalence of bulimia nervosa among Asian school girls. *British Medical Journal*, **297**, 718.

Mumford DB *et al.* (1991). Survey of eating disorders in English-medium schools in Lahore, Pakistan. *International Journal of Eating Disorders*, **11**, 173–84.

Nabakht M and Dezkhan M (2000). An epidemiological study of eating disorders in Iran. *International Journal of Eating Disorders*, **28**(93), 265–71.

Nasser M (1986). Comparative study of the prevalence of abnormal eating attitudes among Arab female students in both London and Cairo Universities, *Psychological Medicine*, **16**, 621–25.

Nasser M (1994). The psychometric properties of the eating attitudes test in a non-western population. *Social Psychiatry & Psychiatric Epidemiology*, **29**, 88–94.

Nasser M (1995). The EAT speaks many languages. Review of the use of the EAT in eating disorders research. *Eating and Weight Disorders*, **2**(4), 174–81.

Nasser M (1997). *Culture and Weight Consciousness*. Routledge, London.

Nasser M (1999). Eating disorders: between cultural specificity and globalization. *Eating Disorders Review*, **9**(5), 1–4.

Nasser (2000). Gender, culture and eating disorder. In J Ushher (eds) *Women's Health, Contemporary International Perspectives*, pp. 379–87. The British Psychological Society, London.

Nasser M and Katzman M (1999). Eating disorders: transcultural perspectives inform prevention. In: N Piran *et al.* (eds) *Preventing Eating Disorders: A Handbook of Interventions and Special Challenges*, pp. 26–44. Brunner/Mazel, London and New York.

Nasser M and Katzman (2003). Sociocultural theories of eating disorders: an evolution in thought. In: J Treasure *et al.* (eds) *Handbook of Eating Disorders*, second edition. pp. 139–51. Wiley, West Sussex.

Nasser M *et al.*(2001). Changing bodies, changing cultures: an intercultural dialogue on the body as the frontal frontier. In: M Nasser *et al.* (eds) *Eating Disorders and Cultures in Transition*, pp. 171–94. Brunner-Routledge (Taylor& Francis Group), London and New York.

Nunes M *et al.* (1991). 'What to think of anorexia nervosa in Brazil, a country of hunger and undernourishment?' Poster presentation at the International Symposium on Eating Disorders, Paris.

Ohzeki T *et al.* (1990). Prevalence of obesity, leanness and anorexia nervosa in Japanese boys and girls aged 12–14 years. *Annals of Nutrition and Metabolism*, **34**, 208–12.

Orbach S (1986). *Hunger Strike: the anorexic struggle as a metaphor for our age*. Norton, New York.

Pok LP and Tian CS (1994). Susceptibility of Singapore Chinese School girls to anorexia nervosa – Part 1 (psychological factors). *Singapore Medical Journal*, **35**, 481–5.

Prince R (1983). Is anorexia nervosa a culture-bound syndrome? *Transcultural Psychiatry Research and Review*, **20**, 299

Pumarino H and Vivanco N (1982). Anorexia nervosa: medical and psychiatric characteristics of 3 patients. *Revista Medica de Chile*, **110**, 1081–92.

Rathner G (2001). Post-communism and the marketing of the thin ideal. In: M. Nasser *et al.* (eds) *Eating Disorders and Cultures in Transition*, pp. 93–111. Brunner-Routledge (Taylor& Francis Group), London and New York.

Rathner G and Messner K (1993). Detection of eating disorders in a small rural town: an epidemiological study. *Psychological Medicine*, **23**, 175–84.

Rathner G *et al.* (1995). Prevalence of eating disorders and minor psychiatric morbidity in Central Europe before the political changes in 1989: a cross cultural study. *Psychological Medicine*, **25**, 1027–35.

Reiss D (1996). Abnormal eating attitudes and behaviours in two ethnic groups from a female British urban population. *Psychological Medicine*, **26**, 289–99.

Russell G (1979). Bulimia nervosa: an ominous variant of anorexia nervosa. *Psychological Medicine*, **9**, 429–48.

Szabo P and Tury F (1991). The prevalence of bulimia nervosa in a Hungarian college and secondary school population. *Psychotherapy and psychosomatics*, **56**, 43–7.

Smith J and Krejci J (1991). Minorities join the majority: eating disturbance among Hispanics and Native American youth. *International Journal of Eating Disorders*, **10**, 179–86.

Silverstein B and Perlick D (1995). *The Cost of Competence: Why Inequality Causes Depression, Eating Disorders and Illness in Women*. Oxford University Press, New York.

Suematsu H *et al.* (1985). Statistical studies of anorexia nervosa in Japan, detailed clinical data on 1,011 patients. *Psychotherapy and Psychosomatics*, **43**, 96–103.

Szabo CP *et al.* (1995). Eating disorders in black South African females. A series of cases. *South African Medical Journal*, **85**, 588–90.

Thomas J and Szmukler G (1985). Anorexia nervosa in patients of Afro-Caribbean extraction. *British Journal of Psychiatry*, **146**, 653–6.

Warczyk-Bisaga K and Dolan B (1996). A two-stage epidemiological study of abnormal eating attitudes and prospective risk factors in Polish school girls. *Psychological Medicine*, **26**, 1021–32.

Weight L and Noakes T (1987). Is running an analog of anorexia? A survey of the incidence of eating disorders in female distance runners, *Medicine and Science in Sports and Exercise*, **19**(3), 213–17.

WHO (1992). *The International Classification of Mental and Behavioural Disorders (ICD-10) Clinical description and diagnostic guidelines*. WHO, Geneva.

Williamson I (1999). Why are gay men a high risk group for eating disorders?. *European Eating Disorders Review*, **7**, 1–4.

CHAPTER 25

Eating disorders: recognition, pathogenesis, classification, management, and services for women with eating disorders

Rebecca Cashmore and Bob Palmer

Eating disorders (EDs)—notably anorexia nervosa (AN)—have been recognized as clinical conditions since the 19th century. However, until the last 40 years, accounts were usually hidden away in the small print of medical textbooks. In contrast, EDs are now much discussed and commented upon even in the lay press. Most people know something about EDs. Many have opinions about them. Nevertheless, some prevalent attitudes tend to play down their importance as a public health problem. Thus, on the one hand, they may be viewed as severe but rare illnesses that mysteriously blight or even snuff out promising young lives. On the other hand, they may be thought of as common but trivial, merely an exaggeration of the shape and weight preoccupations of adolescent girls and of a few narcissists who perseverate such concerns to an age when they should know better. However, complicating matters further, there is sometimes a smidgeon of admiration of the control shown by people with AN evidenced by the quip, so often trotted out as if freshly minted, 'Oh! Anorexia nervosa, I could do with a bit of that'. And sometimes there might be a whiff of misogyny in the downplaying of the problem of EDs which, although males can suffer from them, are clearly in the main afflictions of the female.

Of mental disorders that may affect people of either gender, the EDs have the clearest difference in prevalence between females and males. Studies show a consistent skew with typically a ratio of ten or more females to one male (Hoek and van Hoeken 2003; Button *et al.* 2008). EDs in males are sometimes missed but this is unlikely to be the main explanation. When males do develop EDs, their disorders usually closely resemble those in females (Button *et al.* 2008). So why are women and girls more vulnerable? The answer remains uncertain. Clearly males and females differ in many ways both biologically and psychosocially. It is less clear which of these differences account for the skew in risk of developing EDs.

Pathogenesis

Changes in the incidence and prevalence of EDs over just a few decades suggest that psychosocial issues may be of most immediate relevance. There are data on such changes from richer countries (Hoek and van Hoeken 2003). However, there is little evidence from developing countries although the presence of a few cases in many countries has led to the perception of the EDs as a worldwide problem (see Chapter 24, this volume). The usual interpretation of the evidence available is that AN has been present in the young female population in Europe and North America for over 100 years and that there may have been some increase in prevalence over recent decades. In contrast, bulimia nervosa (BN) seems to be a 'new' disorder that was fully recognized and named only in the 1970s (Russell 1979; Vanderycken 1994). This recognition was probably a consequence of

BN becoming more salient because it was becoming more prevalent. Once a good description and a name were available, more and more cases were diagnosed. Rates of presentation and recognition rose notably during the last two decades of the of the 20th century although there is some suggestions that the peak may have already passed, at least in Europe and North America (Keel *et al.* 2006).

Such changes over decades suggest environmental and most probably psychosocial factors since the genetic vulnerability of a population cannot change over just a generation or so. However, environmental change may expose a newly relevant genetic risk factor and the apparent heritability may rise. Certainly there are data suggesting that EDs run in families in a way that suggests genetic transmission (Strober *et al.* 2000; Fairburn and Harrison 2003). The hunt is on for particular genes importantly affecting risk but as with other disorders, genetics offers the prospect of both greater understanding and therapeutic potency in the future, but such benefits have yet to be delivered.

The most intuitively favoured risk factors for EDs are the social influences that value low weight and a slender form. Research evidence provides some support for this popular view (Fairburn *et al.* 2005). A series of case–control comparisons found that when such ideas are firmly held within the family of origin, they are associated with an increase in the risk of subsequent ED for BN but less so for AN (Fairburn *et al.* 1997, 1999). However, although such ideas—'pressures'—are almost ubiquitous for young women in Western countries, only a small minority develop an ED. There must be other factors involved and for AN, low self-esteem and perfectionism seem to be of importance. Indeed there is evidence supporting an array of risk factors unrelated to weight, shape, or eating. These tend to be associated with increased risk of mental disorder in general including ED (Jacobi 2005).

Thus, the stereotype of a girl or young woman at high risk of ED would depict her as living in a culture or subculture where there was pressure to be slim, as herself feeling personally troubled and having a family history of ED. But why is she at greater risk than her brother? Tentative answers might include the more meaningful and certainly more evident changes in body fat and body shape that signal adulthood and reproductive capacity in the female. It is also plausible that young women have a more challenging journey to adulthood and find themselves in societies with more negative experiences, such as various types of abuse leading to a more delicate sense of self when compared to their male peers. Or the difference might come to be understood biologically. It is certainly possible that the most important risk factors for developing an ED are for the present unknown or neglected.

Diagnosis and classification

Making the diagnosis of ED is not a major problem when the patient is evidently at a low weight and/or she is forthcoming about her thoughts, feelings, and behaviours. Notwithstanding the reputation of ED patients for misleading others, this is usually the case. Many people with EDs seem to be reluctant patients, but most will give a sufficient account of themselves if the clinician is not too pushy and makes room for the expression and exploration of mixed feelings. In the few cases where this is not so, there may be true diagnostic uncertainty. A set of screening questions is available to aid in the detection of ED but in practice the best screen may be thinking of the possibility of ED and asking questions focused on the particular person (Morgan *et al.* 1999). Likewise, self-report questionnaires have their place in monitoring change in individuals and describing populations but rarely add much to clinical assessment. In research, the Eating Disorders Examination (EDE) has come to be the gold standard measure of ED psychopathology (Fairburn and Cooper 1993).

Once the broad diagnosis of an ED is made, the available classifications are seriously flawed. The biggest problem is that a large proportion—sometimes a majority—of people present with a clinical ED fitting neither of the two main diagnostic categories, AN or BN. Within the American DSM-IV system (see Box 25.1), such cases are swept into a residual category with no real criteria namely eating disorders not otherwise specified (EDNOS) (APA 1994). The ICD-10 of the World Health Organization is in practice little better (World Health Organization 1992). Cases of EDNOS cannot be dismissed as mild and unimportant since by definition they are of clinical severity. Indeed they have been shown to be of similar severity to cases of BN (Fairburn *et al.* 2007). The diagnoses fit even less the disorders of younger adolescents and children (Nicholls 2005).

Some respond to this mess by suggesting new categories. The name of purging disorder has been proposed for cases of EDNOS where purging (induced vomiting or laxative abuse) dominates in a normal weight person who does not binge (Keel 2007). Others have advocated a 'transdiagnostic' view which questions the proliferation

Box 25.1 DSM-IV criteria for the eating disorders—slightly simplified

Anorexia nervosa (AN)

- Refusal to maintain body weight at or above a minimally normal weight for age and height

- Intense fear of gaining weight or becoming fat even though underweight

- Disturbance in the way in which one's body weight or shape is experienced, undue influence of body weight or shape on self-evaluation, or denial of the seriousness of the current low body weight

- Amenorrhoea in postmenarcheal females

- Types:

  - Restricting type: no regular binge-eating or purging behaviour

  - Binge-eating/purging type

Bulimia nervosa (BN)

- Recurrent episodes of binge-eating characterized by eating in a discrete period of time an amount of food that is definitely lager than most people would eat under similar circumstances. During the episode there is a sense of lack of control over eating

- Recurrent inappropriate compensatory behaviour in order to prevent weight gain, such as self-induced vomiting, misuse of laxatives, diuretics, enemas or other medications; fasting excessive exercise.

- Binge-eating and compensatory behaviours occur on average at least twice a week for three months.

- Self-evaluation is unduly influenced by body shape or weight.

- The disturbance does not occur exclusively during episodes of anorexia nervosa.

- Types:

  - Purging type: regular use of self-induced vomiting or the misuse of laxatives, diuretics, or enemas.

  - Non-purging type: use of non-purging methods of inappropriate compensation such has fasting or excessive exercise.

Eating disorder not otherwise specified (EDNOS)

- Disorder of eating that does not meet the criteria for any specific eating disorder. The disorder must be of clinical significance and severity.

of categories and emphasizes the similarities between the disorders and the way that an individual may commonly move between categories within an illness career (Fairburn *et al.* 2003). The area remains controversial. It is uncertain what revision will emerge from the classificatory cabal responsible for the DSM-V.

There is a further DSM-IV diagnosis, binge eating disorder (BED) which requires binge eating but without compensatory behaviours and with little specified psychopathology. Strictly BED remains part of EDNOS. The diagnosis is widely criticized but even more widely used (Dingemans *et al.* 2005). In the clinic, BED is associated with overweight but this is less so in community samples (Fairburn *et al.* 1998; de Zwaan 2005). In general the relationship between EDs and obesity is muddled. Obesity as such is traditionally excluded from the ED canon.

Assessment and engagement

People generally seek help because they feel unwell. They worry about their health and want to recover. However, it is more complex for some people presenting with EDs, especially AN. They have mixed, even positive feelings about their state. It is others who worry. The clinician needs to make space to explore these conflicted feelings from the outset. If the patient says that there is nothing wrong but nevertheless keeps the first appointment there is evident ambivalence. The assessor can work with this. Priority should be given to developing a therapeutic dialogue and some initial shared understanding of how the person has reached her current impasse.

Assessment also includes general information gathering, history taking, and mental state examination, encompassing a screen for common comorbidity such as depression, obsessional disorder, substance abuse, and assessment of risk of self-harm. However, there should be special enquiry about the patient's attitude to weight and shape over time and how any changes have related to life events and stressors. How has this person related to her body in the past? Has she ever maintained a stable weight? Or has she battled with her body to maintain a lower than natural weight? What has been the family culture with respect to weight? How have external pressures for slimness been managed? Is there a family history of ED?

Measuring body weight and height with calculation of body mass index (BMI) together with attention to the physical state of the patient are the other necessary components of assessment. Anyone with ED may have physical complications and it is important that someone takes responsibility for the monitoring of the patient's physical state and associated risks and that appropriate collaborations are arranged when the main clinician is not medical. In general the risks are higher in AN and people often look unwell. However, people with BN or EDNOS at normal weight may look well but nevertheless be at risk through biochemical disruption arising from vomiting or otherwise purging on a daily basis. Review of physical symptoms and systems is necessary together with screening investigations usually a full blood count, urea and electrolytes, liver and thyroid function tests. A physical examination and electrocardiogram would be usual for people with AN whose BMI is below 15. A detailed account of the physical issues is beyond the scope of this chapter. See National Collaborating Centre for Mental Health (2004).

As the clinician assesses the patient, the patient will be assessing the clinician, the service, and what is on offer. By the end of assessment, the clinician should be able to provide a provisional formulation that is accessible to the patient. Thus, the account might tentatively suggest aspects of the history, such as personality factors or parental attitudes to weight which may have rendered her vulnerable and events such as bullying or stressful examinations that may have acted as precipitants. Furthermore, information on the physiological and psychological effects of starvation add to the account of how the patient developed an ED and became trapped within it. For example, a patient may be relieved to hear that her preoccupation with food and fear of losing control of eating may to be a response to dietary restraint and that this traps her within a vicious cycle. Thus assessment may often involve psychoeducation and motivational work which is essentially the start of treatment.

But what treatments should be offered? There are useful reviews of research including the guideline published by the National Institute for Clinical Excellence (NICE) which has special importance in the United Kingdom in that it provides guidance for practice within the National Health Service (National Collaborating Centre for Mental Health 2004). However, as a rigorous systematic review it has wider relevance. It is due for updating, but unfortunately advances since its publication have been modest. Evidence-based practice is possible for BN, but is less so for AN where there is a dearth of relevant research. There is even less evidence about the treatment of EDNOS in general with the exception of BED.

Treatment of bulimia nervosa and eating disorders not otherwise specified

There is a substantial evidence base relevant to the treatment of BN and the form of EDNOS known as BED. The 'gold standard' is a specific form of cognitive behavioural therapy known as CBT-BN (Fairburn et al. 1993a). This has been well evaluated and shown to be superior to other treatments with the exception of interpersonal psychotherapy (IPT) although IPT typically takes longer to reach its full effect (Fairburn et al. 1993b, 1995; Agras et al. 2000). Recently Fairburn and colleagues have developed the treatment into CBT-E (e for enhanced) which in one form CBT-Eb (b for broad) incorporates elements of IPT and other less ED-focused therapies (Fairburn 2008; Fairburn et al. in press). These therapies involve about 20 sessions with a trained therapist over about six months. There are group adaptations of both CBT-BN and IPT (Wilfley et al. 2000). Within the trials—and probably in ordinary clinical practice—about half of those having the treatment escape from BN and most remain well. However, half do not. There is little evidence as to what further treatment is best for the unfortunate half but adding antidepressant medication may be helpful. There is extensive evidence that a range of antidepressants and other drugs such as topiramate have some antibulimic effects independent of any effect upon comorbid depression which is, of course, not uncommon (Goldstein et al. 1999; Hoopes et al. 2003). Fluoxetine is the only drug with the licence for BN in the United Kingdom (Fluoxetine Bulimia Nervosa Study Group 1992). Drugs alone are rarely an adequate treatment for BN.

The therapies cited earlier are effective but expensive and adequately trained therapists are scarce. Fortunately there is evidence that some people with BN can benefit from lesser interventions such as the use of self-help books, websites, or DVDs and the like with or without guidance from a professional (Perkins et al. 2006). Offering lesser treatments as a first intervention within a stepped care approach may be sensible (Fairburn and Peveler 1990).

Almost all cases of BN can and should be managed as outpatients although comorbid depression may at times require admission. Furthermore, the not uncommon conjunction of BN and borderline personality disorder with or without recurrent self-harm or substance abuse presents a challenge to most services. Short crisis admissions may be required but there is a widespread impression that long admissions to general psychiatric wards may do more harm than good although special inpatient programmes may have better results (Lacey 1995).

Treatment and management of anorexia nervosa

The treatment of AN is less straightforward and management is more often an issue because of physical risk. A significant minority require more than outpatient contact. There is near consensus and some evidence that various kinds of family therapy are the treatment of choice for teenage patients who are still living with their family (Eisler *et al.* 1997, 2000). The predominant style has come to be known as the 'Maudsley model' in North America (Locke *et al.* 2000). It seeks emphatically to exculpate the parents but nevertheless emphasizes their responsibility to ensure that the young person eats sufficiently to reverse the weight loss. Family counselling where the clinician meets separately with the patient and with the family has been shown to be as effective as the more traditional approach where they all meet together (Eisler *et al.* 2000). Multi-family therapy where several families meet together is being evaluated (Dare and Eisler 2000).

By comparison there is a dearth of evidence for psychological treatment of adults with AN and no gold standard. Some clinicians are purist and offer their favoured therapy model including CBT, IPT, or cognitive-analytic therapy (McIntosh *et al.* 2000; Fairburn *et al.* 2003). However, many clinicians adopt a more eclectic approach combining exploratory approaches with psychoeducation and behavioural techniques, particularly in the initial stages of treatment. In a recent trial, treatment called 'specialized supportive clinical management' proved more effective than CBT or IPT (McIntosh *et al.* 2005).

Good therapy is more than dietary monitoring and encouragement. It also provides a forum for patients to gradually disentangle their emotional issues from food and weight. Therapy should promote better ways of managing emotional states, without resort to the overcontrol of food and weight and in due course become focused upon getting life 'back on track'. Grief work may be useful in recognition of time lost to the illness. In general there is a need for the therapist to be flexible especially with regard to pace. The mixed feelings mentioned earlier may become salient again at any stage.

More intensive treatment for AN usually means going into hospital. People with AN may need admission for three broad reasons. Firstly, their physical state may become too complicated or extreme and admission probably onto a medical ward is necessary to contain and reverse the risk. Secondly, comorbid depression and major suicide risk may require admission, perhaps to a general psychiatric ward. Thirdly, the patient may be stuck despite appropriate treatment as an outpatient and admission to a special ED unit may be offered. In this case—arguably in all cases—the decision to admit is best made collaboratively. Ideally the patient should feel that the time is right. If this is not the case, compulsion is available in the mental health legislation of most countries. However, it is the therapeutic alliance however fragile which remains key in managing AN and compulsion will always complicate, if not compromise, that relationship. There is little evidence on the impact on the use of the legal detention on long-term outcome but many clinicians feel that compulsion should be used only as a last resort (Ramsey *et al.* 1999; Carney *et al.* 2008). There is a danger that battling with the patient may make later treatment more difficult. A clinician who can hold his or her nerve may find advantages in the longer run. The rocky road of weight restoration is better trodden actively, even on ambivalent but acquiescent feet, rather than with feet which are being dragged. The latter may sprint back to the starting point with rapid weight loss, as soon as enforcement is lifted.

The NICE guideline suggests that inpatient treatment regimes should be 'structured . . . symptom-focused with the expectation of weight gain' with 'psychological treatment . . . which has a focus on eating behaviour and attitudes to weight and shape, and wider psychosocial issues'. It advises against 'rigid behaviour modification programmes' (National Collaborating Centre for Mental Health 2004). The content and style of inpatient programmes vary but most include consistent boundaries, clear expectations and an initial giving over of responsibility about diet which is then handed back to the patient gradually later in the admission. Most include a structured therapeutic programme targeting ED psychopathology and involving practical tasks such as shopping, meal preparation, and support in the transition back to independent living. Psychotherapy—individual, group, or family—should continue throughout and ideally after the admission.

Although it may be a relief when a patient in a precarious position agrees to admission, close physical monitoring is required particularly in the early days of refeeding because of potentially dangerous biochemical abnormalities including hypophosphataema due to a carbohydrate-induced intracellular shift of phosphate. There is also a risk of thiamine deficiency, hypomagnesaemia, hypocalcaemia, and hypokalaemia, all of which should also be monitored. The medical management of the refeeding of low weight patients is described elsewhere (NICE 2006; Mehanna *et al.* 2008) Weight restoration can be speedier as an inpatient and may achieve gains as high as 1 kg a week Nevertheless, if the aim is restoration of a normal weight then admission may need to last many months. This is very expensive and long admissions need to be reserved for the most severely afflicted patients. As an unsought consequence inpatient units may come to be full of patients who present especially difficult and challenging problems.

Box 25.2 Components of a comprehensive service for people with eating disorders

Assessment

◆ Diagnosis of ED

◆ Detection and management of psychiatric comorbidity and associated risk

◆ Detection and management of physical complications and associated risk

Treatment

◆ Evidence-based psychological treatment for BN and EDNOS, usually CBT

◆ Preliminary guided self-help for less severe cases

◆ Availability of adjunctive drug treatment

◆ Family treatment for AN in younger people

◆ Sustained psychological treatment for adults with AN

◆ Reassessment and monitoring for people who do not respond

◆ Treatment for comorbid disorders

Management

◆ Availability of more intensive intervention—including admission to hospital—for further treatment of those with AN who have not responded to outpatient treatment

◆ Appropriate admission for the management of high physical or psychiatric risk

◆ Involvement of family where appropriate

◆ Sustained follow-up with monitoring of risks

Services for eating disorders

Special services for EDs are patchily distributed. This remains the case in the United Kingdom although such provision is growing. Overall services need to be comprehensive in scope offering both outpatient and inpatient management although the latter may be supplied through a regional network or referral on to a specialist tertiary unit. There is a tension between the ideal of keeping outpatient services local and the need for a special inpatient unit to be sufficiently large—at least four beds—to sustain an appropriate culture. Furthermore, transitions should be handled with care since arrangements that look satisfactory in planning documents may be experienced by the patient as a disconcerting form of 'pass the parcel'. A move from child and adolescent to adult services may involve shifting from family-orientated practice to one emphasizing personal responsibility. This can be disorientating and unsettling for both patient and family alike. The components of a comprehensive service are summarized in Box 25.2

Conclusions

The EDs are serious mental disorders that should be taken seriously. They are not uncommon and affect at least 2% of most populations of young women in the richer world (Hoek and van Hoeken 2003). Most sufferers recover eventually but EDs afflict and limit people at crucial times in their personal development. For some, perhaps one in ten, their disorder follows a chronic course over decades. A small number meet a premature death through physical consequences or suicide (Neilson S *et al.* 1998). Furthermore, the burden of caring for someone with a severe ED has been shown to be similar to caring for someone with psychosis (Treasure *et al.* 2001). Too often the EDs have been marginalized as a public health problem and patients have been poorly managed as individuals. The disorders have been trivialized or even glamourized. They need to be dealt with as disorders that are important, severe, and *ordinary*.

References

Agras WS *et al.* (2000). A multicenter comparison of cognitive-behavioural therapy and inter-personal psychotherapy for bulimia nervosa. *Archives of General Psychiatry*, **57**, 459–66.

American Psychiatric Association (1994). *Diagnostic and Statistical Manual of Mental Disorders, fourth edition.* American Psychiatric Association, Washington, DC.

Button E *et al.* (2008). Males assessed by a specialised adult eating disorders service; patterns over time and comparison with females. *International Journal of Eating Disorders*, **41**, 758–61.

Carney T *et al.* (2008). Why (and when) clinicians compel treatment of anorexia nervosa patients. *European Eating Disorders Review*, **16**(3), 199–206.

Dare C *et al.* (2000). A multi family group day treatment programme for adolescents with eating disorders. *European Eating Disorders Review*, **8**, 4–18

de Zwaan M (2005). Binge-eating, EDNOS and obesity In: C Norring and B Palmer (eds) *EDNOS: Eating Disorder not Otherwise Specified; Scientific and Clinical Perspectives on the Other Eating Disorders*, pp. 83–113. Routledge, London and New York.

Dingemans AE *et al.* (2005). The empirical status of binge eating disorder. In: C Norring and B Palmer (eds) *EDNOS: Eating Disorder not Otherwise Specified; Scientific and Clinical Perspectives on the Other Eating Disorders*, pp. 63–82. Routledge, London and New York.

Eisler I *et al.* (1997). Family and individual therapy in anorexia nervosa. A five-year follow up. *Archives of General Psychiatry*, **54**, 1025–30.

Eisler I *et al.* (2000). Family therapy for adolescent anorexia nervosa: the result of a controlled comparison of two family interventions. *Journal of Child and Psychology and Psychiatry*, **41**, 727–36.

Fairburn CG (2008). *Cognitive Behavior Therapy and Eating Disorders*. The Guilford Press, New York and London.

Fairburn CG and Cooper Z (1993). The Eating Disorders Examination (12th edition). In: CG Fairburn and GT Wilson (eds) *Binge Eating: Nature, Assessment and Treatment*, pp. 317–60. Guilford Press, New York.

Fairburn CG and Harrison P (2003). Eating disorders. *Lancet*, **361**, 407–16.

Fairburn CG and Peveler RC (1990). Bulimia nervosa and the stepped care approach to management. *Gut*, **31**, 1220–2.

Fairburn CG *et al.* (1993a). Cognitive-behavioral therapy for binge eating bulimia nervosa: A comprehensive treatment manual. In: *Binge Eating: Nature, Assessment and Treatment*, pp. 361–404. Guilford Press, New York.

Fairburn C *et al.* (1993b). Psychotherapy and bulimia nervosa; The longer term effects of interpersonal psychotherapy, behaviour therapy and cognitive behaviour therapy. *Archives of General Psychiatry*, **50**, 419–28.

Fairburn CG *et al.* (1995). A prospective study of outcome in bulimia nervosa and the long term effects of three psychological treatments. *Archives of General Psychiatry*, **52**, 304–12.

Fairburn CG *et al.* (1997). Risk factors for bulimia nervosa: A community based case-control study. *Archives of General Psychiatry*, **54**, 509–17.

Fairburn CG *et al.* (1998). Risk factors for binge eating disorder: A community-based case-control study. *Archives of General Psychiatry*, **55**, 425–32.

Fairburn CG *et al.* (1999). Risk factors for anorexia nervosa: three integrated case comparisons. *Archives of General Psychiatry*, **56**, 468–47.

Fairburn CG *et al.* (2003). Cognitive behaviour therapy for eating disorders: "A transdiagnostic" theory and treatment. *Behaviour Research and Therapy*, **41**, 509–28.

Fairburn CG *et al.* (2005). Identifying dieters who will develop an eating disorder: A prospective, population based study. *American Journal of Psychiatry*, **162**, 2249–55.

Fairburn CG *et al.* (2007). The severity and status of eating disorder NOS; Implications for DSM-V. *Behaviour Research and Therapy*, **45**, 1705–15.

Fairburn CG *et al.* (in press). A new approach to the treatment of outpatients with an eating disorder: A randomised controlled trial. *American Journal of Psychiatry*.

Fluoxetine Bulimia Nervosa Collaborative Study Group (1992). Fluoxetine in the treatment of bulimia nervosa. *Archives of General psychiatry*, **49**, 139–47.

Goldstein D *et al.* (1999). Effectiveness of fluoxetine therapy in bulimia nervosa regardless of co-morbid depression. *International Journal of Eating Disorders*, **25**(1), 19–27.

Hoek HW and van Hoeken D (2003). Review of the prevalence and incidence of eating disorders. *International Journal of Eating Disorders*, **34**, 383–396.

Hoopes S *et al.* (2003). Treatment of Bulimia Nervosa with topiramate in randomised double blind placebo controlled trial. *Journal of Clinical Psychiatry*, **64**, 1335–1341.

Jacobi C (2005). Psychosocial risk factors for eating disorders. In: Wonderlich S, Mitchell J, de Zwaan M and Steiger H (eds) Eating Disorders Review Part 1. pp. 59–85. Academy of Eating Disorders Radcliffe Publishing, Oxford and Seattle.

Keel PK *et al.* (2006). Prevalence of bulimia nervosa in 1982, 1992 and 2002. *Psychological Medicine*, **36**, 119–27.

Keel P (2007). Purging disorder: sub-threshold variant or full-threshold eating disorder? *International Journal of Eating Disorders*, **40**, S89–S94.

Lacey JH (1995). Inpatient treatment of multi-impulsive bulimia nervosa. In: Brownell KD and Fairburn CG (eds) *Eating Disorders and Obesity: A Comprehensive Handbook*. Guilford Press, New York.

Locke J *et al.* (2000). *Treatment Manual for Anorexia Nervosa; A Family Based Approach*. Guilford Press, New York.

Mehanna H *et al.* (2008). Refeeding syndrome what is it and how to prevent and treat it. *British Medical Journal*, **336**, 1495–8.

McIntosh V *et al.* (2000). Interpersonal psychotherapy for anorexia. *International Journal of Eating Disorders*, **27**, 125–39.

McIntosh V *et al.* (2005). Three psychotherapies for anorexia nervosa: a randomised controlled trial. *American Journal of Psychiatry*, **162**, 741–7.

Morgan JF *et al.* (1999). The SCOFF questionnaire: assessment of a new screening tool for eating disorders. *British Medical Journal*, **319**, 1467–8.

National Collaborating Centre for Mental Health (2004). *Eating Disorders: Core interventions in the treatment and management of anorexia nervosa, bulimia nervosa and related eating disorders National Clinical Practice Guideline*

No. CG9. British Psychological Society and Gaskell, London.

NICE (2006). *Nutritional Support in Adults. Clinical Guidance CG32*. NICE, London.

Neilsen S *et al.* (1998). Standardised mortality in eating disorders – a quantitative summary of previously published and new evidence. *Journal of Psychosomatic Research*, **44**, 413–34.

Nicholls D (2005). Eating disorder in children. In: C Norring and B Palmer (eds) *EDNOS: Eating Disorder not Otherwise Specified; Scientific and Clinical Perspectives on the Other Eating Disorders*. Routledge, London and New York.

Perkins SJ *et al.* (2006). Self help and guided self help for eating disorders. *Cochrane Database of Systematic Reviews*, **3**, CD0004191.

Ramsey R *et al.* (1999). Compulsory treatment in anorexia. Short term benefits and long term mortality. *British Journal of Psychiatry*, **175**, 147–53.

Russell GFM (1979). Bulimia nervosa: an ominous variant of anorexia nervosa. *Psychological Medicine*, **9**, 429–48.

Strober M *et al.* (2000). Controlled family study of anorexia nervosa and bulimia nervosa: evidence of shared liability and transmission of partial syndromes. *American Journal of Psychiatry*, **157**, 393–401.

Treasure J *et al.* (2001). The experience of care giving for severe mental illness: A comparison between anorexia nervosa and psychosis. *Social Psychiatry and Psychiatric Epidemiology*, **36**, 343–7.

Vandererycken W (1994). Emergence of bulimia nervosa as a separate diagnostic entity: Review of the literature from 1960 to 1979. *International Journal of Eating Disorders*, **16**, 105–16.

Wilfley D *et al.* (2000). *Interpersonal Psychotherapy for Group*. Basic Books, New York.

World Health Organization (1992). *The ICD-10 Classification of Mental and Behavioural Disorders: Clinical Descriptions and Diagnostic Guidelines*. WHO, Geneva.

PART 3

Special Clinical Topics

CHAPTER 26

Post-traumatic stress disorder

Joanne Stubley

Introduction

This chapter will focus on post-traumatic stress disorder (PTSD) in women. I will begin by giving a brief description of typical trauma presentations that will include an understanding of the spectrum of disorder that may present. The spectrum ranges from a single episode of adult trauma causing a transitory traumatic reaction to a full-blown episode of PTSD; developmental trauma with its variety of psychiatric manifestations in adulthood: and complex trauma including the experience of traumatized refugees and those subject to torture and political persecution. A review of the epidemiology of trauma in relation to women will follow. An overview of current guidelines issued by the National Institute for Clinical Excellence (NICE) for PTSD treatment will be linked with current theoretical views on aetiology. A psychoanalytic model of trauma-focused treatment developed by the Tavistock clinic will also be described.

Clinical presentations

Although the focus of this chapter will be on the specific diagnostic category of PTSD, it is useful to review the spectrum of trauma presentations in women. These have been classified in various ways in different diagnostic systems and some controversy persists as to the overlap with other disorders, e.g. developmental trauma and borderline personality disorder. This is beyond the scope of this chapter but deserves further consideration. The spectrum of trauma presentations includes:

- Transitory traumatic reactions
- PTSD—single-episode adult trauma
- Developmental trauma
- Complex trauma—including refugees, individuals tortured or imprisoned for lengthy periods.

Transitory traumatic reactions

Many people experience traumatic stress symptoms after a traumatic event that settle with time. After a sexual assault, over 90% of women met the criteria for the diagnosis of PTSD (Kessler *et al.* 2005). Recovery for the majority appears to be rapid when prospective studies are reviewed. Galea *et al.* (2003) described PTSD symptoms in New Yorkers after the September 11 attack reducing from 7.5% at one month to 1.6% at four months and 0.6% at six months. This has important implications for treatment in these early stages.

Post-traumatic stress disorder

PTSD occurs after a traumatic event that involved actual or threatened death or serious injury, or a threat to the physical integrity of self or others. The DSM classification also calls for the person to have experienced intense fear, helplessness, or horror when the event occurred. Traumatic events include physical, psychological, and sexual abuse; terrorism and war; domestic violence; witnessing violence against others; and accidents and natural disasters. Approximately 50% of individuals will be exposed to at least one traumatic event in their lifetime. Approximately 8% of survivors will develop PTSD.

Symptoms usually begin within three months of the incident but occasionally emerge years later often via a trigger event—a further blow or another trauma. For the DSM classification, symptoms must have been present for at least one month for the diagnosis.

Symptoms of PTSD come under three main headings of re-experiencing phenomena; avoidance and numbing; and increased arousal. These may be summarized as:

- Re-experiencing phenomena
- Recurrent and intrusive distressing recollections
- Recurrent distressing dreams
- Acting or feeling as if the events are recurring
- Intense psychological distress to cues
- Physiological reactivity to cues
- Avoidance and numbing
- Avoidance of thoughts, feelings, and conversations
- Avoidance of reminders
- Psychogenic amnesia
- Greatly reduced interest in related activities
- Detachment or estrangement feelings
- Restricted range of affect
- Sense of a foreshortened future
- Increased arousal
- Difficulty sleeping
- Irritability or outbursts of anger
- Difficulty concentrating
- Hypervigilance
- Exaggerated startle response.

See Bisson (2007).

Some PTSD symptoms are more common in women than men. Women are more likely than men to be jumpy, to have trouble feeling emotions, and to avoid things that remind them of the trauma. Men are more likely to be angry than women and to have trouble controlling their anger. Women with PTSD may report physical symptoms including headaches, gastrointestinal problems, and sexual dysfunction.

Comorbidity rates are often more than 80%. Forty-four per cent of women with PTSD meet the criteria for three or more other psychiatric diagnoses over their lifetime. (Kessler *et al.* 2005) The most common comorbid conditions are depressive disorders, anxiety disorders, and substance misuse and dependence. Women with PTSD are more likely to become depressed and anxious while men with PTSD are more likely to have problems with drugs and alcohol.

PTSD patients are six times more likely to attempt suicide than the general population (Bender 2004).

Developmental trauma

This includes childhood abuse such as physical, sexual, and emotional abuse as well as other types of traumas of a more discrete episodic nature, such as car accidents, natural disasters, and so on. The impact on the child at the time of the trauma may result in childhood PTSD. There is also an abundance of evidence linking traumatic events in childhood with the development of a number of psychiatric conditions later in life. These include PTSD, anxiety disorders, depressive disorders, and personality disorders, particularly borderline personality disorder (BPD). For example, Zlotnick *et al.* (2001) studied 235 treatment-seeking outpatients with major depression and found that patients reporting sexual abuse were more likely to have a diagnosis of BPD (29% vs 10%) and PTSD (41% vs 11%). These kinds of retrospective studies were used to suggest that BPD could be considered a trauma spectrum disorder. It is important to emphasize that this is an association, not a causative link, and further prospective studies are required.

Complex trauma

This term has been used to differentiate from single-episode or 'simple PTSD' those situations where there is a history of multiple, extreme, or prolonged trauma. In DSM-IV this is referred to as Disorders of Extreme Stress, Not otherwise specified. Examples include domestic violence, political torture, incarceration as a prisoner of war or in a concentration camp, many refugee experiences, and so on.

Herman *et al.* 1992 suggests that alongside the usual PTSD symptoms, complex trauma also presents with dissociation, somatization, re-victimization, affect dysregulation, and disruptions in identity.

Complex trauma reactions (Van der Kolk *et al.* 2005) include presentation of PTSD and depression with common complications, and comorbidity including personality disorders, substance misuse, significant risk of suicide, violence towards others, and self-harm, enduring personality change, significant social problems, and the need for interpreters.

Evaluation instruments for PTSD include the Clinician-Administered PTSD scale (CAPS), the PTSD Symptom Scale, and the Impact of Events Scale-Revised.

Epidemiology

The lifetime prevalence rates of PTSD are found to be 6.8% whilst the 12-month prevalence was 3.5% in a

United States (US) national comorbidity survey (Kessler *et al.* 2005). The lifetime prevalence of PTSD for women—about 10.4%—is more than twice that for men. This is despite the fact that men are more likely to experience trauma than women—60% of men and 51% of women exposed in lifetime to traumatic events (Kessler *et al.* 2005). This raises a number of questions as to why women are more at risk of PTSD. Not everyone who experiences a trauma develops PTSD or even mild stress reactions. Kilpatrick and Resnick (1993) noted in a retrospective study that 35% of rape victims and 39% assault victims report symptoms of PTSD.

The most common trauma for women is sexual assault or child sexual abuse. About one in three women will experience an assault in their lifetime. Rates of sexual assault are higher for women than men. There is some evidence to suggest that sexual assault is more likely to cause PTSD than some other forms of trauma. Women are also more likely to be neglected or abused in childhood, to experience domestic violence or to have a loved one die suddenly (Brewin *et al.* 2000).

Women are more likely to develop PTSD after a traumatic event if they:

◆ Pre-trauma:

• Have a past psychiatric history (e.g. depression or anxiety)

• Do not have good social support

• Are of lower socioeconomic status

• Have minority status race

• Have a family history of psychiatric disorder

◆ Trauma:

• Have experienced a very severe or life-threatening trauma

• Were sexually assaulted

• Were injured during the event

• Had a severe reaction at the time of the event, especially dissociation

◆ Post-trauma:

• Perceived lack of social support

• Experienced other stressful events afterwards.

See Brewin *et al.* (2000) and Ozer *et al.* (2003).

Women have higher rates of PTSD after childhood trauma than men (Breslau *et al.* 1997). They are also more likely to develop PTSD later on in life after a minor event, if they have previously experienced a violent assault (Breslau *et al.* 2007). These kinds of studies lend themselves to the suggestion that prior traumatic events, especially earlier in development, may have a kindling effect on future vulnerability to trauma. This links with neurophysiological and attachment evidence on the impact of developmental trauma and its impact on subsequent resilience to traumatic events.

Neurobiological models

When a traumatic event occurs, the stimulus first reaches the thalamus, a subcortical structure involved in memory and experiences. From here it has two possible pathways. The first goes straight to the amygdala—the powerhouse of emotions, particularly of fear and anger. The amygdala links with the autonomic nervous system responsible for the flight/fight reactions. It is the amygdala that is in a hyperactive state in PTSD, causing a state of vigilance with autonomic overdrive—palpitations, sweating, and gut-churning kinds of symptoms. It is this state that causes alterations in stress hormones and catecholamines—an important area of study in this field.

Several studies had suggested there was evidence for lower cortisol levels being associated with the development of PTSD. However, more recent studies have not supported this finding and instead point to a more complex neuroendocrine aetiology (Young *et al.* 2005). Catecholamine studies have also yielded different results, with some studies suggesting increased catecholamine concentrations in PTSD sufferers may be associated with the consolidation of traumatic memories (Yehuda *et al.* 1992).

This hyperactive state of fight/flight necessitates the individual leading a life centred around the trauma—either by attempts at avoidance aimed at trying to switch the amygdala off or by repetition because there is no verbal, declarative memory of the event stored by the amygdala that would allow one to work it through. This is what the second pathway allows. From the thalamus, an event may be processed through the cortex and the hippocampus as well as going to the amygdala. Thus, the hippocampus, central to declarative or verbal memory allows for symbolization to occur. One can think about the event, and through the involvement of the cortical structures, it is also possible to understand the meaning the event has taken. One can categorize experience, situate it within context, and integrate it into a personal history or narrative.

In PTSD, there is a problem with integrating the event into verbal experience: instead it stays stuck in the primitive powerhouse of the amygdala where there is no sense of time or context. Childhood traumas are also stored in the amygdala and indeed it has been demonstrated that significantly, the amygdala shows functional and anatomical changes when there has been early stressful events.

Hippocampal lesions have been associated with a stronger fear response and smaller hippocampal volume has been associated with PTSD (Bremner *et al.* 1999). Whether this is cause or effect is unknown. Neuroimaging studies have shown reduced activity in anterior cingulated and medial prefrontal areas to be correlated with increased activity in the amygdala. Thus the hypothesis is that a failure of the medial prefrontal and cingulated networks to regulate the amygdala causes hyper-reactivity to threat and is thus the basis of PTSD.

Enhanced negative feedback in the hypothalamic–pituitary–adrenal axis has long been held as a theory that explains the neuron-physiology of PTSD. However, studies are inconsistent when testing PTSD patients for low cortisol levels or an abnormal response to the dexamethasone suppression test (Young *et al.* 2005). PTSD patients have also been found to have increased catecholamine concentrations in some studies and this has led to the theory that an initial adrenergic surge may be associated with the consolidation of traumatic memories (Pitman *et al.* 1991).

Attachment research

John Bowlby recognized that the differences in the security of infant–mother attachment would have long-term implications for later intimate relationships, self-understanding, and psychological disturbance. The impact of trauma and loss on the mother, her bond with her child, and her capacity to reflect on her child's state of mind have been extensively studied in attachment research. The findings to date provide many interesting links and associations with early infant development and areas such as ego resilience, capacity to resolve trauma and loss, and the transgenerational transmission of trauma. Making use of Mary Ainsworth's 'strange situation', the Cassidy and Marvin system, and the Adult Attachment Interview (AAI), researchers have advanced our understanding of trauma in women.

It has been demonstrated that the AAI administered to the mother will predict the type of attachment the infant will demonstrate in the strange situation. Lack of resolution of mourning (unresolved interviews in AAI)

predicts disorganization in infant attachment (van IJzendoorn 1995). The prevalence of disorganized attachment is strongly associated with the presence of family risk factors such as maltreatment, major depressive or bipolar disorder, and alcohol or other substance misuse. Main and Hesse (1990) showed that disorganized attachment behaviour is linked to frightened or frightening care giving: infants who could not find a solution to the paradox of fearing the figures who they wished to approach for comfort in times of distress.

There is general agreement that disorganized infant attachment shifts into controlling behaviour in middle childhood (George and Solomon 1996). The parenting style associated with this behaviour was characterized by a sense of helplessness and even fear of the child whilst the child's play appears to focus on themes of catastrophes, violent fantasies, and helplessness. Disorganized attachment is empirically linked with childhood aggression (Jacobovitz *et al.* 1997).

Individuals with unresolved trauma or loss experiences as measured on the AAI are more prone to dissociative experiences (Hesse and Main 1999). Liotti (1995) showed that individuals with dissociative symptoms were more likely to have parents who suffered a major loss prior to their birth or during the first years of their life.

Disorganized attachment in adulthood is generally linked with AAIs showing the categories of unresolved states of mind (U) or preoccupied overwhelmed by trauma (E3). These categories occur more commonly in groups with severe trauma-related psychopathology (Fonagy *et al.* 1996). They are also more common in women currently involved in a situation of domestic violence. Also mothers who report high levels of domestic violence are likely to have infants with disorganized attachment (Lyons-Ruth and Block 1996).

Attachment may mark changes in neural organizations that are involved in later psychological disturbance. LeDoux (1995) proposed that emotion regulation established in childhood might substantially alter fear-conditioning responses in the amygdala. Schore (1997) suggested connections between the prefrontal cortex and the limbic system may be the major site of potential vulnerability.

There is evidence that infants with disorganized attachment may demonstrate significantly higher levels of cortisol when stressed. Cortisol at high levels may be toxic to the hypothalamus, thus leading to the theory that this early hyperactivity of the autonomic nervous system may cause destruction of brain tissue with a system that then responds to stress in an irregular manner (Spangler and Grossman 1993). Clearly one would expect this to have an impact on the capacity to resolve traumatic experience.

Transgenerational transmission of trauma

Attachment research and neurobiological developments lend further credence to the proposition made by Freud that those who do not remember the past are destined to repeat it, at least with their children. Trauma may thus be transmitted from one generation to the next when the mother has been unable to resolve the traumatic experiences and associated losses. The impact of the Holocaust on second- and third-generation survivors has been described in numerous psychoanalytic writings (Fonagy 2002).

Masud Khan in 1963 described 'cumulative trauma' as the kind of daily, small but persistent traumas a baby faces when exposed to a mother unable to respond to her child's needs. These kinds of microtraumas are particularly described in relation to a mother's difficulty in modulating their baby's states of 'fearful arousal'. The impact of this kind of cumulative trauma has been empirically validated by current Attachment research and developmental neuroscience (Schuder and Lyons-Ruth 2004).

The current evidence base for treatment of PTSD

The National Institute for Clinical Excellence (NICE) has provided guidelines for the treatment of PTSD. The guidelines focus on the current evidence base that at present remains small in terms of the gold standard of randomized controlled trials (RCTs), but is helpful in recognizing the issues for clinical practice and future research needs.

Limitations of NICE guidelines, alongside the limitations of the evidence base, include the patient selection that, inevitably with research trials, is restricted to populations with PTSD without comorbidity or the kinds of complex social situations many patients have. In the majority of the 30 studies reviewed in the meta-analysis on which NICE guidelines are based, only three studies have included patients with more complexity, social and psychological difficulties, and/or comorbidity (Lab et al. 2008).

It is important to remember that these are guidelines for treatment and that evidence is complementary to clinical judgement. Clinical effectiveness is only one dimension in planning psychotherapy services for PTSD. Services must also meet the criteria of being comprehensive, coordinated, user-friendly, safe, and cost-effective (Parry 1996). Empirical research evidence from RCTs tells us what can be achieved under optimum conditions. The evidence is complementary to clinical judgement. A new paradigm of practice-based evidence is well established (Margison et al. 2000). Inferences are drawn from naturalistic unselected clinical populations. Here the samples are often large, with complex clinical cases and outcome monitoring essential.

NICE guidelines recommend that in the initial phases after a trauma, one should adopt a stance of 'watchful waiting'. This is in essence a programme of psychoeducation with the recommendation to make use of current support networks. Formal psychological interventions targeted at everyone involved in traumatic events have been shown to be ineffective (Gaskell and BPS 2005). Some studies have reported negative outcomes in people who receive single-episode, individual critical incident debriefing. This has led NICE to recommend that this kind of intervention should not be used (Bisson et al. 2005).

Complex early interventions have been studied and are generally variations on the cognitive behavioural therapy (CBT) models used in PTSD treatment. These are usually initiated one to three months after the event and are often shorter in duration (Bradley et al. 2005). Basoglu et al. (2007) describe a single session behavioural intervention for survivors of an earthquake in Turkey.

Pharmacological treatment of PTSD is second line according to NICE guidelines. A Cochrane review reported benefits for selective serotonin uptake inhibitors (SSRIs) but no drug satisfied their predetermined threshold for significant clinical improvement (Stein et al. 2006). NICE recommends paroxetine or mirtazapine for general use and states that drug treatments should be considered when the patient expresses a wish not to engage in psychological treatments.

Psychological interventions recommended by NICE guidelines as having the best evidence for the treatment of PTSD are the trauma-focused therapies of trauma-focused cognitive behavioural therapy (tf-CBT) and eye movement desensitization and reprocessing therapy (EMD-R). Both are individual treatments usually provided over the course of up to twelve sessions (Bisson et al. 2005).

The cognitive behavioural approach to treatment has a number of intervention models that focus to a greater or lesser degree on the behavioural and cognitive components. More behavioural emphasis suggests that the original traumatic event results in a learned association of the emotional trauma that has occurred with the stimuli of the event. Future encounters with these triggers activate the traumatic experience, resulting in increased anxiety. Thus exposure with response prevention is necessary, where exposure involves re-experiencing the images for long enough that the patient habituates a fear response and avoidance is prevented (Foa *et al*. 1995). Cognitive techniques address the dysfunctional beliefs that have arisen through the episode and work on cognitive restructuring. Ehlers and Clark (2000) describe a trauma-focused CBT model which incorporates a number of specific interventions reflecting three targets of treatment: elaborating and integrating the trauma memory; modifying problematic appraisals; and dropping dysfunctional behavioural and cognitive strategies.

EMD-R was developed by Shapiro (1989) and it requires the patient to evoke an image of events causing them anxiety, while tracking the therapist's finger as it is moved rapidly and rhythmically from side to side: at the same time they generate cognitive coping statements. Although there is good evidence for the efficacy of EMD-R when contrasted to wait-list or non-specific treatments, within trial contrasts against exposure do not suggest any gains in relation to efficacy (Taylor *et al*. 2003). Whilst dismantling studies which examine the mutative value of the eye movements do not support this theory, they all include a distraction technique and thus do not disprove the notion that there is a benefit to combining exposure with redirection of attention.

There is limited evidence for efficacy of psychodynamic techniques in the treatment of PTSD. Most studies are case reports or open trials and most of the trials have methodological problems and thus contribute to an equivocal picture. There is also considerable variation in the type of treatment studied—group versus individual and length of treatment—and in the patient population with many studies focusing on developmental or complex trauma rather than simple PTSD. Lindy *et al*. (1983) studied 30 survivors of a fire using a brief (six to 12 sessions) manualized psychodynamic therapy. The patients showed significant improvement and were less symptomatic than controls at follow-up. Brom *et al*. (1989) found improvement in patients with PTSD in three treatment groups— psychodynamic psychotherapy, hypnotherapy, and systematic desensitization—compared with controls. The psychodynamic treatment was more effective with avoidance symptoms. Scarvalone *et al*. (1995, cited in Foa and Meadows 1997) contrasted group-based psychodynamic therapy with wait-list controls. The 43 patients had histories of childhood sexual abuse, though not all had PTSD. After treatment, 39% of treatment group met criteria for PTSD and 83% of controls.

The Tavistock model

Caroline Garland and a group of colleagues at the Tavistock Clinic first conceived the Unit for the Study of Trauma and its aftermath in 1987. It grew out of their experience of the *Herald of Free Enterprise* ferry disaster in 1986 and has developed through the clinical application of psychoanalytic theory to work with survivors of trauma. This includes the large, public disasters such as the Kings Cross fire, the Hungerford massacre, the Hillsborough football stadium disaster, the Paddington train crash, September 11, and, more recently, the 2004 Indian Ocean tsunami. It also includes those personal but equally devastating traumatic events of rape, assault, the murder of a loved one and car accidents to name but a few.

Building on this experience, we have developed a model of working based on the notion of a brief, generally four to six session, consultation. Each session is one and a half hours long and is generally two to three weeks apart. We distinguish this from a psychotherapy assessment. These patients are not referred for therapy. They have been sent to the unit for help with an external traumatic experience that for one reason or another they have not been able to recover from using the usual support available to them. This brief contact is therefore aimed at trying to ascertain what has prevented recovery and hopefully provide them with an opportunity to begin to mobilize their own resources.

The therapist works with the traumatized patient in allowing for the focus to become clearer through an unfolding of the transference and countertransference. The focus is in terms of the meaning of the trauma to that individual. The meaning of the trauma is discovered with the patient through the exploration of the links between the event itself, their early object relations, especially linked with a history of trauma and loss and the transference situation. The transference is worked with in relation to this triad of the event, early object relations, and the here and now. Although trauma-focused, there is not the specific intention of retelling the event to process the memories.

Theoretical foundations

Freud described trauma as a piercing of the protective shield around the mental apparatus. With this comes a flooding of the mind so that the usual discriminatory processes that protect the mind from being overwhelmed are lost. One is faced with a barrage of internal anxieties and impulses alongside the excessive external stimulation from the traumatic event itself. Caroline Garland in 1998 described trauma in the following way:

> The breaking down of established defenses which are found to be inadequate to deal with the intensity of the event, the releasing of primitive horrors and the consequent disruption and disintegration of the existing mental organization, with long-lasting consequences for the personality.

Our view of trauma includes the notion of two phases. The first equates with Freud's description of a breach in the psychic shield and is characterized by shock and a disintegration of mental functioning. This phase is common to all and is seen perhaps most vividly on the faces of survivors we see on our television screens—faces full of shock, horror, helplessness, and confusion. This can last for hours to days.

The second phase is often much less visible to the observer. It is the internal response that occurs perhaps whilst externally it can seem life is getting back to normal. The trauma, like any event, is perceived by the mind as attributable to an agent. This is inextricably linked with Melanie Klein's notion of an internal world, populated by objects that are in relationship with one another. With a traumatic event, the mind perceives this in terms of object relationships; a someone or something is responsible for what has happened to me. This results in an enormous sense of persecution—why would anyone do this to me? Alongside these anxieties is a shattering in the trust in the goodness in one's world to protect one from harm, to prevent such things occurring. Meaning and reason have been lost: there are terrible malevolent forces against one and the possibility of protection or safety seems remote.

We make use of Klein's description of the early infantile state of mind to understand the nature of the anxieties the traumatized patient faces and the defences at their disposal. Thus, the trauma results in a reactivation of powerful, infantile anxieties from the paranoid-schizoid position of early infantile life. The patient is overwhelmed by primitive terror and dread, anxieties of disintegration and death predominate. Terrible frightening forces dominate one and there is no sense of protection or trust in the goodness of the world. The worst of infantile and childhood fears are realized.

In the normal course of development, the way an infant attempts to manage unbearable anxieties such as annihilation and disintegration is to split feelings and experiences into categories of very good and very bad. In this way they can feel more manageable and it is only slowly as the mind develops that it can begin to integrate its view of the world. The other defence mechanism that holds sway in these early times is projective identification. What is unbearable is split off and felt to be evacuated or lodged into the mind of another.

From this state, the traumatized mind attempts to find organization and meaning. The infantile experiences and relationships from the paranoid-schizoid position that have been so powerfully reawakened by the trauma are bound to the event itself. This can be understood from Freud's description of the 'excesses of excitation' the traumatic event has caused that need binding for the mind to begin to assimilate the experience. The event itself comes to be understood at an unconscious level as a particular kind of relationship (as a way of giving it meaning—*this is familiar, I have been here before*), and a relationship that confirms the most threatening aspects of early life. We are in the realm of the very bad experiences. At the same time it feels as though there is little hope of believing in the very good. In this way the event undergoes transformation into something recognizable—the template of an early relationship that evoked anxiety and dread.

Aspects of the relationship that emerge in the room between patient and therapist are a reflection of the early experiences that have been taken by the mind to provide meaning for the traumatic event. It is the relationship that is seen as the centre for treatment, not the event itself. By making use of the transference in this way, therapy then offers the hope of some amelioration of both past and present events. Use of the transference relationship enables a deeper and more thorough exploration and understanding of the meaning of the traumatic event for that patient. Discovering the unconscious meaning of the event in this unconscious sense allows the patient to make sense of the way they have responded.

It is in the very nature of trauma that our capacity to symbolize, to use words to describe our experiences, thoughts, and feelings, becomes impaired. When words are no longer available, there is a pressure to act. Although this may take many forms, one important push is to repeat the traumatic experience in some form. Freud described this in terms of the repetition compulsion. One may see this in the way in which traumatized patients make use of the process of identification to re-enact the trauma in some way. This has far-reaching implications in understanding what can happen after a trauma in terms of a person's difficulties and how this impacts in the treatment through the transference.

Freud tells us in 1909 'A thing which has not been understood inevitably reappears; like an unlaid ghost, it cannot rest until the mystery has been solved and the spell broken.'

All trauma involves loss and loss requires mourning if there is to be recovery. Undertaking the work of mourning is an extremely painful and arduous process. When mourning is not possible, recovery—the capacity to get on with life—is impaired. Instead, various pathological solutions, some based on identification within the traumatic event are available. These include melancholia (severe depression), grievance often involving litigation, a persistent victim state, or identification with the aggressor.

Issues for women in treatment

There is to date no clear evidence of the impact of gender on PTSD treatment outcome. However, more general psychotherapy research on therapists' gender and outcome demonstrates that therapist experience is an important variable and that it interacts with gender. Thus the gender of a less experienced therapist may have a more negative impact on outcome than the gender of a more experienced therapist. There are data suggesting that less experienced female therapists do better with women than less experienced male therapists.

Acknowledgements

I would like to thank Caroline Garland for her helpful advice and editing of this paper as well as her support and encouragement in this field over many years.

References

Basoglu M *et al.* (2007). A randomized controlled study of single session behavioral treatment of earthquake-related posttraumatic stress disorder using an earthquake simulator. *Psychological Medicine*, **37**, 203–14.

Bender E (2004). PTSD evaluations in women require delicate balance. *Psychiatric News* **39**(15), 36–8.

Bisson J (2007). Clinical review. Post-traumatic stress disorder. *British Medical Journal*, **334**, 789–93.

Bisson J and Andrew M (2005). Psychological treatment of post-traumatic stress disorder (PTSD). *Cochrane Database of Systematic Reviews*, **2**, CD003388.

Bradley R *et al.* (2005). A multi-dimensional meta-analysis of psychotherapy for PTSD. *American Journal of Psychiatry*, **162**, 214–27.

Bremner JD *et al.* (1999). Neural correlates of exposure to traumatic pictures and sound in Vietnam combat veterans with and without PTSD: a positron emission tomography study. *Biological Psychiatry*, **45**, 806–16.

Breslau N and Anthony JC (2007). Gender differences in the sensitivity to post-traumatic stress disorder: An epidemiological study of urban young adults. *Journal of Abnormal Psychology*, **116**, 607–11.

Breslau N *et al.* (1997). Psychiatric sequelae of post-traumatic stress disorder in women. *Archives of General Psychiatry*, **54**, 81–7.

Brewin CR *et al.* (2000). Meta-analysis of risk factors for post-traumatic stress disorder in trauma-exposed adults. *Journal of Consulting and Clinical Psychology*, **68**, 748–66.

Brom C *et al.* (1989). Brief psychotherapy for PTSD. *Journal of Consulting and Clinical Psychology*, **57**, 607–12.

Ehlers A and Clark DM (2000). A cognitive model of post-traumatic stress disorder. *Behavioral Research and Therapy*, **38**, 319–345.

Foa EB and Meadows EA (1997). The psychosocial treatment of PTSD A critical review. *Annual review of Psychology*, **48**, 449–80.

Foa EB *et al.* (1995). Cognitive behavioral therapy of post-traumatic stress disorder. In: MJ Freidman *et al.* (eds) *Neurobiological and Clinical Consequences of Stress: From Normal Adaptation to PTSD*, pp. 483–94. Raven Press, Philadelphia, PA.

Fonagy P (2002). The transgenerational transmission of holocaust trauma: lessons learned from the analysis of an adolescent with obsessive compulsive disorder. In: C Covington *et al.* (eds) *Terrorism and War*. Karnac, London.

Fonagy P *et al.* (1996). The relation of attachment status, psychiatric classification and response to psychotherapy. *Journal of Consulting and Clinical Psychology*, **64**, 22–31.

Freud 1909. *Analysis of a Phobia in a Five-year-old Boy*. Standard edition 10, pp. 3–149. Hogarth Press, London.

Galea S *et al.* (2003). Trends of probable post-traumatic stress disorder in New York City after the September 11 terrorist attacks. *American Journal of Epidemiology*, **158**, 514–24.

Garland C (ed) (1998). *Understanding Trauma: A Psychoanalytic Approach*. Tavistock Clinic Series, London.

Gaskell BPS (2005). *Post-traumatic stress disorder: the management of PTSD in adults and children in primary and secondary care*. National Collaborating Centre for Mental Health, London/Leicester.

George C and Soloman J (1996). Representational models of relationships: links between caregiving and attachment. *Infant Mental Health Journal*, **17**, 198–216.

Herman J (1992). *Trauma and Recovery*. Basic Books, New York.

Hesse E (1999). The adult attachment interview. In: J Cassidy and PR Shaver (eds) *Handbook of Attachment: Theory, Research and Clinical Applications*, pp. 395–433. Guildford, New York.

Jacobovitz D *et al.* (1997). 'Disorganised mental processes in mothers, frightening/frightened care giving and disoriented/disorganized behavior in infancy.' Paper presented at the Biennial Meeting of the society for research in child development, Washington, DC.

Kessler RC *et al.* (2005a). Lifetime prevalence and age-of-onset distributions of DSM-IV disorders in the national co-morbidity survey replication. *American Medical Association*, **62**, 593–602.

Kessler RC *et al.* (2005b). Prevalence, severity and co-morbidity of 12-moth DSM-IV disorders in the national co-morbidity survey replication. *American Medical Association*, **62**, 617–27.

Khan M (1963). The concept of cumulative trauma. *Psychoanalytic study of the child*, **18**, 286–306.

Kilpatrick DG and Resnick HS (1993). PTSD associated with exposure to criminal victimization in clinical and community populations. In: JRT Davidson and EB Foa (eds) *PTSD in Review: DSM-IV and Beyond*. American Psychiatric Press, New York.

Lab D *et al.* (2008). Treating post-traumatic stress disorder in the "real world": evaluation of a specialist trauma service and adaptations to standard treatment approaches. *Psychological Bulletin*, **32**, 8–12.

LeDoux JE (1995). Emotion: clues from the brain. *Annual Review of Psychology*, **46**, 209–35.

Lindy JD *et al.* (1983). Psychotherapy with survivors of the Beverley Hills supper club fire. *American Journal of Psychotherapy*, **37**, 593–610.

Liotti G (1995). Disorganized/disorientated attachment in the psychotherapy of the dissociative disorders, In: S Goldberg *et al.* (eds) *Attachment theory: Social, Developmental and Clinical Perspectives.* pp. 343–63. Analytic Press, Hillsdale, NJ.

Lyons-Ruth K and Block D (1996). The disturbed care giving system: relations among childhood trauma, maternal care giving and infant affect and attachment. *Infant Mental Health Journal*, **17**, 257–75.

Main M and Hesse E (1990). Parents' unresolved traumatic experiences are related to infant disorganized attachment status: Is frightened and/or frightening parental behavior the linking mechanism? In: M Greenberg *et al.* (eds) *Attachment in the Preschool years: Theory, Research and Intervention*, pp. 161–82. University of Chicago Press, Chicago, IL.

Margison F *et al.* (2000). Evidence based practice and practice based evidence. *British Journal of Psychiatry*, **177**, 123–30.

Ozer EJ *et al.* (2003). Predictors of post-traumatic stress disorder and symptoms in adults: a meta-analysis. *Psychological Bulletin*, **129**, 52–73.

Parry G (1996). *NHS Psychotherapy Services in England*. Department of Health, London.

Pitman RK *et al.* (1991). Psychiatric complications during flooding therapy for PTSD. *Journal of Clinical Psychiatry*, **52**, 17–20.

Schore AN (1997). Early organization of the nonlinear right brain and development of a predisposition to psychiatric disorders. *Development and Psychopathology*, **9**, 595–631.

Schuder MR and Lyons-Ruth K (2004). "Hidden trauma" in infancy: attachment, fearful arousal, and early dysfunction of the stress response system. In: JD Osofsky (ed) *Young Children and Trauma: Intervention and Treatment.* Guilford Press, New York.

Shapiro F (1989). Efficacy of the eye movement desensitisation procedure in the treatment of traumatic memories. *Journal of Traumatic Stress Studies*, **2**, 199–223.

Spangler G and Grossman KE (1993). Biobehavioural organization in securely and insecurely attached infants. *Child Development*, **64**, 1439–50.

Stein DJ *et al.* (2006). Pharmacotherapy for post traumatic stress disorder (PTSD). *Cochrane Database Systematic Review*, **1**, CD002795

Taylor S *et al.* (2003). Comparative efficacy, speed and adverse effects of three PTSD treatments: exposure therapy, EMDR and relaxation training. *Journal of Consulting and Clinical Psychology*, **71**, 330–8.

Van IJzendoorn MH (1995). Adult attachment representations, parental responsiveness and infant attachment: a meta-analysis of the predictive validity of the Adult Attachment Interview. *Psychological Bulletin*, **117**, 387–403.

Yehuda R *et al.* (1992). Urinary catecholamine excretion and severity of PTSD symptoms in Vietnam combat veterans. *Journal of Nervous And Mental Disease*, **180**, 321–5.

Young EA and Breslau N (2005). Cortisol and catecholamines in post traumatic stress disorder: an epidemiological comm unity study. *Archives of General Psychiatry*, **61**, 394–401.

Zlotnick C *et al.* (2001). Clinical features of survivors of sexual abuse with major depression. *Child Abuse and Neglect*, **25**, 357–67.

CHAPTER 27

Self-harm and suicide in women

Judith Horrocks and Allan House

Introduction

This chapter will discuss self-harm and suicide separately: their epidemiology, associated risk factors, theoretical perspectives on causes and meaning, and prevention or treatment. We will also try to show the links between them. We will draw on general research into self-harm and highlight gender differences where they have been found.

Self-harm

Self-harm refers to actions that cause non-fatal, physical harm to the self, regardless of suicidal intent. Conventionally, the term excludes harm resulting from drug or alcohol use or from eating disorders. Self-harm involves either self-poisoning or self-injury. Self-poisoning is roughly synonymous with taking a drug overdose or ingesting substances never intended for human consumption, and self-injury refers to any form of intentional self-inflicted damage including cutting the skin, self-immolation, swallowing objects, hanging, or jumping off buildings. In neither case does the definition depend upon lasting harm being intended.

It is contentious whether 'attempted suicide' should be regarded as a separate phenomenon to 'self-harm' (Walsh and Rosen 1988). Some authors argue that there may be a 'self-harm syndrome' that describes people who cut themselves regularly as a way of coping with emotions rather than as an attempt at suicide (Pao 1969). However, attaching intent to an individual's self-harm is difficult and unreliable. Severity of injury and suicidal intent do not always match (Plutchik et al. 1989). Intent can be transient and complex, making it difficult for people to report when asked. The fact that someone who has harmed themselves has a much higher risk of completed suicide, also suggests that the two are intricately linked and to separate them makes little practical sense except in extreme cases.

Rates and methods

Our understanding of the epidemiology of self-harm relies heavily on data on attendance at Emergency Departments and from those cases referred for assessment by psychiatric services. Another limitation is that most of what we know comes from research in North America and Western Europe. The best current United Kingdom (UK) data came from a three-centre study. The overall proportion of females attending for self-harm was 57% (Hawton et al. 2007). Analysis of first recorded episodes showed markedly higher proportions of females presenting in the under 15, 20–24, 25–29, and 35–39 age groups compared to males. Annual rates of self-harm per 100 000 (age 15 and over) in the three centres of Oxford, Manchester, and Leeds were respectively 342, 587, and 374 for females compared to 285, 460, and 291 for males.

Past literature has often emphasized self-cutting as the main method of self-harm for women yet research has consistently shown that among hospital attenders, a significantly higher proportion of women compared to men self-poison (Horrocks et al. 2002; Hawton et al. 2007).

It is also worth noting that there is no evidence that women self-injure more than men, at least among hospital attendees. More self-injury in women involves cutting, but other methods are more common in males. There is some evidence that women use different drugs in self-poisoning (Hawton et al. 2007). Repetition of self-harm is fairly equal between the genders.

We can be fairly confident that rates of self-harm are much higher (probably at least double) in the general population than we estimate from hospital attendances.

Factors associated with self-harm

Social factors

Social factors associated with repetition of self-harm include current unemployment, lower social class, alcohol or drug misuse, criminality, and debt (Hatcher 1994; House *et al.* 1998).

Results from the WHO/EURO study suggested that in both genders, those with a lower level of education, the unemployed and the disabled were over-represented in people who had attempted suicide when compared with controls (Schmidtke *et al.* 1996).

Although it is accepted that there are strong ecological associations between socioeconomic deprivation, psychiatric morbidity, and attempted suicide (Gunnell *et al.* 1995) it is not clear what role social deprivation has as an independent determinant of self-harm.

Psychiatric aspects

One recent UK study found that 92% of 150 people who presented to a district general hospital in Oxford after self-harm had a diagnosable psychiatric disorder at that time (Haw *et al.* 2001). Affective disorder was the commonest (72%). Women were more likely to have an eating disorder and less likely to be dependent on alcohol than men. However, an earlier study found that although at the time of their self-harm episode 69% of people were measured as having a diagnosable mood disorder, this dropped to 39% a week later (Newson-Smith and Hirsch 1979).

This finding, and the observation of dramatic changes in rates of self-harm over time, suggests that rises in the number of psychiatric diagnoses found in people who self-harm could be due to changes that have occurred in methods of identifying psychiatric disorders and ways of thinking about mental health. Thus, self-harm is less a symptom of pervasive mood disorders and more a response to social circumstances, accompanied by transient states of distress.

Personality

The Oxford study also carried out a follow-up interview of their original sample. They diagnosed a staggering 46% as having a personality disorder and only two of these did not have a co-occurring psychiatric disorder (Haw *et al.* 2001).

It is not only such high rates that raise questions; the very status of personality disorders is a contentious one. For example, Livesley points out that the personality disorders identified by DSM are not clinically useful, since patients usually don't map directly onto one disorder; they are neither mutually exclusive nor exhaustive in their identification of characteristics and traits; they have poor psychometric properties; they draw from a wide variety of theories and historical perspectives which means they lack reliability and validity and behaviours identified within the personality disorders merge with one another and with normality (Livesley 2003).

A comment regarding psychological attributions of self-harm and gender stereotyping: personality disorder as a diagnosis tends to serve as a catch-all for the types of behaviour that society finds unacceptable, so that individuals are pathologized by societal norms. Poor quality studies have led to spurious clusters of people diagnosed with personality disorder, which in turn leads to stereotyping of individuals.

The much higher rates of self-harm in women compared to men that were evident in the 1960s meant that there was a drive to understand 'these women' particularly those that self-harmed more than once (Grunebaum and Klerman 1967; Favazza and Conterio 1989). For example, Graff and Mallin (1967) described the 'typical wrist cutter' using a sample of only 21 patients:

> In summary, the cutter is an attractive, intelligent, unmarried young woman, who is either promiscuous or overly afraid of sex, easily addicted, and unable to relate successfully to others.

The stereotype of the young woman who repeatedly cuts herself, who has suffered childhood abuse, and who is likely to be diagnosed with borderline personality disorder is a common one despite evidence to refute its accuracy. For example a number of studies have shown that relatively equal proportions of men and women cut themselves (Clendenin and Murphy 1971; Horrocks *et al.* 2003; Lilley *et al.* 2008).

Two aspects of self-harm are often neglected as a result of this preoccupation with psychiatric diagnosis. These are: the social context within which the self-harm occurs and self-harm as an adaptive and thus an understandable response to a range of individual situations and histories.

Antecedents of self-harm acts

Although it is not always clear to the individual or to clinicians how an episode of self-harm has occurred, Fig. 27.1 attempts to describe the pathway to self-harm.

Long-term vulnerability factors

Early separation from either parent has been shown to lead to a fourfold increase in risk for further suicidal acts in men, but not for women (Oquendo *et al.* 2007).

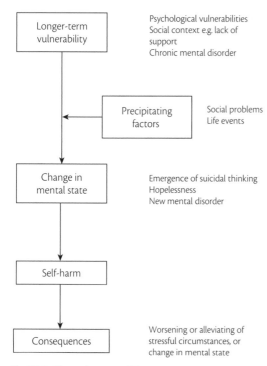

Longer-term vulnerability	Psychological vulnerabilities Social context e.g. lack of support Chronic mental disorder
Precipitating factors	Social problems Life events
Change in mental state	Emergence of suicidal thinking Hopelessness New mental disorder
Self-harm	
Consequences	Worsening or alleviating of stressful circumstances, or change in mental state

Fig. 27.1 The pathway to self-harm.

On the other hand women who perceive themselves as rejected or neglected by either of their parents have been found to be more likely to have made at least one suicide attempt, compared to females without this perception and all men (Ehnvall *et al.* 2008).

One of the more frequent stereotypes of women who self-harm, especially those who do so frequently, is that they have experienced abuse and the presumption is often that this is sexual abuse, though physical and psychological abuse may be as damaging. A community sample in Australia found that boys were more likely to attempt suicide after being sexually abused than girls. After adjustment for depression, hopelessness, and family functioning, the experience of sexual abuse no longer had a significant effect on suicidal behaviour in girls, whilst with boys the increased risk for self-harm and suicide remained (Martin *et al.* 2004).

In another study of antecedents of self-destructive behaviour in 18–34 year olds, histories of physical and sexual abuse, parental neglect, and separation were associated with a range of self-destructive behaviours in adulthood, including suicide attempts and self-cutting (van der Kolk *et al.* 1991). At follow-up, experience of neglect became the most powerful predictor of self-destructive behaviour, leading the authors to suggest

that although trauma was a factor in initiating self-destructive behaviour, experience of neglect appeared to be a factor in maintaining it.

Short-term vulnerability and precipitating factors

Many acts of self-harm have been in response to some immediate emotional or social difficulty that has occurred in the few days immediately before the episode. Examples of such factors include difficulties with partners, parents, children, friends, financial difficulties, anniversaries, bereavement, or other losses (Hawton *et al.* 2003).

These more immediate provocations are most likely to have their effect by interaction with longer-term vulnerabilities—perhaps especially if they mirror or reawaken feelings or dilemmas from those earlier experiences.

Functions of self-harm

Self-harm is often seen as an abnormal behaviour, but it may have an adaptive function.

Early attempts to understand the function of self-harm have derived from accounts from individuals, typically women, who cut themselves and who do so on a frequent basis. As mentioned earlier, this has led to debate about the existence of a separate self-cutting syndrome (Graff and Mallin 1967; Pao 1969; Walsh and Rosen 1988).

Young women's accounts of their self-injury describe it as an expression of emotional distress, such as sadness or anger (Abrams and Gordon 2003); the act of self-injury either communicates this to others or releases emotion and brings calm. Other young women have spoken about the need to turn emotional pain into physical pain, which is easier to deal with (Solomon and Farrand 1996).

The weakness of these studies on subjective experience of self-harm has been that they have been over-generalized to explain other forms of self-harm, which may or may not be repetitive. There is, for example, a strong link between self-cutting and other suicidal behaviour which shows that those who self-injure often also self-poison (Horrocks *et al.* 2003), and there are also people who repetitively self-poison, without specific suicidal intent.

Theoretical models of self-harm

In this chapter we have distinguished between self-reported functions and theoretical accounts of self-harm. Functions relate to the subjective experience and accounts of individuals who self-harm; theory is generated from interpretation, the research evidence and rhetoric.

Suyemoto (1988) has summarized many of the theoretical models associated with 'self-mutilation' and we will not mention all of them here. Although she focuses on explaining repetitive self-injury rather than all self-harm and we would disagree with the terminology, some of the models could also be used to explain other self-harming behaviour.

Environmental model

This model focuses on the two-way interaction between the individual who self-harms and the environment. People who self-harm experience secondary gains from their act, such as care and attention to their needs and this may reinforce or maintain the behaviour. However, the act of self-harm also serves the environment, so, for example, the self-harm act can maintain the status quo of family roles and relationships in a quasi-safe manner. This interaction between environment and individual acts is usually an unconscious one, and in most theories of family function it is seen as especially pertinent to women.

The antisuicide model

A psychodynamic approach sees self-harm as a secondary deviant behaviour that enables women to cope (Maris 1971). Early childhood experiences of neglect, abandonment or abuse lead to low self-esteem. Self-harm allows a woman to partially self-destruct without the finality of suicide, and without dealing with unresolved issues from her childhood. This partial self-destruction actually enables the woman to maintain a veneer of recovery and carry on living. This model sees self-harm as an active coping mechanism used to avoid suicide, rather than as a suicide attempt.

The sexual model

This model relates specifically to women, is based on classical Freudian theory, and focuses on sexual urges and conflicts that arise from repressing them. The theory proposes that women reject the female sexual organs as inferior to the penis because they are internal and therefore not as accessible. This leads to penis envy and a feeling of inferiority. Women become passive and reliant on male penetration for pleasure and internalize their aggression. This aggression may manifest itself in a number of ways, for example, through promiscuity or self-harm.

As with other psychodynamic theories this is difficult to prove or disprove. However, the idea that women are passive sexual beings seems outdated and misogynistic. Although the idea of internalized aggression makes sense, the reasons given for this do not fit well with 21st century sexual politics.

Affect regulation model

This model describes difficulties with tolerating the inner experience of emotions, expressing that emotion, and maintaining emotional equilibrium. Self-harm may be a way of communicating to others feelings of emotional distress. It can also be a way of communicating this to the self, since the act and its consequences can bring emotional distress to the attention of the conscious self. The self-harm either externalizes and releases the emotional pain (for example, through self-cutting) or deadens the emotion, providing escape through self-poisoning.

The dissociation model can be linked with the affect regulation model. Some people who self-harm report feelings of dissociation from their environment; a feeling of separateness or a lack of self. The function of self-harm is often to end that dissociation. Suyemoto (1988) cites other work that suggests that self-harm can also function as a means to *become* dissociated, so as to escape overwhelming emotion.

The boundaries model

This model is based on object-relations theory and has been used to explain self-cutting. Rejection by or loss of someone close, perhaps through relationship breakdown, elicits overwhelming feelings of loss in the person who self-harms. The feelings are so intense that the sufferer feels they are losing themselves. Acts of self-injury reaffirm a sense of self, since the skin represents separateness from others and the scar that is left is a reminder of this distinction.

Cognitive models of self-harm

Cognitive theories have concentrated on styles of thinking that lead to an increased risk of self-harm. Cognitive studies have found that people who self-harm have more passive problem-solving styles than others with solutions being less versatile and less relevant to the problem (Orbach *et al.* 1990). Thus when confronted with a problem, that perhaps has high emotional content, the individual cannot think of a solution other than to harm themselves.

Poor problem-solving leads to hopelessness and/or helplessness, which increase the risk of self-harm (Schotte and Clum 1982). Hopelessness and poor problem-solving ability may, however, act independently of each other to increase risk (Mcleavey *et al.* 1987). There is no evidence that any of these cognitive styles is gender-specific.

Taylor (cited in Jack 1992) complains that theory is fragmented because research has focused on epidemiology, psychiatric diagnosis, and risk. Characteristics or behaviours are dealt with in isolation, rather than drawing on the wider field of suicidal behaviour and thus there is no cohesive theoretical drive to understand suicidal behaviour in all its forms.

Treatment and interventions for self-harm

One of the challenges faced by services wishing to stop people from self-harming is whether it is ethical to do so. If the function of self-harm is to avoid suicide, or to manage overwhelming emotions, then to try and stop it may have more dire consequences, and intervention is likely to be met with resistance and failure because the cause persists. It is therefore essential that treatment programmes attempt to unpick the function of self-harm for the individual or at the very least to provide alternative strategies for coping with emotions or situations that might otherwise lead to self-harm. Another challenge is that self-harm is not in itself a diagnosis; it is a behaviour engaged in by people with a range of diagnosable and non-diagnosable mental health problems.

A review of psychosocial and pharmacological treatments for self-harm (Hawton *et al.* 1998) identified 23 trials. Trials included the following forms of treatment or management: problem-solving therapy, intensive care/outreach, provision of emergency card, dialectical behaviour therapy, inpatient behaviour therapy, continuity of care, hospital admission, drug treatments, and long-term therapy. For most of these interventions, the majority of recipients were women and there is a consensus that women are more easily engaged in treatment after self-harm. The authors noted that both because of small size and the heterogeneity of the samples in the trials, results were unclear. No strong evidence was found for any of the interventions although the evidence was suggestive of benefit for brief problem-oriented psychological interventions. Dialectical behaviour therapy, which was used only with women who had self-harmed more than once, did show some reduction in self-harming behaviour during follow-up.

Goldney's review (1998) notes that interventions do not have a sustained effect. Since suicidal behaviours are often the result of long-term problems, it is necessary to think of long-term solutions, rather than short-term interventions.

Discussion

Epidemiological studies tell us that women self-harm more than men, though in the UK the ratio of women to men has become more equal over the last few decades. The evidence reported here suggests that there are some gender differences in the risk factors for self-harm. Physical and sexual abuse experienced by women in childhood may not lead to suicidal behaviours in the same way that they do for men, whereas neglectful parenting may be more of a risk factor for later self-harm or self-destructive behaviours. We know that anger is a feature of some self-harm in women, but can only hypothesize that the gender difference in rates of self-harm may be due to lack of opportunity and social norms that for women limit the expression of aggression externally, leading to internalized aggression and attacks on the self.

We do not know enough about the functions of self-harm in men or of a range of self-harm in both sexes, to understand where gender differences may lie. The following section on suicide may highlight further areas of difference or similarity that may help with explanations of the gender gap.

Suicide

People who self-harm are at a much greater risk of suicide than any other group of people. However, while there are higher rates of self-harm in women, there are higher rates of suicide in men.

Epidemiology of suicide

Age-standardized rates of suicide for the UK in 2006 show that the rate of suicide for females is 5.3 (per 100 000) and 17.4 for males (ages 15 and over).

In comparison with suicide data from Northern Europe, UK figures are the lowest overall and below the average for the whole of Europe.

There has been a decrease in suicides during both World War I and II; an increase in the 1920s and 1930s when there was severe economic recession, and a further decline in the mid 1960s and early 1970s (Gunnell 2005). The latter may be due to the change in domestic gas to become non-toxic, since the main method of suicide during the early 1960s was by domestic gas poisoning.

In the 1980s there appeared to be an increase in rates for widowed and divorced men and single men but by comparison there was a decrease in rates for widowed and divorced women and single women and the rates for married women remain relatively stable over time (Charlton *et al.* 1993).

A more recent study of suicide in young people between the ages of 15–34 years looked at rates between

1968–2005. By 2005, rates were at their lowest for almost 30 years, for women and men. Worryingly deaths by hanging have increased in young women, and death by overdose has reduced, which may indicate that young women are beginning to choose more lethal and violent methods of suicide (Biddle *et al.* 2008).

Risk factors for suicide

Younger suicides have been characterized by chronic interpersonal difficulties and recent interpersonal problems as well as acute and severe mental disorder (Appleby *et al.* 1999). After controlling for psychiatric history, a number of risk factors remain for men: being single, unemployed, retired, and having higher levels of sickness absence. For women there were no other significant risk factors although one study found a significantly reduced risk of suicide for women who had a child under two years old (Qin *et al.* 2000). This latter finding is consistent with findings that found pregnancy to be a time of reduced risk (Appleby 1991).

Theories of suicide

Biological explanations

Although we briefly mentioned the link between self-harm and aggression earlier in the chapter, it is worth mentioning again. There is biological evidence on the relationship between serotonin function, aggression, and suicidal behaviour (Lidberg *et al.* 2000). In addition, research investigating personality traits has also found low socialization and high impulsive aggression scores in violent offenders (Gunilla Stalenheim 2001). This sheds an interesting light on the male predominance in suicide figures.

Sociological theories

Research on individual risk factors has failed to explain why some people in high-risk groups take their own lives and others do not. Durkheim was interested in the interplay between the individual and the wider community; that this should be a mutually beneficial relationship, maintaining a health balance of individuality and communality. He identified four states that would upset this equilibrium between the individual and the community, leading to a higher probability of suicide within the population of that community. These four states were Altruism, Fatalism, Egoism, and Anomie.

Other sociological explanations also centre around themes of anomie, social integration and isolation, and industrialization and changes in the labour force. Stack's paper (1978) cites the work of Gibbs and Martin (1964) who suggested that those who are divorced,

retired, or have other changes in role, which either do not match with societal expectations or their own, experience role strain. They hypothesized that populations with large proportions of people experiencing this role conflict will have a relatively high rate of suicide. Other work has suggested that female labour force participation may influence suicide rates across countries but there is little evidence to support this (Platt and Hawton 2000).

Psychological theory

Lester (1989) focuses on the presence of depression in those that complete suicide. His theory postulates that events in the lives of depressed individuals have taught them that they cannot influence the outcomes of their own lives (taken from the learned helplessness model of Seligman, 1975). Conversely these same depressed individuals believe they are responsible for their failures (drawn from Beck's work, 1967). This 'depression paradox theory' leads to internal conflict between feelings of helplessness and responsibility. Eventually the individual may feel that the only way out of their situation is suicide (Lester 1989).

Suicide prevention

The World Health Organization strategy for suicide prevention (WHO 2007) sets out a number of objectives. These include:

- Support and treatment of populations at risk (e.g. people with depression, elderly and youth)
- Reduction of availability of and access to means of suicide (e.g. toxic substances, handguns)
- Support/strengthening of networks of survivors of suicide
- Training of primary health care workers and other sectors.

Such steps seem to be logical, yet there is little evidence to support them (Goldney 1998). Some work has already been done on reducing the means to suicide. Changes to the toxicity of the domestic gas supply in the late 1950s and early 1960s coincided with a marked reduction in overall suicide rates. However, there was an increase in the rates of death by overdose from the late 1950s, though this levelled off by the mid 1960s. This could have been partly due to method substitution or the fact that prescribed drugs became both more toxic and more readily available (Gunnell *et al.* 2000). In England and Wales the introduction of catalytic converters in cars had some effect on the overall population suicide rate (all methods). However, there was no over-all change in the suicide rates of young men and women, for whom the rates of hanging increased (Amos *et al.* 2001). Reduction in pack sizes of paracetamol has led to a reduction in deaths by paracetamol overdose (Hawton *et al.* 2004), though data on whether overall suicide rates have simultaneously decreased was not reported.

There is no evidence to guide a suicide prevention policy specifically at women.

Discussion

The work on suicide has consistently shown that in most European countries, and certainly in the UK, suicide rates are higher for men than for women. The usual argument to explain this is that men have access to and choose more violent and therefore lethal means than women. It is unlikely that this is the sole cause for the difference in suicide rates, especially as there is a rise in women hanging themselves. Changes in the last century may shed some light on gender differences. For unmarried women rates of suicide have decreased and this may reflect the change in social norms, where marriage is no longer the overwhelmingly favourable option for women. In contrast the higher rates of suicide in widowed, divorced, and single men may point towards isolation and lack of social support as a key factor in suicide rates. Women are stereotypically more inclined to form supportive social networks than men, whose friendships may be less emotionally supportive. There is little evidence available to support or discount this theory.

It may be that there are more similarities between women and men than there are differences, but research on self-harm and suicide has evolved in such a way that we are unable to determine what gender differences exist. This is partially due to the focus on psychiatric diagnosis, which may be misleading, particularly in relation to personality disorders. We know that women are more likely to receive a diagnosis of borderline personality disorder, but given the lack of reliability of such diagnoses, this is of little help. The fact that subjective experiences, theory generation, and intervention research seem to be studied separately means that often unjustified assumptions are made and little headway is gained in the field of self-harm research as a whole. Given that different methods of self-harm are used by both men and women and that suicide methods may no longer be so gender-specific, research needs to be more encompassing and also specifically look for gender differences, in case gender-specific interventions are needed.

References

Abrams L and Gordon A (2003). Self-harm narratives of urban and suburban young women. *Affilia*, **18**, 429–44.

Amos T *et al.* (2001). Changes in rates of suicide by car exhaust asphyxiation in England and Wales. *Psychological Medicine*, **31**, 935–9.

Appleby (1991). Suicide during pregnancy and in the first postnatal year. *British Medical Journal*, **302**, 137–40.

Appleby L *et al.* (1999). Psychological autopsy study of suicides by people aged under 35. *British Journal of Psychiatry*, **175**, 168–74.

Beck A (1967). *Depression.* Harper & Row, New York.

Biddle L *et al.* (2008). Suicide rates in young men in England and Wales in the 21st century: time trend study. *British Medical Journal*, **336**, 539–42.

Charlton J *et al.* (1993). Suicide deaths in England and Wales: trends in factors associated with suicide deaths. *Population trends*, **71**, 34–41.

Clendenin WW and Murphy GE (1971). Wrist cutting: new epidemiological findings. *Archives of General Psychiatry*, **25**, 465–9.

Ehnvall A *et al.* (2008). Perception of rejecting and neglectful parenting in childhood relates to lifetime suicide attempts for females - but not for males. *Acta Psychiarica Scandinavica*, **117**, 50–6.

Favazza AR and Conterio K (1989). Female habitual self-mutilators. *Acta Psychiatrica Scandinavica*, **79**, 283–9.

Goldney R (1998). Suicide prevention is possible: A review of recent studies. *Archives of Suicide Research*, **4**, 329–39.

Graff H and Mallin R (1967). The syndrome of the wrist cutter. *American Journal of Psychiatry*, **124**, 36–42.

Grunebaum H and Klerman GL (1967). Wrist slashing. *American Journal of Psychiatry*, **124**, 527–34.

Gunilla Stalenheim E (2001). Relationships between attempted suicide, temperamental vulnerability, and violent criminality in a Swedish forensic psychiatric population. *European Psychiatry*, **16**, 386–94.

Gunnell D (2005). Time trends and geographic differences in suicide: implications for prevention. In: Hawton, K (eds) *Prevention and Treatment of Suicidal Behaviour: From Science to Practice*, pp 29–52. Oxford University Press, Oxford.

Gunnell D *et al.* (2000). Method availability and the prevention of suicide – a re-analysis of secular trends in England and Wales 1950–1975. *Social Psychiatry and Psychiatric Epidemiology*, **35**, 437–43.

Gunnell DJ *et al.* (1995). Relation between parasuicide, suicide, psychiatric admissions, and socioeconomic deprivation. *British Medical Journal*, **311**, 226–30.

Hatcher S (1994). Debt and deliberate self-poisoning. *British Journal of Psychiatry*, **164**, 111–14.

Haw C *et al.* (2001). Psychiatric and personality disorders in deliberate self-harm patients. *British Journal of Psychiatry*, **178**, 48–54.

Hawton K *et al.* (1998). Deliberate self-harm: systematic review of the efficacy of psychosocial and pharmacological treatments in preventing repetition. *British Medical Journal*, **317**, 441–7.

Hawton K *et al.* (2007). Self-harm in England: a tale of three cities. *Social Psychiatry and Psychiatric Epidemiology*, **42**, 513–21.

Hawton K *et al.* (2003). *Deliberate Self-Harm in Oxford*. Centre for Suicide Research, Oxford.

Hawton K *et al.* (2004). UK legislation on analgesic packs: before and after study of long term effect on poisonings. *British Medical Journal*, **329**, 1076–9.

Horrocks J *et al.* (2002). *Attendances in the Accident and Emergency Department following Self-harm: A Descriptive Study*. Academic Unit of Psychiatry and Behavioural Sciences, University of Leeds, Leeds.

Horrocks J *et al.* (2003). Self-injury attendances in the accident and emergency department. *British Journal of Psychiatry*, **183**, 34–9.

House A *et al.* (1998). Effective health care: deliberate self-harm. *NHS Centre for Reviews and Dissemination*, **4**, 2–9.

Jack R (1992). *Women and Attempted Suicide*. Lawrence Erlbaum Associates, Hove.

Lester D (1989). A depression paradox theory of suicide. *Personality and Individual Differences*, **10**, 1103–4.

Lidberg L *et al.* (2000). Suicide attempts and impulse control disorder are related to low cerebrospinal fluid 5-HIAA in mentally disordered violent offenders. *Acta Psychiatrica Scandinavica*, **101**, 395–402.

Lilley R *et al.* (2008). Hospital care and repetition following self-harm: a multicentre comparison of self-poisoning and self-injury. *British Journal of Psychiatry*, **192**, 440–5.

Livesley W (2003). Diagnostic dilemmas in classifying personality disorder. In: K Phillips *et al.* (eds) *Advancing DSM: Dilemmas in Psychiatric Diagnosis*, pp 153–90. American Psychiatric Publishers, Inc., Washington, DC.

Maris RW (1971). Deviance as therapy: the paradox of the self-destructive female. *Journal of Health & Social Behavior*, **12**, 113–24.

Martin G *et al.* (2004). Sexual abuse and suicidality: gender differences in a large community sample of adolescents. *Child Abuse and Neglect*, **28**, 491–503.

Mcleavey B *et al.* (1987). Interpersonal problem-solving deficits in self-poisoning patients. *Suicide and Life Threatening Behavior*, **17**, 33–49.

Newson-Smith J and Hirsch S (1979). Psychiatric symptoms in self-poisoning patients. *Psychological Medicine*, **9**, 493–500.

Oquendo M *et al.* (2007). Sex differences in clinical predictors of suicidal acts after major depression: a prospective study. *American Journal of Psychiatry*, **164**, 134–41.

Orbach I *et al.* (1990). Styles of problem-solving in suicidal individuals. *Suicide and Life Threatening Behavior*, **20**, 56–64.

Pao P (1969). The syndrome of delicate self-cutting. *British Journal of Medical Psychology*, **42**, 195–206.

Platt S and Hawton K (2000). Suicidal behaviour and the labour market. In: K Hawton and K Van Heeringen (eds) *Suicide and Attempted Suicide*, pp 303–78. John Wiley & Sons, Chichester.

Plutchik R *et al.* (1989). Is there a relation between the seriousness of suicidal intent and the lethality of the suicide attempt? *Psychiatry Research*, **27**, 71–9.

Qin P *et al.* (2000). Gender differences in risk factors for suicide in Denmark. *British Journal of Psychiatry*, **177**, 546–50.

Schmidtke A *et al.* (1996). Attempted suicide in Europe: rates, trends and sociodemographic characteristics of suicide attempters during the period 1989–1992 Results of the WHO/EURO Multicentre Study on Parasuicide. *Acta Pscychiatica Scandinavica*, **93**, 327–38.

Schotte D and Clum G (1982). Suicide ideation in a college population: a test of a model. *Journal of Consulting and Clinical Psychology*, **50**, 690–6.

Seligman M (1975). *Helplessness: On Depression, Development and Death*. WH Freeman, San Francisco.

Solomon Y and Farrand J (1996). 'Why don't you do it properly?' Young women who self-injure. *Journal of Adolescence*, **19**, 111–19.

Stack S (1978). Suicide: A comparative analysis. *Social Forces*, **57**, 644–53.

Suyemoto KL (1988). The functions of self mutilation. *Clinical Psychology Review*, **18**, 531–54.

Van Der Kolk BA *et al.* (1991). Childhood origins of self-destructive behavior. *American Journal of Psychiatry*, **148**, 1665–71.

Walsh BW and Rosen PM (1988). *Self-Mutilation*. The Guilford Press, New York.

WHO (2007). *SUPRE Prevention of suicidal behaviours: a task for all*. WHO, Geneva.

CHAPTER 28

Medically unexplained symptoms in women

Vedat Şar

The concept of medically unexplained symptoms (MUS) covers a broad range of phenomena. Both subjective complaints (e.g. psychogenic pain) and objective physical (pseudoneurological) symptoms of motor and/or sensory type (conversion disorder) may belong to this spectrum. MUS constitute somatoform disorders in psychiatric nosology. Covering multiple bodily symptoms of both objective and subjective type, somatization disorder is the most severe end of this spectrum. There are also MUS not covered by psychiatric nomenclature, such as irritable bowel syndrome and fibromyalgia (Wessely *et al.* 1999). They are thought to be as physical conditions affected by psychological factors (formerly psychosomatic disorders).

All somatoform disorders are more common among women than men in the general population; in one study, somatization and conversion disorders were seen only among female participants (Faravelli *et al.* 1997). In another study, gender rate of somatoform pain disorder was 2:1 in the general population (Grabe *et al.* 2003a). In a town in western Turkey, the prevalence of conversion disorder was 1.6% among men but 8.9% among women in the general population (Deveci *et al.* 2007). The age group 15–34 and those who had a mother with a psychiatric disorder were at risk in particular. In medical settings, somatoform disorders among internal medical patients are especially prevalent among young women (Fink *et al.* 2004). According to medical public outpatient records in Finland, somatization was associated with female sex, lower educational level, and increased psychiatric morbidity (Karvonen *et al.* 2007). More girls than boys are affected by somatoform disorders also among adolescents (Essau *et al.* 1999). Thus, the predominance of women among subjects with MUS is a common finding shared by studies in diverse cultures, on various age groups, and both in clinical and non-clinical settings.

Epidemiology of medically unexplained symptoms

Various types of MUS are fare from being rare. However, epidemiological studies are faced with methodological difficulties due to the transient nature of the conversion symptoms. The difficulty of a thoroughly medical follow-up to rule out an organic cause while conducting a screening study in the community based on a structured psychiatric interview also contributes to limitations.

Studies in Western Europe and North America have been focused on somatoform disorders in general. One-year prevalence of all DSM-III-R somatoform disorders was 19.9% in the general population in Florence, Italy (Faravelli *et al.* 1997). In Germany, the prevalence of somatoform disorders in the community was 19.7% (Grabe *et al.* 2003b). Representing a problem in psychiatric nosology, most of them were of undifferentiated type.

Among outpatients admitted to a primary health care institution in a semirural area near Ankara, Turkey, the prevalence of conversion symptoms in the preceding month was 27.2% (Sagduyu *et al.* 1997). The lifetime rate increased to 48.2%. A study conducted on women in the general population of Sivas City in central Turkey (a rather non-industrialized region of the country), 48.7% of participants had a lifetime history of a conversion symptom (Şar *et al.* 2009).

Among women in Sivas City, Turkey, dizziness and fainting or loss of consciousness were the most prevalent conversion symptoms, 22.9% and 22.1%, respectively (Şar *et al.* 2009). Non-epileptic seizures or convulsions were reported by 3.8% of the participants. Most of the participants in the conversion group had only one conversion symptom (43.5%), 23.2% of the participants had two, 15.7% had three, and 17.6% of the participants had four or more conversion symptoms. Among subjects with a conversion symptom, 10.5% (n=32) had multiple somatic complaints sufficient to fit the diagnostic criteria of a DSM-IV somatization disorder; i.e. making an overall prevalence of 5.1% in the community. In a psychiatric inpatient setting, however, the most prevalent conversion symptom was pseudoseizure (Şar and Şar 1990).

In a city in western Turkey, the prevalence of DSM-IV conversion disorder was 5.6% in the general population (Deveci *et al.* 2007). In order to fit the diagnostic criteria, these authors eliminated subjects who did not attribute their physical symptoms to a stressful life event. Screening of both genders, a higher average socioeconomic level, and use of the stressful life event criterion seem to be responsible for the lower prevalence obtained in this study. In fact, pseudoseizure patients are less likely than those with epilepsy to see psychological factors as relevant to their symptoms; they are more likely to deny that they have suffered from life stress (Stone *et al.* 2004).

Psychological trauma, health status, and medically unexplained symptoms

In a study on a large group of women in Norway (Eberhard-Gran *et al.* 2007), all somatic symptoms and several diseases were significantly more common in women exposed to physical/sexual violence as compared to non-exposed women. The impact of violence on somatic symptoms and diseases remained after controlling for depression and sociodemographic factors. The same study documented that 18% of the studied population reported exposure to physical violence and 3% had been forced into sexual intercourse as an adult.

Several studies suggest that not only traumatic experiences in adulthood, but traumatic experiences in childhood also affect both psychiatric and overall health throughout whole life. In evaluation of data collected in the National Comorbidity Survey (Sachs-Ericsson *et al.* 2005), childhood sexual and physical abuse were

associated with one-year prevalence of serious health problems for both men and women. Participants' psychiatric disorders partially mediated the effects of childhood trauma on adult health; however, childhood abuse continued to independently influence health status after the authors controlled for psychiatric disorders. There is a strong relationship between adverse childhood experiences and adolescent pregnancy (Hillis *et al.* 2004). Moreover, the negative psychosocial sequelae and fetal deaths commonly attributed to adolescent pregnancy seem to result from underlying adverse childhood experiences rather than adolescent pregnancy per se.

MUS are also frequently associated with a history of traumatization. Chronic pain was associated with childhood physical abuse among women in the community (Walsh *et al.* 2007). In a chronic pelvic pain population, women with self-reported sexual or physical abuse histories were found to have significantly higher dissociation, somatization, and substance abuse scores than women without such a history. Although a high rate (86%) of traumatic life events are reported by patients with irritable bowel syndrome, only a small percentage of them (7.8%) met criteria of post-traumatic stress disorder (PTSD), a rate close to that in the general population (Cohen *et al.* 2006). However, high rates of somatization, obsessive–compulsive behaviour, interpersonal sensitivity, and anxiety symptoms were seen among them. There is a strong association between sexual trauma exposure and somatic symptoms, illness attitudes, and healthcare utilization in women (Stein *et al.* 2004). In this study, sexual assault was associated with a significant increase in somatization scores, physical complaints across multiple symptom domains, and health anxiety. Sexual assault was also a significant statistical predictor of having multiple sick days in the prior six months and of being a high utilizer of primary care visits in the prior six months. Childhood abuse or neglect was associated with increased vasomotor symptom reporting among midlife women (Thurston *et al.* 2008).

Among women attending a primary care clinic, traumatic events were reported by 81% of the subjects (Escalona *et al.* 2004). The lifetime prevalence of PTSD was 27%; this rate was 19% for somatization. PTSD was the best predictor of somatization after control for demographic variables, veteran status, and other anxiety and mood disorders. Psychological numbing symptoms of PTSD emerged as a particularly strong predictor of somatization. Somatoform symptoms are more prevalent in traumatized psychiatric patients compared with non-traumatized patients (Sack *et al.* 2007). There were specific elevations of symptom frequencies for pseudoneurological (conversion) symptoms and symptoms associated with discomfort and dysfunction in sexual organs.

Overall, there is an association between lifelong traumatic experiences and health status including MUS. While being associated with a higher prevalence of MUS compared to men, female gender also constitutes a predisposition for various kinds of psychological trauma in the community (Brand 2003).

Childhood trauma, dissociation, and somatization

Conversion, somatization, and dissociative disorders have a common historical and theoretical origin (Freud 1895/1974; Harris 2005). Among women in the general population in Turkey, 26.5% of the subjects with a conversion disorder had a concurrent DSM-IV dissociative disorder (Şar *et al.* 2009). In clinical settings, 30.1–50.0% of patients with a conversion disorder had a concurrent DSM-IV dissociative disorder (Litvin and Cardena 2000; Tezcan *et al.* 2003; Şar *et al.* 2004). Taking this overlap and the common ground into consideration, several authors suggest that conversion disorder should be classified among dissociative disorders, as in ICD-10 (Bowman 2006; Brown *et al.* 2007). Moving forward, Nijenhuis *et al.* (1999) conceptualize conversion phenomena themselves as a kind of somatoform dissociation, in contrast to psychological dissociation. In fact, they are correlated with each other (Nijenhuis *et al.* 1998). This notion is in accordance with the BASK model of dissociation which points out not only the disconnection between behaviour (B), affect (A), and knowledge (K), but also between them and sensation (S) (Braun 1988).

MUS are extremely common in patients with complex dissociative disorder such as dissociative identity disorder, many of whom also meet diagnostic criteria for somatization disorder (Saxe *et al.* 1994). Somatoform dissociative phenomena (e.g., anaesthesias, seizures, paralysis, dysphagia) are significantly more common in patients with dissociative disorders than in psychiatric controls and the severity of these symptoms is also correlated with the complexity of the dissociative disorder (Nijenhuis *et al.* 1999). Significant positive correlations were found between reports of both dissociation and somatization with maladaptive coping strategies and among dissociation, somatization, and substance abuse (Badura *et al.* 1997).

Although somatization can not be reduced to a dissociative origin, it has a strong link to dissociation. Modern studies demonstrate that patients who have conversion, somatization, and dissociative disorders report childhood abuse and/or neglect frequently (Morrison 1989; Roeloff *et al.* 2002; Şar *et al.* 2004, 2007a, 2007b, 2009). In a sample of low-income African-American women, dissociation was related to childhood trauma exposure and mental health symptoms (Banyard *et al.* 2001).

Physical abuse and life threat posed by a person predict somatoform dissociation best (Nijenhuis *et al.* 2003). In one study, women with conversion disorder or chronic pelvic pain did not demonstrate a relationship between childhood trauma and dissociation in general; however, somatoform dissociation was related to physical abuse in childhood (Spinhoven *et al.* 2004). Women with conversion symptom history report all types of childhood abuse and neglect more frequently than non-conversion subjects (Şar *et al.* 2009). In multivariate analysis, only childhood physical abuse predicted a conversion symptom significantly. Effects of childhood neglect and emotional and sexual abuse, on the other hand, were mediated by lifetime major depression and/or dissociative disorder comorbidity which were two further predictors of a conversion symptom.

Dissociation is a problem for a substantial segment of patients with fibromyalgia and it is related to certain physical symptoms of the disorder (Leawitt and Katz 2003). In a group of female patients, fibromyalgia was associated with increased risk of victimization (Walker *et al.* 1997). Sexual, physical, and emotional traumas were important factors in the development and maintenance of this disorder and its associated disability in many patients. According to one study, although dissociation, somatization, alexithymia, and depression were distinct syndromes they correlate to a considerable extent (Lipsanen *et al.* 2004). Proposing a new category of 'complex' PTSD, Van der Kolk *et al.* (1996) underlined that PTSD, dissociation, somatization, and affect dysregulation represent a spectrum of adaptations to trauma; i.e. they often occur together, but traumatized individuals may suffer various combinations of symptoms over time.

Family relationships, insecure attachment, and affect dysregulation

One reason to focus on dissociation while inquiring about somatization is its relationship with developmental traumas, dysfunctional attachment, and affect dysregu-lation. These phenomena appear as significant factors repetitively in empirical studies on MUS. Somatoform disorders are associated with affect dysregulation, including a proneness to experience undifferentiated affects alongside with alexithymia (Waller *et al.* 2004). Fearful and preoccupied attachment styles are both associated with symptom reporting via a negative model of the self and increased negative affectivity, but alex-ithymia was an additional predictor of symptom report-ing in individuals with fearful attachment. This difference is thought to be linked to the model of others developed in early interactions with caregivers (Wearden *et al.* 2005).

For women, childhood trauma influences adult levels of somatization by fostering insecure adult attachment (Waldinger *et al.* 2006). Families of pseudoseizure subjects are more troubled and may unwittingly contribute to the symptom through family distress, criticism, and tendencies to somatize (Wood *et al.* 1998). Many patients with somatization disorder are raised in an emotionally cold, distant, and unsupport-ive family environment characterized by chronic emo-tional and physical abuse (Brown *et al.* 2005). In a large female sample, patients with preoccupied and fearful attachments had the highest symptom reporting; how-ever, they were in the opposite ends of healthcare utili-zation spectrum, i.e. patients with fearful attachment had the lowest healthcare costs (Ciechanowski *et al.* 2002).

Recent studies document that childhood trauma and dysfunctional attachment may underline the syndrome entitled borderline personality disorder in DSM-IV (American Psychiatric Association 1994); i.e. emotion-ally unstable personality as its equivalent in ICD-10 (World Health Organization 1992). In fact, there is a large overlap between dissociative disorders and bor-derline phenomena in clinical and non-clinical popula-tions (Şar *et al.* 2003, 2006) and many of these subjects have also multiple somatoform symptoms (Saxe *et al.* 1994; Hudziak *et al.* 1996). Both dissociative and bor-derline phenomena are reported to be more common among women then men (Akyüz *et al.* 1999; Şar *et al.* 2003, 2006). Curiously, this gender difference is more prominent in clinical settings than in the community (Tutkun *et al.* 1998). Differences in trauma history, health-seeking behaviour, and symptomatology seem to be responsible for the preponderance of women in clinical settings with this condition including cultural factors (Lewis-Fernández *et al.* 2007; Martínez-Taboas *et al.* 2009).

Medically unexplained symptoms and psychiatric comorbidity

Evidence from several studies demonstrates that patients with pseudoneurological symptoms often experience other MUS. Mace and Trimble (1996) followed-up a group of pseudoneurological patients and found that 64% met criteria for somatization disor-der ten years later, even though only 4% received that diagnosis at the outset. Similarly, patients with large numbers of MUS across multiple bodily systems had pseudoneurological complaints as their predominant symptoms (Swartz *et al.* 1986). Patients with pseudone-urological symptoms have numerous symptoms encompassing multiple systems (Gara *et al.* 1998).

Patients with pseudoneurological symptoms have overall psychiatric symptom scores close to those of the general psychiatric patients, suggesting high general psychiatric comorbidity (Spitzer *et al.* 1999). In a two-year follow-up, 89.5% of patients with pseudoneuro-logical symptoms had at least one other psychiatric diagnosis (Şar *et al.* 2004). In a primary health care centre in Turkey, conversion symptoms were more fre-quently observed among subjects who had an ICD-10 (World Health Organization 1992) diagnosis depres-sion, generalized anxiety disorder, and neurasthenia being the most prevalent psychiatric disorders (Sagduyu *et al.* 1997). In the community, the conversion-symp-tom group had significantly higher comorbidity for lifetime and current major depression, dissociative dis-orders, and borderline personality disorder than the non-conversion group (Şar *et al.* 2009). They also reported more suicide attempts and self-mutilation. These features were significantly more prominent in the subgroup with somatization disorder than the conversion disorder group, highlighting a more severe clinical condition.

In an effort to develop a strictly medical model of psychiatric disorders, the so-called Saint Louis school, a research group from Washington University, St. Louis, adopted the earlier work of French physician Pierre Briquet and redefined hysteria (Briquet's syn-drome) as a chronic disorder with multiple somatic complaints, a precursor of today's somatization disor-der (Hudziak *et al.* 1996). Researchers following this tradition have also investigated possible genetic links among somatization disorder, antisocial personality disorder, and alcoholism. Although those cases exist, only 10.5% of the participants with a conversion symp-tom had a DSM-IV somatization disorder in an epide-miological study (Şar *et al.* 2009). Thus, for a majority of subjects, somatoform symptoms are not part of a fully developed somatization disorder or they may coexist with another psychiatric disorder. Conversion group reported a higher frequency of childhood trauma than non-conversion subjects and the rate of childhood trauma was highest in the somatization disorder group (Şar *et al.* 2009).

Among patients with a dissociative disorder, alongside being an indicator of general severity of the disorder, somatization disorder was also a predictor of suicidal ideation (Öztürk and Şar 2008).

Among patients with conversion disorder, a concurrent dissociative disorder predicts higher psychiatric comorbidity more generally, including somatization disorder, dysthymic disorder, major depression, borderline personality disorder, self-destructive behaviour, suicide attempts, and childhood traumas (Şar *et al.* 2004). In a group of patients with irritable bowel syndrome, the abused group had substance abuse, dysthymia, and generalized anxiety disorder more frequently than the non-abused patients (Blanchard *et al.* 2004). Some patients with conversion and dissociative disorders may even decompensate in a dissociative psychotic breakdown when in crisis due to trauma-related intrapsychic factors, interpersonal conflicts, or environmental stress (Şar and Öztürk, 2008, 2009).

Childhood trauma is usually correlated with higher psychiatric comorbidity in many clinical samples (Şar and Ross 2006). Thus, in consideration of this phenomenon, Ross (2007) proposed a trauma model of psychopathology covering several diagnostic categories such as dissociative disorders, somatoform disorders, borderline personality disorder, eating disorders, substance abuse, and even a trauma-related dissociative subtype of schizophrenia. Beside a history of developmental traumas, these patients usually have suicidality, self-mutilative behaviour, dissociative experiences, and a high number of descriptive psychiatric comorbidity in common, leading to a challenge for current psychiatric nosology and classification (Zoroglu *et al.* 2003; Akyüz *et al.* 2005; Ross 2007). Patients who fit to this model are less suitable to respond to biological treatment modalities while they usually benefit from psychotherapeutic intervention. These patients remain treatment-resistant for a long time and have complications added if their needs are not handled by mental health delivery system appropriately.

Conclusions

Data do not support the view that various somatoform syndromes are distinct entities (Nimnuan *et al.* 2001).

Thus, a dimensional classification rather than defining diverse syndromes has been proposed (Wessely *et al.* 1999). We conclude that MUS may be part of a larger complex of psychopathology with temporary predominance of somatization disorder, major depression, dissociative disorder, PSTD, or any combination of them. Beside a broad range of psychiatric comorbidity, episodes of major depression and suicide attempts may be complications throughout the natural course of this process if there is a lack of appropriate psychiatric or psychotherapeutic treatment in particular. It is noteworthy that, in one screening study, only 24.5% of women with a conversion symptom had received psychiatric treatment (Şar *et al.* 2009). Although most adolescents with somatoform disorders are psychosocially impaired, only a small proportion of them receive treatment (Essau *et al.* 1999). Thus, the majority of the cases in the community remain unrecognized and untreated except for visits to emergency psychiatry wards when in a crisis situation (Şar and Koyuncu *et al.* 2007). Given the subjects' reports of substantial childhood adversity, high psychiatric comorbidity, and chronicity, we conclude that MUS warrant a multidimensional treatment strategy. A full investigation on reasons of preponderance of MUS among women exceeds the boundaries of this study; however, a gender-sensitive approach is warranted while considering this reality with a long past in the history of mental health.

References

Akyüz G *et al.* (1999). Frequency of dissociative identity disorder in the general population in Turkey. *Comprehensive Psychiatry*, **40**, 151–9.

Akyüz G *et al.* (2005). Reported childhood trauma, attempted suicide and self-mutilative behavior among women in the general population. *European Psychiatry*, **20**, 268–73.

American Psychiatric Association (1994). *Diagnostic and Statistical Manual of Mental Disorders, fourth edition*, American Psychiatric Press, Washington, DC.

Badura AS *et al.* (1997). Dissociation, somatization, substance abuse, and coping in women with chronic pelvic pain. *Obstetrics and Gynecology*, **90**, 405–10.

Banyard VL *et al.* (2001). Understanding links among childhood trauma, dissociation, and women's mental health. *American Journal of Orthopsychiatry*, **71**, 311–21.

Blanchard EB *et al.* (2004). The role of childhood abuse in Axis I and Axis II psychiatric disorders and medical disorders of unknown origin among irritable bowel syndrome patients. *Journal of Psychosomatic Research*, **56**, 431–6.

Bowman ES (2006). Why conversion seizures should be classified as a dissociative disorder. *Psychiatric Clinics of North America*, **29**, 185–211.

Brand B (2003). Trauma and women. *Psychiatric Clinics of North America*, **26**, 759–79.

Braun BG (1988). The BASK (behavior, affect, sensation, knowledge) model of dissociation. *Dissociation*, **1**, 4–23.

Brown RJ *et al.* (2005). Dissociation, childhood interpersonal trauma, and family functioning in patients with somatization disorder. *American Journal of Psychiatry*, **162**, 899–905.

Brown RJ *et al.* (2007). Should conversion disorder be re-classified as a dissociative disorder in DSM-V? *Psychosomatics*, **48**, 369–78.

Ciechanowski PS *et al.* (2002). Attachment theory: a model for health care utilization and somatization. *Psychosomatic Medicine*, **64**, 660–7.

Cohen H *et al.* (2006). Post-traumatic stress disorder and other co-morbidities in a sample population of patients with irritable bowel syndrome. *European Journal of Internal Medicine*, **17**, 567–71.

Deveci A *et al.* (2007). Prevalence of pseudoneurologic conversion disorder in an urban community in Manisa, Turkey. *Social Psychiatry and Psychiatric Epidemiology*, **42**, 857–64.

Eberhard-Gran M *et al.* (2007). Somatic symptoms and diseases are more common in women exposed to violence. *Journal of General Internal Medicine*, **22**, 1668–73.

Escalona R *et al.* (2004). PSTD and somatization in women treated in a VA primary care clinic. *Psychosomatics*, **45**, 291–6.

Essau CA *et al.* (1999). Prevalence, comorbidity, and psychosocial impairment of somatoform disorders in adolescence. *Psychology Health & Medicine*, **4**, 169–80.

Faravelli C *et al.* (1997). Epidemiology of somatoform disorders: a community survey in France. *Social Psychiatry and Psychiatric Epidemiology*, **32**, 24–9.

Fink P *et al.* (2004). The prevalence of somatoform disorders among internal medical inpatients. *Journal of Psychosomatic Research*, **56**, 413–18.

Freud S (1895). *Studien über Hysterie. [Studies on hysteria.]* Fischer Taschenbuch Verlag, München.

Gara MA *et al.* (1998). A hierarchical classes analysis (HICLAS) of primary care patients with medically unexplained somatic symptoms. *Psychiatry Research*, **81**, 77–86.

Grabe HJ *et al.* (2003a). Somatoform pain disorder in the general population. *Psychotherapy and Psychosomatics*, **72**, 88–94.

Grabe HJ *et al.* (2003b). Specific somatoform disorder in the general population. *Psychosomatics*, **44**, 304–11.

Harris JC (2005). A clinical lesson at the Salpêtrière. *Archives of General Psychiatry*, **62**, 470–2.

Hillis SD *et al.* (2004). The association between adverse childhood experiences and adolescent pregnancy, long-term psychosocial consequences, and fetal death. *Pediatrics*, **113**, 320–7.

Hudziak JJ *et al.* (1996). Clinical study of the relation of borderline personality disorder to Briquet's syndrome (hysteria), somatization disorder, antisocial personality disorder, and substance abuse disorders. *American Journal of Psychiatry*, **153**, 1598–606.

Karvonen JT *et al.* (2007). Somatization symptoms in young adult Finnish population-associations with sex, educational level and mental health. *Nordic Journal of Psychiatry*, **61**, 219–24.

Leawitt F and Katz RS (2003). The dissociative factor in symptom reports of romatic patients with and without fibromyalgia. *Journal of Clinical Psychology in Medical Settings*, **10**, 259–66.

Lewis-Fernandez R *et al.* (2007). The cross-cultural assessment of dissociation. In: JP Wilson and CC So-Kum Tang (eds) *Cross-Cultural Assessment of Trauma and PTSD*, pp. 289–318. Springer, New York.

Lipsanen T *et al.* (2004). Exploring the relations between depression, somatization, dissociation, and alexithymia-overlapping or independent constructs. *Psychopathology*, **37**, 200–6.

Litwin R and Cardeña E (2000). Demographic and seizure variables, but not hypnotizability or dissociation, differentiated psychogenic from organic seizures. *Journal of Trauma Dissociation*, **1**, 99–122.

Mace CJ and Trimble MR (1996). Ten-year prognosis of conversion disorder. *British Journal of Psychiatry*, **169**, 282–8.

Martínez-Taboas A*et al.* (2009). Cultural aspects of psychogenic non-epileptic seizures. In: SC Schachter and WC LaFrance, Jr (eds) *Gates and Rowan's Non-Epileptic Seizures*, third edition, pp. 121–30. Cambridge University Press, Cambridge.

Morrison J (1989). Childhood sexual histories of patients with somatization disorder. *American Journal of Psychiatry*, **146**(2), 239–41.

Nijenhuis ERS *et al.* (1998). Degree of somatoform and psychological dissociation in dissociative disorder is correlated with reported trauma. *Journal of Traumatic Stress*, **11**, 711–30.

Nijenhuis ERS *et al.* (1999). Somatoform dissociation discriminates among diagnostic categories over and above general psychopathology. *Australian and New Zealand Journal of Psychiatry*, **33**, 511–20.

Nijenhuis ER *et al.* (2003). Evidence for associations among somatoform dissociation, psychological dissociation and reported trauma in patients with chronic pelvic pain. *Journal of Psychosomatics Obstetrics and Gynaecology*, **24**, 87–98.

Nimnuan C *et al.* (2001). How many functional somatic syndromes? *Journal of Psychosomatic Research*, **51**, 549–57.

Öztürk E and Şar V (2008). Somatization as a predictor of suicidal ideation in dissociative disorders. *Psychiatry and Clinical Neurosciences*, **62**, 662–8.

Roelofs K *et al.* (2002). Childhood abuse in patients with conversion disorder. *American Journal of Psychiatry*, **159**, 1908–13.

Ross CA (2007). *The Trauma Model. A Solution to the Problem of Comorbidity in Psychiatry*. Manitou Communication, Richardson, Texas.

Sachs-Ericsson N *et al.* (2005). Childhood sexual and physical abuse and the 1-year prevalence of medical problems in the National Comorbidity Survey. *Health Psychology*, **24**(1), 32–40.

Sack M *et al.* (2007). Trauma prevalence and somatoform symptoms. Are there specific somatoform symptoms related to traumatic experiences? *Journal of Nervous and Mental Disease*, **195**, 928–33.

Sagduyu A *et al.* (1997). Saglik ocagina basvuran hastalarda dissosiyatif (konversiyon) belirtiler (Prevalence of conversion symptoms in a primary health care center). *Turkish Journal of Psychiatry*, **8**, 161–9.

Şar V and Öztürk E (2008). Psychotic symptoms in complex dissociative disorders. In: A Moskowitz, I Schaefer, M Dorahy (eds) *Psychosis, trauma and dissociation: emerging perspectives on severe psychopathology*, pp. 165–75. Wiley Press, New York.

Şar V and Öztürk E (2009). Psychotic presentations of dissociative identity disorder. In: P Dell and J O'Neil (eds) *Dissociation and Dissociative Disorders: DSM-V and Beyond*, pp. 535–45. Routledge Press, New York.

Şar V and Ross CA (2006). Dissociative disorders as a confounding factor in psychiatric research. *Psychiatric Clinics of North America*, **29**, 129–44.

Şar I and Şar V (1990). Konversiyon bozuklugunda belirti dagilimi. [Symptom patterns in conversion disorder.] *Journal of Uludag University Faculty of Medicine*, **17**, 67–74.

Şar V *et al.* (2000). Differentiating dissociative disorders from other diagnostic groups through somatoform dissociation in Turkey. *Journal of Trauma and Dissociation*, **1**, 67–80.

Şar V *et al.* (2003). Axis-I dissociative disorder comorbidity of borderline personality disorder among psychiatric outpatients. *Journal of Trauma and Dissociation*, **4**, 119–36.

Şar V *et al.* (2004). Childhood trauma, dissociation, and psychiatric comorbidity in patients with conversion disorder. *American Journal of Psychiatry*, **161**, 2271–76.

Şar V *et al.* (2007a). Prevalence of dissociative disorders among women in the general population. *Psychiatric Research*, **149**, 169–76.

Şar V *et al.* (2007b). Dissociative disorders in the psychiatric emergency ward. *General Hospital Psychiatry*, **29**, 45–50.

Şar V *et al.* (2009). The prevalence of conversion symptoms in women from a general Turkish population. *Psychosomatics*, **50**(1), 50–8.

Saxe GN *et al.* (1994). Somatization in patients with dissociative disorders. *American Journal of Psychiatry*, **151**, 1329–34.

Spinhoven P *et al.* (2004). Trauma and dissociation in conversion disorder and chronic pelvic pain. *International Journal of Psychiatry in Medicine*, **34**, 305–18.

Spitzer C *et al.* (1999). Dissociative experiences and psychopathology in conversion disorders. *Journal of Psychosomatic Research*, **46**, 291–4.

Stein MB *et al.* (2004). Relationship of sexual assault history to somatic symptoms and health anxiety in women. *General Hospital Psychiatry*, **26**, 178–83.

Stone J *et al.* (2004). Illness beliefs and locus of control. A comparison of patients with pseudoseizures and epilepsy. *Journal of Psychosomatic Research*, **57**, 541–7.

Swartz M *et al.* (1986). Somatization disorder in a US Southern community: Use of a new procedure for analysis of medical classification. *Psychological Medicine*, **16**, 595–609.

Tezcan E *et al.* (2003). Dissociative disorders in Turkish inpatients with conversion disorder. *Comprehensive Psychiatry*, **44**, 324–30.

Thurston RC *et al.* (2008). Childhood abuse or neglect is associated with increased vasomotor symptom reporting among midlife women. *Menopause*, **15**, 16–22.

Tutkun H *et al.* (1998). Frequency of dissociative disorders among psychiatric inpatients in a turkish university clinic. *American Journal of Psychiatry*, **155**, 800–5.

Van der Kolk BA *et al.* (1996). Dissociation, somatization, and affect dysregulation: the complexity of adaptation to trauma. *American Journal of Psychiatry Supplementum*, **153**, 83–93.

Waldinder RJ *et al.* (2006). Mapping the road from childhood trauma to adult somatization: the role of attachment. *Psychosomatic Medicine*, **68**, 129–35.

Walker EA *et al.* (1997). Psychosocial factors in fibromyalgia compared with rheumatoid arthritis: II. Sexual,physical, and emotional abuse, and neglect. *Psychosomatic Medicine*, **59**, 572–7.

Waller E and Scheidt CE (2004). Somatoform disorders as disorders of affect regulation. A study comparing TAS-20 with non-self report measures of alexithymia. *Journal of Psychosomatic Research*, **57**, 239–47.

Walsh CA *et al.* (2007). Child abuse and chronic pain in a community survey of women. *Journal of Interpersonal Violence*, **22**(12), 1536–54.

Wearden AJ *et al.* (2005). Adult attachment, alexithymia, and symptom reporting.An extention to the four category model of attachment. *Journal of Psychosomatic Research*, **58**, 279–88.

Wessely S *et al.* (1999). Functional somatic syndromes: one or many? *Lancet*, **354**, 936–9.

Wood BL *et al.* (1998). Factors distinguishing families of patients with psychogenic seizures from families of patients with epilepsy. *Epilepsia*, **39**(4), 432–7.

World Health Organization (1992). *International Classification of Diseases*, 10th edition. World Health Organization, Geneva.

Zoroglu SS *et al.* (2003). Suicide attempt and self-mutilation among Turkish high-school students in relation with abuse, neglect and dissociation. *Psychiatry and Clinical Neurosciences*, **57** (1), 119–26.

PART 4

Parental Psychiatric Disorders

Michael Göpfert

CHAPTER 29

Maternal stress, anxiety, and depression during pregnancy: effects on the fetus and the child

Vivette Glover, Kieran O'Donnell, and T.G. O'Connor

Introduction

The mental health of a woman can be important not only for herself but also for her child. This is especially so during pregnancy and the early postnatal period. While postnatal maternal depression can impair her mothering and thus affect the child via psychological mechanisms, changes in her mood during pregnancy can change her physiology, and this in turn can affect fetal development.

Symptoms of anxiety and depression are frequent during pregnancy. Indeed, they occur more frequently in late pregnancy than in the postpartum period (Heron *et al.* 2004). Lee *et al.* (2007), in a Hong Kong sample, found that more than half the women had symptoms of anxiety and one-third had symptoms of depression on at least one antenatal assessment. Pregnancy is also a period in which major life events cluster, as women, and their partners, begin to adjust to a major life transition. Several studies show that domestic violence in pregnancy is common (Chhabra 2007; Macy *et al.* 2007).

There is very strong evidence from animal studies that maternal stress in pregnancy has a long-term effect on the neurodevelopment of the offspring (Weinstock 2001). With animals it is possible to cross foster the prenatally stressed pups to control mothers after birth, and thus establish the timing of the exposure. Prenatal stress in animal models has been linked with a wide range of outcomes, including altered cerebral laterality

and abnormal sexual behaviour (Weinstock 2001). However, the most widely reproduced effects are on cognition, including reduced memory and attention, and increased anxiety and emotional dysregulation. Work with non-human primates has identified brain structures altered by prenatal stress. For example, Coe *et al.* (2003) have shown that exposure to unpredictable noise, either early or late in pregnancy, resulted in reduced volume of the hippocampus in the offspring. This is a part of the brain that is important for memory. The responsiveness of the hypothalamic–pituitary–adrenal axis (HPA) which produces the stress hormone cortisol, was also increased in the offspring. Other experiments have shown that the effects of prenatal stress may be moderated and even reversed by positive postnatal rearing. This suggests that although there may be persisting effects of prenatal stress, it is not inevitable (Maccari *et al.* 1995). One notable result with the animal studies is that the effects of prenatal stress on male and female offspring are often different (Weinstock 2007). Learning deficits are more readily seen in prenatally-stressed males, while anxiety, depression, and increased response of the HPA axis to stress are more prevalent in females.

In this chapter we will discuss the evidence that maternal mood during pregnancy can affect the outcome for her child. We will particularly focus on neurodevelopmental outcomes that have implications for psychology and psychiatry, although there is evidence that antenatal maternal stress and anxiety can also have other adverse effects such as causing preterm labour (Homer *et al.* 1990; Wadhwa *et al.* 2001)

Effects of maternal emotional disturbance during pregnancy on the child

There is now good evidence that if a mother is stressed or anxious while pregnant, her child is substantially more likely to have emotional, behavioural, or cognitive problems, including an increased risk of symptoms of attention deficit/hyperactivity, anxiety, or language delay (Van den Bergh *et al.* 2005; Talge *et al.* 2007). These findings are independent of effects due to maternal postnatal depression and anxiety.

An immediate link between antenatal maternal mood and fetal behaviour is well established, from 27–28 weeks of pregnancy onwards (Van den Bergh *et al.* 2005). For example, if the mother carries out a stressful task such as mental arithmetic or the Stroop test, the heart rate of her fetus changes, especially in more anxious women (Monk *et al.* 2003). The mechanisms underlying this are not known.

An early observational study linking antenatal stress with longer term effects on the child was published by DH Stott in 1973. Information was collected from 200 women in Scotland in 1965–6, at the end of their pregnancy. The questions asked of the mother concerned her physical and mental health, the course of the pregnancy, and her social circumstances. The health, development, and behaviour of the child were followed for the next four years. Stott's major conclusion was that stresses during pregnancy involving severe and continuing personal tensions, in particular marital discord, were closely associated with child morbidity in the form of ill health, neurological dysfunction, developmental delays and behaviour disturbance (Stott 1973). Another early study was that of Meijer (1985) which examined the outcome for two cohorts of boys, one group consisting of those born in the year of the Israeli Six-Day War and a second group born two years later. The children from the 'war-exposed pregnancies' had significant developmental delays and showed regressive behaviour. However, these studies, although pioneering, did not control for possible confounding factors such as smoking or postnatal mood.

In the last ten years, several independent prospective, and better controlled, studies have examined the effects of antenatal stress, anxiety, or depression on social/emotional and cognitive outcomes during childhood. Even though these studies used a wide range of different methods, both for measuring antenatal stress or anxiety, and for assessing the child, they all support a link between prenatal mood and the development of the fetal brain. These studies are mainly European with two in North America (Field *et al.* 2003; Laplante *et al.* 2004); none are from developing countries or countries at war, where one might predict that the effects would be even more marked.

A wide range of different outcomes can be affected by prenatal stress. Several studies have shown links between antenatal stress/anxiety and behavioural/emotional problems in the child. The most consistent adverse outcome is in symptoms of attention deficit hyperactivity disorder (ADHD) (O'Connor *et al.* 2002b; Van den Bergh and Marcoen 2004; Rodriguez and Bohlin 2005), but an increase in anxiety is also often observed (O'Connor *et al.* 2002b; Van den Bergh and Marcoen 2004). Other studies show an effect of prenatal stress or anxiety on the cognitive development of the child, as assessed by scores on the Bayley Mental developmental Index (MDI) (Huizink *et al.* 2003; Bergman *et al.* 2007) or language development (Laplante *et al.* 2004).

Three studies have shown an association between antenatal anxiety or stress and more mixed handedness in the child (Obel *et al.* 2003; Glover *et al.* 2004; Gutteling *et al.* 2007). Atypical laterality has been found in children with autism, learning disabilities, and other psychiatric conditions, including problems with attention as well as in adult schizophrenia. There is anecdotal evidence for a link between antenatal maternal stress and both autism and dyslexia, in addition to the evidence discussed already for ADHD (O'Connor *et al.* 2002b). It is an interesting possibility that many of these symptoms or disorders, which are associated with mixed handedness, share some neurodevelopmental components in common, which may be exacerbated by antenatal maternal stress or anxiety.

Different studies have examined the child at different ages, from newborn to adolescence. The newborn studies show effects that must be independent of postnatal experience; those with adolescents show the persistence of impairment (Van den Bergh *et al.* 2005; Talge *et al.* 2007). Two studies found impairment in the newborn using the Brazelton scale (Brouwers 2001; Field *et al.* 2002) and one study used the Prechtl neurological assessment (Lou *et al.* 1994). Field *et al.* (2002) reported that the newborns of mothers with high anxiety had greater relative right frontal brain activation (as measured by electroencephalogram) and lower vagal tone.

The babies also spent more time in deep sleep and less time in quiet and active alert states, and showed more state changes and less optimal motor maturity, autonomic stability, and withdrawal. Lou *et al.* (1994) proposed there may be a 'fetal stress syndrome' analogous to the 'fetal alcohol syndrome', on the basis of their study which showed that antenatal life events resulted in a smaller head circumference, lower birthweight, and lower neurological scores on the Prechtl scale. O'Connor *et al.* showed a continuity of effects from four to seven years old (O'Connor *et al.* 2003), while Van den Bergh and colleagues (2007) have found links between antenatal anxiety and child depression in adolescence.

More needs to be understood about the exact period of gestation which is most important for all the effects described here. Different studies have found different periods of vulnerability. What is clear is that the effects are not confined to the first trimester. Although the basic body structures are formed early, the brain continues to develop, with neurons making new connections, throughout gestation, and indeed after birth. In the study of O'Connor *et al.* (2002b) anxiety was measured only at 18 and 32 weeks' gestation, and the associations were stronger with the latter time point. It remains possible that the effects were actually maximal at midgestation, for example, about 24 weeks. It is also likely that the gestational age of sensitivity is different for different outcomes. Brain systems underlying different aspects of cognition or behaviour mature at different stages.

The size of the effects found in many of these studies is considerable, although it is important to emphasize that most children are not affected. In the general population study of O'Connor *et al.* we found that women in the top 15% for symptoms of anxiety at 32 weeks' gestation had double the risk of having children with behavioural problems at four and seven years of age, even after allowing for multiple covariates (O'Connor *et al.* 2002b). It raised the risk for a child of this group of women having symptoms of ADHD, anxiety, depression, or conduct disorder, from 5% to 10%. These results imply that the attributable load in behavioural problems due to antenatal anxiety is of the order of 15% (Talge *et al.* 2007). Other studies have also found that antenatal maternal stress or anxiety accounted for 10–20% of the variance depending on the particular outcome studied (Laplante *et al.* 2004; Van den Bergh and Marcoen 2004; Bergman *et al.* 2007).

These are substantial effects, but there remains considerable variation across children. Bergman *et al.* (2007), for example, have found that although antenatal maternal stress increased the risk for both cognitive delay and raised anxiety, these did not necessarily occur in the same children. It is likely that the particular outcome affected depends on the timing of the stressor but also on the specific genetic vulnerabilities of the child. There is now some evidence for gene/environment interactions with respect to the postnatal development of psychopathology (Caspi *et al.* 2003); it is probable that the same occurs prenatally.

Some have suggested that the observed associations between maternal mood in pregnancy and child outcome are actually due to genetic factors or the postnatal environment; a mother prone to be stressed or anxious may pass these genes on to her child which in turn makes them more likely to be anxious or have other behavioural or cognitive problems. She may also show impaired postnatal parenting. Although both genetics and parenting certainly can contribute to child outcome the evidence suggests that there is also a direct contribution from antenatal maternal mood. The associations have been found with antenatal stress or anxiety independent of postnatal maternal mood or exposure to life events (e.g. O'Connor *et al.* 2002a; Bergman *et al.* 2007). If the association between mother and child were genetic one would predict as strong an association with postnatal factors. The animal evidence also shows that maternal stress during pregnancy can have long-term effects on fetal development, independent of the postnatal environment or genetics.

The nature of the risk

The evidence shows that the effects described earlier are not specific to one type of stress or anxiety. It also seems that many neurodevelopmental effects can be observed with relatively low levels of anxiety or stress (O'Connor *et al.* 2002b). Most of the studies have used maternal self-rating questionnaires, some using anxiety questionnaires, and others measures of stress (O'Connor *et al.* 2002b; Van Den Bergh and Marcoen 2004). Some studies assessed daily hassles (Huizink *et al.* 2003), whereas others focused on life events (Lou *et al.* 1994; Bergman *et al.* 2007), perceived stress (Rodriguez and Bohlin 2005), or pregnancy-specific worries. Some have used exposure to an external trauma, such as a severe Canadian ice storm (Laplante *et al.* 2004), the Chernobyl disaster (Huizink *et al.* 2007), or September 11 (Yehuda *et al.* 2005).

In contrast to most of the findings, one study has found, in cohort of financially and emotionally stable women, that there was a small but significant positive association between antenatal stress and both the mental and physical development of the child (DiPietro *et al.* 2006). The authors suggest that a small to medium amount of antenatal stress may actually be helpful for the development of the child, although this remains to be confirmed.

Little is known about the types of anxiety or stress which may be most harmful for fetal development. Generalized anxiety, panic, specific phobia, post-traumatic stress, acute stress, and obsessive–compulsive disorders may involve quite different, or even opposite, physiological processes (Tsigos and Chrousos 2002). It is notable that whereas maternal anxiety has been found to be associated with raised cortisol in the child (O'Connor *et al.* 2005), maternal exposure to the trauma of September 11 was found to be associated with low cortisol levels in the infant (Yehuda *et al.* 2005).

It is interesting that the life events found in one study to be most linked with both low scores on the Bayley MDI and increased fear reactivity, were 'separation/divorce' and 'cruelty by the partner' (Bergman *et al.* 2007). This finding is similar to the conclusion by Stott (1973) that continuing personal tensions (in particular, marital discord) were a particular risk factor for later 'neurological dysfunction, developmental delays and behaviour disturbance' in the child.

The high co-occurrence of symptoms of anxiety and depression raise questions about the specific predictions from maternal anxiety. There is some evidence that the effect on the child derives more from prenatal anxiety than depression. O'Connor *et al.* (O'Connor *et al.* 2002b) found that although antenatal depression was associated with child behavioural problems in a similar way to prenatal anxiety, the effect was smaller; furthermore, when prenatal anxiety was included as a covariant, the association with depression was not significant. In contrast, the prediction from prenatal anxiety to child behavioural problems was substantial and not reduced when prenatal depression was covaried. The authors also found that the link between antenatal anxiety and child behavioural problems was separate and additive to the effects of postnatal depression (O'Connor *et al.* 2002a).

Thus the current evidence suggests that the risk most closely linked with adverse child outcomes is maternal anxiety/stress. There is also evidence that the effects on the child are not restricted to extreme anxiety or stress in the mother, but can occur along a continuum of stress or anxiety (O'Connor *et al.* 2002a).

Underlying mechanisms

The mechanisms underlying these effects have only just started to be studied in humans. In animal models,

increased fetal exposure to glucocorticoids such as cortisol has been found to be one mechanism for such fetal programming (Weinstock 2001; Schneider *et al.* 2002) although many other systems, such as those involving dopamine and serotonin, have also been shown to be involved.

In humans, maternal anxiety during pregnancy has been associated with reduced blood flow to the baby through the uterine arteries (Teixeira *et al.* 1999), but we do not know whether this is of clinical significance. We have started to test the hypotheses that maternal anxiety is associated with raised maternal cortisol, that this in turn is related to increased fetal exposure to cortisol, and that this can affect fetal neurodevelopment. The maternal HPA axis becomes desensitized to stress as gestation increases (Kammerer *et al.* 2002) and the association between maternal anxiety and cortisol level is weak, especially in the second half of gestation (Sarkar *et al.* 2006), so the first part of this hypothesis remains to be proven. We know that there is a strong correlation between maternal and fetal levels of cortisol (Sarkar *et al.* 2007), suggesting that there is passage of cortisol across the placenta, at least from 18 weeks' gestation. This correlation is increased with higher maternal anxiety (Glover *et al.* 2009), suggesting that placental function can be affected by the emotional state of the mother, and regulate the amount of cortisol that reaches the fetus. However, much remains to be understood with respect to the mediating mechanisms.

Conclusions

The clinical implications of this research are that the emotional state of the woman during pregnancy should receive much more attention, both for the sake of the woman herself, and for the development of her future child. Most antenatal anxiety and depression are currently undiagnosed and untreated.

One small randomized, controlled trial of 16 sessions of interpersonal psychotherapy for antenatal depression has been conducted (Spinelli and Endicott 2003). It was found to be successful in reducing the depression, and the authors recommend it as a first line of antidepressant treatment during pregnancy. A meta-analysis of treatments for depression in both pregnancy and postpartum (Bledsoe and Grote 2006), conclude that a range of treatments can be effective, with cognitive behavioural therapy producing the largest effect sizes. A recent study has shown the efficacy of cognitive behavioural therapy in reducing antenatal anxiety (Austin *et al.* 2008).

Effective interventions to reduce maternal stress and/or anxiety during pregnancy should help to decrease the incidence of cognitive and behavioural problems in children. The evidence shows that it is not only extreme levels of stress and anxiety that need attention, but possibly the most affected 15% of the population. Also, it is not only clinically diagnosed mental illness that is important here, but stress due to other factors too, especially the relationship with the partner.

References

Austin MP *et al.* (2008). Brief antenatal cognitive behaviour therapy group intervention for the prevention of postnatal depression and anxiety: A randomised controlled trial. *Journal of Affective Disorders*, **105**, 35–44.

Bergman K *et al.* (2007). Maternal stress during pregnancy predicts cognitive ability and fearfulness in infancy. *Journal of the American Academy of Child and Adolescent Psychiatry*, **46**, 1454–63.

Bledsoe SE and Grote NK (2006). Treating depression during pregnancy and the postpartum: a preliminary analysis. *Research on Social Work Practice*, **16**, 109–20.

Brouwers E *et al.* (2001). Maternal anxiety during pregnancy and subsequent infant development. *Infant Behaviour and Development*, **24**, 95–106.

Caspi A *et al.* (2003). Influence of life stress on depression: moderation by a polymorphism in the 5-HTT gene. *Science*, **301**, 386–9.

Chhabra S (2007). Physical violence during pregnancy. *Journal of Obstetrics and Gynaecology*, **27**, 460–3.

Coe CL *et al.* (2003). Prenatal stress diminishes neurogenesis in the dentate gyrus of juvenile Rhesus monkeys. *Biological Psychiatry*, **54**, 1025–34.

DiPietro JA *et al.* (2006). Maternal psychological distress during pregnancy in relation to child development at age two. *Child Development*, **77**, 573–87.

Field T *et al.* (2002). Prenatal anger effects on the fetus and neonate. *Journal of Obstetrics and Gynaecology*, **22**, 260–6.

Field T *et al.* (2003). Pregnancy anxiety and comorbid depression and anger: effects on the fetus and neonate. *Depression and Anxiety*, **17**, 140–51.

Glover V *et al.* (2004). Antenatal maternal anxiety is linked with atypical handedness in the child. *Early Human Development*, **79**, 107–18.

Glover V *et al.* (2009). Association between maternal and amniotic fluid cortisol is moderated by maternal anxiety. *Psychoneuroendocrinology*, **34**, 430–5.

Gutteling BM *et al.* (2007). Prenatal stress and mixed-handedness. *Pediatric Research*, **62**, 586–90.

Heron J *et al.* (2004). The course of anxiety and depression through pregnancy and the postpartum in a community sample. *Journal of Affective Disorders*, **80**, 65–73.

Homer CJ *et al.* (1990). Work-related psychosocial stress and risk of preterm, low birthweight delivery. *American Journal of Public Health*, **80**, 173–7.

Huizink AC *et al.* (2007). Chernobyl exposure as stressor during pregnancy and behaviour in adolescent offspring. *Acta Psychiatrica Scandinavica*, **116**, 438–46.

Huizink AC *et al.* (2003). Stress during pregnancy is associated with developmental outcome in infancy. *Journal of Child Psychology and Psychiatry*, **44**, 810–8.

Kammerer M *et al.* (2002). Pregnant women become insensitive to cold stress. *BMC Pregnancy and Childbirth*, **2**, 8.

Laplante DP *et al.* (2004). Stress during pregnancy affects general intellectual and language functioning in human toddlers. *Pediatric Research*, **56**, 400–10.

Lee AM *et al.* (2007). Prevalence, course, and risk factors for antenatal anxiety and depression. *Obstetrics and Gynecology*, **110**, 1102–12.

Lou HC *et al.* (1994). Prenatal stressors of human life affect fetal brain development. *Developmental Medicine and Child Neurology*, **36**, 826–32.

Maccari S *et al.* (1995). Adoption reverses the long-term impairment in glucocorticoid feedback induced by prenatal stress. *Journal of Neuroscience*, **15**, 110–6.

Macy RJ *et al.* (2007). Partner violence among women before, during, and after pregnancy multiple opportunities for intervention. *Women's Health Issues*, **17**, 290–9.

Meijer A (1985). Child psychiatric sequelae of maternal war stress. *Acta Psychiatrica Scandinavica*, **72**, 505–11.

Monk C *et al.* (2003). Effects of women's stress-elicited physiological activity and chronic anxiety on fetal heart rate. *Journal of Developmental and Behavioral Pediatrics*, **24**, 32–8.

O'Connor TG *et al.* (2002a). Antenatal anxiety predicts child behavioral/emotional problems independently of postnatal depression. *Journal of the American Academy of Child and Adolescent Psychiatry*, **41**, 1470–7.

O'Connor TG *et al.* (2002b). Maternal antenatal anxiety and children's behavioural/emotional problems at 4 years. Report from the Avon Longitudinal Study of Parents and Children. *British Journal of Psychiatry*, **180**, 502–8.

O'Connor TG *et al.* (2003). Maternal antenatal anxiety and behavioural/emotional problems in children: a test of a programming hypothesis. *Journal of Child Psychology and Psychiatry*, **44**, 1025–36.

O'Connor TG *et al.* (2005). Prenatal anxiety predicts individual differences in cortisol in pre-adolescent children. *Biological Psychiatry*, **58**, 211–7.

Obel C *et al.* (2003). Psychological factors in pregnancy and mixed-handedness in the offspring. *Developmental Medicine and Child Neurology*, **45**, 557–61.

Rodriguez A, Bohlin G (2005). Are maternal smoking and stress during pregnancy related to ADHD symptoms in children? *Journal of Child Psychology and Psychiatry*, **46**, 246–54.

Sarkar P *et al.* (2006). Maternal anxiety at amniocentesis and plasma cortisol. *Prenatal Diagnosis*, **26**, 505–9.

Sarkar P *et al.* (2007). Ontogeny of foetal exposure to maternal cortisol using midtrimester amniotic fluid as a biomarker. *Clinical Endocrinology (Oxford)*, **66**, 636–40.

Schneider ML *et al.* (2002). The impact of prenatal stress, fetal alcohol exposure, or both on development: perspectives from a primate model. *Psychoneuroendocrinology*, **27**, 285–98.

Spinelli MG and Endicott J (2003). Controlled clinical trial of interpersonal psychotherapy versus parenting education program for depressed pregnant women. *American Journal of Psychiatry*, **160**, 555–62.

Stott DH (1973). Follow-up study from birth of the effects of prenatal stresses. *Developmental Medicine and Child Neurology*, **15**, 770–787.

Talge NM *et al.* (2007). Antenatal maternal stress and long-term effects on child neurodevelopment: how and why? *Journal of Child Psychology and Psychiatry*, **48**, 245–61.

Teixeira JM *et al.* (1999). Association between maternal anxiety in pregnancy and increased uterine artery resistance index: cohort based study. *British Medical Journal*, **318**, 153–7.

Tsigos C and Chrousos GP (2002). Hypothalamic-pituitary-adrenal axis, neuroendocrine factors and stress. *Journal of Psychosomatic Research*, **53**, 865–71.

Van den Bergh BR *et al.* (2004). High antenatal maternal anxiety is related to ADHD symptoms, externalizing problems, and anxiety in 8- and 9-year-olds. *Child Development*, **75**, 1085–97.

Van den Bergh BR *et al.* (2005). Antenatal maternal anxiety and stress and the neurobehavioural development of the fetus and child: links and possible mechanisms. A review. *Neuroscience and Biobehavioral Reviews*, **29**, 237–58.

Van den Bergh BR *et al.* (2007). Antenatal maternal anxiety is related to HPA-axis dysregulation and self-reported depressive symptoms in adolescence: a prospective study on the fetal origins of depressed mood. *Neuropsychopharmacology*, **33**, 536–45.

Wadhwa PD *et al.* (2001). The neurobiology of stress in human pregnancy: implications for prematurity and development of the fetal central nervous system. *Progress in Brain Research*, **133**, 131–42.

Weinstock M (2001). Alterations induced by gestational stress in brain morphology and behaviour of the offspring. *Progress in Neurobiology*, **65**, 427–51.

Weinstock M (2007). Gender differences in the effects of prenatal stress on brain development and behaviour. *Neurochemical Research*, **32**, 1730–40.

Yehuda R *et al.* (2005). Transgenerational effects of posttraumatic stress disorder in babies of mothers exposed to the World Trade Center attacks during pregnancy. *Journal of Clinical Endocrinology and Metabolism*, **90**, 4115–8.

CHAPTER 30

Depressed mothers and their children: attachment issues

Antonia Bifulco

Introduction

Depression is a common psychological disorder in mothers. This is not only because female rates are nearly double male rates at different life stages (Nolen-Hoeksema 1990), but also because motherhood confers added risk (Bebbington *et al.* 1991). This results in dual social and psychological problems: first around the health and lack of well-being of mothers who suffer the depression, and second around the health and development of their children on whom it impacts. Thus women's quality of life, intergenerational transmission of risk, and obstacles to a child's healthy development become inter-related problems linked to maternal depression. Parenting and attachment style are both implicated.

Maternal depression

Rates of major depression in inner-city working class mothers are quoted as 15% yearly, with 10% new onsets (Brown *et al.* 1990). This is similar to the 10–15% rates for women in the six-month postnatal period (Boyce 2003). Whilst depressive disorder can encompass bipolar and psychotic varieties, these are substantially less common than major depression (for example, psychotic depression affecting 1 in 1000 women after childbirth). Major depression is the focus of this chapter, defined by the *Diagnostic Statistical Manual of Mental Disorders* (DSM) as a series of symptoms, of which depressed mood or loss of interest are crucial, and others include weight loss or gain, insomnia/hypersomnia, agitation or retardation, fatigue or energy loss, feelings of worthlessness, diminished ability to think, concentrate, or make decision, and recurrent thoughts of death or suicide plans or attempts. Clinical level disorder is signified by the overlap of five such symptoms

which need to occur, most of the time, for a minimum of two weeks with significant distress or impairment to functioning (American Psychiatric Association 1997).

Despite the high prevalence of such disorder, treatment for mothers is by no means easily available or accessed. For example it is estimated that 40–50% of episodes of postnatal depression go undetected in the United Kingdom (Seeley *et al.* 1996) with similar estimates for depression at other life stages (Paykel *et al.* 1997). This is due to a variety of reasons: stigma associated with depression, mistrust of medication, constraints around help-seeking, fear of having a child taken away, and high waiting lists for counselling services in primary care. Identifying the causes and correlates of maternal depression can aid in the public understanding of the disorder to help with detection and service-access.

Depression is a culmination of social adversity and psychological vulnerability compounded by recent stressors to provoke an onset (Brown *et al.* 1990). A hostile relationship with partner, lack of support from close others, and low self-esteem, constitute the proximal vulnerability factors which increase risk of disorder (Brown *et al.* 1990). This vulnerability is primed by more distal early life history of neglect and abuse in the woman, together with adverse adolescent and early adult experiences (Harris *et al.* 1987; Bifulco *et al.* 2000). Thus an episode of depression in the mother carries with it an accumulation of vulnerability and stressors and all can impact on her child.

Maternal depression and childcare

Mechanisms by which maternal depression can have an impact on offspring are numerous. Those researched include parenting behaviour, attachment behaviour, and stress responses. Whilst genetic factors have also been identified (Caspi *et al.* 2003; Wilhelm *et al.* 2006), these are not as yet implicated in parenting behaviour. Depressive disorder can impede mother–child interactions and the quality of care provided in infancy (Murray *et al.* 2003), in later childhood (Belsky and Vondra 1989; Hammen 1992; Murray *et al.* 2003), in adolescence (Kestler and Lewis 2006), and in relation to child safeguarding services (Cleaver *et al.* 1999). However, studies increasingly show that other factors causally related to depression may have greater impact. The medicalization of risk transmission by identifying depression as the source of the problem, masks a more complex model which involves social and psychological life-course issues in mothers, transmitted to their offspring through parenting, attachment, and social adversity, including the behaviour of partners.

There have been a number of studies showing the negative impact of maternal postnatal depression on the mother–infant relationship. Thus depressed mothers' engagement with their infants is characterized by hostile intrusive behaviour or withdrawal and disengagement (Cohn *et al.* 1990; Field *et al.* 1990). These maternal interactive profiles are accompanied by distinctive styles of infant disturbance, including distress and avoidance. Depressed mothers are less sensitively attuned to infants, less affirming, and more negating (Murray *et al.* 2003). However, the studies also show the impact of social factors: first the negative effects on infants are significantly associated with the mother's life events and difficulties as well as her disorder (Murray *et al.* 2003). Second, among depressed populations who are *not* disadvantaged, extreme forms of infant disturbance do not occur (Field 1992).

In older children, the parenting task is identified in terms of the provision of adequate care and control, attunement to the child's capabilities, and development. Poor parenting is determined by the quality of marital relationships, work, and social networks (Belsky and Vondra 1989), and these are influenced over the life course by prior developmental history and experiences. Stress factors emerge as more important than maternal disorder in relating to parenting outcomes (Shaw *et al.* 1994).

Maternal depression and partner relationships

The marital or partner relationship is seen as key to parenting success. In mothers, conflict in the partner relationship is associated with critical parenting and with low emotional responsivity, and this together with powerlessness in the marital relationship lead to conduct problems in children (Webster Stratton and

Hammond 1999). Similar findings are shown for fathers, but here marital powerlessness does not add. The quality of relationship with a partner is also central to models of women's affective disorder. Negative effects on the women can occur through a number of mechanisms, such as the increased burden of sole parenting when partner is absent (Brown and Moran 1997), or through the impact of partners' violence or other unpredictable behaviour related to alcohol use, antisocial disorder, and poor work history (Andrews and Brown 1988). It is also clear from examining accounts of childhood experience of the next generation that the absence of the father, family discord, violence involving the father, and abuse from the father are key for disorder in the offspring (Bifulco *et al.* 2009). The marital/partner relationship is a critical candidate in the transmission of risk simultaneously to mothers and offspring. This can also be protective—studies of young women with an institutional care background have better parenting behaviour if living with a socialized partner with no obvious psychopathology (Quinton *et al.* 1985).

Attachment theory

Attachment theory provides a powerful framework for understanding and investigating parent–child interaction (Bowlby 1969, 1973, 1980). However, it has a wide remit and it also explains relationship patterns in general (for example, partner relating, support-access, and parenting capacity) as well as providing linkages with early life parenting experiences and risk of psychological disorder. It also illuminates the intergenerational transmission of risk. Attachment style has been investigated across the lifespan, including in perinatal investigation (Fonagy *et al.* 1991), parenting of children and adolescents (Shapiro and Levendosky 1999), and neglect/abuse of children (Crittenden 1997). It has also been examined in relation to the quality of marital/partner relationships (Hazan and Shaver 1994), accessing support (Larose and Bernier 2001), and mental health (Hammen *et al.* 1995; Sable 1997; Dozier *et al.* 1999; Muller and Lemieuz 2000). Thus within the attachment framework, parenting, partnerships, support, and depression are all implicated. All can be shown to converge on mother–child interactions.

The tenets of attachment theory hold that inconsistent, uncaring, or hostile parenting in the early years of life have long-lasting consequences for future relating style and adjustment. This occurs through 'internal working models' or cognitive structures developed in early years to create a template for future expectations of relationships (Fraley and Waller 1998). These working models are expressed in terms of secure or insecure styles of relating to others. Those with secure styles have a positive expectation of support, care, and warmth from those who are close to them. Those with insecure styles have expectations of harm, rejection, abandonment, betrayal, or unreliable support or care. Such styles have implications for the care of children intergenerationally, as experiences of poor parenting in early life can be repeated (van IJzendoorn 1995), but they also have other implications such as negatively influencing the choice of partner or support figures and failure to access emotional support (Rholes et al. 1998).

Attachment research on parenting has typically involved closely observed interactions between parent and infant in representative samples to examine normative experience (Ainsworth et al. 1978; de Wolff and van IJzendoorn 1997). However, the extension of attachment research to families living in more extreme social conditions, in relation to neglect, abuse, and maternal disorder, has moved the study of attachment further into the fields of child safeguarding (Crittenden 1988; Howe 2003) and psychopathology (Dozier et al. 1999). Insensitive parenting in the child's early years may, under certain adverse conditions, become implicated in maltreatment further down the line. Thus, models of parenting that involve social deprivation, marital disharmony, parents' work life, social isolation, and parents' early life history are gradually becoming incorporated into the attachment approach (Belsky and Vondra 1989; Shaw et al. 1994).

Most of the research on attachment and parenting has utilized the Adult Attachment Interview (AAI) for parents, together with the Strange Situation test (SST) for assessing infant style. However, more contemporary instruments include the Attachment Style Interview (ASI) which is a support-based assessment of attachment style used for parents which has examined mothers in relation to parental support context, depression, and parenting of adolescent children. The two instruments and relevant research will be examined in turn.

The Adult Attachment Interview

The Adult Attachment Interview (George et al. 1984) is a well-established research tool for assessing attachment style in adults, based upon questions about childhood and early life experience, with discourse analysis of transcripts to ascertain cognitive features related to attachment such as coherence, idealization, derogation,

and recall. These are used to derive attachment style categories in terms of autonomous–secure, dismissing–insecure, and preoccupied–insecure style in addition to 'unresolved loss' (Prior and Glaser 2006). The measure has been particularly orientated towards parenting style and the transmission of attachment patterns from mother to child. Thus, the AAI has been used in mother–infant pairs to examine similarity of style in the dyads, where attachment style in the infants is determined by the SST (Ainsworth et al. 1978). In this paradigm, the interaction within mother–child dyads plays out the expression of the internalized secure, anxious–ambivalent or avoidant working models of attachment in both participants (Main et al. 1985). The transmission of attachment insecurity across generations is argued to be through maternal insensitivity, intrusiveness or detached interaction, and poor emotional regulation when in contact with the child (de Wolff and van IJzendoorn 1997). This is indicated by significant concordances shown between mother and infant of around 65–72% (van IJzendoorn 1995). The consistency of mother–infant attachment categories also holds prospectively; for example, from maternal antenatal assessments of attachment style, to child attachment behaviour in the SST at three months (Fonagy et al. 1991), and later at 12–18 months of age (Steele et al. 1996). Reviews of the literature show a consistent association of maternal depression with insecurity in the child (Martins and Gaffan 2000) with lifetime maternal depression similarly predicting poor mother–infant interactions and insecure infant attachment (Carter et al. 2001).

Family systems approaches have added to the parent–child focus on intergenerational transmission by examining the contribution of either parents' attachment style, as well as the effects of the relationship between parents, on children's development and disorder. Studies by Cowan and colleagues have specifically explored the quality of the parents' relationship as partners, their attachment styles, and problem behaviour in their preschool-age children (Cowan et al. 1996). In a sample of couples and their first-born child, the AAI was administered to both mothers and fathers, together with assessments of marital quality, parenting style, and child problem behaviour—both internalizing and externalizing. While no direct associations were found between parents' attachment scores and the child's problem behaviour, path analytic models showed different outcomes for mothers' and fathers' behaviour and for type of disorder outcome. The models showed that mothers' attachment representations, quality of marital relationship, and parenting style provided the best fit for explaining internalizing behaviour in the child, while for fathers, attachment representations followed a similar model but for externalizing behaviour. For mothers, the quality of marriage was found to be independent of adult attachment status with positive marital functioning acting as a buffer, protecting the child against the negative impact of insecure attachment in one or both parents.

The Attachment Style Interview

The social psychological approach to measurement of adult attachment style is built around support, and typically includes a set of questions about relationships with romantic partners and close support figures (Hazan and Shaver 1994; Mickelson *et al.* 1997). The Attachment Style Interview (ASI) is one of the few interviews measures that provides such contextual information while also coding attachment style categorizations (Bifulco *et al.* 2002a). This instrument assesses the quality of close relationships in adulthood (with partner and other adults named as very close) as well as attitudes indicative of both secure and insecure styles (e.g. Enmeshed, Fearful, Angry–Dismissive, and Withdrawn) (Bifulco *et al.* 2002b). Insecure attachment style has been shown to mediate between childhood neglect/abuse and onsets of depression in mothers (Bifulco *et al.* 2006a) with evidence emerging that parenting of the next generation is also implicated.

Findings similar to those reported by Cowan and colleagues concerning mothers were found in a study of intergenerational transmission to adolescent offspring. Mothers' insecure attachment style was assessed with the ASI in relation to her history of partner relationships, her parenting competence, and emotional disorder in her adolescent offspring (Bifulco *et al.* 2009). The sample comprised 146 high-risk, mother–adolescent offspring pairs in London, who were recruited on the basis of the mothers' psychosocial vulnerability for depression. Interviews were undertaken independently with mother and offspring. A path model was developed which showed that while mothers' insecure attachment style had no direct link to her offspring's report of maternal neglect/abuse, or to the young persons' disorder, indirect links occurred through mothers' incompetent parenting, partners' problem behaviour and marital adversity. Mother's lifetime depression, although common in this series, did not add to risk in her offspring.

The ASI has also been utilized across European and United States centres to assess its utility as a risk marker for maternal perinatal disorder (Bifulco *et al.* 2004).

The study showed insecure attachment related to lower social class position, more negative social context, and major or minor depression both antenatally and postnatally. A specific association of Enmeshed or Fearful styles and postnatal disorder was found. Other findings from the same study showed poor partner support in pregnancy was related to poor mother–baby interaction at six months, with no effect from maternal depression (Gunning *et al.* 2004). Evidence is also emerging that insecure attachment style antenatally also related to the mothers' insensitive interaction with the baby at six months (Bifulco *et al.* 2006b). A Portuguese study showed insecure attachment style using the ASI was also related to teenage pregnancy and depression during pregnancy (Figueirido *et al.* 2006). Pregnant teenagers were found to be nearly three times more likely to have an insecure attachment style than adults. Enmeshed style and poor partner support provided the best model for depression in both teenagers and comparison adult mothers.

These studies all indicate that an ecological approach (emphasizing social adversity and different role domains), and a lifespan approach (emphasizing a history of adverse relationships at different life stages) can be used in an attachment framework to indicate mechanisms of transmission of risk to the next generation.

Discussion

The negative impact of maternal depression on infant health and development is increasingly shown to work through associated problems in relating, compounded by social adversity. These can be encompassed by attachment and social ecological approaches, to show effects on the children. This has important implications for preventative and early intervention work with families. The recent government agenda has highlighted children's development and well-being in its Every Child Matters legislation (www.everychildmatters.gov.uk). Whilst this approach is child-centred, the promotion of parenting programmes for mothers is also advocated, although the emphasis on the *mothers* themselves and their psychosocial risks receives less attention.

The use of the ASI or similar assessments for health visiting services, or to use alongside parenting assessments, may prove useful for intervention work. This is already happening in the adoption–fostering field to gauge carer vulnerability or resilience (Bifulco *et al.* 2008). Given health and care services working jointly with education to focus on children in schools, this may also be an opportunity to capture mothers vulnerable to disorder in these contexts for intervention. Thus parenting programmes could be geared not only to care provision and mother–child interaction, but also to maternal help for depression and associated vulnerability. Research needs to examine whether parenting programmes may serve not only to improve mother–child interaction, but also improve mother's psychosocial risk and disorder.

Depression is a very treatable disorder, with both therapeutic approaches and medications shown to have significant beneficial effects, whether treated in general practice (Schulberg *et al.* 1995; Rost *et al.* 2000) or in the postnatal period (O'Hara *et al.* 2000; Stuart *et al.* 2003). Problems arise when depression is undetected and access to services restricted. Whilst screenings in the antenatal period are common, these can miss psychosocial vulnerability. Depression is known to be increasing with much still undetected, despite its causes being known and treatments available. It is perhaps partly due to the scale of the problem that there is insufficient proactive work in the area. The Layard report has indicated the large size of the cognitive behavioural therapy workforce required to tackle the scale of the problem (Layard 2006). Whether treatments for depression will also tackle the underlying psychosocial risks which affect parenting and children's development is unclear. Both aspects need to be tackled in order to improve well-being in families.

Problems in parenting and family life need to be seen in the context of social adversity. Disadvantage, stress, failed relationships, and loss of support are all key to understanding negative impact on children and mothers. Intervention is important at different points, both in the child's development—infancy, mid-childhood, and adolescence—but also at different stages in the development of maternal risk. Tackling maternal depression is rather late in the evolution of these problems. Whilst depression itself must be treated, earlier solutions for resolving problems would ensure less suffering and cascading of risk factors. This should be the aim of multiple agencies working with children and families.

References

Ainsworth MDS *et al.* (1978). *Patterns of Attachment: A Psychological Study of the Strange Situation*. Lawrence, Erlbaum, Hillsdale, NJ.

American Psychiatric Association (1997). *Diagnostic and Statistical Manual of Mental Disorders. Fourth edition, text revision*. American Psychiatric Association, Washington, DC.

Andrews B and Brown GW (1988). Marital violence in the community: A biographical approach. *British Journal of Psychiatry*, **153**, 305–12.

Bebbington PE *et al.* (1991). Gender, parity and the prevalence of minor affective disorder. *British Journal of Psychiatry*, **158**, 40–5.

Belsky J and Vondra J (1989). Lessons from child abuse: the determinants of parenting. In C Cicchetti and V Carlson (eds) *Handbook of Child Maltreatment: Theory and Research*, pp 153–202. Cambridge University Press, Boston, MA.

Bifulco A *et al.* (2000). Lifetime stressors and recurrent depression: preliminary findings of the Adult Life Phase Interview (ALPHI). *Social Psychiatry and Psychiatric Epidemiology*, **35**, 264–275.

Bifulco A *et al.* (2002a). Adult attachment style. I: Its relationship to clinical depression. *Social Psychiatry & Psychiatric Epidemiology*, **37**, 50–9.

Bifulco A *et al.* (2002b). Childhood adversity, parental vulnerability and disorder: examining inter-generational transmission of risk. *Journal of Child Psychology and Psychiatry*, **43**, 1075–86.

Bifulco A *et al.* (2004). Maternal attachment style and depression associated with childbirth: Preliminary results from a European/US cross-cultural study. *British Journal of Psychiatry (Special supplement)*, **184**, 31–7.

Bifulco A *et al.* (2006a). Adult attachment style as a mediator of childhood neglect/abuse and adult depression and anxiety. *Social Psychiatry & Psychiatric Epidemiology*, **41**, 796–805.

Bifulco A *et al.* (2006b). *Examining maternal insecure attachment style antenatally and mother infant interactions at 3–6 months in four European sites.* Conference presentation, The Marce Society International Biennial Conference, September 2006, Keele University, UK.

Bifulco A *et al.* (2008). The Attachment Style Interview (ASI) as an assessment of support capaity: exploring its use for adoption-fostering assessment. *Adoption and Fostering*, **32**, 33–45.

Bifulco A *et al.* (2009). Problem partners and parenting: Exploring linkages with maternal insecure attachment style and her neglect/abuse of children. *Attachment and Human Development*, **11**, 69–85.

Bowlby J (1969). *Attachment and Loss (Volume 1). Attachment.* Basic Books, New York.

Bowlby J (1973). *Attachment and Loss (Volume 2). Separation: Anxiety and Anger.* Basic Books, New York.

Bowlby J (1980). *Attachment and Loss (Volume 3). Loss: Sadness and depression.* Basic Books, New York.

Boyce P (2003). Risk factors for postnatal depression: a review and risk factors in Australian populations. *Archive of Women's Mental Health*, **6**, s43–s50.

Brown G and Moran P (1997). Single mothers, poverty and depression. *Psychological Medicine*, **27**, 21–33.

Brown GW *et al.* (1990). Self-esteem and depression: III. Aetiological issues. *Social Psychiatry and Psychiatric Epidemiology*, **25**, 235–43.

Carter A *et al.* (2001). Maternal depression and comorbidity: predicting early parenting, attachment insecurity and toddler social-economic problems and competencies.

Journal of the American Academy of Child & Adolescent Psychiatry, **40**, 18–26.

Caspi A *et al.* (2003). Influence of life stress on depression: moderation by a polymorphism in the 5-HTT gene. *Science*, **301**, 386–9.

Cleaver H *et al.* (1999). *Chidren's Needs – Parenting Capacity. The impact of mental illness, problem alcohol and drug use, and domestic violence on children's development.* The Stationery Office, London.

Cohn JF *et al.* (1990). Face to face interactions of postpartum depressed and non-depressed mother-infant pairs at two months. *Developmental Psychology*, **26**, 15–23.

Cowan P *et al.* (1996). Parents' attachment histories and children's externalising and internalising behaviours: Exploring family systems models of linkage. *Journal of Consulting and Clinical Psychology*, **64**, 53–63.

Crittenden PM (1988). Relationships at risk. In: J Belsky and T Nezworski. *Clinical Implications of Attachment.* Laurence Erlbaum, Hillsdale, NJ.

Crittenden PM (1997). Toward an integrative theory of trauma: A dynamic-maturation approach. In: D Cicchetti and SL Toth (eds) *Developmental Perspectives on Trauma: Theory, Research and Intervention*, pp. 33–84. University of Rochester, Rochester, New York.

de Wolff M and van IJzendoorn M (1997). Sensitivity and attachment: A meta-analysis of parental antecedents of infant attachment. *Child Development*, **68**, 571–591.

Dozier M *et al.* (1999). Attachment and psychopathology in adulthood. In: J Cassidy and PR Shaver (eds) *Handbook of Attachment: Theory, Research, and Clinical Applications*, pp. 497–519. Guilford Press, New York.

Field T (1992). Infants of depressed mothers. *Development and Psychopathology*, **4**, 49–66.

Field T *et al.* (1990). Behaviour-state matching and synchrony in mother-infant interactions in non-depressed versus depressed dyads. *Developmental Psychology*, **26**, 7–14.

Figueirido B *et al.* (2006). Teenage pregnancy, attachment style and depression: A comparison of teenage and adult pregnant women in a Portuguese series. *Attachment and Human Development*, **8**, 123–8.

Fonagy P *et al.* (1991). Maternal representations of attachment during pregnancy predict the organisation of infant-mother attachment at one year of age. *Child Development*, **62**, 891–905.

Fraley RC and Waller NG (1998). Dismissing-avoidance and the defensive organization of emotion, cognition, and behavior. In: A Simpson and WS Rholes (eds) *Attachment Theory and Close Relationships*, pp 77–114. Guilford Press, London.

George C *et al.* (1984). *Attachment Interview for Adults.* University of California, Berkeley, CA.

Gunning M *et al.* (2004). Measurement of mother-infant interactions and the home environment in a European setting: preliminary results from a cross-cultural study. *British Journal of Psychiatry (Supplement)*, **46**, s38–44.

Hammen C (1992). Cognitive, life stress, and interpersonal approaches to a developmental psychopathology model of depression. *Development and Psychopathology*, **4**, 189–206.

Hammen CL *et al.* (1995). Interpersonal attachment cognitions and prediction of symptomatic responses to interpersonal stress. *Journal of Abnormal Psychology*, **104**, 436–43.

Harris TO *et al.* (1987). Loss of parent in childhood and adult psychiatric disorder: The role of social class position and premarital pregnancy. *Psychological Medicine*, **17**, 163–83.

Hazan C and Shaver PR (1994). Attachment as an organizational framework for research on close relationships. *Psychological Inquiry*, **5**, 1–22.

Howe D (2003). Attachment disorders: Disinherited attachment behaviours and secure base distortions with special reference to adopted children. *Attachment and Human Development*, **5**, 265–70.

Kestler L and Lewis M (2006). 'Early Attachment, Maternal Depression, and Adolescent Maladjustment' *Paper presented at the annual meeting of the XVth Biennial International Conference on Infant Studies, Westin Miyako, Kyoto, Japan*, 19 June 2006.

Larose S and Bernier A (2001). Social support processes: mediators of attachment state of mind and adjustment in late adolescence. *Attachment and Human Development*, **3**, 96–120.

Layard R (2006). *The Depression Report: A New Deal for Depression and Anxiety Disorders.* Mental Health Policy Group, London.

Main M *et al.* (1985). Security in infancy, childhood and adulthood: a move to the level of representations. Growing points of attachment theory. In: I Bretherton and E Waters (eds) *Monographs of the Society for Research in Child Development*, **50**, 66–104.

Martins C and Gaffan E (2000). Effects of early maternal depression on patterns of infant-mother attachment: A meta-analytic investigation. *Journal of Child Psychology and Psychiatry*, **41**, 737–46.

Mickelson KD *et al.* (1997). Adult attachment in a nationally representative sample. *Journal of Personality and Social Psychology*, **73**, 1092–106.

Muller RT and Lemieuz KE (2000). Social support, attachment, and psychopathology in high risk formerly maltreated adults. *Child Abuse and Neglect*, **24**, 883–900.

Murray L *et al.* (1996). The role of infant factors in postnatal depression and mother-infant interactions. *Developmental Medicine and Child Neurology*, **38**, 109–19.

Murray L *et al.* (2003). Mental health of parents caring for infants. *Archives of Women's Mental Health*, **6**, s71–7.

Nolen-Hoeksema S (1990). *Sex Differences in Depression.* Stanford University Press, Stanford, CA.

O'Hara MW *et al.* (2000). Efficacy of interpersonal psychotherapy for postpartum depression. *Archive of General Psychiatry*, **57**, 1039–45.

Paykel ES, Tylee A, Wright A, Priest RG, Rix S, and Hart D (1997). The Defeat Depression Campaign: psychiatry in the public arena, *American Journal Psychiatry*, **154**, 59–65.

Prior V *et al.* (2006). *Understanding Attachment and Attachment Disorders*. Jessica Kingsley Publishers, London.

Quinton D *et al.* (1985). Institutional rearing, parenting difficulties, and marital support. *Annual Progress in Child Psychiatry and Child Development*, 173–206.

Rholes WS *et al.* (1998). Attachment orientations, social support and conflict resolution in close relationships. In: JA Simpson and WS Rholes (eds) *Attachment Theory and Close Relationships*. Guilford Press, New York.

Rost K *et al.* (2000). Designing and implementing a primary care intervention trial to improve the quality and outcome of care for major depression. *General Hospital Psychiatry*, **22**, 66–77.

Sable P (1997). Disorders of adult attachment. *Psychotherapy*, **34**, 286–96.

Schulberg HC *et al.* (1995). Major depression in primary care practice. Clinical characteristics and treatment implications. *Psychosomatics*, **36**, 129–37.

Seeley S *et al.* (1996). The detection and treatment of postnatal depression by health visitors. *Health Visit*, **64**, 135–8.

Shapiro DL and Levendosky AA (1999). Adolescent survivors of childhood sexual abuse: The mediating role of attachment style and coping in psychological and interpersonal functioning. *Child Abuse and Neglect*, **23**, 1175–91.

Shaw D *et al.* (1994). Chronic family adversity and early child behaviour problems: A longitudinal study of low income families. *Child psychology and psychiatry*, **35**, 1109–22.

Steele H *et al.* (1996). Associations among attachment classifications of mothers, fathers and their infants. *Child Development*, **67**, 541–55.

Stuart S *et al.* (2003). The prevention and psychotherapeutic treatment of postpartum depression. *Archives of Women's Mental Health*, **6**, s57–69.

van IJzendoorn MH (1995). Adult attachment representations, parental responsiveness and infant attachment: A meta-analysis of the predictive value of the Adult Attachment Interview. *Psychological Bulletin*, **117**, 387–403.

Webster Stratton C and Hammond M (1999). Marital conflict management skills, parenting style, and early-onset conduct problems: Processes and pathways. *Journal of Child Psychology and Psychiatry and Allied Disciplines*, **40**, 917–27.

Wilhelm K *et al.* (2006). Life events, first depression onset and the serotonin transporter gene. *British Journal of Psychiatry*, **188**, 210–15.

CHAPTER 31

Women, neglect and abuse, and the consequences

Patricia Moran

Introduction

There are many factors that influence our ability to manage and enjoy the role of parenting, but there is nothing that quite prepares us for it. Many people will seek advice and help about parenting from family and friends, and some will seek more formal forms of support from services. Over 5000 calls a month, for example, are received by the 'Parentline Plus' telephone help-line in the United Kingdom (UK) from parents asking for advice about managing their children (Boddy et al. 2004). Around three-quarters of callers are female, reflecting the predominance of women as main carers of children. The adult-focused issue callers identify as contributing most to their parenting difficulty is their own mental health. Surveys indicate that many more parents struggle to care for their children but do not engage with formal support services due to fears around confidentiality, stigmatization, and being labelled a failure (National Family and Parenting Institute 2006). In a significant minority of cases, involving several thousands of parents in the UK, parenting difficulties cross the threshold into child maltreatment requiring statutory intervention for the protection of children. For some, this intervention either arrives too late or else fails, with official statistics showing that every ten days in England and Wales one child is killed at the hands of their parent (Coleman et al. 2007).

There is an over-representation of parents with mental health difficulties and substance misuse among families in which child maltreatment occurs, and a significant proportion of these parents will themselves have been the victim of neglect and abuse. Working with women in psychiatric and psychotherapeutic settings therefore necessitates an understanding of their context, including their role as parents, and an understanding of child protection issues (Royal College of Psychiatrists 2002). It also involves consideration of their adult relationships, attachment style, and supportive context, and of their own history of neglect and abuse, since these are factors that are likely to influence their ability to cope as parents, and influence continuity of risks to the next generation (Bifulco et al. 2009).

The aim of this chapter is to develop understanding of neglect and abuse in terms of its contexts, its impact on women, and its relation to mental illness. Rates of various forms of maltreatment and the gender of its victims and perpetrators are described. The contexts in which child maltreatment is most likely to occur are examined, and in particular the relationship between parental mental health and parenting. The consequences of neglect and abuse for life-course development are considered, including the intergenerational risk for neglect, abuse, and mental illness. Finally, some implications for intervention with women and families are outlined.

Neglect, abuse, and gender

Child maltreatment is typically defined with reference to four categories: neglect, physical abuse, sexual abuse, and emotional or psychological abuse (Department of Health 2006). Estimates of incidence and prevalence rates for these forms of maltreatment vary according to differences in the definitions and threshold adopted, the sample studied, and data collection approaches. Of the several forms of child maltreatment, neglect stands out as one of the most difficult to define and yet the most common. It is often chronic in nature, and is characterized by acts of omission rather than commission. Neglect involves the persistent failure to meet a child's basic physical and/or psychological needs likely to result in the serious impairment of the child's health or development (Department of Health 2006). Official statistics for England show that neglect is the most frequent reason for registering a child as 'at risk', present in 44% of registered child protection cases (Department for Children, Schools and Families 2007). Findings from a random, community-based survey of 18–24-year-olds in the UK also confirm the predominance of this form of parenting difficulty, with 18% having experienced absence of care in childhood, and 20% having experienced inadequate supervision (Cawson *et al.* 2000).

Gender differences in exposure to neglect are less well investigated, but there may be differences in rates when specific forms of neglect are considered. It has been suggested that boys may be permitted greater freedom and are exposed to less intensive supervision, reflecting gender-specific cultural norms in parenting practice (Cawson *et al.* 2000). In contrast, girls may be more likely to be exposed to educational neglect (by being absent from school), as in some cultures girls are either not allowed to receive schooling or else are kept at home to take on domestic responsibilities (World Health Organization 2000). In terms of perpetrators, neglect has traditionally been viewed as a failure of maternal rather than paternal responsibility, as there is a gender-stereotypical expectation of mothers as providers of care within the home (Turney 2005).

Physical abuse involves hitting, shaking, throwing, poisoning, burning or scalding, drowning, suffocating, or otherwise causing physical harm to a child (Department of Health 2006). Analysis of physical abuse in relation to victims and perpetrators shows that in many countries boys are more likely to be the victim than girls, although this is not the case in UK studies. In the United States (US), for example, Scher *et al.* (2004) report a rate of 17% among females and 21% among males, while in the UK, Cawson *et al.* (2000) report rates of 20% and 21% for females and males, respectively. When we consider the perpetrators of physical abuse, it appears there may be higher rates committed by mothers compared to fathers (Cawson *et al.* 2000), but when the severity of physical abuse is taken into account, fathers or male carers are more likely to carry out attacks of greater severity (Bifulco and Moran 1998).

Sexual abuse involves forcing or enticing a child or young person to take part in sexual activities, whether or not the child is aware of what is happening (Department of Health 2006). Prevalence rates for sexual abuse vary according to differences in definition, including factors such as whether physical or non-physical contact are involved, and age differences between perpetrator and victim. Reviews of sexual abuse studies suggest prevalence rates of around 9–10% for boys and 19–20% for females (Finkelhor 1994; Bolen 2001), but rates are reduced to 2% among boys and 5% among girls when more limited definitions are used, involving a minimum of five years' age difference between the people involved, and including only penetration or coerced masturbation (Kelly *et al.* 1991). Figures show that perpetrators are predominantly male and, unlike other forms of child maltreatment such as neglect, most sexual abuse does not involve parents as perpetrators (Bifulco and Moran 1998; Cawson *et al.* 2000).

Emotional or psychological abuse has more recently begun to be investigated and is a complex phenomenon to define and measure (Moran *et al.* 2002). It is defined by the Department of Health (2006) as the persistent emotional maltreatment of a child such as to cause severe and persistent adverse effects on the child's emotional development. It involves a variety of parental behaviours including conveying to a child that they are worthless, unloved, or inadequate, causing a child to feel frightened or in danger, or the exploitation or corruption of a child. It may feature as a component of other forms of maltreatment but it also occurs alone. Due to wide variation in definitions, the reported prevalence rates for emotional abuse also vary quite considerably, for example, from 1–26% in the US (Fortin and Chamberland 1995). In the UK, Cawson *et al.* (2000) report a rate of 6%, while prevalence rates among a community-based study of women selected for their psychosocial vulnerability to depression were found to be 16% (Moran *et al.* 2002). There do not appear to be marked gender differences in rates of experiencing emotional abuse (Doyle 1997), or gender differences in perpetrators (Bifulco and Moran 1998), although further studies are needed to confirm this.

As many as a third of women experience either neglect or physical or sexual abuse in childhood, and these experiences significantly raise their risk of developing psychiatric disorders in adulthood (Bifulco and Moran 1998). Childhood maltreatment is therefore not uncommon, which suggests that there are many parents whose context—psychological, interpersonal, social, or material—may impede their ability to do the best for their children. Understanding the context in which neglect and abuse occur has important implications for early intervention in order to prevent or limit its damaging consequences.

The context of neglect and abuse

Much of what is known about the context that gives rise to difficulties in parenting comes from studies of families who access family support services (e.g. Gardener 2003), or else encounter statutory intervention in relation to protection of their children (e.g. Masson *et al.* 2008), as well as from community-based studies of 'normative' parenting (e.g. Ghate *et al.* 2003). These studies provide a fairly consistent picture of the circumstances associated with the neglect and abuse of children. They include: parents or carers on low incomes or unemployed; young parents; socially isolated parents; lone parents; large/unplanned families; lack of cohesion in the family; domestic violence or high levels of conflict; maternal low self-esteem; parents' own childhood maltreatment; parents' insecure attachment; maternal unresponsiveness to child; parental mental health problems including maternal depression; and parental substance misuse.

These factors are markers of increased risk for neglect and abuse rather than predictors, as many families with these characteristics do not maltreat their children. It is likely that neglect and abuse arise from the complex interplay of multiple risk factors rather than single risk factors (Crittenden 1999), and it is the accumulation and interaction of risk factors that is particularly damaging for children's outcomes (Rutter 1987). Among these factors, some are more directly causally involved than others, and it is important to distinguish between risk indicators and risk mechanisms. Crittenden (1999), for example, suggests that poverty and child neglect are associated via their links with parents' difficulties in sustaining interpersonal relationships. Interpersonal relationships are a significant component of maintaining family life, in getting and keeping a job, and in obtaining help from others. Neglectful parents struggle to understand social relationships and the caring role, and this may arise as a consequence, for example, of their mental health needs.

The quality of relationships and attachment are central to understanding the causes of child maltreatment, as many of the risk factors for child maltreatment are associated with disrupted attachment processes. Research into child neglect, for example, indicates that neglectful mothers are more likely to have a history of unstable, hostile, and non-nurturing relationships in childhood (Stevenson 1998), disrupted or conflictful relationships in adulthood (Horwath 2007), and to be less sensitive and less responsive in interactions with their children (Crittenden 1993). A lifespan model of these types of relational factors has been examined in a retrospective, intergenerational study of community-based women. It suggests that women's difficulties in parenting arise from their insecure attachment style and their partner's history of mental health difficulties,

criminality, or violence (Bifulco *et al.* 2009). However, the study found that women's insecure attachment style per se was not directly related to the neglect or abuse of their children. Insecure attachment style may lead to selection of 'problem' partners that contribute to difficulties in parenting. From a psychotherapeutic perspective, one of the implications of this study is that enabling women to develop more secure attachment style and supportive close relationships may reduce risks for the next generation.

Parental psychiatric disorder and parenting

The most common mental health difficulties among the British population are neurotic disorders involving anxiety and depression, and these are more common among women, and also among lone parents, who are predominantly female (Singleton *et al.* 2001). Specific figures for the number of people experiencing psychiatric disorders who are also parents are not known. Estimates put the figure at between 20–50% of patients attending adult psychiatric settings (Royal College of Psychiatrists 2002; Seeman and Göpfert 2004).

Parental mental health is a significant contributory factor in child maltreatment. A recent study of a random selection of 386 care proceeding cases brought under the 1998 Children Act for the protection of children found that maternal mental health problems, maternal drug abuse, and maternal alcohol abuse featured in 32%, 39%, and 25% of cases, respectively (Masson *et al.* 2008). More than half of mothers were also experiencing domestic violence, and in a fifth of cases fathers had no involvement with their children. It is also significant to note that there was a lack of cooperation with services (either Children's Services, or Adult Social Care and the Health Service) in 72% of cases, indicative of the challenge for services in engaging with these parents. Other studies involving statutory services provide a similar picture of parental mental health difficulties, with high rates of depression, personality disorders, suicide attempts, and substance misuse among child protection cases (Falkov 1997).

Falkov (1998) describes the impact of mental illness on parenting capacity in terms of a number of dimensions of parenting. These include: parents' ability to provide physical care, which may be affected by their lack of energy, poor concentration, altered belief systems, and fear of going out; parents' capacity to manage children's behaviour, which may be affected by parents' excessive emotional lability, poor concentration, distorted thinking, and despair; parents' capacity to respond emotionally in order to support and contain children, which may be affected by parents' self-preoccupation and their own needs for emotional support; and parents' capacity to develop self-confidence in parenting, which can be undermined by symptoms that lead to feelings of failure as a parent, and can generate further anxiety, guilt, and low self-esteem that exacerbates symptoms. Duncan and Reder (2000) discuss the way in which specific mental illnesses may impact on parenting, and show how the impact may differ according to the age and developmental needs of the child. However, they also suggest that the most useful way of understanding the impact of disorders on parenting is to consider the parental behaviour rather than their diagnosis (Duncan and Reder 2000). They draw on research into children of psychiatric patients such as the study carried out by Rutter and Quinton (1984), which showed that outcomes for the children were associated with relational and social functioning of the family (including conflict and marital disharmony) rather than the parents' psychiatric diagnosis per se.

In terms of the risk for disorder among the children of parents with mental illness, several studies show intergenerational associations. It has been suggested that girls are especially vulnerable to increased risk of depression and anxiety if they have a depressed parent, especially a depressed mother, and boys are more likely to develop oppositional defiant disorder and conduct disorder when raised by a depressed mother and alcoholic father (Foley et al. 2001). Maternal emotional disorders have also been shown to be associated with persistence of children's conduct disorder, although the direction of the causal relationship is unclear (Meltzer et al. 2003). Recent evidence suggests that there may be gender differences in genetic and shared environmental contributions to the development of callousness and conduct disorder, with a greater contribution from environmental factors for girls (Viding et al. 2007). Boys and girls may therefore require highly tailored approaches to interventions aimed at enabling them to develop empathy and reduce risk for conduct disorder.

The significance of the psychosocial context of parents with psychiatric disorder for outcomes for children has been shown by several studies (e.g. Emery et al. 1982; Rutter and Quinton 1984). Relationship factors such as domestic conflict or lack of support play an important role, independent of parental diagnosis. Recent support for this conclusion comes from a study of the impact of maternal vulnerability to depression on the childhood experience and mental health outcomes of their young adult offspring (Bifulco et al. 2002b). The offspring of women with psychosocial vulnerability to depression (conferred by low self-esteem, and conflictful or inadequate supportive context) were four times more likely to have a disorder in the preceding 12 months (involving depression, anxiety, or substance abuse/dependence) compared to the offspring of a representative series of women. Such disorder among the offspring was not directly associated with their mothers' depression, but with mothers' psychosocial vulnerability and their offspring's childhood risk of neglect and abuse. This study draws attention to the role of mothers' psychosocial vulnerability to depression, rather than the disorder itself, as a marker of the adverse family context for risks for neglect and abuse and disorder among children. Hence the transmission of parental psychiatric risk for disorder to children may be through a number of routes within the family context.

The consequences of child abuse and neglect

Child maltreatment has the potential to impact on all of the developmental needs of a child, and consequently is associated with multiple, wide-ranging negative outcomes. One of the effects of childhood maltreatment that has been the focus of recent research is the detrimental effect of maltreatment on the developing brain, particularly during infancy. Studies show that the way in which an infant's brain develops is influenced by caregiving experiences and particular forms of stimulation and environmental conditions (Schore 2002). Chronic, severe, or unpredictable stressors such as neglect and abuse, especially within the first three years of life, can alter brain physiology and have a damaging effect on the development of cognitive and emotional abilities and personality. This has implications for the development of the attachment system. With neglectful or abusive early experience, the infant's brain may not develop sufficient capacity for positive emotional development and bonding. Insecure attachment to caregivers as a result of hostile or neglectful parenting may lead to internal models of relationships in which others are viewed as unreliable and threatening (Bowlby 1973). Such internal models and attachment patterns may persist into adulthood, where studies indicate that insecure attachment is a predictor of mental health problems such as depression (Bifulco et al. 2002a).

During mid to later childhood and teenage years, maltreated children are more likely than other children to experience feelings of shame, loneliness, and helplessness (Bifulco and Moran 1998), lack social skills (Hildyard and Wolfe 2002), have difficulty in peer relationships (Young *et al.* 1994), experience educational failure (Erikson and Egeland 2002), as well as higher rates of mental health difficulties, including internalizing and externalizing disorders (Smith *et al.* 2005). Hence the need for early intervention approaches such as home visiting, begun prenatally or during infancy, to prevent or minimize risks and enhance parents' strengths and coping.

Studies show that abused or neglected children experience a raised risk of negative outcomes in adulthood compared to their non-maltreated peers. As in childhood, relationship difficulties are more likely, with isolation or else problematic relationships involving frequent crises and break-ups (Horwath 2007), as well as greater risk of teenage pregnancy or domestic violence (Bifulco and Moran 1998). In terms of mental health outcomes, childhood maltreatment has been associated with raised risk for a range of disorders in adulthood including depression, anxiety, suicide, substance misuse, eating disorders, self-harm, personality disorders, post-traumatic stress disorder and psychotic disorders (e.g. see McClelland *et al.* 1991; Greenfield *et al.* 1994; Fergusson *et al.* 1996; Rodriguez *et al.* 1996; Bifulco and Moran 1998; Minzenberg *et al.* 2008). There may be some gender-specific differences in the consequences of childhood maltreatment in relation to these disorders, which may have implications for intervention. For example, there is some evidence that sexual abuse is linked to suicidal thoughts and suicide attempts in boys, even in the absence of depression, while for girls this relationship is mediated by depression (Martin *et al.* 2004). Childhood experience of neglect or abuse also relates to physical ill-health and disability in adulthood, and this pattern is more pronounced in women than men (Chartier *et al.* 2007). The cost of child maltreatment is therefore considerable in terms of human suffering and in terms of the economic costs of support services.

Parenting and intergeneration risk

As described earlier, maltreated children are more likely than their non-maltreated peers to experience poor outcomes in a range of areas across their life course. These outcomes are likely to place them at a distinct disadvantage as adults when they themselves become parents, since they are at greater risk of finding themselves in circumstances that are associated with neglect and abuse of their own children. However, we know that many maltreated children do not become maltreating parents. Estimates suggest that around a third of parents who have been abused or neglected go on to abuse or neglect their own children (Oliver 1993). Intergenerational transmission of neglect and abuse is therefore not inevitable.

A number of factors are likely to play a role in breaking the cycle of neglect and abuse and risks for mental illness across generations. Just as an accumulation of risk factors increases chance of negative outcomes, so an accumulation of opportunities and protective factors can increase the chances of positive outcomes. In particular, resilience factors have been identified which promote positive adaptation in the face of severe adversity (Rutter 1987). A resilient child is less likely to succumb to the effects of a stressor, and is more likely to cope successfully with traumatic events (Newman 2004). Hence these factors have important implications for interventions aimed at enhancing children's emotional well-being, and breaking cycles of disorder. Resilience factors have been identified at the level of the individual child, parent, and community (for a summary see Department for Education and Employment 2001). Factors that relate to parenting and promotion of resilience include: secure early relationships for the child; at least one good parent–child relationship; affection; support for education; supportive long-term family relationships characterized by the absence of severe discord; and clear, firm, and consistent discipline. The role of parenting strategies in the reduction of childhood risk for disorders has been demonstrated in a community-based sample of over 10 000 children in Great Britain, which investigated the relationships between parental psychopathology, parenting strategies, and mental health outcomes for children. High reward, non-punitive parenting strategies were associated with an absence of disorder in children (Vostanis *et al.* 2006). This has implications for the development of parenting support and education programmes.

Implications for intervention

The evidence regarding the relationship between neglect and abuse and mental illness strongly suggests that clinicians need to be aware of the broader context of their patients' lives, and specifically their role as parents (Royal College of Psychiatrists 2002). Mental health service users report that psychiatric services are not well equipped to do this (Göpfert *et al.* 1999). The roles of patient and parent appear to involve conflicting qualities of dependency and responsibility that do not sit easily with the traditional helping role of the professional

(Göpfert *et al.* 2004). Knowledge of child protection issues and skills in assessment of parenting are also important for clinicians working with parents in order to reduce risk of neglect, abuse, and disorder among children. A collaborative relationship between adult and children's services is required to provide a cohesive response to the families' needs. Traditionally, adult and children's services have not been set up in a way that addresses the needs of mothers and fathers and their children in an integrated way (McLean *et al.* 2004). Providing integrated family services may involve a complex balancing of parent and children's needs without compromising the duty of care to either, but where conflicts arise, the needs of the child are paramount.

Since a woman's psychosocial context may be a more significant contributing factor to her parenting difficulties than her psychiatric diagnosis, these circumstances also need to be assessed. The quality of her close relationships, and especially the support received from a partner, or the lack of it, will be highly significant. Practitioners need to be aware of relationship difficulties such as domestic violence or high levels of conflict, or else absence of close relationships and support that exacerbate symptoms and undermine parenting, and to liaise with relevant agencies that can provide additional support in these areas. Multidisciplinary, multi-agency joined-up working is needed to enable patients to manage their lives and not just their symptoms.

Early intervention with children and families is important for limiting the damage that inadequate parenting can lead to. There are now several evaluated parent support and education programmes that can improve outcomes for families (Moran *et al.* 2004), and some are being developed in culturally sensitive ways (Barlow *et al.* 2004). Given the centrality of attachment processes to both mental health and parenting, attachment-based interventions can be offered to parents, children, and families. Interventions that are likely to impact on attachment processes include those in which practitioners can provide a 'secure base'; increase the sensitivity, availability, and responsiveness of carers; increase the trust, attunement, and understanding between parents and children; and increase factors such as self-esteem, and capacity for empathy (Howe *et al.* 1999).

Men's responsibility to their children also needs to be more widely recognized by services. Although there is increasing awareness of the beneficial influence of fathers for children's outcomes (Sarkadi *et al.* 2008), responsibility for parenting still falls disproportionately upon women. Practitioners and service providers need to examine their own gender stereotype assumptions about women and men as carers, and develop ways of working more closely with fathers. There is now a growing practice-based knowledge regarding ways of working with and engaging fathers with services to improve outcomes for children (Burgess and Bartlett 2004).

In the current policy climate, parents are increasingly being held to account for a variety of social ills perpetrated by children and young people, evidenced, for example, by the introduction of Parenting Orders in England and Wales. More often than not, this accountability and its accompanying burden of blame falls on mothers rather than fathers. While increased debate and scrutiny of the role of parenting is to be welcomed, it is also vital to finds ways of working with parents that do not disempower them. In the words of John Bowlby: 'If a community values its children it must cherish their parents' (Bowlby 1951, p. 84).

References

Barlow J *et al.* (2004). *Parenting Programmes and Minority Ethnic Families: Experience and Outcomes.* Joseph Rowntree Foundation, York.

Bifulco A and Moran P (1998). *Wednesday's Child: Research into Women's Experience of Neglect and Abuse in Childhood, and Adult Depression.* Routledge, London.

Bifulco A *et al.* (2002a). Adult attachment style. 1: Its relation to clinical depression. *Social Psychiatry and Psychiatric Epidemiology*, **37**, 50–9.

Bifulco A *et al.* (2002b). Childhood adversity, parental vulnerability and disorder: examining inter-generational transmission of risk. *Journal of Child Psychology and Psychiatry*, **43**, 1075–86.

Bifulco A *et al.* (2009). Problem partners and parenting: Exploring linkages with maternal insecure attachment style and adolescent offspring internalising disorder. *Attachment and Human Development*, **11**, 69–85.

Boddy B *et al.* (2004). *Evaluation of Parentline Plus.* Home Office Online Report 33/04. Available from: http://www.homeoffice.gov.uk/rds/pdfs04/rdsolr3304.pdf (Accessed 15 February 2008.)

Bolen RM (2001). *Child Sexual Abuse: Its Scope and Our Failure,* Kluwer Academic/Plenum Publishes, New York.

Bowlby J (1951). *Maternal Care and Mental Health.* World Health Organization Monograph (Serial No. 2), Geneva.

Bowlby J (1973). *Attachment and Loss (Vol. 2), Separation: Anxiety and Anger.* Routledge, London.

Burgess A and Bartlett D (2004). *Working with Fathers. A Guide for Everyone Working with Families.* Fathers Direct (now the Fatherhood Institute), London.

Cawson P *et al.* (2000). *Child Maltreatment in the United Kingdom. A Study of the Prevalence of Child Abuse and Neglect.* NSPCC, London.

Chartier MJ *et al.* (2007). Childhood abuse, adult health, and health care utilization: results from a representative community sample. *American Journal of Epidemiology*, **165**, 1031–8.

Coleman K *et al.*(2007). *Homicides, firearms offences and intimate violence 2005/2006. Supplementary volume 1 to Crime in England and Wales 2005/2006.* Home Office, London. Available from: http://www.homeoffice.gov.uk/rds/pdfs07/hosb0207.pdf (Accessed 15 February 2008.)

Crittenden P (1993). An information processing perspective on the behaviour of neglectful parents. *Criminal Justice and Behaviour*, **20**, 27–48.

Crittenden P (1999). Child neglect: Causes and contributors. In: H Dubowitz (eds) *Neglected Children: Research, Practice and Policy*, pp. 47–68. Sage, Thousand Oaks, CA.

Department for Children, Schools and Families (2007). *Referrals, Assessments and Children and Young People who are the subject of a Child Protection Plan or are on Child Protection Registers, England - year ending 31March 2007. Statistical First Release 28/2007.* DCSF, London. Available from: http://www.dcsf.gov.uk/rsgateway/DB/SFR/s000742/SFR28–2007.pdf (Accessed 15 October 2007.)

Department of Health (2006). *A Guide to Inter-agency Working to Safeguard and Promote the Welfare of Children.* TSO, London.

Department for Education and Employment (2001). *Promoting Children's Mental Health within Early Years and School Settings. DfEE (0121/2001)*, DfEE Publications, Nottingham.

Doyle C (1997). Emotional abuse of children: issues for intervention. *Child Abuse Review*, **6**, 330–42.

Duncan S and Reder P (2000). Children's experience of major psychiatric disorder in their parent. An overview. In: P Reder *et al.* (eds) *Family Matters: Interfaces Between Child and Adult Mental Health*, pp. 83–95. Routledge, London.

Emery R *et al.* (1982). Effects of marital discord on the school behavior of children of schizophrenic, affectively disordered, and normal parents. *Journal of Abnormal Child Psychology*, **10**, 215–28.

Erickson MF and Egeland B (2002). Child neglect. In: JEB Myers *et al.* (eds) *The APSAC Handbook on Child Maltreatment*, pp. 13–20. Sage, Thousand Oaks, CA.

Falkov A (1997). *Parental Psychiatric Disorder and Child Maltreatment: Part II: Extent and Nature of the Association. Highlight 149.* National Children's Bureau, London.

Falkov A (1998). *Crossing Bridges. Training Resources for Working with Mentally Ill Parents and Their Children.* Pavilion Publishing, Brighton.

Fergusson DM *et al.* (1996). Childhood sexual abuse and psychiatric disorder in young adulthood: II. Psychiatric outcomes of childhood sexual abuse. *Journal of the American Academy of Child & Adolescent Psychiatry*, **35**, 1365–74.

Finkelhor D (1994). The international epidemiology of child sexual abuse. *Child Abuse and Neglect*, **18**, 409–17.

Foley DL *et al.* (2001). Parental concordance and comorbidity for psychiatric disorder and associated risks for current psychiatric symptoms and disorders in a community sample of juvenile twins. *Journal of Child Psychology and Psychiatry*, **42**, 381–94.

Fortin A and Chamberland C (1995). Preventing the psychological maltreatment of children. *Journal of Interpersonal Violence*, **10**, 275–95.

Gardner R (2003). *Supporting Families: Child Protection in the Community.* Chichester, Wiley.

Ghate D *et al.* (2003). *Parents, Children and Discipline: Key Findings.* Policy Research Bureau/NSPSCC, London.

Göpfert M *et al.* (1999). *Keeping the Family in Mind; Participative Research into Mental Ill-Health and how it Affects the whole Family.* Liverpool Save the Children, Barnardos, Imagine, and North Mersey Community Trust.

Göpfert M *et al.* (2004). The construction of parenting and parenting and its context. In: M Göpfert *et al.* (eds) *Parental Psychiatric Disorder. Distressed Parents and their Families*, pp. 62–84. Cambridge University Press, Cambridge.

Greenfield SF *et al.* (1994). Childhood abuse in first-episode psychosis. *British Journal of Psychiatry*, **164**, 831–4.

Hildyard C and Wolfe D (2002). Child neglect: developmental issues and outcomes. *Child Abuse and Neglect*, **26**, 679–95.

Horwath J (2007). *Child Neglect: Identification and Assessment.* Palgrave Macmillan, Hampshire.

Howe D *et al.* (1999). *Attachment Theory, Child Maltreatment and Family Support.* Erlbaum, Mahwah, NJ.

Kelly L Regan *et al.* (1991). *An Exploratory Study of the Prevalence of Sexual Abuse in a Sample of 16–21 year olds*, Child and Woman Abuse Studies Unit, London Metropolitan University, London.

Martin G *et al.* (2004). Sexual abuse and suicidality: gender differences in a large community sample of adolescents. *Child Abuse and Neglect*, **28**, 491–503.

Masson J *et al.* (2008). *Care Profiling Study.* Ministry of Justice. Available at:.http://www.justice.gov.uk/docs/care-profiling-summary.pdf (Accessed 1 March 2008.)

McClelland L *et al.* (1991). Sexual abuse, disordered personality and eating disorders. *British Journal of Psychiatry*, **158**, 63–8.

McLean D *et al.* (2004). Are services for families with a mentally ill parent adequate? In: M Göpfert *et al.* (eds) *Parental Psychiatric Disorder. Distressed Parents and their Families*, pp. 333–44. Cambridge University Press, Cambridge.

Meltzer H *et al.* (2003). *Persistence, Onset, Risk Factors and Outcomes of Childhood Mental Disorders.* TSO, London.

Minzenberg MJ *et al.* (2008). A neurocognitive model of borderline personality disorder: Effects of childhood sexual abuse and relationship to adult social attachment disturbance. *Development and Psychopathology*, **20**, 341–68.

Moran P *et al.* (2002). Exploring psychological abuse in childhood: 1. Developing a new interview scale. *Bulletin of the Menninger Clinic*, **66**, 213–40.

Moran P *et al.* (2004). *What Works in Parenting Support? An International Review of Literature.* DfES, London.

National Family and Parenting Institute (2006). *Where Do Parents Turn For Advice? An Overview of Research Findings at the National Family and Parenting Institute*, NFPI. Available from: http://www.familyandparenting.org/surveys#1 (Accessed 20 February 2008.)

Newman T (2004). *What Works in Building Resilience?* Barnardos, Ilford.

Oliver JE (1993). Intergenerational transmission of child abuse: rates, research, and clinical implications. *American Journal of Psychiatry*, **150**, 1315–24.

Rodriguez N *et al.* (1996). Posttraumatic stress disorder in a clinical sample of adult survivors of childhood sexual abuse. *Child Abuse and Neglect*, **20**, 943–52.

Royal College of Psychiatrists (2002). *Patients as Parents. Council Report CR105*. Royal College of Psychiatrists, London.

Rutter M (1987). Psychosocial resilience and protective mechanisms. *American Journal of Orthopsychiatry*, **57**, 316–31.

Rutter M and Quinton D (1984). Parental psychiatric disorder: effects on children. *Psychological Medicine*, **14**, 853–0.

Sarkardi A *et al.* (2008). Fathers' involvement and children's developmental outcomes: a systemic review of longitudinal studies. *Acta Paediatrica*, **97**, 153–8.

Scher C *et al.* (2004). Prevalence and demographic correlates of childhood maltreatment in an adult community sample. *Child Abuse and Neglect*, **28**, 167–80.

Schore AN (2002). Dysregulation of the right brain: a fundamental mechanism of traumatic attachment and the psychopathogenesis of post-traumatic stress. *Australian and New Zealand Journal of Psychiatry*, **36**, 9–30.

Smith CA *et al.* (2005). Adolescent maltreatment and its impact on young adult antisocial behaviour. *Child Abuse and Neglect*, **29**, 1099–119.

Seeman MV *et al.* (2004). *Parental Psychiatric Disorder, Distressed Parents and their Families*. Cambridge University Press, Cambridge.

Singleton N *et al.* (2001). *Psychiatric Morbidity Among Adults living in Private Households, ONS, 2000*. HMSO, London.

Stevenson O (1998). *Neglected Children: Issues and Dilemmas*. Blackwell Science, Oxford.

Turney D (2005). Who cares? The role of mothers in cases of child neglect. In: J Taylor and B Daniel (eds) *Child Neglect: Practical Issues for Health and Social Care*, pp. 249–62. Jessica Kingsley, London.

Viding E *et al.* (2007). Aetiology of the relationship between callous–unemotional traits and conduct problems in childhood. *British Journal of Psychiatry*, **190**, s33–38s.

Vostanis P *et al.* (2006). Relationship between parental psychopathology, parenting strategies and child mental health: Findings from the GB national study. *Social Psychiatry and Psychiatric Epidemiology*, **41**, 509–14.

World Health Organization (2000). *World Report on Violence and Health*. World Health Organization, Geneva. Available at: http://whqlibdoc.who.int/publications/2002/9241545615_chap3_eng.pdf (Accessed 14 February 2008.)

Young RE *et al.* (1994). Comparison of the effects of sexual abuse on male and female latency-aged children. *Journal of Interpersonal Violence*, **9**, 291–306.

Women and Learning Disability

Jane McCarthy

Women with intellectual disability and mental health problems: the invisible victims

Jane McCarthy

Introduction

Intellectual disability (ID) includes the presence of impaired intelligence reducing the ability to understand new or complex information (low intelligence is taken to be an intelligence quotient score below 70), with impaired social functioning, that is, reduced ability to cope independently, and disorder that presented before adulthood with a lasting effect on development. People with ID are amongst the most socially excluded and vulnerable groups. Very few have jobs and live in their own homes. Many have few friends outside their families and those paid to care for them. Recent national documentation in the United Kingdom (UK), *Valuing People: A New Strategy for Learning Disability for the 21st Century* (Department of Health 2001) makes no reference to the different roles in society of men and women and how these roles impact on the lives of people with intellectual disability.

There has been an increase in the literature on women with ID over the past decade (Burns 2000). Researchers have not previously wanted to acknowledge gender in the lives of people with ID and assumed people with ID to be asexual and genderless individuals (Burns 1993). The issues for which feminists have worked for, such as women not to be defined sexually and for the rights to roles other than mothers, appears to be the opposite of what disabled women demand (Kallianes and Rubenfeld 1997). It may be that having ID is a more important determinant than gender on the living conditions for people with ID. A study in Sweden of people with ID looking at living conditions of adults with ID from a gender perspective (Umb-Carlsoon and Sonnander 2006) found women and men with ID participated to about the same extent in recreational and cultural activities. These findings contrast with women and men in the general population were there were clearly gender-related differences in the involvement in a number of these activities.

Recognition of mental health problems in women with intellectual disability

Our understanding of the nature and cause of mental illness in people with ID have increased over the past 20 years (Bouras and Holt 2007). However, how gender impacts on the presentation and rates of mental health problems has only recently been addressed in the literature. As in the general population, certain risk factors may have a particular impact on women. The recognition of mental health problems in women with ID has not kept up with the growth in the study of the mental health needs of women in the wider population (Lunksy and Havercamp 2002). Recent national policy in the UK does recognize that women with ID are a more vulnerable group within mental health services (Department of Health 2002). This consultation document focused on a strategy to address inequalities in the delivery of mental health services and to tackle discrimination and disadvantage of women in mental health services. The document lists certain groups of women who may be particularly vulnerable to mental illness, one being women with ID. At that time there was serious criticism of mixed-sex acute inpatient care, community residential, and secure care in relation to women's safety. Concerns focused on the vulnerability of women patients to harassment, intimidation, violence, and abuse by other patients, visitors, intruders, or staff members. Many women were reported as experiencing women-only services as safer services and more attuned and responsive to their needs. How much these concerns are relevant to the lives of women with ID and mental health problems are unknown. Women with ID and mental health problems are the invisible victims both in the delivery of services and the research literature.

The relationship between biological and social factors and their effect on prevalence of mental health problems is one area that is increasingly studied in the general population but little has been looked at for women with ID. In order to recognize mental health problems in women with ID, there is a need to understand the way disorders may present and whether that will be different in people with ID and specifically in women with ID. Assessment of mental health problems is more difficult in people with ID than the general population due to a number of factors including communication difficulties.

The literature on women with ID has mainly focused on physical health needs, vulnerability to abuse, and their role as parents. The focus of this chapter will be on needs of women with ID and the prevalence of mental health problems with reference to social, psychological, and biological risk factors. Recognition of mental health problems in women with ID through detection and appropriate assessment will be discussed. The treatment of mental health problems in women with ID will be reviewed briefly along with service provision. The impact of being a parent, the ethnicity of women with ID, and those who offend will be highlighted as there is some evidence that their experiences within services may be different to that of men.

Prevalence of mental health problems in women with intellectual disability

Research on the prevalence of mental health problems has largely overlooked gender issues in people with ID. Taylor et al. (2004) did find that women had higher scores than men on the affective/neurotic disorders subdomain of the Psychiatric Assessment Schedule for Adults with Intellectual Disability (PAS-ADD) Checklist but not on their two other subdomains of organic and psychotic disorders. Lunsky (2003) conducted structured interviews with 99 men and women with ID. She found that women were more likely to report depression,

loneliness, and stress. However, Rojahn and Ebensen (2005) reviewing the literature felt the evidence for increased rates of depression in women with ID was inconsistent. Higher rates of substance abuse in men as compared to women with ID have also been found (Taggart et al. 2006).

A recent large-scale population study of adults with ID in Scotland (Cooper et al. 2007) showed variation in the point prevalence of mental health problems with gender. Case notes were reviewed and a face-to-face assessment was completed with each participant supported by a paid or family carer. Those suspected of a psychiatric disorder were then assessed by a specialist psychiatrist who also accessed their mental health notes, if available. The assessment included detailed clinical assessments of each participant supported by a carer, the use of several semi-structured instruments, and interviews with relevant others. This study cast a wide net to obtain a population-based sample, finding a point prevalence of mental ill health of 40.9–35.2% using clinical diagnostic criteria with lower rates when using research diagnostic criteria of 16.6–15.7%. The study identified similarities with the general population in terms of the factors independently associated with mental ill health: high number of preceding life events, a higher number of preceding general practitioner or family physician consultations, being a smoker, and being female, but also some differences in that there was no association with living in a more deprived area, not having a daytime occupation, marital status, or epilepsy. Women were more likely than men to show mental ill health than men, with an odds ratio of 1.3 when considering clinical diagnosis excluding specific phobias and autism spectrum disorders. The overall gender pattern of mental health problems was similar to that reported in the general population although eating disorders, mainly pica, was more common in men (2.5% vs 1.3%).

A very different study to that of Cooper et al. (2007) is one of consecutive clinical referrals to a specialist mental health service in London (Tsakanikos et al. 2006). This was a retrospective study. The study looked at 295 men and 295 women over a 20-year period. Eligibility for the study required an intelligence quotient score below 70 and significant social impairment. Clinical assessments were made by a psychiatrist following clinical interviews with the clients and key informants. Only ICD-10 diagnoses were made and problem behaviours were not assessed which was a different approach to the study of Cooper and colleagues (2007).

This study of referrals to a specialist mental health service in South London showed men were more likely to be referred to the service (Tsakanikos *et al.* 2006). There was significant difference in care pathways by gender with a large proportion of women being referred through primary care, and a large proportion of men were referred from generic mental health services. There were no gender differences in terms of ID level to account for these different referral pathways.

There were also differences in terms of psychiatric diagnoses between men and women. More men had a personality disorder and more women had an adjustment reaction and dementia. There was no significant difference in terms of depression, anxiety, schizophrenia, or epilepsy. There was no gender difference in terms of admission to a psychiatric unit or use of medication.

Risk factors for mental health problems

Social issues

Social and economic factors influence the prevalence of mental health problems, 70% of the world's poor are girls and women with two-thirds of the world illiterate being women (UNIFEM 2003). Economic factors such as poverty, low social support, and unemployment are all more common in the lives of people with mild ID and mental health problems (Emerson 2007), but the interaction between these factors and gender is unknown.

Abuse and domestic violence is more common among people with ID (O'Callaghan *et al.* 2003). Normal adult and sexual roles may not be offered and adult women are expected to live with men who are not family, friends, or lovers. Few report experiencing sexual pleasure. Most able-bodied women experience problems in being treated as sex objects, whereas many disabled women experience being treated as asexual objects (Burns 2000). One-third of women worldwide suffer abuse simply because they are female (UNIFEM 2003). The relationship between abuse and mental health problems is strong in the general population (Kohen 2000). Women with ID are more likely to be abused physically and sexually than women in the general population: they are also at greater risk than men with ID. Men with ID are more likely than women with ID to be believed when they report having been sexually abused (McCarthy and Thompson 1997). Women are the main recipients of domestic violence and it has been suggested that it is common among women with mild to moderate ID who may not be confident to complain

(Walsh and Murphy 2002).There is also a link identified between mental health symptoms and abuse in people with ID (Sequeria *et al.* 2003). Flynn and colleagues (2002) found evidence suggesting a link between childhood abuse and later personality disorder in adults with ID. Treatment for problems related to abuse is often unavailable, inaccessible, or inappropriate for people with ID.

Whilst women with ID fare better than their male counterparts in terms of social supports, they report fewer social supports than non-disabled women and tend to cite paid carers and family members as their main social supports. Also women with ID are more likely than men with ID to be carers and this may be an opportunity to be seen as an adult and so gain new respect and opportunities.

Biological issues

The influence of hormones throughout the life of women with mental health problems is well recognized (Scott 2000). How changes in the endocrine system affect the rates of mental illness in women with ID is unknown. This includes menstruation, pregnancy, birth, and menopause where there is no evidence available (Ditchfield and Burns 2004). The mainstream area of research into the menstrual cycle has hardly penetrated the ID literature. Many women with ID view menstruation entirely negatively, are ill-prepared for the menarche, and ill-informed as to what it is and its relationship with fertility (McCarthy 2000). Women with ID go through the menopause earlier, especially women with Down syndrome (Schupf *et al.* 1997). As a result, women with ID may be at increased risk of physical health problems due to early onset of menopause. For example, an increased risk for fractures and osteoporosis with fractures occurring at a young age (Scrager *et al.* 2007). There is evidence that women with Down syndrome or autism spectrum disorder appear to have a higher rate of period pain than women in the general population, but the presence of pain had to be deduced from behavioural changes (Kyrkou 2005). How painful menstruation and an early menopause affects the emotional well-being of women with ID is unknown.

Psychological issues

Due to cognitive immaturity people with ID may find it more difficult to modulate emotions in reaction to events in their lives and this may lead to a lack of sense of self. This results in low self-esteem, poor sense of identity, and poor coping skills. Women with ID when faced with conflict or interpersonal stress may internalize the frustration and cope poorly. Also, women with ID live longer than men so more likely to experience more episodes of loss. All of these psychological factors increase the risk for women with ID for mental illness.

Detection and assessment of mental health problems

In the general population, making a psychiatric diagnosis depends primarily on the account given by the patient. Many psychiatric diagnoses rely on patients describing complex internal subjective feelings or cognitions. Whilst many people with mild ID will be able to describe such phenomena, those with more severe intellectual disability may either not have had such experiences or be able to adequately describe them. Assessment of the person's communication ability is necessary at the outset of the assessment with the use of appropriate language and to avoid the use of leading questions. An interdisciplinary approach to the assessment, diagnosis, treatment, and management of mental health problems in people with intellectual disability is the accepted approach (O'Hara 2007). The detection of mental health in people with ID does commonly depend on others such as family and day or residential care staff providing reliable information. However, people with mild ID do present themselves to services.

Assessment of a woman with ID should include a full psychiatric history including past experiences, social history, menstrual history, and parenting. During the assessment, consideration needs to be given to social, psychological, and biological risk factors as described earlier.

Treatment and management

There is a lack of all types of psychological therapies available for people with ID. Until recently, behavioural interventions have been the key approach to reducing maladaptive behaviours and improving daily living and social skills of people with ID. Psychosocial interventions, including cognitive behavioural therapy, are becoming increasingly available for people with ID but there is a limited evidence base on their use (Dagnan 2007). There is some evidence that psychodynamic treatment is an effective and useful tool for people with ID (Parkes and Hollins 2007). Psychodynamic psychotherapy has been effective in improving self-esteem, reduction in distress, and problem behaviours. There are few services in the UK offering psychodynamic

treatment for adults with ID and none that focus specifically on the needs and experiences of women with ID within the National Health Service (NHS). As with the general population, neuroleptic medication can cause weight gain, menstrual disturbances, and tardive dyskinesia in women with ID although there is little or no research to support these clinical observations. These side effects can be distressing for women and reduce treatment compliance.

Women who are parents

Forty to sixty per cent of children born to parents with ID are taken into care (Booth 2000). Losing a child to fostering or adoption can be devastating. O'Hara and Martin (2003) found high levels of psychiatric symptoms and behavioural disturbance in mothers with ID in East London even when their children remained at home. Mental health problems are more common in mothers with ID than in fathers (McGaw *et al.* 2007). Tymchuk (1994) reported that 39% of mothers with ID had depression compared to 13% of mothers without ID from the same socioeconomic background and locality. Such mental health problems will impact on parenting, and are associated with mental health problems in their children. Parental mental health problems are frequently cited as contributory factors in the permanent removal of children from their families (Booth and Booth 2005).

Practice in the past has been to control the fertility of women through a number of ways dating back through many decades into the early part of the last century (Walmsley 2000). A recent study of referrals for sterilization to the High Court in England and Wales over a ten-year period from 1988 showed almost all were for women with ID with only 5% being for men with ID. The ages of the women were between 21–41 years and nearly three-quarters did not have partners so were unlikely to have had or will have a sexual relationship in the future (Stansfield *et al.* 2007).

Ethnicity and gender

There is a very limited literature on the impact of ethnicity and culture in women with disabilities with almost no literature on women with ID (Traustadothir and Johnson 2000). This pervasive invisibility is apparent throughout the literature in the needs of women with ID. The 2006 national census of inpatients in mental health and learning disability services in England and Wales (Count Me In 2007) found significant differences between admission rates within ethnic groups for gender. Admission rates were significantly lower than average among all Asian groups. Admission rates from the Indian and Pakistani groups were significantly lower than the average with no women inpatients from the Bangladeshi group. Also the uptake of day services are low in the South Asian community as parents felt these were not appropriate to the cultural and religious needs of their daughter (Raghavan and Waseem 2007). As a solution, females were accessing support workers from a voluntary organization for people from the South Asian community rather than use the statutory services.

Women who show offending behaviour

There are few reports on female offenders with ID (Holland *et al.* 2002). A study of a cohort of offenders in Scotland showed that females constitute a low number of referrals to services of less than 10% (Lindsey *et al.* 2004). The suggested explanation is that women with ID do not show the same levels of sexually abusive or aggressive behaviours which are the most common reasons for referral of a man with ID. However, the women with ID were found to have higher levels of mental illness, higher levels of sexual abuse, and lower levels of re-offending. There is some evidence that within health and social care services, women whose behaviour is illogical or antisocial receive different treatment from men, and are more likely to receive intrusive interventions such as punishment or medication (Scotti *et al.* 1999).Within specialist health services, women may be particularly vulnerable to sexual abuse by staff and other service users (Williams *et al.* 1993).

Women with ID form a very small subgroup of the prison population and little is known about them. As with their non-disabled counterparts, women with ID in prison have a high rate of mental illness, greater than their male counterparts with ID (Hayes 2007). Many have been victims of physical, emotional, or sexual abuse (Hayes 2007). They are, again, invisible victims being overlooked and devalued.

Gender-specific services

Gender specific services understand women in the context of their lives, including hormonal and reproductive changes, parenting/caring roles and their need to keep safe due to past experience of abuse. In the general population the voluntary sector leads in the provision of community based women-only services including services for women who experience violence and abuse. Howlett and Danby (2007) reported on a pilot scheme in Newcastle where women with ID are enabled by being supported to get to counselling sessions and to access a mainstream rape crisis centre that offers counselling to women who have been abused at any time in their lives. Self-advocacy groups have helped many women. Such groups may focus on a particular issue such as abuse, parenting, and health. Some have been set up by paid workers, others by women with ID, sometimes with the support of paid workers. Women without ID tend to act as supporters rather than as participants. Women-only groups may be less embarrassing and intimidating than mixed-sex groups for some women, and be perceived as safer and more appropriate for the discussion of some issues.

The private sector leads in the provision of women-only secure services and there are secure NHS inpatient facilities for women with ID, for example, in North East England. These gender-specific services are rare resources but for women with ID may offer greater safety and privacy. The creation of a safe environment has particular relevance to women with ID who have commonly experienced violence and abuse and may be sexually more vulnerable when suffering from mental illness.

Conclusions

There is little research in this area with gender differences not being satisfactorily investigated in people with ID. Epidemiological studies on prevalence risk factors and presentation of disorders which have a focus on gender will help build up a picture of the mental health needs of women with ID. Inclusion of women into research of both pharmaceutical and psychological interventions needs to address if the benefits and risks are similar for women and men with ID. The experience of mental health services by women with ID needs to be understood, including aspects of privacy and safety. This increasing evidence will make the lives of women with ID more visible in the eyes of practitioners and the commissioners of services so leading to improved outcomes and well-being for this vulnerable group of the population.

References

Booth T and Booth W (2000). Growing up with parents who have learning difficulties. *Mental Retardation*, **38**, 1–14.

Booth T and Booth W (2005). Parents with learning difficulties in the child protection system: experiences and perspectives. *Journal of Intellectual Disabilities*, **9**, 109–29.

Bouras N and Holt G (2007). *Psychiatric and Behavioural Disorders in Intellectual and Developmental Disabilities*, second edition. Cambridge University Press, Cambridge.

Burns J (1993). Invisible women: women who have learning disabilities, *The Psychologist Bulletin of the British Psychological Society*, **6**, 102–105.

Burns J (2000). Living on the edge: women with learning disabilities. In: JM Ussher (ed) *Women's Health: Contemporary International Perspectives*, pp. 196–203. Wiley-Blackwell, London.

Cooper SA *et al.* (2007). Mental ill-health in adults with intellectual disabilities: prevalence and associated factors. *British Journal of Psychiatry*, **190**, 27–35.

Count Me In (2007). *Commission for Healthcare Audit and Inspection: Results of the 2006 National Consensus of Inpatients in Mental Health and Learning Disability Services in England and Wales*. Department of Health, London.

Dagnan D (2007). Psychosocial interventions for people with intellectual disabilities. In: N Bouras and G Holt (eds) *Psychiatric and Behavioural Disorders in Intellectual and Developmental Disabilities*, second edition, pp. 330–8. Cambridge University Press, Cambridge.

Department of Health (2001). *Valuing People: A New Strategy for Learning Disability for the 21st Century*. Available at: http://www.dh.gov.uk

Department of Health (2002). *Mainstreaming Gender and Women's Mental Health: Implementation Guidance*. Available at: http://www.dh.gov.uk

Ditchfield H and Burns J (2004). Understanding our bodies, understanding ourselves: the cycle, mental health and women with learning disabilities. *Tizard Learning Disability Review*, **9**, 24–32.

Emerson E and Hatton C (2007). Poverty, socio-economic position, social capital and health of children and adolescents with intellectual disabilities in Britain: a replication. *Journal of Intellectual Disability Research*, **51**, 866–74.

Flynn A *et al.* (2002). Validity of the diagnosis of personality disorder in adults with learning disability and severe behavioural problems. *British Journal of Psychiatry*, **180**, 543–6.

Hayes SC (2007). Women with learning disabilities who offend: what do we know? *British Journal of Learning Disabilities*, **35**, 187–91.

Holland T *et al.* (2002). Prevalence of 'criminal offending' by men and women with intellectual disability and the characteristics of 'offenders': implications for research and service development. *Journal of Intellectual Disability Research*, **46**, 6–20.

Howlett S and Danby J (2007). Learning Disability and sexual abuse: use of a women-only counselling service by women with a learning disability: A pilot study. *Tizard Learning Disability Review*, **12**, 4–15.

Kallianes V and Rubenfeld P (1997). Disabled women and reproductive rights. *Disability and Society*, **12**, 203–22.

Kohen D (2000). *Women and Mental Health*, Routledge, London.

Kyrkou M (2005). Health issues and quality of life in women with intellectual disability. *Journal of Intellectual Disability Research*, **49**, 770–2.

Lindsay WR *et al.* (2004). Women with intellectual disability who have offended: characteristics and outcome. *Journal of Intellectual Disability Research*, **48**, 580–90.

Lunsky Y and Havercamp SM (2002). Women's mental health. In: PN Walsh and T Heller (eds) *Health of Women with Intellectual Disabilities*, pp. 59–75. Blackwell Publishing Company, Oxford.

Lunksy Y (2003). Depressive symptoms in intellectual disability: does gender play a role. *Journal of Intellectual Disability Research*, **45**, 417–27.

McCarthy M (2000). Sexual experiences of women with mild and moderate intellectual disabilities (abstract). *Journal of Intellectual Disability Research*, **44**(suppl. 1), 384

McCarthy M and Thompson D (1997). A prevalence study of sexual abuse of adults with intellectual disabilities referred for sex education. *Journal of Applied Research in Intellectual Disability*, **10**, 105–24.

McGaw S *et al.* (2007). Prevalence of psychopathology across a service population of parents with intellectual disabilities and their children. *Journal of Policy and Practice in Intellectual Disabilities*, **4**, 11–22.

O'Callaghan AC *et al.* (2003). The impact of abuse on men and women with severe learning disabilities and their families. *British Journal of Learning Disabilities*, **31**, 175–80.

O'Hara J and Martin H (2003). Parents with learning difficulties: a study of gender and cultural perspectives in East London. *British Journal of Learning Disabilities*, **31**, 18–24.

O'Hara J (2007). Inter-disciplinary multi-modal assessment for mental health problems in people with intellectual disabilities. In: N Bouras and G Holt (eds) *Psychiatric and Behavioural Disorders in Intellectual and Developmental Disabilities*, second edition, pp. 42–61. Cambridge University Press, Cambridge.

Parkes G and Hollins S (2007). Psychodynamic approaches to people with intellectual disabilities: individuals, groups/ systems and families, In: N Bouras and G Holt (eds) *Psychiatric and Behavioural Disorders in Intellectual and Developmental Disabilities*, second edition, pp. 339–52. Cambridge University Press, Cambridge.

Raghavan R and Waseem F (2007). Services for young people with learning disabilities and mental health needs from South Asian communities. *Advances in Mental Health and Learning Disabilities*, **1**, 27–31.

Rojahn J and Ebensen AJ (2005). Epidemiology of mood disorders in people with mental retardation. In: P Sturmey (ed) *Mood Disorders in People with Mental Retardation*, pp. 123–38. NADD Press, Kingston, NY.

Schupf N *et al.* (1997). Early menopause in women with Down's syndrome. *Journal of Intellectual Disability Research*, **41**, 264–7.

Scott LV (2000). A physiological perspective, In: D Kohen (eds) *Women and Mental Health*, pp. 17–38. Routledge, London.

Scotti *et al.* (1991). A meta-analysis of intervention research with problem behaviour: treatment validity and standards of practice. *American Journal on Mental Retardation*, **96**, 233–56.

Scrager S *et al.* (2007). Prevalence of fractures in women with intellectual disabilities: a chart review. *Journal of Intellectual Disability Research*, **51**, 253–9.

Sequeria H *et al.* (2003). Psychological disturbance associated with sexual abuse in people with learning disabilities: a case control study. *British Journal of Psychiatry*, **183**, 451–6.

Stansfield AJ *et al.* (2007). The sterilisation of people with intellectual disabilities in England and Wales during the period 1988 to 1999. *Journal of Intellectual Disability Research*, **51**, 569–79.

Taggart L *et al.* (2006). An exploration of substance misuses in people with intellectual disabilities. *Journal of Intellectual Disability Research*, **50**, 588–97.

Taylor JL *et al.* (2004). Screening for psychiatric symptoms: PAS-ADD Checklist norms for adults with intellectual disabilities. *Journal of Intellectual Disability Research*, **48**, 37–41.

Traustadottir R, Johnson K (2000). *Women with Intellectual Disabilities: Finding a Place in the World*. Jessica Kingsley Publishers, London.

Tsakanikos E *et al.* (2006). Psychiatric co-morbidity and gender differences in intellectual disability. *Journal of Intellectual Disability Research*, **50**, 582–7.

Tymchuk AJ (1994). Depression symptomatology in mothers with mild intellectual disability. An exploratory study. *Australian and New Zealand Journal of Developmental Disabilities*, **19**, 111–19.

Umb-Carlsson O and Sonnander K (2006). Living conditions of adults with intellectual disabilities from a gender perspective. *Journal of Intellectual Disability Research*, **50**, 326–34.

Unifem (2003). United Nations Development Fund for Women Annual Report 2002/2003, *Working for Women's Empowerment and Gender Equality*. Unifem, New York. http://www.umifem.org

Walmsley J (2000). Women and the Mental Deficiency Act of 1913: citizenship, sexuality and regulation. *British Journal of Learning Disabilities*, **28**, 65–70.

Walsh PN, Murphy GH (2002). Risk and vulnerability: dilemmas for women. In: PN Walsh and T Heller (eds) *Health of Women with Intellectual Disabilities*, pp. 154–69. Blackwell Publishing, Oxford.

Williams J *et al.* (1993). *Purchasing Effective Mental Health Services for Women: A Framework for Action*. Centre for the Applied Psychology of Social Care (Tizard Centre), Canterbury.

CHAPTER 33

Affective disorders in women with intellectual disabilities

Alaa Al-Sheikh and Dimitrios Paschos

Introduction

The issue of gender and depression within the general population has been given substantial research attention and an association between female gender and increased risk for depression is established. Adverse childhood experiences, sociocultural roles, and vulnerability to life events are thought to increase the prevalence, incidence, and morbidity risk of depressive disorders in females. Biological factors seem to play a less important role in the emergence of gender differences (Piccinelli *et al.* 2000).

Affective disorder, and in particular depression, is more common in people with intellectual disabilities (ID). Higher rates of physical illness including epilepsy, socioeconomic adversity, past experience of abuse, and reduced life supports are thought to be relevant risk factors (Richards *et al.* 2001; Lunsky 2003; De Collishaw and Maughan 2004). When people with ID become depressed, all psychological and somatic symptoms of depression can be observed, but changes are often subtle and develop over time. Depression in this population often remains undiagnosed, atypical symptoms are common, and self-injurious or aggressive behaviour may dominate the clinical picture of people with more severe ID (Gravestock *et al.* 2005).

In the Diagnostic Criteria for Psychiatric Disorders for use with Adults with Learning Disabilities/Mental Retardation (DC-LD) (Royal College of Psychiatrists 2001) the following disorders are classified under affective disorders:

1. Depressive episodes in recurrent depressive disorder and bipolar affective disorder

2. Manic episodes in bipolar affective disorder

3. Other affective disorder.

In this chapter, we will discuss the presentation of two major disorders, depression and bipolar affective disorder in women with ID. We will highlight epidemiological studies that have taken gender issues into account and explore gender-related risk factors. The assessment of females with ID and affective disorder will be discussed, as well as diagnostic, treatment, and service delivery issues for this highly vulnerable group.

Epidemiology

Few studies have presented results separately for men and women with ID and affective disorder. In contrast to the wealth of gender-related research in the general population, there is a continuing lack of evidence base and robust epidemiological data regarding this population. However, several studies documented that depressive disorders are more common in woman than in men with ID (Hastings *et al.* 2004; Lunsky and Palucka 2004; Lunsky and Canrinus 2005; Cooper *et al.* 2007).

Cooper *et al.* (2007), in a population-based study of 1023 adults with an ID, found a 3.8% point prevalence of affective disorder, which was higher than that of the general population. Comprehensive individual assessments with each person with ID were conducted and DC-LD diagnostic criteria were employed. A point prevalence of 0.6% was yielded for mania. Additionally, 1.0% of the sample had bipolar disorder currently in remission, and 0.1% had previous episode of mania currently in remission. There was no conclusion, however, regarding potential risk factors that could explain the gender differences. Indeed, whether higher rates of depression in females with ID are owing to biological or psychosocial influences remains relatively unexplored (Stavrakaki and Lunsky 2007).

A population-based study by Hastings *et al.* (2004) of over 1000 adults with ID demonstrated a significantly higher rate of affective symptoms in women than in men, as measured by the PAS-ADD Checklist (Moss *et al.* 1998). One recent study examined gender differences in people with ID admitted to inpatients units. In this study, Lunsky *et al.* (2009) compared 1971 men and women with and without ID, admitted to psychiatric units, in terms of diagnosis and clinical issues. Amongst inpatients with ID (126 females and 243 males), females were more likely to have a diagnosis of affective disorder and a past history of sexual abuse. Men were more likely to misuse substances, show aggressive behaviour and have forensic issues. Gender difference patterns found for persons with ID and affective disorder were similar to gender differences in inpatients without ID.

Women and men with ID seem to present equal rates of bipolar affective disorder, as in general population studies. However, a later onset of bipolar illness has been suggested for females with ID (Glue 1989; Vanstraelen and Tyrer 1999). Cain *et al.* (2003) reviewed four groups of people with ID and additional diagnoses of bipolar affective disorder, depression, psychotic depression, schizophrenia, or psychosis not otherwise specified. Females with ID represented 53% of the major depression group and 38% of the bipolar affective disorder group. Subjects of the latter group had significantly more mood-related symptoms, as well as functional impairments, compared to individuals from the other groups. Behavioural profiles of the bipolar group patients differed significantly from the other three groups adding to the evidence that bipolar disorder can be reliably identified in persons with ID. Mixed affective disorders, persistent affective disorders, dysthymia, cyclothymia, and their relation to gender has not been systematically studied in people with ID.

Risk factors

In the general population, several risk factors for affective disorder have been examined including stress, life events, low socioeconomic status, lack of social support, and female gender. A review of epidemiological studies on mental health problems of adults with ID showed that these risk factors are shared by people with ID, who may be further disadvantaged by their limited coping skills, experiences of discrimination, rejection, stigma, and abuse (Smiley 2005).

Using logistic regression analysis, Cooper *et al.* (2007) investigated factors associated with depression in persons with ID. Higher number of consultations with general practitioner in the last year, having experienced a life event in the last year, being a smoker, and being a female were all found to be associated independently with depression.

Biological risk factors in relation to women with ID experiencing mental health problems have not been studied in detail. However, syndrome-specific research (e.g. Down syndrome, Prader–Willi syndrome) has highlighted relevant hormonal differences between women with and without ID (Lunsky and Havercamp 2002). Both depression and menstrual cycles in woman with ID are associated with self-injurious behaviour (SIB). According to DC-LD, an onset of, or increase in, problem behaviours such as aggression or SIB are common in depressive episodes (Royal College of Psychiatrists 2001).

In a small study of records analysis of nine women with ID who exhibited SIB for six months, an attempt was made to determine any association between phases of the menstrual cycle and rates of SIB. Menstrual cycles were divided into four phases: (1) menses and early follicular phase; (2) late follicular phase; (3) early luteal phase; and (4) late luteal or premenstrual phase. Analysis showed that the highest frequency of SIB occurred in the first two phases: 43.5% during early follicular phase and 47.3% in the late follicular phase. Seven of the nine women manifested identical phase/SIB relations (Taylor *et al.* 1993).

Tsakanikos *et al.* (2007) examined 281 consecutive referrals to a community mental health and ID service in South East London for the impact of exposure to life events on mental health. Logistic regression analysis demonstrated that single exposure to life events was significantly associated with female gender, schizophrenia, personality disorders, and depression, with females being more likely to have been exposed to at least one life event. The authors did not find overall higher rates of depression in women with ID but found significantly higher rate of adjustment disorder in reaction to an identifiable stressor within the previous three months.

Lunsky (2003) recruited and interviewed 99 adults with borderline to moderate ID (51 men and 48 women) from community services in Ontario, Canada. Different scales and measures were used including one specific to depression. The ratings for women on the depression measures were higher than those of men. Informants' ratings reported no gender differences. Women with higher scores in the depression measures reported significantly fewer coping strategies, lower socioeconomic status, and more stressful relationships.

Women with ID are more vulnerable to be abused than women in the general population and men with ID. There is ample research evidence demonstrating the high prevalence of sexual abuse among women with ID (McCarthy and Thompson 1997; McCarthy 2000; Lunsky 2003). In the general population a history of sexual abuse is well recognized as a significant factor for major depression, suicide attempts, personality disorder, substance misuse, and social anxiety (Nelson *et al.* 2002). In a United Kingdom (UK) case–control study, looking at the association between sexual abuse of persons with ID and psychological disturbance, more individuals from the abused group were meeting diagnostic criteria for depression and anxiety disorders as assessed by the PAS–ADD checklist (Sequeira *et al.* 2003). Other forms of abuse such as physical, emotional abuse, and neglect are prevalent among people with ID. However, no gender-specific studies explored in detail the effects of other types of abuse on the mental health of people with ID.

Loss of a family member, friend, or significant other, including staff members in residential homes, is a common experience for people with ID. There has been limited gender-specific research conducted in the area of bereavement and loss. However, when Hollins and Esterhuyzen (1997) compared the bereavement process in 22 females and 28 males with ID with a matched control group, they found a higher rate of depression, anxiety, and adjustment disorders in the bereaved group.

Pregnancy, birth, and parenting

The association between pregnancy, birth, and the postpartum period and depression has not been widely explored in women with ID. General population studies of affective disorders associated with the postpartum period have not included those with diagnosis of ID. It is generally believed that pregnant women with ID have the disadvantage of poor social support which renders them more vulnerable to affective disorder. A large proportion of mothers with ID experience further traumatization by the removal of their children by child welfare agencies in cases of serious concerns about their ability to provide safe parenting.

Tymchuk (1994) investigated depression in mothers with ID and found significantly more depressive symptoms in comparison to a control group of women of the same socioeconomic background. National data from French and Belgian mother and baby unit admissions revealed that women with psychiatric disorder or ID remained hospitalized longer, improved less, were more often separated from their babies, or discharged with supervision, than women admitted with other diagnoses (Glangeaud-Freudenthal 2004). In the UK, the increased number of children of people with ID removed from the care of their parents is thought to be in breach of Human Rights legislation and this has led to calls for positive corrective action by the Department of Health (House of Lords 2007).

Special considerations

Suicide in adults with ID has been reported, but very few in-depth studies have been undertaken (Lunsky 2004; Merrick *et al.* 2006). Most of the literature agrees that suicide rates in people with ID are lower than those seen in the general population and suicide among those with more severe intellectual impairments is extremely rare. There is lack of evidence base on the relationship between gender and risk of suicide in people with ID. However, the majority of case studies of attempted and completed suicide in ID have focused on men, therefore further research is warranted (Lunsky and Canrinus 2005).

A recent study looked at affective disorder or related disorders in women with ID who are in contact with the criminal justice system. Lindsay *et al.* (2004) studied characteristics and outcome of female offenders with ID by examining referrals to a community service for offenders with ID in the UK during an 11-year period. They found that females accounted for 9% of referrals to the service: 61% of female offenders had suffered sexual abuse and 66% were identified as having a significant mental illness (schizophrenia, bipolar disorder, or major depression).

Autism is common in people with ID. Depression is probably the most common psychiatric disorder seen in individuals with autism. Lainhart and Folstein (1994) found an excess of females in their review of published reports of affective disorder in people with autism. However, Ghaziuddin *et al.* (2002) argue that it remains unknown whether depression is more common in females than in males with autism, because most of the existing literature reports on samples which are drawn from specialist clinics.

Assessment and diagnosis

Diagnosing mental health problems in women with ID can be a complex process. In many ways, the assessment of this population follows the same principles of the psychiatric assessment for women without ID.

Referral pathways, however, seem to be different as it is very rare for women with ID to initiate a mental health referral themselves. In most cases they rely on family or residential staff to identify the problem, with the most common reason for referral (for both genders) being behavioural disturbance. Subtle or slowly developing changes in mood, sleep, or appetite are less likely to be detected in busy residential homes. Subjective states of depressed mood or hopelessness require adequate cognitive and verbal skills in order to be expressed. Women with more severe ID are less likely to poses those skills; therefore reliance on behavioural equivalents or informants' reports is necessary. The DC-LD criteria for depressive and manic episodes are shown in Boxes 33.1 and 33.2.

It is important to understand the mental health problems of both females and males with ID as a synthesis of vulnerability, precipitating, and maintaining factors (biological, psychological, social, and environmental) This is a complex task and requires a coordinated multi-modal and interdisciplinary approach to assessment (O'Hara 2007).

The initial assessment interview is generally best conducted at the person's home where observations can be made about the living environment and family or care home dynamics. The length and style of the interview must also be flexible to accommodate for memory or attention span problems, suggestibility, or acquiescence in some people with ID.

The issue of 'diagnostic overshadowing' is of great importance when assessing affective symptoms. Symptoms such as apathy, decreased verbal output, slowness, low initiative, and other depressive symptoms may be erroneously attributed to the ID, especially when little effort is made to document the person's baseline of mood, affect, and functioning. Also, developmentally appropriate phenomena, such as talking to oneself or with imaginary friends, should be distinguished from psychotic phenomena, such as auditory

---

Box 33.1 DC-LD diagnostic criteria for depressive episode

According to DC-LD a diagnosis of depressive episode in adult with ID requires that:

1. Symptoms are present daily for at least 2 weeks

2. They are not the direct consequence of drugs or physical disorders

3. The criteria for mixed affective episodes or schizoaffective episodes are not met

4. There is a change of individual premorbid state

5. Either of the following are present and prominent:

   ◆ Depressed or irritable mood

   ◆ Loss of interest or pleasure in activity

6. Some of the following symptoms must be present (four in total from items 5 and 6):

   ◆ Loss of energy

   ◆ Loss of confidence

   ◆ Increased tearfulness

   ◆ Onset or increase in somatic symptoms

   ◆ Reduce ability to concentrate

   ◆ Increase in specific problem of behaviour increase motor agitation or retardation

   ◆ Onset or increase in appetite disturbance or weight changes

   ◆ Onset or increase in sleep disturbance.

Box 33.2 DC-LD diagnostic criteria for manic episode

According to DC-LD a diagnosis of a manic episode in adult with ID requires that:

1. Symptoms present daily for at least 1 week

2. They must not be direct consequence of drugs or physical disorders

3. The criteria for mixed affective episodes or schizoaffective episodes are not met

4. A change of individual premorbid state

5. Elevated or irritable mood must be present

6. Some of the following symptoms must be additionally present:

   ◆ Onset or increase of overactivity

   ◆ Flight of ideas

   ◆ Increased talkativeness

   ◆ Loss of usual social inhibition

   ◆ Reduced sleep

   ◆ Increase in self-esteem/grandiosity

   ◆ Reduced concentration

   ◆ Reckless behaviour

   ◆ Increased libido or sexual indiscretions.

hallucinations (Hurley and Silka 2003; Pickard and Paschos 2005).

A crucial aspect of the initial assessment is to exclude any physical cause for the affective symptoms such as endocrine and metabolic conditions, epilepsy, or other neurological conditions which are seen more commonly in people with ID. A full physical examination, blood investigations, imaging, and referral for other consultations should also be considered. A thorough assessment of physical health is more important for people with ID, who often have significant physical health needs (US Public Health Service 2002; Kerr 2004; NHS Scotland 2004). Several studies reported inequalities in accessing healthcare for people with ID as well as lower proportions of women with ID receiving cervical and breast screening compared to women without ID (DRC 2007).

It is expected that an assessment of a woman with ID should include a full psychiatric history, family and personal history, social history, relationships, menstrual history, pregnancies, and parenting experiences. A comprehensive risk assessment estimating the risk to self and/or others, as well as the risk of self-neglect, abuse, and exploitation, should also be a routine component of the assessment pathway.

Diagnostic instruments

In the past two decades, a number of screening, assessment, diagnostic, and monitoring instruments have been developed for people with ID (Mohr and Costello 2006). Although not a substitute for a thorough clinical assessment they can help increase the correct identification of mental health problems in this population.

The PAS-ADD checklist (Moss *et al.* 1998; Moss 2002) has recently had its psychometric properties independently assessed. It is a screening tool that can be used by untrained people to identify persons with ID with a possible psychiatric disorder. It contains 29 items concerning common psychiatric symptoms, split into five scales. These scales combined produce three total scores for: (1) affective/neurotic disorder; (2) possible organic disorder; and (3) psychotic disorder. The affective/neurotic disorder scale includes items on depression and hypomania. Sturmey *et al.* (2005) replicated the psychometric properties of the PAS-ADD in a sample of 226 persons with ID who were referred over a three-year period to a specialist service. Total scores on the affective/neurotic disorders scale had alpha values equal to or greater than 0.7. Internal consistency was found to be similar to that reported by Moss *et al.* (1998). There was

also a significant difference in scores between participants who had depressive disorder and those with no diagnosis.

Instruments such as the PAS-ADD checklist cover a wide range of psychiatric conditions with affective disorders being only part of the schedule. However, the Glasgow Depression Scale for people with a Learning Disability (GDS-LD), was specifically developed for the assessment of affective disorders. The scale contains 20 items based on DC-LD diagnostic criteria. Focus groups (consisting of people with mild to moderate ID) data analysis provided the language often used to describe affect and emotions in this population. The developers of the scale demonstrated differentiation between depression and non-depression groups, correlation with the Beck Depression Inventory-II, good test–retest reliability (r=0.97) and internal consistency (Cronbach's α=0.90), and 96% sensitivity and 90% specificity (Cuthill *et al.* 2003).

It is worth noting none of the diagnostic instruments reported in ID literature take into account any gender related issues.

Pharmacotherapy

The treatment of females with ID with psychotropic (including antidepressant) medication and relevant issues are discussed in depth on Chapter 34. Basic principles on best prescribing practices for people with ID include a thorough physical, psychological, social, and behavioural assessment before prescribing, and also a date for reviewing the need for medication (Einfeld 2001). To maximize effectiveness, treatment with medication should be part of a broader and holistic treatment plan. Polypharmacy should be avoided, and clear guidelines are needed regarding the use of 'as required' medication. Although there is a significant association between affective disorders (depression and hypomania) and challenging behaviour (Moss *et al.* 2000); this relationship is likely to be complex and where medication failed to control symptoms and behaviours, other interventions may be more effective, as shown in Case vignette 1.

Case vignette 1

Ms Mary is a 40-year-old woman with a moderate ID, severe autism, and behaviour disturbance including physical aggression and repeated self-injury. She has an additional diagnosis of bipolar affective disorder. She had spent her entire life in care settings. In the past year, her self-injurious behaviour deteriorated, she presented with depressed and irritable mood, poor sleep and appetite, and needed admission to an inpatient unit. On some weeks over 100 instances of difficult behaviours were documented in the unit. She was prescribed a depot antipsychotic injection, two anticonvulsants for mood stabilization, and benzodiazepines, both regular and 'as required'. Four previous trials of antidepressants, lithium, and other antipsychotic medication did not improve her symptoms.

Following a year-long admission she was transferred to a secure small residential unit for people with autism and challenging behaviour. In just over two months, a significant improvement in her mood and behaviour was noted. There were no changes in her medication but all care staff in the unit had formal training in Positive Behaviour Support and special training and experience in autism. Ms Mary is now attending a day centre in the community and her medication is being reduced.

Psychological interventions

Large-scale provision of psychotherapy for people with ID has been slow to emerge, because of previous assumptions about the suitability of this group for talking treatments and the predominance of behavioural therapy. There is now a growing awareness that, with appropriate adaptations, most available psychological therapies can benefit people with ID, their families, and staff (Hurley 2005). Two recent meta-analyses of a small number of controlled studies have shown at least moderate benefit from engagement in a wide range of psychological treatments with schema-focused cognitive work appearing to have a lasting effect on a sample of people with moderate ID (Prout and Nowak-Drabik 2003; Royal College of Psychiatrists 2004).

Despite limited evidence base on the use of cognitive behavioural therapy (CBT) for people with ID (Dagnan and Jahoda 2006; Dagnan 2007), several models have been developed to treat depression and anxiety disorders, to teach assertiveness and social skills, and to inform anger management interventions. Role play and use of non-verbal materials, drawings, photographs, and picture storybooks are commonly employed to enhance CBT techniques.

There is some evidence that psychodynamic treatment can improve self-esteem and reduce distress and problem behaviours in persons with ID (Beail et al. 2005; Parkes and Hollins 2007). Like men, women with ID may find it difficult to express negative feelings, such as anger, towards people on whom they depend. It is theorized that verbalization of such unacknowledged feelings can result in therapeutic benefit. The effect the primary disability has on the person's self-image (the 'secondary handicap') is also considered in psychodynamic therapy with people with ID (Hollins and Sinason 2000). Issues around sexuality, sexual abuse and other trauma, dependency needs, illness, and death can be difficult to discuss for many women with ID and a sensitive approach and a safe environment are required. Gender matching of the therapist should also be considered, especially when depression is linked to past experiences of abuse. Female-only support groups for women with ID who have been sexually abused and also providing support to access relevant mainstream counselling services have been found to be beneficial (Howlett and Danby 2007; Peckham et al. 2007).

Non-directive counselling or person-centred therapy can be a powerful approach for people with ID whose personal experiences are often ignored or discounted (Oliver and Smith 2005). Other forms of therapy such as dialectical behaviour therapy for people ID have also been described (Lew et al. 2006). Art, drama, and music therapy have all been used with people with ID and with people who have autism. The use of various media and communication alternatives is thought to allow choice and foster the growth of self-esteem. There is, however, a lack of controlled studies regarding these less structured interventions.

Presently, no particular model or approach seems to be superior and availability of local resources sometimes determines what type of therapy is provided. Although specialist skills will be required to work with some women with ID, a large number should be able to benefit from mainstream psychotherapy services (Royal College of Psychiatrists 2004).

Social interventions and supports

Social and environmental risk factors for depression are well documented in the general population. People with ID may have an increased risk of depression because of higher rates of physical illness, socioeconomic adversity, experience of abuse and reduced life supports (Richards et al. 2001; Lunsky 2003; De Collishaw and Maughan 2004). Thus, a treatment package for females with ID and depression should consider a review of her housing situation, daily activities, and life and social opportunities. A safe environment and extra social supports may be necessary to achieve or maintain positive change in mental health.

Service provision

Gender differences in patterns of service utilization and delivery have been documented among people with ID receiving specialist services; however, the focus of studies has not been solely affective disorders. Tajuddin, *et al.* 2004 carried out a retrospective note review of all admissions to a specialist ID mental health inpatient unit over a period of two years. People with mild and moderate ID made up over 90% of a sample of 72 people. More men with ID tended to be hospitalized than women with ID. The most common reason for admission for females with ID was behavioural disorder, followed by schizophrenia, personality disorder, depression, and bipolar affective disorder. In a review of a consequent referrals to a community mental health and ID specialist team, Tsakanikos *et al.* (2006) found that in a sample of 295 men and 295 women with ID and psychiatric problems, women with ID were more likely to be referred by their primary care physician, but men were more likely to be referred from generic mental health services. Finally, in a pattern similar to that seen in the general population, women with ID were found to be less likely to have forensic issues or to be placed in secure units (Beer *et al.* 2005).

Following de-institutionalization and the move to the community there has been little consensus as to who should provide services for people with ID and mental or behavioural disorders (Bouras and Holt 2004). As a general rule, the shape of services tends to reflect historical, political, and economic realities of the areas they serve. There has been a large geographical variation of the type, capacity, and functions of available services, sometimes even within the same country or region. Even though women with ID may be more likely to experience violence and abuse and become particularly vulnerable when they are mental ill, there have been no systematic efforts to address this issue. Services for people with ID and in particular inpatient provision have been criticized for continuing to be delivered in 'gender blind' manner (Kohen 2004).

Conclusions

There is little research in the area of gender differences in people with ID who experience affective disorders. Females with ID follow a pattern seen in the non-ID population and tend to experience higher rates of depression than males with ID. Their increased vulnerability to depression seems to be related to adverse life experiences, abuse and neglect, increased ill health, social isolation, and lack of support to meet culturally expected roles. The assessment of possible affective disorder in females with ID is similar to that for females without ID. Particular attention should be given to gender-specific issues and histories of abuse. The treatment should be holistic and take into account the need for a safe environment and space to talk about painful emotions. Despite a growing awareness of these issues, specialist ID services continue to be delivered with little regard to gender issues. Epidemiological studies on prevalence, risk, and protective factors for affective disorders will need to have a focus on gender to help understand better the mental health needs of women with ID. Providing that the right safeguards are in place, it is important that females with ID are included in trials of medication that could prove beneficial to them. In addition, more studies should concentrate on evaluating interventions and models of service delivery. The development of research networks which are not attached to a particular theoretical school and can evaluate different interventions based on holistic, gender-sensitive, and integrated models should be a future priority.

References

Beail N *et al.* (2005) Naturalistic evaluation of the effectiveness of psychodynamic psychotherapy for people with intellectual disabilities. *Journal of Applied Research in Intellectual Disabilities*, **18**, 245–51.

Beer D *et al.* (2005) Low secure units: factors predicting delayed discharge. *Journal of Forensic Psychiatry & Psychology*, **16**(4), 621–37.

Bouras N and Holt G (2004) Mental health services for adults with learning disabilities. *British Journal of Psychiatry*, 184, 291–29.

Cain NN *et al.* (2003) Identifying bipolar disorders in individuals with intellectual disability. *Journal of Intellectual Disability Research*, **47**, 31–8.

Cooper SA *et al.* (2007) An epidemiological investigation of affective disorders with a population-based cohort of 1023 adults with intellectual disabilities. *Psychological Medicine*, **37**(6), 873–82.

Cuthill F *et al.* (2003) Development and psychometric properties of the Glasgow Depression Scale for people with a Learning Disability. Individual and carer supplement versions. *British Journal of Psychiatry*, **182**, 347–53.

Dagnan D and Jahoda A (2006) Cognitive-behavioural intervention for people with intellectual disability and anxiety disorders. *Journal of Applied Research in Intellectual Disabilities*, **19**(1), 91–7.

Dagnan D (2007) Psychosocial interventions for people with intellectual disabilities. In: N Bouras and G Holt (eds) *Psychiatric and Behavioural Disorders in Intellectual and Developmental Disabilities*, 2nd edition. pp. 330–8. Cambridge University Press, Cambridge.

De Collishaw S and Maughan J (2004) Affective problems in adults with mild learning disability: the roles of social disadvantage and ill health. *British Journal of Psychiatry*, **185**, 350–1.

Disability Rights Commission (2007) Equal Treatment: Closing The Gap. http://83.137.212.42/sitearchive/DRC/library/health_investigation.html (Accessed May 2008.)

Einfeld SL (2001) Systematic management approach to pharmacotherapy for people with learning disabilities. *Advances in Psychiatric Treatment*, **7**, 43–9.

Gravestock S *et al.* (2005) Psychiatric disorders in adults with learning disabilities. In: G Holt *et al.* (eds) *Mental Health in Learning Disabilities: A Reader*, pp. 7–17. Estia Centre & Pavilion Publishing, Brighton.

Ghaziuddin M *et al.* (2002) Depression in persons with autism: implications for research and clinical care. *Journal of Autism and Developmental Disorders*, **32**(4), 299–306.

Glangeaud-Freudenthal NMC (2004) Mother-Baby psychiatric units (MBUs): national data collection in France and in Belgium (1999–2000). *Archives of Women Mental Health*, **7**(1), 59–64.

Glue P (1989) Rapid cycling affective disorders in the mentally retarded. *Biological Psychiatry*, **26**(3), 250–6.

Hastings RP *et al.* (2004) Life events and psychiatric symptoms in adults with intellectual disabilities. *Journal of Intellectual Disability Research*, **48**, 42–6.

Hollins S and Esterhuyzen A (1997) Bereavement and grief in adults with learning disabilities. *British Journal of Psychiatry*, **170**, 497–501.

Hollins S and Sinason V (2000) Psychotherapy, learning disabilities and trauma: new perspectives. *British Journal of Psychiatry*, **176**, 32–6.

House of Lords (2007) House of Commons. Joint Committee on Human Rights. A Life Like Any Other? Human Rights of Adults with Learning Disabilities. Seventh Report of Session 2007–08. http://www.publications.parliament.uk/pa/jt200708/jtselect/jtrights/40/4002.htm.

Howlett S and Danby J (2007) Learning disability and sexual abuse: use of a women-only counselling service by women with a learning disability: a pilot study. *Tizard Learning Disability Review*, **12**, 4–15.

Hurley AD (2005) Psychotherapy is an essential tool in the treatment of psychiatric disorders for people with mental retardation. *Mental Retardation*, **43**(6), 445–8.

Hurley AD and Silka VR (2003) Identification of hallucinations and delusions in people with intellectual disability. *Mental Health Aspects of Developmental Disabilities*, **6**, 153–7.

Kerr M (2004) Improving the general health of people with learning disabilities. *Advances in Psychiatric Treatment*, **10**, 200–6.

Kohen D (2004) Mental health needs of women with learning disabilities: services can be organized to meet the challenge. *Learning Disability Review*, **9**, 12–19.

Lainhart JE and Folstein SE (1994) Affective disorders in people with autism: a review of published cases. *Journal of Autism and Developmental Disorders*, **24**, 587–601.

Lindsay WR *et al.* (2004) Women with intellectual disability who have offended: characteristics and outcomes. *Journal of Intellectual Disability Research*, **48**, 580–90.

Lunsky Y *et al.* (2009). Gender differences in psychiatric diagnoses amongst inpatients with and without intellectual disabilities. *American Journal on Intellectual and Developmental Disabilities*, **114**, 52–60.

Lunsky Y and Canrinus M (2005) Gender issues, mental retardation and depression. In: P Sturmey (ed) Mood Disorders in People with Mental Retardation, pp. 113–29. NADD Press, Kingston, NY.

Lunsky Y and Havercamp SM (2002) Women's mental health. In: PN Walsh and T Heller (eds) Health of Women with Intellectual Disabilities, pp. 59–75. Blackwell Publishing Company, Oxford.

Lunsky Y (2004) Suicidality in a clinical and community sample of adults with mental retardation. *Research in Developmental Disabilities*, **25**, 231–43.

Lunsky Y and Palucka A (2004) Depression and intellectual disability: a review of current research. *Current Opinion in Psychiatry*, **17**, 359–63.

Lunsky Y (2003) Depressive symptoms in intellectual disability: does gender play a role? *Journal of Intellectual Disability Research*, **47**, 417–27.

McCarthy M (2000) Sexual experiences of women with mild and moderate intellectual disabilities. *Journal of Intellectual Disability Research*, **44**(1), 384

McCarthy M and Thompson D (1997) A prevalence study of sexual abuse of adults with intellectual disabilities referred for sex education. *Journal of Applied Research in Intellectual Disability*, **10**, 105–24.

Mohr C and Costello H (2006) Mental health assessment and monitoring tools for people with intellectual disabilities. In: N Bouras and G Holt (eds) *Psychiatric and Behavioural Disorders in Intellectual and Developmental Disabilities*, second edition. pp. 24–41. Cambridge University Press, Cambridge.

Moss SC *et al.* (2000) Psychiatric symptoms in adults with learning disability and challenging behaviour. *British Journal of Psychiatry*, **177**, 452–6.

Moss S *et al.* (1998) Reliability and validity of the PAS–ADD Checklist for detecting psychiatric disorders in adults with intellectual disability. *Journal of Intellectual Disability Research*, **42**, 173–83.

Moss S (2002). The PAS–ADD Checklist (revised). Pavillion Publishing, Brighton.

Merrick J *et al.* (2006) A Review of Suicidality in Persons with Intellectual Disability. *Israel Journal of Psychiatry and Related Sciences. Jerusalem*, **43**(4), 258–65.

NHS Health Scotland (2004) People with learning disabilities in Scotland. NHS Health Scotland, Glasgow.

Nelson EC *et al.* (2002) Association between self-reported childhood sexual abuse and adverse psychosocial outcomes: results from a twin study. *Archives of General Psychiatry*, **59**, 139–45.

O'Hara J (2007) Inter-disciplinary multi-modal assessment for mental health problems in people with intellectual disabilities. In: N Bouras and G Holt (eds) *Psychiatric and Behavioural Disorders in Intellectual and Developmental Disabilities*, second edition. pp. 42–61. Cambridge University Press, Cambridge.

Oliver B, Smith P (2005) Psychological interventions for people with learning disabilities. In: G Holt *et al.* (eds) *Mental Health in Learning Disabilities: A Reader*, pp. 41–8. Estia Centre & Pavilion Publishing, Brighton.

Parkes G, Hollins S (2007) Psychodynamic approaches to people with intellectual disabilities: individuals, groups/systems and families. In: N Bouras and G Holt (eds) *Psychiatric and Behavioural Disorders in Intellectual and Developmental Disabilities*, second edition. pp. 339–52. Cambridge University Press, Cambridge.

Peckham NG *et al.* (2007) Evaluating a survivors group pilot for women with significant intellectual disabilities who have been sexually abused. *Journal of Applied Research in Intellectual Disabilities*, **20**, 308–22.

Pickard M and Paschos D (2005) Pseudohallucinations in people with intellectual disabilities: two case reports. *Mental Health Aspects of Developmental Disabilities*, **8**(3), 91–3.

Piccinelli M and Wilkinson G (2000) Gender differences in depression. Critical review. *British Journal of Psychiatry*, **177**, 486–92.

Prout HT and Nowak-Drabik KM (2003) Psychotherapy with persons who have Mental Retardation: An Evaluation of Effectiveness. *American Journal on Mental Retardation*, **108**(2), 82–93.

Richards M *et al.* (2001) Long-term affective disorder in people with mild learning disability. *British Journal of Psychiatry*, **179**, 523–7.

Royal College of Psychiatrists (2001) Diagnostic Criteria for Psychiatric Disorders for Use with Adults with Learning Disabilities/Mental Retardation (DC-LD). Gaskell, London.

Royal College of Psychiatrists (2004) Psychotherapy and Learning Disability. Council Report CR116. College Research Unit, London.

Sequeira H and Hollins S (2003) Clinical effects of sexual abuse on people with learning disability: critical literature review. *British Journal of Psychiatry*, **182**, 13–18.

Smiley E (2005) Epidemiology of mental health problems in adults with learning disability: an update. *Advances in Psychiatric Treatment*, **11**, 214–22.

Stavrakaki C and Lunsky Y (2007) Depression, anxiety and adjustment disorders in people with intellectual disabilities. In: N Bouras and G Holt (eds) *Psychiatric and Behavioural Disorders in Intellectual and Developmental Disabilities*, second edition, pp. 42–61. Cambridge University Press, Cambridge.

Sturmey P.*et al.* (2005) The PAS-ADD checklist: independent replication of its psychometric properties in a community sample. *British Journal of Psychiatry*, **186**, 319–23.

Tajuddin M *et al.* (2004) A study of the use of an acute inpatient unit for adults with learning disability and mental health problems in Leicestershire, UK. *British Journal of Developmental Disabilities*, **98**, 59–68.

Taylor DV.*et al.* (1993) Self-injurious behavior within the menstrual cycle of women with mental retardation. *American Journal of Mental Retardation*, **97**(6), 659–64.

Tsakanikos E *et al.* (2006) Psychiatric co-morbidity and gender differences in intellectual disability. *Journal of Intellectual Disability Research*, **50**, 582–7.

Tsakanikos E *et al.* (2007) Multiple exposure to negative life events and clinical psychopathology in adults with intellectual disability. *Social Psychiatry and Psychiatric Epidemiology*, **42**(1), 24–8.

Tymchuk AJ (1994) Depression symptomatology in mothers with mild intellectual disability: An exploratory study. *Journal of Intellectual & Developmental Disability (Previously published as: Australia and New Zealand Journal of Developmental Disabilities)*, **19**(2), 111–19.

Vanstraelen M and Tyrer P (1999) Rapid cycling bipolar affective disorder in people with intellectual disability: a systematic review. *Journal of Intellectual Disability Research*, **43**, 349–59.

US Public Health Service (2002) Closing the Gap: a national blueprint for improving the health of individual with mental retardation. Report of the Surgeon General's Conference on Health Disparities and Mental Retardation. US Department of Health and Human Services, Washington, DC.

CHAPTER 34

Psychopharmacology in women with learning disabilities

Gregory O'Brien and Geetha Kumeravelu

Introduction

This chapter outlines some of the main issues concerning psychopharmacology in women with learning disabilities. Review of recent literature shows that women's mental health has been explored increasingly closely over the last 30 years but for the most part women with learning disabilities unfortunately have been excluded from these studies. This is despite women with learning disabilities having different needs and challenges, due to their particular situation and unique mental health needs (Romans 1998). The following chapter briefly reviews these matters, and gives practical guidance to a pragmatic approach to psychiatric drug prescribing for this high profile patient group.

The chapter opens with an overview of general issues concerning gender, health, and psychotropic prescribing for women with learning disability. A brief summary of general guidelines to be followed in prescribing psychotropics for this population closes the chapter. Throughout the chapter, advice on common clinical scenarios is presented in the form of 'practice points'.

Gender, health, and psychotropic medication for women with learning disability

Historically, clinical practice in the psychiatry of learning disability has been largely centred on the male population (Aman 1983). Meeting the health needs of women with learning disabilities requires consideration of the interactions between their experiences and needs at each stage of the life span and the interface with social, economic, and cultural environments, including gender-specific issues, in addition to those which are common across both genders. Meeting the health needs of women with learning disabilities, including a rational approach to their psychopharmacology entails consideration of their sexual development, sexuality, the menstrual cycle, aspects of contraception, fertility, reproduction, puerperium, and menopause: all of which are unique to women, or are at least gender-specific.

To date, however, little attention has been paid to addressing gender-specific issues relating to the health needs of women with learning disabilities (Ayd 1991). The reasons for this are numerous, including a long tradition of a lack of attention being paid to the needs of women in learning disability services, a lack of appreciation of the reproductive healthcare needs of women with learning disability, and a general lack of interest in gender-specific issues with respect to pharmacological interventions.

On the positive side, there is evidence of some shift in contemporary approaches to the predicament of women with learning disabilities, which signify that there are initiatives in progress to redress these inequalities. For example, the general shift towards a health service which aims to reduce all health inequalities has direct relevance to the situation of women with learning disabilities, and consequentially to prescribing of psychotropic medication for them. In face of this, it is now incumbent upon us to consider whether there are any such inequalities which are gender-specific, to address these, and to ensure that women's needs in this respect are met. One of the issues highlighted by the recent report by Mansell (Department of Health 2007) concerns drug prescribing for behaviour disorder. In common with a number of previous documents, it is highlighted here that many people with severe learning disabilities—and especially women—are likely to receive drug treatment for behaviour disorders and self-injurious behaviour. This is therefore one of a set of contemporary documents which emphasizes the need to consider other strategies, and where possible, avoid getting into a trap of inappropriate psychotropic prescribing in women with learning disabilities who have challenging needs.

At present the literature is sparse on topics related to psychopharmacology for women with learning disabilities. Research on the prevalence of mental health problems in individuals with learning disabilities has largely overlooked the issue of gender, and there is a tendency for women's physical health problems to go unrecognized and untreated, due to diagnostic overshadowing—even more than among men with learning disabilities (Kohen 2001). Some of the confounding factors include biological predisposition to certain illnesses, and the social circumstances of this extremely vulnerable group of people.

Reproductive and physical health

Reproductive and physical health has direct relevance to the prescribing of psychotropic medication. Standard guidelines and formularies for drug prescribing are substantially geared towards otherwise healthy individuals, while also taking account of health conditions and intercurrent prescribing thereof. Compared with women in the general population, women with learning disabilities have several characteristics that increase their risk for reproductive and physical health conditions. These include higher rates of hypogonadism and failure to menstruate, early menopause, and high levels of comorbid conditions such as epilepsy, hypothyroidism, and obesity (Carr and Hollins 1995). In addition to this set of factors, there are the general observations that there is a high frequency of psychotropic medication in this population, and that these women tend to have a relatively sedentary lifestyle. Also, among women with learning disabilities, the average age at onset of menarche is similar to that of women in the general population. Taken together, these interplaying factors highlight the need for a careful, cautious approach to initiating and psychotropic prescribing in women with learning disabilities, where there is such a high rate of comorbidity, and need to be aware of any intercurrent prescribing.

Prescribing psychotropic medication for women with learning disability

When the physician embarks on psychotropic drug prescribing in women with learning disabilities, care is required in selection, introduction, and manipulation of dose and other aspects of drug treatment, in order to maximize efficacy and minimize side effects and toxicity, which can readily occur in this population (Arnold 1993). This entails consideration of pharmacokinetics, drug interactions, and treatment/compliance monitoring—and how these relate to the special needs of women with learning disabilities (O'Brien 2002).

Pharmacokinetics

Pharmacokinetics refers to the process of distributions of drugs within the body and their concentration within various body tissues. It encompasses drug absorption, excretion, and metabolism. Appropriate dosage regimens for starting medication in women with learning disabilities often vary from the general population—the cautious approach to be taken in clinical practice is to start at lower dosage, and to increase dose slowly. Other considerations can then be made, depending on the characteristics of the individual patient, and the specific drug.

Body composition and pharmacokinetics

Gender differences in body composition, weight, and physiology affect drug absorption, distribution, biotransformation, and excretion. Crucially, women have 11% more body fat than men and this results in initially lowered serum levels of most psychopharmacological agents. Certain other key differences between the physiology of women and men are also of direct relevance to psychotropic prescribing. In comparison with men, women have lower bone mass and lower muscle mass. Males and females also have structural differences in various organs including heart, brain, and gastrointestinal system, in addition to the different sexual organs and respective sexual hormonal systems. The sex hormones (oestrogens and androgens) are physically important in both males and females, and play an important role at various stages in a person's development. They are vital in the sexual differentiation prenatally, during the maturation phase in adolescence, in menstruation and pregnancy. Oestrogen and progesterone significantly drop at menopause in women and there is a gradual decline in testosterone with ageing in both men and women.

Practice point

For the most part, starting doses of psychopharmaco-logical agents do not vary between the sexes. However, women whose body mass vary substantially from the norm, can show significant changes in pharmacokinetics. In those psychopharmacological agents in which serum level of drug is crucial, special caution must be initiated in monitoring dose levels, and in manipulating these over the course of therapy – especially in lithium, carbamazepine, and other agents where serum level of active ingredient is crucial for effective psychopharmacological intervention.

Cardiovascular system

The blood pressure is 5–10 mmHg lower in women than men. This difference disappears after menopause. The average heart rate is higher in women than age-matched men. Furthermore, the QT interval is found to be longer in women than among men—these factors need to be taken into account when initiating treatment with any medication which can alter QT interval, especially antipsychotic medication, and also some antidepressant drugs.

Practice point

Certain antipsychotics and antidepressants have a significant impact on Q–T interval. It is crucial, in preparing to prescribe these agents for women with learning disabilities, that the full pretreatment investigation protocol should be carried out, including electrocardiogram investigation.

Renal system

The glomerular filtration rate is slightly lower in young women than age-matched men. It may decline more rapidly with aging in men than women. This clearly has implications on the blood levels of various psychopharmacological agents. For the body concentration of many agents—notably antipsychotic and sedatives—may all too quickly become toxic, with disastrous consequences for the general health and well-being of women with learning disabilities. It is therefore important that, particularly among older subjects, such women be monitored by specialist physicians who are familiar with the change in renal function of older people, and understand the needs for careful manipulation of drug dosage. This needs to be routinely accompanied by monitoring of kidney function, in addition to monitoring of serum levels of those psychopharmacological agents where this is appropriate and available.

Practice point

In prescribing psychopharmacological agents in women with learning disabilities, it is important to bear in mind the reduced glomerular filtration rate and renal function in the elderly, to monitor for any signs of toxicity, utilizing serum level of drug where available.

Hepatobiliary system

Gender differences have been noted in rates of hepatic metabolism, possibly due to the inhibitory effect of oestrogen on some hepatic microsomal enzymes. By delaying gastric emptying time, progesterone may influence drug absorption. Oestrogen and progesterone, both highly protein-bound, may compete with psychotropic medications for protein binding sites. Free, unbound levels of medications may vary with reproductive hormone levels. Competitive binding and microsomal enzyme induction are therefore routine matters to be addressed in all psychopharmacological prescribing, in balancing maximal efficacy with minimal side effects and toxicity. In practice among women with learning disabilities, the physician must give careful attention to the measurable health and body function indices, through routine investigations, in order to clarify the precise internal biochemical milieu of the patient.

Practice point

The prescribing physician must take account of the effects of hepatic metabolism on bioavailability of psychopharmacological agents, especially in the presence of other drugs, notably those affecting sex hormone functioning.

Side effects of psychopharmacological agents: recognition and management

Women with learning disabilities are likely to experience the same spectrum of adverse effects from psychotropic drugs as does the general population. In addition, these women may be at increased risk of experiencing side effects which may be unrecognized or ignored, for various reasons. For example, in a person with moderate learning disabilities with communication difficulties, the sedating signs resulting from toxicity of many psychotropic agents may be difficult to distinguish from pre-existing functional disability. Women with learning disabilities in the mild to moderate range potentially may be able to describe some problems which are drug side effects, but they may not be able to attribute these adverse effects as being drug-induced. People with severe to profound learning disability may be unable to recognize or report side effects because of impairments or deficits in speech.

Individual variation in medication response is greater in people with learning disabilities, due to the impact of brain development on the pharmacodynamics of a given medication. Also, such is the tolerability of antipsychotic drugs among women, that extrapyramidal and anticholinergic reactions are more often experienced by them. Furthermore, psychotropic drugs are among the most common groups of drugs to adversely affect sexual and reproductive function. However, sexual side effects caused by psychotropic drugs tend to be underestimated, because some patients are reluctant to report such intimate issues and indeed other have such major communication difficulties. Moreover, vulnerability to sexual dysfunction caused by psychotropic medication generally increases with age. These effects need to be borne in mind by the prescribing physician, who needs to routinely monitor the effects of medication on sexual functioning.

Practice point

In prescribing psychopharmacological agents, the physician should be aware of the higher incidence of the common extrapyramidal and anticholinergic side effects among women, of the impact of medication on sexual functioning, and that the patient will frequently not identify these health problems as drug side effects.

Old age and women with learning disabilities

With improved longevity in the learning disabled population, we need to consider the impact of ageing on psychopharmacological prescribing in women with learning disability. Despite it being a common experience, very little attention has been paid to the menopause among women with learning disabilities. Also in this population, the drug treatment of dementia and mental health problems poses special challenges. Great care is required in selection, introduction, and manipulation of dose and other aspects of drug treatment of these patients, in whom side effects and toxicity frequently occur. Staff caring for people in this spectrum require training and awareness of the additional problems faced with advancing age. Again the increasing rates of physical morbidity in older women with learning disabilities need to be addressed accordingly.

Prescribing for certain disorders

Gender difference in mental illness

Gender is a critical determinant of mental health and mental illness. Gender determines the differential power and control men and women have over the socioeconomic determinants of their mental health and lives, their social position, status and treatment in society, and their susceptibility and exposure to specific mental health risks.

Depression and anxiety

Gender differences occur particularly in the rates of common mental disorders—depression, anxiety, and somatic complaints. These disorders, in which women predominate, affect approximately one in three people in the community and constitute a serious public health problem. Depression is not only the most common women's mental health problem but may be more persistent in women than men. Depression is found to be twice as common in women than men in the general population (McGrath *et al.* 1990). A study by Hastings *et al.* (2004) of a population based sample of over 1000 adults with learning disabilities showed a significantly increased rate of affective and neurotic symptoms in women than men. Apart from the well-recognized risk factors like stress, life events, female gender, low socioeconomic status, lack of social support, and old age, people with learning disabilities are further disadvantaged by their limited coping skills, experiences of discrimination, stigma, and abuse.

Schizophrenia and paranoid psychoses

There are no marked gender differences in the rates of severe mental disorders such as schizophrenia. From time to time, minor gender differences have been reported in age of onset of symptoms, frequency of psychotic symptoms, course of disorder, subsequent social adjustment, and long-term outcome of disease, but despite these debates, there remain no significant gender differences here. In the general population, the course of schizophrenia is more favourable in women, who tend to have a later onset of the illness, fewer negative symptoms, more prominent mood symptoms, and a better treatment response to the illness than men (Seeman and Fitzgerald 2000). For these reasons, women tend to be diagnosed with schizophrenia at a later stage as they are often misdiagnosed as having a mood disorder (Castle 2000). There is very little research in this area on women with learning disabilities in particular.

Eating disorders

Eating disorders are more common in women than men. Anorexia nervosa and Bulimia nervosa occur much more frequently in women than men (10:1) (Romans 1998). The extent to which this is common in people with learning disabilities is yet to be fully ascertained. More often, in this population, it is postulated that weight loss is likely to be secondary to other problems such as depression or adverse life events, rather than a wish to become thin.

Additional research is needed in this area to understand more about these issues and the role of increased awareness of such issues as well-being and body image among women with learning disability.

Principles of prescribing among women with learning disabilities

General

Women with learning disabilities have the right to be given information about what is happening to their bodies, and to learn about the experiences of other women. There is a need to support them in a proactive manner. The use of accessible audio-visual aids can facilitate their understanding of these matters, as can targeted staff training and support. Working in partnership with families and professional carers can be pivotal in improving compliance with medication. Encouraging women to live a healthy lifestyle and ensuring access to primary healthcare is the bedrock of a holistic approach to the management of the mental health of women with learning disabilities.

Prescribing according to psychiatric diagnosis

When possible, prescribing of drugs should be based on clinical diagnosis. Psychiatric disorders are relatively common in this population and there is a wide scope for pharmacological interventions; however, many of the behavioural constellations do not constitute diagnosable psychiatric disorders (Eaton and Menolascino 1982). In this situation, prescribing may be informed by the responsiveness of individual behaviour types to certain drugs.

Prescribing according to the evidence base

The evidence base for psychopharmacological agents in the mental health and behaviour problems of women with learning disabilities is sparse. Current prescribing practice in learning disabilities largely draws on evidence from the general population and adjustments are to be made on an individual basis.

Initiating treatment

A conservative approach to the use of medication is required. Most behavioural problems in this clientele do not merit drug treatment, particularly those that are brief, self-limiting, caused by intercurrent physical health problems, or caused by environmental stressors.

However, certain diagnosable disorders such as depression merit prompt rather than last-resort drug therapy.

Dose regimen

This should be guided by a simple rule—'start low, go slow'. An initial dose of one-half of the adult dose is usually recommended to minimize side effects. Increases to the full dose should be undertaken over twice the period of time used in mainstream practice.

Polypharmacy

It is very important to avoid polypharmacy due to the potential adverse interactions between various agents. However, if the individual patient needs a mixture of medication, it is good practice to document the need and to monitor side effects accordingly and to work closely with the pharmacists.

Consent

Under the Capacity Legislation, it is recognized that each individual should be free to make personal choices for themselves, according to their capacity to understand the choice made and the implications of that choice. This is a crucial matter for those with learning disability—especially where choices concerning medication have to be made. When a person is assessed to be unable to make such an informed choice, then all relevant professionals concerned in their care must act in their 'best interests', while making every effort to ascertain their wishes (Mental Capacity Act 2007). The UN Convention on the Rights of Persons with Disabilities (December 2006) highlights the following as some of the salient recommendations to be addressed: equality between men and women, equality of opportunity, respect for individual autonomy and dignity and inclusion in society.

Conclusion

Psychotropic prescribing in the care of women with learning disabilities needs to be planned and implemented as part of a holistic care plan. In general, a conservative approach towards psychotropic drug prescribing is advisable, in which other non-drug interventions are explored before any inception of psychopharmacological agent. More research is needed to explore possible gender differences in the manifestation of mental illness among people with learning disability, and the implications of this on pharmacological management. The development of person-centred planning, partnerships between various agencies, and evidence-based practice provide a strong foundation for further positive changes in the provision of care for women with learning disabilities, particularly where any gender specific interventions might be planned accordingly.

References

Aman MG (1983) Psychoactive drugs in mental retardation. In: JL Matson and F Andrasik (eds) *Treatment and Innovations in Mental Retardation*, pp. 455–513. Plenum Press, New York.

Arnold LE (1993) Clinical pharmacological issues in treating psychiatric disorders of patients with metal retardation. *Annals of Clinical Psychiatry*, **5**, 189–98.

Ayd FJ (1991) The early history of modern psychopharmacology. *Neuropsychopharmacology*, **5**, 71–84.

Carr J *et al.* (1995) Menopause in women with learning disabilities. *Journal of Intellectual disability Research*, **39**(2), 137–9.

Castle DJ (2000) Women and schizophrenia: an epidemiological perspective. In: D J Castle *et al.* (eds) *Women and Schizophrenia*, pp.19–34. Cambridge University Press, Cambridge.

Department for Constitutional Affairs (2007) Mental Capacity Act 2005 Code of Practice. The Stationery Office, London.

Department of Health (2007) Services for people with learning disability and challenging behaviour or mental health [Mansell Report]. http://www.dh.gov.uk/en/Publicationsandstatistics/Publications/PublicationsPolicyAndGuidance/DH_080129.

Eaton L and Menolascino F (1982) Psychiatric disorders in the mentally retarded: types, problems, and challenges. *American Journal of Psychiatry*, **139**, 218–30.

Hastings RP *et al.* (2004) Life events and psychiatric symptoms in adults with intellectual disabilities. *Journal of Intellectual Disability Research*, **48**, 42–6.

Kohen D (2001). Psychiatric services for women. *Advances in Psychiatric Treatment*, **7**, 328–34.

McGrath E *et al.* (1990) *Risk Factors and Treatment Issues*. American Psychological Association, Washington, DC.

O'Brien G (2002) Psychopharmacological interventions. In: G O'Brien (ed) *Behavioural Phenotypes in Clinical Practice*, pp 123–36. Clinics in Developmental Medicine, Mac Keith Press, London.

Romans SE (1998) Gender differences in psychiatric disorder. In: S.E. Romans (ed) *Folding Back The Shadows: A Perspective on Women's Mental Health*, pp. 43–62. University of Otago Press, New Zealand.

Seeman MV and Fitzgerald P (2000) Women and schizophrenia: clinical aspects. In: DJ Castle *et al.* (eds) *Women and Schizophrenia*, pp. 35–50. Cambridge University Press, Cambridge.

United Nations (2006; implemented 2008). 'Final report of the ad hoc committee on a convention on the protection and promotion of the rights and dignity of persons with disabilities'. General Assembly of UN: A/61/611. United Nations, Geneva, Switzerland. http:www.un.org/disabilities/convention/conventionfullshtml.

PART 6

Legislation and Policy

Dora Kohen

Building on or building in? The contribution of policy and the law to women's mental health

Karen Newbigging and Jenifer Paul

Introduction

Women's mental health and the provision of appropriate services have been the focus of attention for many years. In the 1990s, concerns about the safety of women in mental health services (Gorman 1992) and a growing body of literature that described the needs of women, illustrating how mental health services failed women, led to a call for changes in provision (Williams *et al.* 1993; Parry-Crooke *et al.* 2000). Despite this, the influence on statutory mental health service provision appeared to be minimal, although the government acknowledged that mental health services were not always sensitive to the needs of women (Davies and Waterhouse 2005). Women's mental health therefore became a focus for policy development following the publication of the *National Service Framework for Mental Health* (DH 1999). The publication of *Into the Mainstream: Strategic Development of Mental Health Care for Women* (Department of Health 2002) set out to tackle the key issue for mental health services of how to shape and deliver a response, building on an understanding of the underlying causes of women's distress, the contribution of these underlying causes to the expression of distress, and enabling women to tackle these issues through providing gender-specific and gender-sensitive services.

More recently there have been legislative developments that include provisions to tackle unlawful discrimination on the basis of gender (Equality Act 2006) requiring public bodies, including Primary Care (PCTs),

Mental Health Trusts, and Local Authorities, to assess the gender impact of major policies and service developments. The purpose of this chapter is to provide an overview of the contribution of these legislative and policy developments; to demonstrate how they can support improvements in women's mental health and mental health service provision, and to review the progress made in this arena, concluding with implications for further development. We draw on our experience of commissioning and providing mental health services and job-sharing a national post with responsibility for leading the implementation and development of the women's mental health strategy across England.

The starting point

By the end of the last century, the need to understand and provide differentiated mental health services for women was evident (Department of Health 1998). The starting point for this was twofold. First, the body of evidence, which demonstrated the gender differences in expression and experience of mental distress, pathways into care and preferences in relation to the nature of treatment and support, as summarized in Table 35.1.

The link between women's expression of distress and their disadvantageous social circumstances and the way in which their distress is conceptualized has been a major theme within this (Busfield 1996). Further inequalities in the treatment of women and men by mental heath services, and the way that mental health services were consistently failing women by ignoring the sources

Table 35.1 Gender differences relvant to mental health service provision

	Women	Men
Life experiences	Sexual, physical abuse Domestic violence Caring responsibilities	Accidents Victims and perpetrators of violence
Socioeconomic realties	Poverty Pay Isolation Juggling the demands of work and caring Backbone of caring services but minority in leadership positions	Full-time employment Unemployment Retirement
Expression of mental distress	Depression Anxiety Eating disorders Self-harm Perinatal mental health Borderline personality disorder	Early-onset psychosis Suicide Substance misuse Antisocial personality disorder
Pathways into services	Primary care Community services Maternity services	Accident & Emergency department Drug/alcohol-related services Via criminal justice routes
Treatment needs and responses	Community-based, informal Gender-specific services	Assertive outreach Early intervention

Sourced from *Into the Mainstream* (Department of Health 2002) and *Mind Your Head: Men, boys and mental wellbeing* (Men's Health Forum 2006).

of their distress and medicalizing their social difficulties, and place them at risk through exposure to abusive treatment either at the hands of male service users or staff, has also been highlighted.

Feminists' critiques, viewing gender as a social construct, rather than objective fact, locate these differences in the social control of women by psychiatry and the medicalization of women's unhappiness (Wright and Owen 2001). More generally, they are seen as a complex interplay of factors including role and responsibilities in relation to caring, low social status and value, social isolation and poverty, childhood sexual abuse, domestic violence, and sexual violence (Jacqui Smith, the Health Minister in the foreword to *Into the Mainstream*, Department of Health 2002).

Second, increasing concern about the safety of women and appropriateness of care for women, particularly in inpatient and secure settings, was evident as highlighted by the MIND campaign (Gorman 1992) and WISH (Parry-Crooke *et al.* 2000). Together these described and illustrated the diverse needs of women, placed an emphasis on safety within mental health services, and demonstrated that the focus should be on need not numbers of women in the service system.

These concerns were particularly evident in secure settings, where women were always in a minority in mixed sex environments. Further it was apparent that

they were often inappropriately placed at higher levels of security for less serious problems than men; that the regimes of care in secure settings were not consistent with social values regarding equality; and that the women in secure settings had high levels of abuse histories (Bartlett and Hassell 2008). Box 35.1, with voices from women in secure settings, illustrates that there was a clear need to redefine what security meant; to provide care that was gender specific; and to address issues relating to abuse (Department of Health 2002).

Box 35.1 Women's voices from secure services

'There's sixteen of them and they dominate. I'm always having to stand up for myself and then I explode. The staff then say I'm violent and threatening.'

Men get away with it. If women do something they get a harder time'

'I was severely abused as a child so I did not want to go and talk to a sixty-year-old man.'

'No-one has ever discussed why I did my crime. To try and understand why I did it. I'd like someone to talk to.'

Good girls surviving the secure system: A consultation with women in high and medium secure settings (Parry-Crooke *et al.* 2000).

Policy and legislative context for achieving change

Power and influence as manifested by legislation and policy development are factors in the successful implementation of change. They are key elements in protecting rights and setting equality parameters for how society meets the needs of all citizens.

Awareness of the issues and of the need for change in relation to women's mental health was apparent considerably in advance of policy and legislative support. Why was this? Women are, numerically, a very large 'minority' and not an homogeneous group, their needs therefore feel hard to define and contain; women lack socioeconomic power and hence influence, therefore their voices are not readily heard. Campaigns for change may also have been perceived as feminist, and therefore either radical in nature, implicitly linking women's health, including mental health, to structures of patriarchal disadvantage (Carpenter 2000), or 'old-fashioned' (Squires 2008). Further, there was also concern about the experience of men within the mental health system, and particular groups of men—the high rate of suicide for young men; the high rates of compulsory detention and treatment and deaths in care of men from black and minority ethnic (BME) communities. The drive therefore at the end of the last century was to achieve universal improvements in service provision.

Policy developments: A women's mental health strategy

The National Service Framework (NSF) for mental health (Department of Health 1999), described as 'a landmark' in mental health policy (McCulloch *et al.* 2003), articulated the need for services to be well suited to those who use them and to be non-discriminatory. It drew attention to providing safe care for women in mixed sex accommodation as a priority and consistent with broader Department of Health policy (HSC (97)1), which had highlighted the commitment to eliminate mixed sex accommodation.

Following on from this, work started on developing a women's mental health strategy and the Department of Health commissioned expert briefings and undertook a series of listening events with women who used mental health services. The results of these events indicated that women wanted mental health services that (Davies and Waterhouse 2005, p. 259.):

- Ensured their safety
- Promoted empowerment, choice, and self-determination
- Placed importance on the underlying causes and context of women's distress in addition to their symptoms
- Addressed important issues relating to women's roles as mothers, and the need for accommodation and work
- Valued women's strengths and abilities and potential for recovery.

The resulting consultation document, Into the Mainstream, was broadly welcomed, viewed as providing a much needed, indeed overdue, focus on women's mental health (Department of Health 2003a). However, there was widespread concern about the lack of focus on implementation. This led to the publication of the implementation guidance (Department of Health 2003b); the development of a national programme for women's mental health; leads identified within each of the NIMHE Regional Development Centres; and the inclusion of indicators for the development of women's mental health services in the annual self-assessment process in relation to the NSF. This was supplemented by the commissioning guidance on women-only day services Supporting Women into the Mainstream (Department of Health 2006). Table 35.2 provides a summary of these and other key reports that have focused on issues of concern to women. There has been further guidance published by the National Institute for Mental Health England and professional bodies on key issues: see, for example, Butler and Kousoulou (2006) on women in contact with the criminal justice system and the Royal College of Psychiatry (2007) on sexual boundary issues in psychiatric settings. Whilst reports from voluntary organizations have continued to highlight unmet needs, for example, MIND's report (2006) on postnatal depression.

An important element of Department of Health policy and associated guidance was the provision of gender-specific support and *Mainstreaming Gender and Women's Mental Health* recommended extending women-only provision to include women-only inpatient services, women-only community-based acute care teams, women's secure services, and women-only community day services, following on from a commitment made in the NHS Plan (NHS Executive 2000). The importance of mainstreaming women's mental health was also emphasized as the mechanism by which mental health service provision that is sensitive to the specific needs of women can be developed:

> Mainstreaming gender and the needs of women service users are as much to do with making adjustment to existing structures and processes that are consistent and sustainable
> (Department of Health 2003, p. 9)

Table 35.2 Policy developments and key reports since 1998

Policy development	Key messages	Implications
Safety, Privacy and Dignity in Mental Health Units: Guidance on Mixed Sex Accommodation for Mental Health Services (NHS Executive 2000)	Specified the type and nature of separate physical facilities in inpatient environments	The needs of women inpatients for single-sex accommodation—private, public, children visiting, and outside space became an objective for providers
Into the Mainstream: Strategic Development of Mental Health Care for Women (Department of Health 2002).	Articulation and advocacy for the needs of women from diverse backgrounds and in diverse settings	Establishment of national programme to support development of women's mental health services
Mainstreaming Gender and Women's Mental Health: Implementation Guidance (Department of Health 2003).	Key principles described actions and approaches to implement *Into the Mainstream* Key areas for development included workforce development, governance, service evaluation, and monitoring	Provided tools and guidance, including service specifications for women-only acute in-patient, secure and community-based day services to organizations to improve services for women
Kerr Haslam Report (HM Government 2005)	Health organizations must have policy on handling allegations or disclosures of sexualized behaviour. Robust recruitment and appointment practices for all clinicians	Gender power relations (male doctors, female nurses) to be taken account of in responding to complaints. Female complainants must be treated seriously. Sexual Offences Act 2003 enacted
Delivering Race Equality Action Plan (Department of Health 2005)	Experience and expressions of distress are specific to different cultures; services must provide care that meets culturally-specific needs	Establishment of national programme with associated funding and description of 12 service characteristics. Asserts that the needs of BME women must be addressed
Tackling the Health and Mental Health Effects of Domestic and Sexual Violence and Abuse (Itzin 2006)	Root causes of physical and mental ill-health must be addressed. Staff need to be equipped to respond and intervene therapeutically	Women's experience of physical and sexual violence and abuse, either as an adult and/or as a child, is highlighted. Training for staff to address underlying causes
Supporting Women into the Mainstream (Department of Health 2006)	Commissioning guidance for appropriate day services for women, taking into account needs described in strategy	Provision of gender-specific community-based support improving choice and control, safety, and security. Development of 3rd sector provision. Stressed staff skills to support 'time to talk'
With Safety in Mind: Mental Health Services and Patient Safety (National Patient Safety Agency 2006)	Incidence of safety events around falls, self harm, violence, sexual safety, medication analysed	Staff need to be aware of women patients' sexual vulnerability. Reports of sexual harassment must be taken seriously. Access to sexual and reproductive health advice is required
Antenatal and Postnatal Mental Health (National Institute for Health and Clinical Excellence 2007)	Clinical management and service guidance on the prediction, detection, and treatment of mental disorders in women during pregnancy and the first year postpartum	Coherent, multi-agency service will address needs holistically. Skilled staff to support women, their carers, and their babies through pregnancy and postnatal period
The Corston Report: A Review of Women with Particular Vulnerabilities in the Criminal Justice System (Home Office 2007)	Women need a distinct approach. Social factors predominant cause of offending. Increased availability of community disposals.	Women no longer in a system designed for and run by men. Women supported to address offending behaviour. The majority of women need to remain in the community and with their families
Informed Gender Practice: Mental Health Acute Care that Works for Women (NIMHE, RCN and CSIP, 2008)	This guidance describes how women's needs are different from men's and how this can be addressed through gender informed practice across the acute care pathway	Positive staff attitudes and understanding of women's mental health issues, improvements in physical environment and whole system pathways are all needed to improve the experience of acute care for women

This means commissioning, developing, and providing mental health services that are built on an understanding of the social context of women's mental distress including structural inequalities; that have staff with the skills and knowledge in relation to key issues that affect women's mental health, in particular violence and abuse, parenting and caring roles, and poverty and isolation, and are accessible and provide a feeling of safety, avoiding further retraumatization of the women using them.

The Commissioning Framework for Health and Wellbeing (Department of Health 2006) introduces values, structure, and methodology that should support the appropriate development of services for women. The aim is to enable a shift towards services that are personal, sensitive to individual need, and refocus investment towards health promotion and well-being. The key themes of choice, voice, and control echo policy recommendations for women's services and women service user requirements. An emphasis on personalization should, by definition, address the needs of the individual woman as will an assessment and care plan that addresses all health and social care needs in an holistic way focused on health promotion.

The Commissioning Framework sets out the requirement for Joint Strategic Needs Assessment as the main method for identifying the needs of local populations.

It is expected that this will be achieved by active commissioner consultation with local groups, of which many will be women's groups. Again the influence of power is a factor that commissioners must be aware of. The trick will be to listen hard to the marginalized and least powerful and not be overly influenced by the most vocal, well connected, vested interest groups. If this is successful there is a real opportunity for the needs of the disempowered to be represented when investment decisions are made.

Legislative developments: achieving gender equality

In the last ten years a legislative framework for addressing equality issues, including gender, has been developed. Table 35.3 provides an overview of the legislation. The Equality Act (2006) introduced the Public Sector Gender Duty requiring public bodies to undertake a gender impact assessment to ensure that polices and major service developments do not unlawfully discriminate on the basis of gender. The implementation of the Act will be monitored by the Equalities and Human Rights Commission Equality Bill (2009), whose role is described in Box 35.2. The Equality Bill (2008) brings together existing Equalities legislation and extends protection to gender reassignment, age, religion or belief and sexual orientation.

Table 35.3 A legislative framework for equalities

Legislation	Key messages	Implications
Human Rights Act 1998	Strengthens the UK application of 15 Rights of European Convention of Human Rights including: ◆ Right to respect for private and family life ◆ Right not to be discriminated against in respect of rights and freedoms	Right for families to live together (single parents, asylum seekers) Right of self determination ◆ Choose sexual identity ◆ Choose how you look and dress Equal access to Convention Rights irrespective of differences of status
Race Relations (Amendment) Act 2000	Elimination of unlawful racial discrimination Promotion of racial equality	Services must be appropriate to the needs of different ethnic communities and for women and men from these communities
Gender Recognition Act 2004	Provides trans people with legal recognition of their acquired gender	Postoperative trans people can marry in their acquired gender and found a family Continuity of parental rights in original gender
Equality Act 2006, Part 4	Creates a specific gender equality duty on public bodies to eliminate unlawful discrimination and to promote equality of opportunity between women and men in both services and employment.	Organizations will be in breach of the law if they are not providing services which are appropriate to the needs of women and men; this encompasses the physical environment, staff skills, and treatment options
Equality Bill 2008	Promoting equality is essential for individuals to fulfil their potential and for the creation of a cohesive society and for a strong economy. This bill simplifies and extends existing equalities legislation to cover age, gender reassignment, religion or belief and sexual orientation	Places a new equality duty on public bodies, which brings together the three existing duties (in relation to gender, race and disability) and extends to age, gender reassignment, sexual orientation and religion or belief

Box 35.2 The role of the Equality and Human Rights Commission

The Equality and Human Rights Commission was established in 2007 under the Equality Act. It has brought together the work of three separate commissions with the objective of taking a whole system approach to inequality by addressing all strands of equalities – gender, race, disability, age, sexual orientation, religion or belief. In doing so it has had to allay concerns that it may lead to a dilution of focus on specific issues. It is a public body, independent of government and its role is to eliminate discrimination, reduce inequality, protect human rights, and to build good relations. The Commission has extensive legal powers and can challenge infringements in the law as well as enforcing equalities duties and will contribute to the development of law and policy. See http://www.equalityhumanrights.com for more information.

The past five years have also seen developments in mental health legislation. The Mental Health Capacity Act 2005 asserts that capacity is presumed unless medical examination proves inability to make a decision and/or inability to communicate a decision. The issue is particularly relevant to women who currently make up 60% of clients of the Court of Protection, a disproportionately higher percentage than in the general population. It supports the ability to exercise choice and make decisions, including their reasonably foreseeable treatment options, care arrangements, close relationships, sexual relations, having a baby. The Mental Health Act 2007 introduced Supervised Community Treatment, access to independent advocacy, and speedier access to Mental Health Review Tribunals. This should provide opportunities for improved advocacy of women's needs.

The Sexual Offences Act 2003 is not specific to mental health but does contain sections that prohibit any sexual activity between any member of care staff and a patient with a mental disorder placed in a relationship of care with that person. This adds legislative rigour to professional standards and supports the voices of women patients who have been sexually abused while in the health and social care system.

Making progress with implementation

The success of policy in building on gender-specific provision and building in gender sensitivity with regard to women has not yet been fully evaluated.

A survey of the experience of 73 women using mental health services in Brent by Brent Mental Health User Group and members of the Local Implementation Team sub-group, confirmed that the improvements that these women wanted to see were consistent with the areas for action highlighted in *Into the Mainstream* (Brent Mental Health User Group 2006). The survey indicated that care planning was weak and typically did not include the issues, which were of most concern to women. Safety was also identified as a significant issue with only a minority of women having felt safe during a recent admission to psychiatric hospital with 'violence and aggression, illegal drugs, disturbed and difficult service users and men "trying it on"' as reasons for feeling unsafe (Brent Mental Health User Group 2006, p. 63). It was also evident that access to a range of services was patchy, with limited choices available. The focus was on mental illness rather than recovery and resilience and medication was the most frequently used treatment. The critical role that staff throughout mental health services play was reinforced, particularly the importance of understanding issues related to women's mental health and the disposition and ability to work in partnership with women.

It is clearly early days in the introduction of a gendered approach within mental health services and the impact on the direct experience of women is not necessarily going to be immediate. *Mainstreaming Gender and Women's Mental Health* recommended the identification of senior leadership with a commitment to addressing gender and the specific needs of women and the development of a multi-agency steering group to lead the local development of services in line with the guidance. Two surveys of Mental Health Trusts have therefore been undertaken by the National Programme for Gender Equality and Women's Mental Health to ascertain what progress is being made. The first in 2006, in collaboration with the National Mental Health Partnership, aimed to identify what action had been taken to implement *Into the Mainstream* and to prepare for the forthcoming Public Sector Gender Duty (Gregoire *et al.* 2006), and the second in 2007 to identify the progress being made on priority areas for implementation identified by the National Programme (NMHDU, in press) and activity in relation to the Public Sector Gender Duty.

It was evident from the 2006 survey that progress was being made in some areas. Increase in women-only provision, either secure provision or inpatient care were identified by those Trusts that responded as the major area of development. Table 35.4 provides a summary of all the areas identified in rank order of frequency.

A notable omission is initiatives in relation to women from BME communities, despite the publication of *Delivering Race Equality in Mental Health Care* (Department of Health 2005) the previous year. Nearly all of the Trusts that responded had an identified lead for women's services, typically a management lead with approximately half also identifying a clinical lead. There were examples of strategy development and workforce development, through the provision of training in gender awareness, although these initiatives were far from universal. The most commonly cited barriers to change were competing priorities and/or a lack of resources, particularly in relation to the development of gender-specific acute care provision.

The 2007 survey generated responses from nearly 70% of the total number of Mental Health Trusts in England. As with the 2006 survey, this provides evidence of activity in relation to the development of gender-specific services, particularly in relation to acute care and psychological therapies; the development of services and partnership working to improve the response and support of women experiencing violence and abuse, and the development of perinatal services. It is clear that the third sector is playing an important role in the provision of gender-specific services; private organizations in respect of the development of secure care and the voluntary sector in relation to day services. The position of the voluntary sector remains a cause for concern. Whilst providing informal, highly valued, accessible woman-centred care, a lack of secure funding continues to negatively affect sustainability and the capacity of these organizations to work in partnership with the statutory sector. As with the 2006 survey, the extent of activity to meet the diverse needs of specific groups of women, for example, women from BME communities, women in contact with the criminal justice system, lesbians, or older women, was much more limited. Further there was little, if any mention of a gendered approach in the introduction of new service models, such as crisis resolution or early intervention teams.

Discussion

The need for change to enable mental health services to meet the needs of women is established. Policy and related reports help enormously by providing rationale, authority, and guidance to planners, commissioners, and providers and provide the opportunity for synergy with dedicated clinicians and managers. The information currently available suggests that there have been significant strides in building on gender sensitive provision to existing services as a result of *Into the Mainstream.* However, it is not yet evident whether this has also involved a radical rethink of the underlying model of care and therefore the way in which services are provided, including the dynamics of the relationship between provider and service user (Knowles *et al.* 2005).

Indeed the evidence to indicate that a whole system approach to meet the needs of women has been adopted is scant. It is not uncommon for good services, for

Table 35.4 Initiatives undertaken by Mental Health Trust members of NMHP (Gregoire *et al.* 2006)

Rank order	Development identified	Examples
1	Single sex provision	Inpatient wards, psychiatric intensive care units, high dependency areas, medium secure units, women only crisis houses, dedicated services for women with a diagnosis of bipolar disorder
2	Single gender provision within a mixed sex environment	Women-only group work or sessions, women-only services within day services, provision for younger women with dementia
3	Perinatal mental health service development	Specialist perinatal mental health services, strengthening partnership working, capacity building, pathway development
4	Training and development	Women's mental health, child protection, vulnerable adults, women and equality, self-harm, eating disorders, and childhood sexual abuse
5	Violence and abuse	Department of Health sexual assault pilot programme, training and protocol development in relation to domestic violence
6	Strengthening the involvement of service users	In strategy and service improvement groups
7	Other	Choice of care coordinators monitoring standards for inpatient care

example, in relation to acute inpatient care, to coexist with very limited provision in respect of other needs, for example, perinatal mental health services, and for partnership working with the voluntary sector to be underdeveloped. It is also not clear whether the specific needs of women are being considered in the development of NSF teams. Crisis resolution teams, for example, are grounded in an assumption that home is preferred to inpatient admission. However, as Patiniotis (2005) makes clear, the role of women within the home and/or the risk of abuse or domestic violence at home challenge this assumption. Further the diverse range of needs of women are often not being systematically taken into account, as witnessed by the relatively limited focus on the specific needs of women from BME communities.

The importance of staff training and development in gender equality is universally highlighted. This has a number of aspects from increasing awareness of key issues directly influencing individual care and the choices offered (Brent Mental Health User Group 2006) through to a lack of awareness about gender inequality, reflected in personal attitudes, impacting negatively on the priority afforded this agenda. However, there appear to be few examples of a strategic approach to workforce development, although there are examples of positive initiatives being taken, for example, in relation to responding to sexual abuse and domestic violence (Itzin 2006).

Monitoring and audit are useful tools for highlighting gaps and increasing compliance. The Healthcare Commission Audit of Violence 2006–7, conducted by the Royal College of Psychiatrists, gives information on incidence, progress, and areas for development for inpatient wards. Similarly, the findings of the Healthcare Commission (2008b) acute inpatient mental health service review provides the best opportunity in recent years to work with the worst performing trusts towards better service provision for women.

It is evident that if further progress is to be made then this agenda has to be mainstreamed and built into the commissioning and provision of mental health services. The Equality Act 2006 provides a major opportunity to drive this forward by providing the requirement that this work is undertaken, a methodology for it—equality impact assessments—and an independent body with powers of scrutiny. The requirement, introduced by the Equality Act, to undertake a Equality Impact Assessment (EIA), including gender, for all new policy has already begun to make a difference. The review of the care programme approach (Department of Health 2008) was subject to an EIA at the consultation stage to the benefit of the final document (National Institute for Mental Health England 2008).

In leading the implementation and development of the women's mental health strategy across England we have drawn heavily on the leverage that this legislation and policy provide. They are not, however, the sole mechanism for effecting change. A multi-faceted approach is likely to produce the best results. The existence of a national programme and leadership and the network of regional gender equality and women's mental health leads have been influential, just as concerted leadership and multi-agency groups at a local level have worked hard to bring about positive change in women's mental health.

Implications for the future

For progress on women's mental health to be sustained, the implementation of the Equality Act is key. It relocates women's mental health within a postmodern discourse of gender, which takes account of the structured diversity of experiences among women and men as well as between them (Carpenter 2000), and within a broader equality and diversity agenda. The challenges of this agenda are not to be underestimated. It brings with it opportunities to refresh and sustain significant developments in this area as well as concerns about the risk of a loss of focus on the needs of women. Squires (2008) argues that mainstreaming has transformative potential but that to realise this, it has to be more than a technocratic tool. She advocates the central role of deliberative democracy, i.e. inclusive and democratic participation of diverse interests in policy formation if the potential of mainstreaming is to be fully realised. This has far-reaching implications for commissioners, mental health providers, and, above all, those involved in further policy development in relation to women's mental health.

Finally, it is evident that a broad range of factors, many of them out of the jurisdiction of mental health policy or legislation, have an impact on women's mental health. This calls for a across-governmental approach in order to take action on the underlying causes of women's distress. The mental health agenda must therefore be clearly linked with broader priorities, for instance, those highlighted by the Minister for Women, which emphasize action in key areas of women's lives—within their families, as victims of abuse, offenders, and contributing to community cohesion, especially in BME communities.

Conclusion

A good momentum for change has been generated since the publication of the women's mental health strategy. For this to impact significantly it is important to sustain that momentum, using the current equalities legislative framework to drive a systematic and deliberately inclusive approach to mainstreaming a gendered approach in order to comprehensively improve mental health service provision for women and, indeed, for men and transgendered people.

References

Bartlett A and Hassell Y (2008) Do women need special secure services? *Advances in Psychiatric Treatment*, **7**, 302–9.

Brent Mental Health User Group (BUG) (2006). *Women into the mainstream: Survey of women using services to deal with mental health issues – or to deal with issues which affect their mental health – in Brent.* BUG, London.

Busfield J (1996). *Men, Women and Madness: Understanding Gender and Mental Disorder.* Macmillan Press Ltd, London.

Butler P and Kousolou D (2006). *Women at Risk: The mental health of women in contact with the judicial system.* London Development Centre; CSIP, London.

Carpenter M (2000). Reinforcing the pillars. In: E Annandale and K Hunt (eds) *Gender Inequalities in Health*, pp. 36–63. Open University Press, Buckingham.

Davies J and Waterhouse S (2005). Do women need specific services? In: M Nasser *et al.* (eds) *The Female Body in Mind – The Interface between the Female Body and Mental Health*, pp. 255–65. Routledge Publishing, Hove.

Department of Health (1998). *Modernising Mental Health Services: Safe, Sound and Supportive.* HMSO, London.

Department of Health (1999). *National Service Framework for Mental Health.* HMSO, London.

Department of Health (2000). *The NHS Plan: A Plan for Investment; a Plan for Reform.* Department of Health. http://www.dh.gov.uk/prod_consum_dh/groups/dh_digitalassets/@dh/@en/documents/digitalasset/dh_4055783.pdf

Department of Health (2002). *Women's Mental Health: Into the Mainstream: Strategic Development of Mental Health Care for Women.* Department of Health, London.

Department of Health (2003a). *Mainsteaming Gender and Women's Mental Health: Implementation Guidance.* Department of Health, London.

Department of Health (2003b). Feedback from consultation events on *Into the Mainstream*. http://www.dh.gov.uk

Department of Health (2005). *Delivering race equality in mental health care: an action plan for reform inside and outside services: and the Government's response to the independent inquiry into the death of David Bennett.* Department of Health, London.

Department of Health (2006). *The Commissioning Framework for Health and Wellbeing.* Department of Health, London.

Department of Health (2008). *Refocusing the Care Programme Approach.* Department of Health, London.

Gorman J (1992). *Out of the shadows – stress on women.* MIND, London.

Gregoire A *et al.* (2006). *Promoting gender equality and women's mental health.* National Mental Health Partnership, London.

Healthcare Commission (2008). *The Pathway to Recovery: A review of NHS acute inpatient mental health services.*

Healthcare Commission and Royal College of Psychiatrists (2008). *Healthcare Commission National Audit of Violence 2006–7.* http://www.rcpsych.ac.uk/PDF/OP%20Nat%20Report%20final%20for%20Leads.pdf

HM Government (2005). *Kerr Haslam Inquiry Final Report.* HMSO, London.

HM Government (2008). *Framework for a Fairer Future – The Equality Bill.* http://www.equalities.gov.uk/pdf/FrameworkforaFairerFuture.pdf

Home Office (2007). *The Corston Report: A review of women with particular vulnerabilities in the criminal justice system.* Home Office, London.

Itzin C (2006). *Tackling the Health and Mental Health Effects of Domestic and Sexual Violence and Abuse.* Department of Health and National Institute for Mental Health in England in partnership with the Home Office, London.

Knowles K *et al.* (2005). *Women and Mental Health: Turning rhetoric into reality – sharing practice and perspectives and strategies for action on women's mental health.* Social Perspectives Network, London.

McCulloch A *et al.* (2003). The National Service Framework for Mental Health: Past, Present and Future. *Mental Health Review*, **8**, 7–17.

Men's Health Forum (2006). *Mind Your Head. National Men's Health Week: Policy Report.* www.menshealthforum.org.uk

MIND (2006). *Out of the blue? Motherhood and depression.* MIND, London.

National Institute for Health and Clinical Excellence (2007). *Antenatal and Postnatal Mental Health: Clinical Management and Service Guidance. NICE Clinical Guideline 45.* National Institute for Health and Clinical Excellence, London.

National Institute for Mental Health England (2007). *Single Equality Impact Assessment Report: Care Programme Approach Review.* http://www.nimhe.csip.org.uk/cpaseia

National Mental Health Development Unit (in press). *Working Towards Women's Well-being.*

National Patient Safety Agency (2006). *With Safety in Mind: Mental Health Services and Patient Safety.* NPSA, London.

Newbigging K and Abel K (2006). *Supporting Women into the Mainstream: Commissioning Women Only Day Services.* Department of Health, London.

NHS Executive (2000). *Safety, Privacy and Dignity in Mental Health Units: Guidance on Mixed Sex Accommodation for Mental Health Services.* NHS Executive, London.

Parry-Crooke G *et al.* (2000). *Good Girls Surviving the Secure System: A Consultation with Women in High and Medium Secure Settings.* WISH, London.

Patiniotis (2005). *Who's listening? Gender Sensitive Mental Health Service Provision: Key Issues from the Perspectives of Service Users. A report on consultation with women service users of Mersey Care NHS Trust.* PPI Forum for Mersey care, Liverpool.

Royal College of Psychiatrists (2007). *Sexual Boundary Issues in Psychiatric Settings.* Royal College of Psychiatrists, London.

Squires J (2008). *Equality and Diversity: A New Equality Framework for Britain?* www.bath.ac.uk/esml/Library/pdf-files/squires.pdf.

Williams J *et al.* (1993). *Purchasing effective mental health services for women: a framework for action; guidance for mental health purchasers and providers.* University of Kent, Canterbury.

Wright N and Owen S (2001). Feminist conceptualisations of mental illness. *Journal of Advanced Nursing,* **36**, 143–50.

Afterword

Mary V. Seeman

Quite a few books about women's mental health have been published in the last 10 years because the issue is important to a range of disciplines, from basic science to psychology, sociology, psychiatry, obstetrics and gynaecology, nursing, social work, nutrition, rehabilitation science, education, and the history of medicine. This book, under the editorial guidance of Professor Dora Kohen, has attempted to encompass all these disciplines and to present the subject from many points of view.

Focusing on women's mental health suggests that women's cognitions, affects, and behaviours are essentially different from those of men. Essentialist thinking about women is often disparaged because of the inference that a woman's destiny is fixed at birth, determined by her two X chromosomes and nothing else. The term 'sex differences' is said to refer to such fixed and invariable points of contrast between men and women. In Chapter 3, 'Mind the gender gap: mental health in a post-feminist context', David Pilgrim ably discusses the many faces of essentialism. Environmentalists can be accused of it as readily as biologists when implying false dichotomies: women poor, men rich; women powerless, men authoritarian; women victims, men perpetrators.

Arbitrary divisions such as these are made in the name of 'gender differences' rather than 'sex differences'—a constructionist viewpoint that accords with Simone de Beauvoir's credo, 'one is not born, but *becomes* a woman'. Social critics view the 'becoming' as forced moulding by a patriarchal power that turns girls, and later women, into objects of oppression—sexual objects, objects exploited for reproduction and child rearing, objects fashioned to care for and minister to the needs of men, objects of domestic violence, coerced into lives of submission, poverty, and second class citizenship. This is reductionistic since women differ, as do men, in their character and experience, in their achievement of status, personal wealth, and authority.

They also differ in their mental health. The recent interest in women's health (and mental health) is one small step toward individualizing health for all. Rather than accepting that human health can be defined universally, individuals need to define the condition for themselves, and identify subjective goals for well-being. Opinions on what constitutes categories of illness such as depression or anxiety, for instance, vary widely, as do ideals of shape and weight, estimates of what is 'natural', or tolerance of perceptions and beliefs not universally shared. Use of stimulants or relaxants is also perceived differently in different cultures and among individuals.

Male/female disparity constitutes a clustering of individual differences, and this book speaks to those differences. There is, of course, infinite variation among women which, one day, can be more finely addressed when medicine has become more personalized, less wed to a common and collective view of what it is to be either ill or illness-free. For now, we need to start with less fine distinctions and that is why discussions such as the ones in this book are so very useful. We need to know that, for starters, mental health for half the population—women—differs significantly from mental health of the other half.

There are several ways in which mental illnesses assume different forms in women and men. An important way is that women, as a group (although this is very dependent on age, culture, and social class) are exposed to an environment that is far from identical to that of men. The example I like to cite, because it is so remarkable and so unusual, is the neuropsychiatric illness called kuru, which means 'trembling fear'. It is (or rather *was*, because it has almost completely disappeared) a brain disease with neurological and psychological manifestations, characterized by truncal ataxia, headaches, joint pains, limb tremor, and pathologic bursts of laughter. It is a progressive illness that leads to death.

In the 1950s, before the Western world had heard of kuru, two husband–wife teams of anthropologists first reported that the Foré, a linguistic tribe living in Papua New Guinea, practised ritual cannibalism. When a person died, the maternal relatives cooked and ate the muscles and internal organs of the deceased. The men of the community, who believed that eating human flesh made them vulnerable to enemies, did not take part in the feast. But the women and children did eat, and the brain was considered a special delicacy. The practice probably started shortly after the turn of the 20th century, when the illness, kuru, first emerged and spread among successive generations of the tribe. The Foré thought it was an affliction caused by sorcery. They noticed that it affected mainly women and they blamed it on sorcerers from other tribes who were trying to interfere with the fertility of Foré women. The cannibalism rite was intended to counteract the sorcery and thereby increase fertility. Since dead bodies fertilized the ground when buried, the Foré reasoned that eating corpses would serve the analogous purpose.

In 1963, Carlton Gajdusek, an American paediatrician studying kuru in New Guinea, demonstrated that, in adulthood, 14 women were affected to every man. Over the age of 40, the ratio became 72 women to every man. His first impression was that hormones were somehow involved. He also considered an autoimmune aetiology and looked for genetic mechanisms that could affect women and children of both sexes but spare adult men. Reading the anthropologists' reports, Gadjusek began to search for an infective causal agent and ultimately found that prions were involved, unconventional infectious agents composed of misfolded protein. For this discovery, he was awarded the Nobel Prize.

The pathologic prions were being passed from generation to generation by the eating (mainly by women) of infected brains.

This is an unusual example of a well-known phenomenon, differential exposure by sex or gender role. By virtue of custom, culture, and circumstance, men and women are differentially exposed to substances of abuse, to domestic violence, to sexual abuse, to peer pressure with respect to body shape, to reproductive hazards, and to hormonal fluctuations, among other biologic and environmental sex-specific exposures.

As Mervat Nasser notes in Chapter 4 in this book, the prevalence of eating disorders can be explained by the influence of Western cultural norms on girls and women. Jona Lewin, in 'Depression in women' (Chapter 11), while acknowledging the complexity of aetiology in depression, discusses the role of the exposure of women to changing hormone levels after puberty and also explores the disproportionate exposure of girls and women to sexual and physical abuse (child sexual abuse, rape, and male partner violence). We learn in this chapter that young married women looking after small children are at particular risk for depression, which suggests a gender-specific exposure to the downsides of childcare.

Clearly, in most psychiatric disorders, aetiology is not as straightforward as attributing everything to a prion. Most disorders result from a complex interweaving of genetic and environmental factors of such complexity that any one explanation can only hope to apply to a minority of individuals. More is becoming known about genetic factors, although this field is still largely awash in mystery.

The genetics of autism, a male-prevalent condition, remain largely unexplained; some syndromes that fit into the autistic spectrum, however, have been identified and their genetic causes are being unravelled. An interesting example is Rett syndrome, which, contrary to most early developmental illnesses, is almost exclusive to girls. It occurs in 1 in 10 000 girls, whereas it is all but non-existent in boys. German paediatrician Andreas Rett was the first to describe the syndrome. He was struck by the sight of two young girls, sitting in the waiting room of his outpatient clinic for neurologically disabled children, constantly wringing their hands. The mothers of both girls told him that their daughters had initially developed normally but, after a year, had begun to regress intellectually; the continuous hand wringing started subsequently. Rett made a film of the girls and, in 1966, he published his findings. Because the syndrome was seen in girls only, the speculation was that it was a genetic X-linked disorder, but so lethal that it brought about uterine death in boys, who lacked the protection of a healthy allele on a second X chromosome. By 1998, three groups had localized the Rett gene to the Xq28 region. The laboratory of Huda Zoghbi identified the gene, MECP2, in 1999.

In girls suffering from Rett syndrome, one of the X chromosomes, usually the one inherited paternally, contains a de novo mutation (more than 300 different mutations have so far been identified) of the MECP2 gene. Because it is the paternal X that is most vulnerable to mutation, boys (who receive their X from their mothers) are not affected. Since one of the X chromosomes in all female cells is randomly inactivated, half of the cells in Rett girls contain the mutant gene. Skewed (non-random) X-inactivation that results in more than

50% of the mutant chromosomes being inactivated can so spare a woman from the effects of mutant MECP2 that she may have no symptoms at all. Such women can pass on the mutant X-chromosome to both daughters and sons and, more recently, a number of males with MECP2 mutations have been identified. All of them show signs of intellectual disability, autism, or other psychiatric disorder.

This is because the MECP2 gene is a member of a family of proteins containing a domain that binds to methylated DNA. This is an epigenetic process that, when disrupted, can interfere with the transcriptional silencing of other genes and result in abnormal chromatin assembly. Through their effects on the three-dimensional folding of chromatin, MECP2 mutations are thought to contribute not only to classical Rett syndrome but also to various autistic spectrum disorders, various forms of mental retardation, and, even, various forms of psychosis. Fresh mutations on paternal chromosomes, X-linkage, X-inactivation, skewed inactivation of the X chromosome, and disruptions of chromatin assembly are all recently discovered genetic mechanisms that may eventually help to explain sex differences in susceptibility, progression, and outcome of a variety of diseases other than Rett syndrome. The fact is, however, that, in 2009, too little is known about the link between mental health and genetic mechanisms to do more than to speculate.

It is well known that boys, rather than girls, populate child psychiatry clinics but that, roughly at the age of puberty, this ratio is suddenly reversed and psychiatric services become mainly women-oriented because more women than men come seeking help. As Pilgrim elaborates in his chapter, women present themselves more readily than men for assessment and diagnosis and this fact could explain many gender differences in lifetime prevalence of conditions such as depression and anxiety. In other words, women, as a group, may not actually suffer more from these conditions than men but they are perhaps more likely than men to seek help for them.

Gender-role socialization is the usual explanation for the help-seeking disparity between women and men. In Western cultures, men want to be seen as self-sufficient, not 'wimpy' or 'unmanly'. Help-seeking puts the seeker, at least temporarily, into a dependent role, which is an uncomfortable one for many men. The masculine ideal in the West is to be emotionally unexpressive, to show a high threshold for pain, and to be interpersonally 'on top', i.e. to be sensitive to perceived power in all relationships, including those between patient and healthcare provider. Many men view help-seeking as antithetical to the traditional male role in that it means showing vulnerability and relinquishing power to another. Many men prefer to self-treat stress with alcohol because that is more socially compatible with the gender role they perceive as culturally appropriate. This masculine ideal varies widely by personality, life experience, traditional background, socioeconomics, and age and is best captured by the title of a 2005 paper in *Social Science and Medicine*: '"It's caveman stuff, but that is to a certain extent how guys still operate": men's accounts of masculinity and help seeking' (O'Brien *et al.* 2005)

One of the reasons why boys present more at clinic than girls is thus explained by the fact that mothers are more likely to seek treatment for sons because their behaviour at home (externalizing behaviour) disturbs mothers more than the relatively quiet internalizing behaviour of their daughters, however pathological.

Another quite different explanation lies in the possibility that pregnant women 'attack' their male fetuses by mounting an immune response to the H-Y antigen. H-Y antigen is a histocompatibility antigen of the cell membrane, with a gene locus on the Y chromosome that mediates testicular organization in the male. The male fetus, by virtue of this antigen that is foreign to his mother, is exposed to the mother's H-Y antibodies and therefore experiences greater risk in the uterine environment than does a female fetus. We know that more male than female fetuses die *in utero* and it has been proposed that the high male to female ratio of autism, attention deficit disorder, stuttering, delayed speech, learning disability, and conduct disorder may be attributable to this more difficult uterine transit for males. Maternal antibodies can cross the placenta and attack the cells of the son. Conversely, the son's cells can cross the placenta in the other direction and create a state of fetal microchimerism in the mother, which has been implicated in the aetiology of autoimmune disease.

In 1996, Lee Nelson first proposed that fetal microchimerism might partly explain the high rates of autoimmune disease in women. Her group discovered elevated levels of fetal cells in the blood of women with scleroderma and systemic lupus erythematosus (SLE). Depression often accompanies autoimmune disorders. Experimental mice data have linked the depression that occurs in SLE with antiribosomal P, a protein autoantibody associated with the central nervous system. Several studies show an association between thyroid autoimmunity and depression. Microchimerism leading to autoimmunity is an intriguing new mechanism that might one day deepen our understanding of the excess prevalence of certain psychiatric disorders in women.

Clues to sex differences in disease have been looked for in functions that are unique to one sex, such as hormones and their organizing effects on brain structures. For instance, why is it that neurofibrillary pathology in the hypothalamus occurs in 90% of men with Alzheimer's disease and in only 8–10% of age-matched women? Is that because of hypothalamic differences established before birth? Why is it that men with schizophrenia show significantly larger ventricles than do healthy men, whereas no such relative enlargement is seen in women with schizophrenia? Does that help to explain sex differences in age of onset, symptoms, and time course, as described by Anita Riecher-Rössler in Chapter 12 on schizophrenia?

After puberty, activating hormones play an important role in the manifestations of mental illness in men and women. For instance, days 10–19 postpartum are associated with the greatest risk of readmission for mothers with a prior history of psychiatric illness. Pregnancy is associated with the least risk. It is tempting to attribute this to the brain protective action of oestrogens during pregnancy and to oestrogen withdrawal effects postpartum. The role of hormones in women's mental health is well covered in this book in Chapter 5 by Peter Fitzgerald and Timothy Dinan. How then to explain the high rate of postpartum depression in fathers? It has been estimated that approximately 14% of women experience postpartum depression and that 10% of men do—an almost equal amount. There must be more to the link between the transition to parenthood and depressed affect than hormones (although a role for hormone alterations in fathers has been postulated).

The father's intense empathy with his pregnant, labouring, and postpartum partner is an interesting phenomenon with a long history. It has been studied by historians and anthropologists for centuries. It is called couvade, from the French 'to hatch' (*couver*). Couvade means that fathers undergo some or all of the symptoms of pregnancy: cravings, nausea, breast augmentation, insomnia, and, sometimes, an expanding abdomen. They can then go on to postpartum depression, more than twice as common in new fathers as depression in the general adult male population. This has been attributed to the dramatic change in family structure that occurs when a new baby is born. The mother is preoccupied with the infant; the father is faced with new caretaking and economic responsibilities at a time when he is not sleeping adequately, probably not eating adequately, and,

perhaps, coping with in-laws and other household intruders. Maternal depression is apparently the strongest predictor of paternal depression during the postpartum period, which means either a contagion of depression or the father's response to the considerable added burden of providing care to a depressed new mother.

An important issue in women's mental health is the stress of caretaking, a stress that falls overwhelmingly on women in most cultures. The stress also appears to affect women more than it does men. In almost all studies of the psychiatric burden of caregiving, women caregivers report more psychiatric symptoms (usually depression and anxiety) than men caregivers.

A last example of a woman-specific pathway to mental illness is blood loss. Menstruating women lose, on average, 20 mg of iron a month. Any woman who loses more than 60 mL of blood with every cycle is iron-depleted. This has important effects on the brain because iron is an essential cofactor for tyrosine hydroxylase, the rate-limiting enzyme for dopamine synthesis.

Restless legs syndrome (RLS) is a neuropsychiatric condition first described in the 17th century and believed to be twice as common in women as in men. It is characterized by an irresistible urge to move one's legs in an effort to stop uncomfortable peripheral sensations such as burning, itching, or tickling. It used to be considered a form of 'hysteria' or 'neurasthenia'. The condition worsens with rest and with pregnancy and has been linked to fibromyalgia and to depression.

The reduction of brain iron in RLS is visible on brain imaging, and is proportionate to the severity of symptoms. Iron supplements appear to help 60% of sufferers. Low iron levels are sometimes risk factors in fibromyalgia or depression whether or not these are accompanied by restlessness.

But women's mental health is a larger topic than the narrow focus on diseases and treatments permits. It encompasses gender economics, workplace stress, work–family conflicts, and so much more. It is distinct in many ways from the mental health of men, a fact that this book firmly establishes. This is a good initial step toward the eventual realization of individual mental health and person-customized interventions, both preventive and therapeutic.

References

O'Brien R *et al.* (2005) 'It's caveman stuff, but that is to a certain extent how guys still operate': men's accounts of masculinity and help seeking. *Social Science and Medicine*, **61**, 503–16

Index

BRITISH LEPROSY ASSOCIATION

WITHDRAWN
FROM LIBRARY